NCLEX-RN® Review

1,000 Questions to Help You Pass

Patricia McLean Hoyson, Ph
Youngstown State University
Youngstown, Ohio

Kimberly A. Serroka, MSN, RN
Youngstown State University
Youngstown, Ohio

JONES AND BARTLETT PUBLISHERS
Sudbury, Massachusetts
BOSTON   TORONTO   LONDON   SINGAPORE

World Headquarters
Jones and Bartlett Publishers
40 Tall Pine Drive
Sudbury, MA 01776
978-443-5000
info@jbpub.com
www.jbpub.com

Jones and Bartlett Publishers Canada
6339 Ormindale Way
Mississauga, Ontario L5V 1J2
Canada

Jones and Bartlett Publishers International
Barb House, Barb Mews
London W6 7PA
United Kingdom

Jones and Bartlett's books and products are available through most bookstores and online booksellers. To contact Jones and Bartlett Publishers directly, call 800-832-0034, fax 978-443-8000, or visit our website www.jbpub.com.

Substantial discounts on bulk quantities of Jones and Bartlett's publications are available to corporations, professional associations, and other qualified organizations. For details and specific discount information, contact the special sales department at Jones and Bartlett via the above contact information or send an email to specialsales@jbpub.com.

The authors, editor, and publisher have made every effort to provide accurate information. However, they are not responsible for errors, omissions, or for any outcomes related to the use of the contents of this book and take no responsibility for the use of the products and procedures described. Treatments and side effects described in this book may not be applicable to all people; likewise, some people may require a dose or experience a side effect that is not described herein. Drugs and medical devices are discussed that may have limited availability controlled by the Food and Drug Administration (FDA) for use only in a research study or clinical trial. Research, clinical practice, and government regulations often change the accepted standard in this field. When consideration is being given to use of any drug in the clinical setting, the health care provider or reader is responsible for determining FDA status of the drug, reading the package insert, and reviewing prescribing information for the most up-to-date recommendations on dose, precautions, and contraindications, and determining the appropriate usage for the product. This is especially important in the case of drugs that are new or seldom used.

Additional credits appear on page viii, which constitutes a continuation of the copyright page.

Production Credits
Executive Editor: Kevin Sullivan
Acquisitions Editor: Emily Ekle
Associate Editor: Amy Sibley
Editorial Assistant: Patricia Donnelly
Production Director: Amy Rose
Production Editor: Carolyn F. Rogers
Senior Marketing Manager: Katrina Gosek
Associate Marketing Manager: Rebecca Wasley
Manufacturing and Inventory Coordinator: Amy Bacus
Composition and Interior Design: Arlene Apone
Cover Design: Kristin E. Ohlin
Cover Image: © ErikN/ShutterStock, Inc.
Interactive Technology Manager: Dawn Mahon Priest
Printing and Binding: Malloy, Inc.
Cover Printing: Malloy, Inc.

Library of Congress Cataloging-in-Publication Data
NCLEX-RN review : 1,000 questions to help you pass / [edited by] Patricia McLean Hoyson, Kimberly A. Serroka.
    p. ; cm.
Includes bibliographical references.
ISBN-13: 978-0-7637-4096-2 (pbk. : alk. paper)
ISBN-10: 0-7637-4096-9 (pbk. : alk. paper)
   1. Nursing--Examinations, questions, etc. 2. National Council Licensure Examination for Registered Nurses. I. Hoyson, Patricia McLean. II. Serroka, Kimberly A.
   [DNLM: 1. Nursing--Examination Questions. WY 18.2 N33655 2008]
RT55.N732 2008
610.73076--dc22
                        2007020363

6048

Printed in the United States of America
12 11 10 09   10 9 8 7 6 5 4 3

Dedication

This book is dedicated to all of those who have chosen to be a part of the most rewarding profession there is; to my mother, Thelma McLean, who instilled in me a great appreciation for and love of education; and to Rick, my husband and best friend, whose love and support helps to make all things possible.

Patricia McLean Hoyson

This book is dedicated to the love of my life, my husband Dave Serroka, for it was he who supported me in so many ways to achieve the success that I have enjoyed in life. The sudden loss of this dear man has only validated the love that we shared. I know that someday he will have a clever word to tell me that he was my inspiration to attempt this project. To my children, Kristin and Paul, I am forever thankful for their strength that they give to me to continue on each day. To my dear mother, Nancy Hudy, I thank her for encouraging me to continue to pursue higher levels of learning. I share this text with all these special people in my life and will always carry a place for each of them in my heart.

Kimberly A. Serroka

Contents

Contributors

Louise Aurilio, PhD, RNC, CNA
Youngstown State University
Youngstown, OH

Cheryl L. Brady, MSN, RN
Kent State University
Kent, OH

Angela T. Douglass, MSN, RN, CHN
Kent State University
Kent, OH

Mada Hodgson Janosik, MSN, RN
Youngstown State University
Youngstown, OH

Richard J. Hoyson, MSEd, Doctoral Candidate
Jefferson Area Local Schools
Jefferson, OH

Nora Lipscomb, MSN, RN
Youngstown State University
Youngstown, OH

Susan A. Lisko, MSN, RN
Youngstown State University
Youngstown, OH

Patricia A. McCarthy, PhD, RN, BCAPN
Youngstown State University
Youngstown, OH

Diane R. McDougal, MNEd, RN
Youngstown State University
Youngstown, OH

Dottie McLean, MSN, RN
Homecare with Heart, LLC
Youngstown, OH

Renee L. McManus, MSN, RN
Youngstown State University
Youngstown, OH

Nancy Mosca, PhD, RN
Youngstown State University
Youngstown, OH

Molly Roche, MSN, RN
Youngstown State University
Youngstown, OH

Valerie O'Dell, MSN, RN
Youngstown State University
Youngstown, OH

Cynthia M. Shields, MSN, RN
Youngstown State University
Youngstown, OH

Tracy Skripac, MSN, RN, AOCN, CHPN
Indiana Wesleyan University
Marian, IN

Claudia Swantek, MSN, RN, CNS
Humility of Mary Health Partners
Youngstown, OH

Lisa L. Taafe, MSN, CNS, CDE, CPNP
Akron Children's Hospital
Akron, OH

Patricia Testa, MSN, RN
Youngstown State University
Youngstown, OH

Nancy Wagner, MSN, RN
Youngstown State University
Youngstown, OH

Amy Weaver, MSN, RN
Youngstown State University
Youngstown, OH

Kimber L. Zolnier, BSN, RN, OCN, CPN
Forum Health
Youngstown, OH

Acknowledgments

We thank all the contributors of this NCLEX-RN® review text for their dedication and hard work that was put forth to create a text that will help nursing students to prepare for the NCLEX-RN® Licensure Exam. With much appreciation, we sincerely thank each author for the expertise and diligence that has been shown throughout the development of this book.

Photo Credits

Page 13: © Photos.com

Pages 134 and 136: From *Arrhythmia Recognition: The Art of Interpretation*, courtesy of Tomas B. Garcia.

Pages 156 and 221: © Elena Kalistratova/ShutterStock, Inc.

Unit 1 • Introduction

Introduction

Congratulations! If you are reading this book, chances are you have completed or are nearing completion of your formalized preparation for becoming a registered nurse (RN). Whether you have attended a diploma program, an associate degree program, or are receiving your bachelor's degree, you all share some things in common. First, you have completed a rigorous program designed to prepare you for one of the most exciting and rewarding careers a person can embark upon. Second, before you can become licensed as an RN you must successfully take the National Council Licensure Examination for Registered Nurses (NCLEX-RN®) exam and achieve a passing score. This is the last hurdle you must negotiate before you begin your career as an RN. Naturally, a test of this importance carries with it a considerable amount of potential anxiety. This book is designed to help you develop the confidence which comes with knowing that you have taken the steps necessary to best prepare yourself for this exam.

As nursing faculty we have watched as students at the end of their senior year began to prepare for the NCLEX-RN® exam. We know that our students (as well as those of you who are at the end of your formalized preparation) had completed a curriculum of both course work and clinical experiences that contains everything necessary to successfully pass the NCLEX-RN® exam. Several years ago we were looking for ways to better prepare our senior-level students for their upcoming NCLEX-RN® exam. As a result we developed a senior-level course which is offered during the last semester of a nursing student's senior year. This course is designed to help students identify areas of strengths they have developed over the course of their preparation for becoming an RN. It is also designed to help them identify areas in which they need to concentrate their efforts to help them achieve the best possible results on the NCLEX-RN® exam. In addition, students in our class are taught test preparation strategies and test-taking strategies designed to maximize their efforts. It has been our experience that students who have applied the self-assessment strategies they have learned, in addition to the test preparation and test-taking techniques from our course, show significantly higher success rate on the NCLEX-RN® exam than those who do not employ these strategies.

How to Use This Review Book to Guide Your Study

This review book will help you to prepare for the National Council of State Boards of Nursing Licensing Examination for Registered Nurses (NCLEX-RN®) and/or other nursing exams you may take in nursing school. The configuration of this review book includes 1,000 questions in both print and CD-ROM versions. Each question is written in a format that you will find on the NCLEX-RN® exam. We have done this so that you can become familiar with the types of questions you will be answering on the exam. The questions in this book may be taken in pencil/paper format and be completed anywhere when you have some extra time to complete review questions. The CD-ROM included with this book allows you an opportunity to practice test-taking on the computer. It is recommended that you at least become familiar with answering questions using a computer format prior to the day of your exam. You can use these resources in any combination as you study and prepare for your NCLEX-RN® exam.

This book is organized into seven units. In Unit I you will learn how to use this review book and the accompanying CD-ROM to prepare for your NCLEX-RN® examination. Also, licensure requirements for RNs will be discussed. The NCLEX-RN® Test Plan will be explored along with identification of the format of the examination and content areas found on the exam. You will complete a comprehensive self-assessment of your learning needs designed to help begin your study preparation. After identifying your areas of content strengths and learning needs, you will develop your plan for preparing for the exam. You will prioritize your content areas for study and develop a timeline and study plan to organize your preparation for the exam. Finally, you will learn how to psychologically prepare yourself for this very important test and will also learn some effective strategies to use in order to manage any test anxiety you may experience prior to or during the examination.

The next five units (II–VI) contain questions and rationales organized according to the following content areas:

- Unit II—Specific Aspects of Care: Includes questions on safety, communication, fundamental nursing skills, and medication administration principles
- Unit III—Managing Client Care: Includes questions on delegation and prioritization of care and questions associated with bioterrorism and disaster nursing
- Unit IV—Adult Nursing: Contains questions on physiological disorders and associated nursing care activities organized according to body systems
- Unit V—The Client Having Surgery: Includes pre-operative and post-operative care, nutrition, and TPN/IV therapy questions
- Unit VI—Nursing Care of Specific Groups: Includes questions on maternity, female reproductive and women's health nursing, and child and adolescent health, as well as psychiatric mental health nursing questions.

This book also contains two comprehensive tests that will allow you to take timed tests that follow the NCLEX-RN® test plan. You will find a pretest at the beginning of the book, and a posttest after the last unit. The questions in these comprehensive exams also contain rationales for the correct and incorrect responses. As you answer the questions in this review book, it is important that once you finish answering the questions and calculate your score that you spend some time reading the rationales for each of the answers. There is much information included in the written rationales that is an excellent "mini content review" for you as you prepare to take the NCLEX-RN® examination. In addition to the written rationales, each answer contains a reference that you can refer to for additional reading and/or review if you find the content of the question to be an area in which you need additional study. If you do not have the text listed as a reference for the question, you can use any of your nursing textbooks to further review the content area.

The National Council Licensure Examination (NCLEX®)

The NCLEX-RN® examination, developed by the National Council of State Boards of Nursing, Inc., is designed to test knowledge, skills, and abilities essential to the safe and effective practice of nursing at the entry level. NCLEX® examination results are an important measure used by boards of nursing to make decisions about granting or not granting nursing licensure. The use of a standardized examination by all jurisdictions (50 states in the United States, the District of Columbia, and United States Possessions) facilitates licensure by endorsement from one jurisdiction to another.

Computer Adaptive Testing

The NCLEX-RN® examination uses Computerized Adaptive Testing (CAT) to administer the examination. CAT means that the examination is created as the candidate test taker answers each question. The first questions are relatively easy, with subsequent questions being targeted to the candidate's ability. CAT re-estimates the candidate's ability after each question is answered. If the candidate selects a correct response, the computer searches the question bank for a more difficult question. If the candidate answers the question incorrectly, the computer selects an easier question for the next question, this process continues throughout the examination. The CAT format re-estimates the candidate's ability every time a question is answered and each question has a degree of difficulty that is approximately equal to that ability estimate. After answering a question, the computer re-estimates the candidate's ability and selects the next question for the candidate. This testing process continues until the candidate's ability is either above or below the passing standard with a 95% certainty.

About the Exam

The NCLEX-RN® examination consists of between 75 and 265 questions with a maximum time limit of six (6) hours. The six (6) hour time limit includes any time that the candidate takes for a break or breaks during the examination. Included in the questions the candidate answers are fifteen (15) questions designated as "pretest items." These pretest items are test questions that NCLEX® is testing for use on future examinations and are not included in the scoring of the candidate's examination. The candidate has no way of identifying which of the questions are the fifteen (15) pretest questions and which are actual exam questions. For this reason it is important to do your best on every test question/item during the examination. On the NCLEX-RN® examination there is only one correct response for each question. There is no credit given on this examination for the second best answer.

The computer screen will display one question at a time. You will need to answer the question by selecting what you identify as the correct response and verifying your response before moving on to the next question. After you verify your response, the computer will move to the next question. You cannot go back and change an answer to a question after the computer has moved on to the next question. You may not skip a question; you must select an answer to each question before moving on to the next question. There is no penalty for guessing on this examination. If you are not certain of an answer to a question, try to eliminate responses that you know are not correct, and then use your nursing knowledge to make an educated guess as to the correct response.

Scoring

To pass the NCLEX-RN® exam your performance must be above the passing standard. The computer will stop testing when it is 95% certain that the candidate's ability is either above or below the passing standard. If the candidate's score is above the passing standard, the candidate passes. If the score is below the passing standard, the candidate fails the exam. If the computer is not able to determine clearly whether the candidate has passed or failed because the candidate's ability is close to the passing standard, then the computer continues asking questions. If the exam ends before the candidate completes the entire 265 exam questions, it means the candidate has not demonstrated with absolute certainty that they are clearly above or below the passing standard. If this happens, the computer will review the candidate's performance during testing and specifically the last 60 questions answered. If the candidate's ability was consistently above the passing standard on the last 60 questions, the candidate passes. If the candidate's ability falls to or below the passing standard, even once, the candidate fails the exam. If the candidate takes the maximum number of questions (265), the computer will make a decision as to whether the candidate passes or fails the exam. The computation will be based on the candidate's final ability level based on every question answered. The computer will compare this computed score with the passing standard. If the ability level is above the passing standard, the candidate passes. If the ability level is not above the passing standard, the candidate fails.

Analysis Results

The testing center will transmit your results to Pearson Vue, which then transmits the results to your state board of nursing. Your board of nursing will send you the results of your examination in about 2 to 4 weeks. At the end of the examination, you will be given information about how to obtain your results within 48 hours of your exam. There is a small fee to obtain results by the Internet or telephone.

If you do not successfully pass the NCLEX-RN® exam, you will receive a Candidate Performance Report (CPR) in the mail. The CPR provides the number of items administered to the candidate and a summary of the candidate's strengths and weaknesses based on the test plan. This information can be very helpful to guide study before retaking the examination.

The NCLEX-RN® Test Plan and Distribution of Content

The NCLEX-RN® exam tests knowledge the newly licensed entry-level registered nurse must have and activities that a newly licensed entry-level registered nurse must be able to perform to provide clients with safe effective nursing care. The questions are written to address the levels of cognitive ability, client needs, and integrated processes as identified in the test plan developed by the National Council of State Boards of Nursing (NCSBN). The questions test the candidate's comprehension, application, and analysis of nursing knowledge.

Cognitive Levels of Testing

The NCLEX-RN® examination includes questions from various cognitive levels grouped according to Bloom's Taxonomy. The cognitive level of a question varies depending on the type of mental activity required to answer the question and these levels are ranked according to the cognitive ability required to answer the question. The lowest level is the knowledge level. At this level the candidate is asked to recall facts, define, or identify facts about concepts or procedures. The next level, comprehension, requires an understanding of data. Questions at the comprehension level ask the candidate to interpret, explain, or predict a response. The third level is application. At the application level the questions involve using new information in situations. The candidate at this level will be asked to solve problems, modify plans, manipulate data, and demonstrate use of information. The next level is analysis which requires recognizing relationships. The client answering questions at this level will be asked to analyze, evaluate, differentiate, or interpret data from a variety of sources and to set priorities. The highest level is synthesis. At this level the candidate will put data together in new meaningful ways. The majority of questions on the NCLEX-RN® examination are written at the cognitive level of application and analysis.

Client Needs Categories

The NCLEX-RN® Test Plan is organized into four major client needs categories. Two of these four categories are further divided into subcategories. The percentage of test questions in each of the categories and subcategories are as follows:

Client Needs Categories	Percent of Questions on NCLEX-RN®
(1) Safe and Effective Care Environment	
A. Management of Care	13%–19%
B. Safety and Infection Control	8%–14%
(2) Health Promotion and Maintenance	6%–12%
(3) Psychosocial Integrity	6%–12%
(4) Physiological Integrity	
A. Basic Care and Comfort	6%–12%
B. Pharmacological and Parenteral Therapies	13%–19%
C. Reduction of Risk Potential	13%–19%
D. Physiological Adaptation	11%–17%

(1) Safe and Effective Care Environment

A. Management of Care (13%–19% of the test): Providing integrated, cost-effective care to clients by coordinating, supervising, and/or collaborating with members of the multidisciplinary healthcare team. Related content includes but is not limited to:

Advanced directives	Ethical principles
Advocacy	Incident/irregular occurrence/
Case management	variance reports
Client rights	Informed consent
Collaboration with multidisciplinary team	Legal rights and responsibilities
Concepts of management	Organ donation
Confidentiality	Performance improvement
Consultation	Referrals
Continuity of care	Resource management
Delegation	Staff education
Establishing priorities	Supervision

B. Safety and Infection Control (8%–14% of the test): Protecting clients and healthcare personnel from environmental hazards. Related content includes but is not limited to:

Accident prevention	Reporting of incident/event/
Disaster planning	irregular occurrence/variance
Emergency response plan	Safe use of equipment
Error prevention	Security plan
Handling hazardous and infectious materials	Standard/transmission based/
Injury prevention	other precautions
Medical and surgical asepsis	Use of restraints/safety devices
Home safety	

(2) Health Promotion and Maintenance (6%–12% of the test): The nurse provides and directs nursing care of the client and family/significant others that incorporates expected growth and development principles, prevention, and early detection of health problems, and strategies to achieve optimal health. Related content includes but is not limited to:

Aging process	Health promotion programs
Ante/intra/postpartum and newborn care	Health screening
Developmental stages and transition	High risk behaviors
Disease prevention	Human sexuality
Expected body image changes	Immunizations
Family planning	Lifestyle choices
Family systems	Principles of teaching and learning
Growth and development	Self-care
Health and wellness	Techniques of physical assessment

(3) Psychosocial Integrity (6%–12% of the test): The nurse provides and directs nursing care that promotes and supports the emotional, mental, and social well-being of the client and family/significant others experiencing stressful events, as well as clients with acute and chronic mental illness. Related content includes but is not limited to:

Abuse/neglect	Crisis intervention
Behavioral interventions	Cultural diversity
Chemical dependency	End of life
Coping mechanisms	Family dynamics
Grief and loss	Stress management
Mental health concepts	Support systems
Psychotherapy	Therapeutic communication
Religious and spiritual influences on health	Therapeutic environment
Sensory/perceptual alterations	Unexpected body image changes
Situational role changes	

(4) Physiological Integrity: The nurse promotes physical health and well-being by providing care and comfort, reducing client risk potential, and managing the client's health alterations.

   A. Basic Care and Comfort (6%–12% of the test): Providing comfort and assistance in the performance of activities of daily living. Related content includes but is not limited to:

Alternative and complementary therapies	Nutrition and oral hydration
Assistive devices	Palliative/comfort care
Elimination	Personal hygiene
Mobility/immobility	Rest and sleep
Nonpharmacologic comfort interventions	

   B. Pharmacological and Parenteral Therapies (13%–19% of the test): Managing and providing care related to the administration of medications and parenteral therapies. Related content includes but is not limited to:

Adverse effects/contraindications & side effects	Parenteral fluids
Blood and blood products	Pharmacologic agents/actions
Central venous access devices	Pharmacologic interactions
Dosage calculation	Pharmacologic pain management
Expected outcomes/effects	Total parenteral nutrition
Intravenous therapy	Medication administration

C. Reduction of Risk Potential (13%–19% of the test): Reducing the likelihood that clients will develop complications or health problems related to existing conditions, treatments, or procedures. Related content includes but is not limited to:

Diagnosis tests	Potential for complications from
Laboratory values	surgical procedures and health
Monitoring conscious sedation	alterations
Potential for alterations in body systems	System specific assessments
Potential for complications of diagnostic	Therapeutic procedures
tests/treatments/procedures	Vital signs

D. Physiological Adaptation (11%–17% of the test): Managing and providing care for clients with acute, chronic, or life-threatening physical health conditions. Related content includes but is not limited to:

Alterations in body systems	Medical emergencies
Fluid and electrolyte imbalances	Pathophysiology
Hemodynamics	Radiation therapy
Illness management	Unexpected response to therapies
Infectious diseases	

Source: Used with permission of the National Council of State Boards of Nursing, Inc., Chicago, IL.

Integrated Processes

There are four (4) processes identified as being fundamental to the practice of nursing which are integrated throughout the NCLEX-RN® examination. The processes are as follows:

1. Caring—The interaction of the nurse and client in an atmosphere of mutual respect and trust. The nurse provides encouragement, hope, support, and compassion to help achieve desired goals and outcomes.
2. Communication & Documentation—The verbal and nonverbal interactions between the nurse and client/significant others/healthcare team members. Events and activities associated with client care reflect standards of practice and accountability and are documented in patient records.
3. Teaching/Learning—Facilitation of the acquisition of knowledge, skills, and attitudes promoting a change in behavior.
4. Nursing Process (described in the next section)

These processes are integrated throughout the client needs categories (discussed in the previous section) found in the NCLEX-RN® examination.

Nursing Process

The nursing process is a scientific problem-solving approach to client care that is integrated throughout the questions on the NCLEX-RN® examination. The NCLEX-RN® Test Plan includes questions from all five (5) steps in the nursing process. Each step is represented by an equal number of test questions on the exam. The steps in the nursing process are as follows:

(1) Assessment

Assessment is the first step in the nursing process. This first step involves gathering subjective and objective data about the client. The client may be an individual patient, family, or community. This data may include physiological, psychological, developmental, sociocultural, or environmental information. After the data is gathered the nurse organizes the data to begin the next step in the process.

(2) Analysis

Analysis involves clustering or grouping the collected data and comparing the collected data with norms. During this phase the nurse identifies and interprets actual or potential health-care needs or problems of the client based on the assessment data.

(3) Planning

Planning begins with developing and setting goals and outcomes for meeting the needs of the client. In this phase the selected goals are then used by the nurse and client to develop a plan of action in order to meet the identified outcomes and goals. In developing the plan, the nurse and client will identify client actions as well as nursing interventions that will be completed in order to meet the identified outcomes and goals.

(4) Implementation

Implementation involves initiating the nursing actions necessary to carry out the plan to meet the outcomes and goals. This may involve organizing and/or managing care, counseling, teaching, and supervising care of the client.

(5) Evaluation

Evaluation involves determining the effectiveness of nursing care and assessing whether or not the goal(s) have been met. The identified goal(s) may have been met and the problem(s) may be resolved, be in the process of being resolved, or be unresolved. Evaluation may indicate that the assessment, analysis, planning, and intervention were effective and the problem(s) is/are resolved. Evaluation may also indicate a need for a change in the plan. Perhaps the assessment was not complete and after further assessment, a change is needed in the plan. Maybe the goal(s) were not appropriate or the interventions were not what was needed. This step in the nursing process will identify the areas where a change or modification is indicated as being necessary. Evaluation is the final step in the nursing process as well as an on-going component of each of the other four steps in the nursing process. Evaluation should be occurring at all steps throughout the nursing process. With on-going evaluation, changes and/or modifications can be made at any time and at any step in the nursing process.

Types of Test Questions/Test Items

There are a variety of types of questions or test items found on the NCLEX-RN® examination. The types of questions you will find include multiple-choice, multiple-response, fill-in, prioritizing (ordered response) and identify-a-location questions using the mouse to point and click at a specific area/location for the correct response. In this section of the book you will become familiar and comfortable with the various question formats you can expect to encounter on the test. An example of each of the question types has been provided for you.

Multiple-choice

Multiple-choice questions include a patient situation or scenario followed by a question and four (4) possible options or responses. With the multiple-choice option there is only one correct option/response. You will want to carefully read the information presented in the situation or scenario as the question will relate to the information presented in the situation/scenario. The stem of the question is where the question is asked that poses the problem to be solved. There will be four (4) possible answers/options/responses to the question. For each question, there is only one correct response.

Sample question:
An irregularly irregular cardiac rhythm characterized by absence of a P wave and an erratic, undulating baseline is identified as which of the following?

1. Atrial fibrillation
2. Atrial flutter
3. Paroxysmal atrial tachycardia
4. Premature atrial contraction

Correct response: 1

Rationale: In atrial fibrillation, totally disorganized electrical activity of the atrial myocardium results in no effective contraction, only fibrillation. The electrocardiogram reveals an erratic, undulating baseline with no P wave present. Ectopic atrial foci produce between 400 and 700 impulses per minute. In atrial flutter "saw tooth" flutter waves are present and in paroxysmal atrial tachycardia and premature atrial contraction P waves are present.

Multiple-response

A multiple-response question is similar in structure to the multiple-choice question except that there may be more than four (4) options/responses, and more than one may be correct. This type of question may ask the candidate to "select all that apply". This may indicate that more than one of the options/responses should be included when selecting the correct answer to the question. The candidate must select all of the correct options/responses in order to be given credit for answering the question correctly. There is no partial credit for selecting some of the correct options/responses with this type of question.

Sample question:
An 18-year-old patient has been admitted to the hospital with a diagnosis of new onset Type 1 diabetes mellitus. During the admission history and physical assessment the nurse would expect to find which of the following?

Select all that apply:
☐ 1. Increased thirst
☐ 2. Frequent urination
☐ 3. Weight gain
☐ 4. Cool, moist skin
☐ 5. Increased hunger

Correct response: 1, 2, 5
☒ 1. Increased thirst
☒ 2. Frequent urination
☐ 3. Weight gain
☐ 4. Cool, moist skin
☒ 5. Increased hunger

Rationale: Symptoms of Type 1 diabetes mellitus are attributed to decreased or absent insulin levels causing increased blood glucose levels. Three of these are classic signs/symptoms of Type 1 diabetes that include polyuria (increased urination), polydypsia (increased thirst), and polyphagia (increased hunger). In addition weight loss not weight gain is associated with Type 1 diabetes mellitus. Cool and moist skin is symptomatic of hypoglycemia rather than the hyperglycemia associated with new onset Type 1 diabetes mellitus.

Prioritizing (Ordered Response)

Prioritizing or ordered response questions require you to look at the options/responses and put them in correct sequence or order. You may be asked to determine the sequence or order (1st, 2nd, 3rd) in which you would complete a specific nursing action or prioritize some information/data according to importance or priority (first priority/most important to last priority/least important).

To be scored as correct, all the option/responses must be in the correct order. There is no partial credit for having some of the option/responses in correct orders with this type of question.

Sample question:
In observing the EKG strip of her client the nurse identifies the client is in atrial fibrillation. List in order of priority the following actions that should be taken by the nurse:

1. Defibrillate the client
2. Check the client for a patent airway
3. Palpate for a carotid pulse
4. Assess for breathing

Correct response: 4, 1, 3, 2

Rationale: Ventricular fibrillation is uncoordinated activity of the heart. Immediate defibrillation is performed after assessment of the ABCs of cardiopulmonary resuscitation (CPR). The ABCs of CPR are (A) airway, (B) breathing, and (C) circulation.

Fill-in

Fill-in the blank questions typically involve calculations and/or require you to type in your answer. You are permitted to use the drop-down calculator on the computer in answering these questions. If the question involves some type of measurement such as milliliter (ml), ounce (oz), centimeter (cm), or inch (in), the measurement unit will be identified in the stem of the question.

Sample question:
A nurse hangs a 1000 cc IV of D5NS to infuse at a rate of 125 ml/hr. How many hours will it take for the entire IV to infuse?

Answer: _____

Correct response: 8 hours

Rationale: The following formula and calculation

$$\frac{\text{Total volume to infuse}}{\text{ml/hr}} = \text{Infusion time} \qquad \frac{1000 \text{ ml}}{125 \text{ ml}} = 8 \text{ hours}$$

Select-an-answer/area (Point & Click)

The select-an-answer/area (point & click) question will ask you to answer a question based on some illustration, chart, table, or figure. You may be asked to "identify a specific location" on a figure or illustration. To answer this type of question, you will need to select the correct area and identify the area by pointing and clicking the mouse to mark the location with an "x" or use the mouse to point at a "hot spot" on the diagram that represents the correct response.

Sample question:

A nurse is performing infant cardiopulmonary resuscitation (CPR). Identify where the nurse should assess the pulse on the infant.

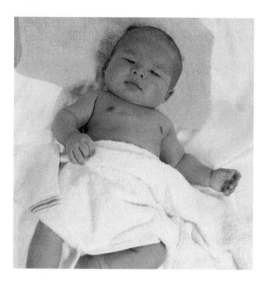

Correct response:

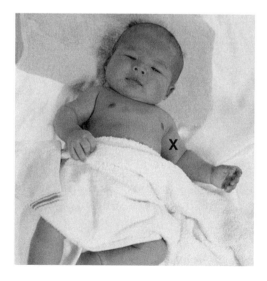

Rationale: The brachial pulse should be assessed when performing CPR. A carotid pulse is difficult to locate and assess on an infant because infants have a very short neck. A carotid pulse is the pulse to assess when performing CPR on a child and/or adult victim.

Developing Your Individualized Study Plan

Just as no two people are the same, no two people have the exact same learning experiences or learn in the same manner. People have different strengths and weaknesses and no two individuals' nursing preparation experiences are exactly the same. For that reason this section is designed to help you develop a plan of study tailored uniquely for your individualized preparation for the NCLEX-RN® examination. This section contains a step by step guide to help you assess your learning needs and strengths in order to develop a proactive individualized plan designed to maximize your effort on preparing for and successfully completing the NCLEX-RN® examination.

Individualized Self-Assessment

You will begin with an individualized self-assessment. In your self-assessment, you will assess three different areas in preparation for your study plan. The first area of assessment is of your content knowledge, the second is of your study methods and skills, and the last area for you to assess is your test-taking skills.

Content Knowledge Assessment

In this section you will learn how to perform a self-assessment to identify your content knowledge areas of strength and areas needing additional study and review. The outline/form on pages 27–29 will help guide you in this process. You can either tear the form out of the book or make a copy of the page for your use. The form is also available electronically at www.nursing.jbpub.com (search "Hoyson") for easy downloading and printing.

To begin your self-assessment, this book contains a 92-question pretest to assist you with this process. In addition to taking the pretest, you should reflect back over your years of nursing education—the content areas you did very well in and those content areas in which you had more difficulty learning and remembering the concepts. Another good self-assessment measure is the results of any assessment tests you took while in nursing school. Hopefully you have saved this information and can retrieve it now to begin your self-assessment process. If you do not have any prior assessment testing information available to you, do not be concerned, this book is designed to be a resource for you even without any prior assessment information. After you complete the pretest and as you begin to take the practice tests in this book you will be able to identify your specific content areas of strength and areas where you need further study and review.

Content Knowledge Assessment—Initial Pretest (Step 1)

Complete the pretest found on page 31 which has been developed following the same format as the NCLEX-RN® examination. This will help you initially to become familiar with the types of questions asked on the NCLEX-RN® exam as well as help to identify content areas you feel very comfortable with and content areas where you feel you need more study/review. The questions in the pretest are taken directly from the subject-specific units in the book. For this reason, answers and rationales are not provided for the pretest.

Determining your score on the sample practice tests

In order to most accurately determine how well you did on a practice test we will show you a simple way to calculate your score. If you receive a score of 75%–80% or above on any of the practice exams you should feel confident about your performance in that content area. If you receive a score lower than this, do not despair, you have identified an area in which you need to focus your attention and efforts. The following is the quickest and most accurate way to determine a score.

To determine your score you need to know two numbers. The first number is the number of questions you answered *correctly*. The second number is the total number of questions on the sample test. The next thing you need to do is divide the number of questions answered correctly by the number of possible questions. Your answer will be in the form of a number following a zero and decimal point. To obtain your percentage score you need to multiply the number by 100 or simply drop the zero and the decimal point and you have your percentage score.

Example one:
You answered 27 questions correctly out of a possible 30 questions.
27 divided by 30 = 0.90
Drop the zero and the decimal point (multiply by 100) and you have a score of 90%.

Example two:
You answered 32 questions correctly out of a possible 50 questions.
32 divided by 50 = 0.64
Drop the zero and the decimal point (multiply by 100) and you have a score of 64%.

If you end up with a number with more than three places after the decimal point take the third number and round up if it is greater than five.

Example one:
Your score after dividing is 0.867 = 87%

Example two:
Your score after dividing is 0.723 = 72%

As with any of the practice tests you complete during your study process, if you scored 75%–80% or above—congratulations! You are on your way to NCLEX-RN® success. If you scored less than 75%–80% on the test—do not despair! This gives you a starting point in your review process. One word of caution though—no one test is a perfect predictor of success or failure . . . so on to more testing, let's continue!

Content Knowledge Assessment—Historical Review (Step 2)

If you have retained any data from your years in nursing school, it is now time to take a look at this information. At this time you should review your old test scores and determine how you did on your physical assessment, pharmacology, fundamental nursing, medical/surgical, pediatric, obstetric, and psych/mental health nursing exams. This reflection will help you identify areas of strengths and areas needing more review and study. Also, take a look at your scores on any assessment tests you may have taken over the years. Some schools give paper/pencil assessment tests after completion of course content. Other schools may have an on-line testing program that students participated in. If you have this information from school, now is the time to retrieve these test results. There is an area on the self-assessment plan/form for you to write in this information. If you do not have testing information available, look back at old report cards and/or your grade transcripts. This will give you some information on courses you did well in and those in which you had more difficulty. You may find that the content you have most recently covered is most fresh in your memory and that content covered earlier in your nursing program are content areas requiring review. Reviewing this information can also give you some idea of your areas of strength and where you need some additional study/review.

Content Knowledge Assessment—Prioritization of Your Data (Step 3)

Now that you have some information/data on paper, it is time to prioritize your study plan according to content areas. From your list of content areas, go through and number them starting with number one (1) being the content area where you feel you did the best and have the most knowledge to the last number being the area where you feel you need the most review/study. After you have your content areas numbered, you need to reverse the list when developing your study plan. The area you identified as number one (1) on your list now will become the last area on your list for study and review and the last numbered content area will now become the first area for you to begin your study plan. There are a couple of good reasons to do this which are discussed below.

You want to start your study with the content that is most difficult for you and/or the content in which you feel you need the most review. One reason for this is that you will be the most refreshed when beginning your study for NCLEX-RN®. This is the best time in which to begin to study the content which is most difficult for you and where you require more time or emphasis. Another reason is there is the potential you may feel rushed for time at the end of your study plan due to circumstances beyond your control. If this is the case, you have saved the material you're most confident of until the last to review and if you do not have time for review, it should not pose a problem. What you do not want to happen is to not have enough time to study in an area in which you need a great deal of review.

You have now completed a thorough assessment of your nursing knowledge, identified your content areas of strength and areas needing more study and review, and have prioritized your content areas for study. If you have not already written this information on the study plan worksheet on page 27, do so at this time.

Remember, as with any assessment process, as you gather more data you may need to revise your plan. When completing your review/practice questions, pay particular attention to questions you answer incorrectly. Did you miss a question because you did not read the question carefully or due to a lack of content knowledge? As you begin to answer review questions, you may find your initial assessment of your knowledge level in a specific content area may change. If you find this happens, you will easily be able to modify and revise your plan and change your prioritized list of content to study.

Congratulations! You have now completed the most difficult and time-consuming area (content knowledge) in the self-assessment process. The next area to look at is your study methods & skills in preparation for developing your study plan for NCLEX-RN® success.

Study Methods & Skills

Begin to think about how you studied and prepared for the nursing exams you have taken. How did you prepare for the tests in which you scored the highest? What study strategies did you use? Where and when do you study best? Some of the following techniques/methods may have been methods you used successfully in your nursing program and may be helpful as you prepare for the NCLEX-RN® exam.

- Review and highlight your class notes. As you review class notes make yourself notes on the page or in the margins to aid your study. You may find it helpful to highlight (in another color) information that you find you need to spend more time reviewing.

- Outline content in your nursing texts and/or review books. Highlight those areas that you want to review in more detail.
- Make study notecards/flashcards of important and/or difficult content. You can use these to help you review and refresh these concepts.
- Make tape recordings of content and listen to the tapes while doing other activities. This is especially helpful if you are an auditory learner. For some individuals hearing the information aids in the learning process. Some individuals also find the recording of the study tapes is a method of learning. They learn better by reading or saying aloud the information.
- Think of examples that illustrate the key concepts and principles of the content.
- Make meaningful associations—tie new or difficult concepts with familiar concepts. The goal is to use what you already know to help you to make memorable what you want to remember by creating associations.
- Answer the review/practice questions in the text and look up and read the rationale for both correct and incorrect responses. Do not try to memorize review/practice questions. You should be reading the question rationales for comprehension and review. The rationales will explain and reinforce content material.
- Look up unfamiliar terminology and or unfamiliar concepts or content. Remember you cannot learn something you do not understand. You must read to understand the content before you can learn the material.
- Identify what time of day that is best for you to study. Every individual has a certain time of day when they are at their peak for performance and concentration. For some individuals it is early in the morning, others may be afternoon, and for some later in the day or evening hours are peak times. Your peak time is the ideal time for you to set aside for your study and review time. If it is not possible for you to study at this time, you still need to pick a designated time and set aside this time for NCLEX-RN® preparation.
- If you study better with another person or group of persons, you should try to identify a study-buddy to study with in preparation for the NCLEX-RN® exam. With another person, you can take turns quizzing each other over content material. Another potential benefit is that each of you will possibly have different areas of content strengths and weaknesses. In reviewing more difficult concepts you can help each other.

You now have some ideas about what you will do and how you will structure your study for the NCLEX-RN® exam. Take some time now and reflect on what have been successful study strategies that you have used in the past when you scored well on nursing exams. On the study plan worksheet on page 28, identify some of the specific strategies you are going to use in your study and review of the content in preparing for the NCLEX-RN® examination.

Congratulations, you have now completed two (content knowledge and study skills) of the three areas of assessment in the self-assessment process. The next areas to look at are the location(s) you will use for study and the development of your timeline in preparation for the NCLEX-RN® examination.

Study Location

It is important that you identify an area where you will study. The area you select should be quiet and have plenty of room for your books and class notes and papers. It will be more time efficient for you if you do not have to pull your study materials out and clean them up after each of your study sessions. This study space could be in your home, at a bookstore, or in a library setting. You need to turn off your cell phone and allow the voicemail and/or answering machine to pick up phone calls when you are studying. It is also important that your family members and friends understand the importance of you having this uninterrupted time for study and review.

In addition, you will want to take advantage of the free time you have when available. Review questions can be completed while waiting in the doctor's office, at the beauty/barber shop, waiting for a parking spot, waiting in traffic, between classes, or at the ball field. These times present an opportunity for completing the pencil/paper review questions such as those found in this text. Use this time to your advantage by completing questions and reading and studying the information found in the rationales. You will be surprised at how many questions you will be able to complete during these times. On the study plan worksheet on page 28, identify the specific locations where you will plan to study and review content in preparation for the exam.

Study Timeline

The last step in developing your study plan is the very important step of developing a study timeline designed to effectively implement your study plan. After assessing your content areas of strength, areas where you feel you need more review, and your study skills, it is time to develop a consistent plan of study. Allow yourself adequate time for content review as well as answering test review questions. If you schedule study time on a regular basis this will increase your commitment to study preparation. Frequent shorter periods of study are more effective than periodic lengthy study sessions. You should attempt to block one or two hours a day for NCLEX-RN® study and review questions. On page 29 is a sample one page calendar for you to use in developing your study schedule. You can photocopy additional pages of the calendar depending on how many days or weeks you are away from your examination date. To assure your commitment to a study plan, schedule appointments with yourself on a daily basis. It is important that you keep your study appointments with yourself. Remember the time you invest now in NCLEX-RN® preparation will reward you with the feeling of confidence of knowing you prepared yourself to the best of your ability for this very important exam.

Completing Your Study Plan

You have now completed all the steps in the self-assessment process and have the information needed to develop your individualized self study plan. You have a thorough assessment of your nursing knowledge and have prioritized content areas for study. Your preparation for the exam will begin with those content areas needing more study and review and will finish with those content areas which you have identified as your strongest areas of knowledge. You have identified study strategies that have proven to be successful for you in the past and have identified those you will use for your study plan. In addition, you have identified where and when you will schedule study time and are ready to complete your study plan. If you have not already written this information on the study plan worksheet on pages 27–29, do so at this time.

Congratulations! Your individualized NCLEX-RN® study plan is now complete. You have developed your blueprint or your roadmap to take you to NCLEX-RN® success. It is crucial at this point to be certain to adhere to your plan. The time you invest now in preparation for the NCLEX-RN® examination is well worth the reward of being able to successfully pass the NCLEX-RN® examination on your first attempt. This is the last and final step in the process you began many years ago upon beginning your educational program in nursing. So on to NCLEX-RN® success!

Preparation for Your NCLEX-RN® Examination

Nursing students know the nursing material on which they are being tested but sometimes have difficulty preparing for taking and passing examinations. This section offers suggestions to help you to be at your best on the day of your examination.

Application Process

Submit your application to the board of nursing in the state or territory in which you wish to be licensed. Be sure you meet the board of nursing's deadline for application. You may register for the NCLEX-RN® examination by mail, by telephone, or on the web site. There is an application you must complete and a registration fee for the examination.

Scheduling Your Exam

After your board of nursing declares you are eligible to take the NCLEX-RN® examination, you will receive your authorization to test (ATT). At this time you will call the Pearson Professional Center at which you would like to take your examination. When scheduling your appointment, you should plan for a six (6) hour examination. Make your appointment to test as soon as possible after receiving your ATT even if you do not want to test immediately. The schedules at the test centers tend to fill up quickly and waiting to make your call may limit the dates the center has available.

The Week Before the Exam

- Drive to your testing site and identify parking areas. Time how long it took you to drive to the site so you will know how much time to allow on the day of your test.
- Identify your travel route and check construction schedules. Identify an alternate route in case of construction on your route the day of your exam.
- Get adequate sleep the week before the test. You want to be well rested for the exam.
- Eat a well balanced diet the week before the exam.
- Continue any regular exercise activity schedule you may follow.
- Practice your anxiety management/relaxation techniques.

The Night Before the Exam

- Do not spend the evening studying, plan to be prepared by this time.
- Do something relaxing that takes your mind off your upcoming exam. Go to a movie, rent a movie, or read a book (not a nursing text!).
- Do not drink alcoholic beverages. You do not want to have a sluggish and slow start the morning of the exam.
- Get a good night's sleep the night before the test.
- Set an additional back-up alarm for the morning of the test. This is especially important if you have an early morning testing appointment.

The Day of the Exam

- Have a well-balanced breakfast. Limit your caffeine intake. Remember, caffeine is a diuretic and your breaks during the examination count against your total testing time.
- Allow yourself plenty of time to arrive at the testing site. You need to arrive at least thirty (30) minutes before your examination start time/appointment.

- Dress comfortable and wear layers. It may be excessively warm or cool at the test site. You want to be able to remove or add layers of clothing.
- If you have something you wear that you consider to be "lucky" test taking clothes, wear them to your test.
- Drive yourself to the testing site or if someone drives you to the testing site plan to call for your ride when you finish the examination. Do not have someone drive you to the test and wait for you. Knowing someone is waiting for you will add additional pressure that you do not want on this day.

What to Expect at the Exam Site

The following information is provided to you to answer questions you may have about what to expect at the examination site on the day you are scheduled to take your NCLEX-RN® examination.

- Plan to arrive at the Pearson's Professional Center for your test at least 30 minutes before your testing time.
- If anyone travels with you to the testing center, they will not be able to wait at the center.
- You will need to present your ATT to test and a photo identification that includes your signature.
- Upon arrival at the testing site you will be fingerprinted and have your picture taken prior to starting your test.
- You will not be able to take anything in to the testing room with you. Secure storage will be provided for personal belongings but the testing center is not responsible for personal belongings.
- You will be given an erasable note board that you may take into the testing center. You will turn in the note board when you leave the examination.
- You will have up to six hours to complete the examination. Total examination time will include a short tutorial, two programmed optional breaks, and any unscheduled breaks you may take.
- The first pre-programmed break is offered after two (2) hours of testing and the second is offered after three and one-half (3½) hours of testing. Remember all breaks count against testing time.
- If you take a break you must leave the testing room.
- The testing associate will give you a short orientation and will then escort you to a testing terminal. You must remain in your seat during the exam unless authorized to leave by the testing center staff. If you need assistance or would like to take a break, you need to raise your hand.

Test Taking Strategies/Skills

Knowing how to successfully take a test is important in ensuring NCLEX-RN® examination success. The following are some test taking skills/strategies that are helpful in improving test scores and contributing to successful test results.

- Make certain you are comfortable with the computer testing format. Earlier in this text you read about the computerized NCLEX-RN® testing procedure. Included with this text also is a CD-ROM containing test questions. Use this CD to practice taking tests on the computer. One important feature in the computerized testing process is the use of a drop down calculator. Practice using this calculator on your home computer or a computer at school or at the library. You want to be able to use this drop down calculator quickly and efficiently the day of the test.

- Understand the various types of test questions that you will see in the NCLEX-RN® examination. The formats will include multiple choice, multiple response multiple-choice, fill-in-the-blank, and select-an-answer questions. These types of questions were discussed in more detail earlier in this unit. You will find examples of these various types of questions throughout this text as you complete the review questions in this book.

- Read each question completely and carefully before attempting to answer the question. Be certain you clearly understand what the question is asking. If you are not certain of what the question is asking, take time to read the question again.

- Sometimes the question will contain information that is really not significant in answering specifically what the question is asking. For example a question may ask about a patient with celiac disease that has just been given pre-operative medications. Upon reading the question your initial reaction might be that you do not remember anything about celiac disease. When you finish the entire question, you realize the correct response to what the question is asking is to assure the side rails are up and the patient call light is within reach. Therefore knowledge of celiac disease is not relevant in choosing the correct response.

- Other times there will be information in the question that is relevant to the correct response. For example often when the age of the client/patient is given it is important to the correct response. An example would be identifying appropriate play therapy for a child. The correct response would vary greatly for a one (1) year and a nine (9) year old child.

- You will need to determine which type of client need the question is addressing. Are you being asked to determine the nurse's best initial response or to select the nursing action that is best? When asked for the best initial nursing action a good way to determine the correct response is to review and use Maslow's Hierarchy of Needs. In using Maslow's Hierarchy of Needs to prioritize the initial need is physiologic (air, food, water); followed by safety and security needs; loving and belonging needs; self-esteem needs; with the top of the pyramid being self actualization.

Maslow's Need Hierarchy

Self Actualization
Self Esteem
Love and Belonging
Safety and Security
Physiologic

- Remember the NCLEX-RN® examination is a test of nursing practice. This means that rarely will your best response be to notify the physician or to call the doctor. The correct response is one of dealing with a nursing action. Your answers should be based on your nursing knowledge. Remember you have learned the information you need during your nursing education that you need to answer the questions on this examination.

- Another important concept you will utilize during the exam is that of the nursing process. It is important to identify and understand which area of the nursing process is being tested in the question. As you remember the steps in the nursing process are: Assessment, Diagnosis, Planning, Implementation, and Evaluation. You need to determine whether the question is asking you to assess, diagnose, plan (set priorities), implement (nursing action), or evaluate (judge outcomes). Oftentimes when the question asks for an initial nursing action, you should look for an option that is related to assessment of the client. Remember assessment is the first step in the nursing process and nurses will not take action unless there is enough patient data on which to plan or implement an action.

- Look for key words in questions that can provide clues to the correct response. Key words that can change the meaning of a question are the words except, only, not, never, least, unacceptable, and unrelated. These words are negative and when found in the stem of a question are asking you to identify an exception, detect an error, or identify a nursing action that is not warranted/indicated or one which is unacceptable. Other words to look for in the options/responses of each question are the words always, never, all, none. As you know in nursing there are very few things that are entirely one way or the other. There is very little in nursing that is totally black or white. There are many exceptions or lots of shades of gray in the nursing profession. Because of this the words that convey a sense of absoluteness tend to make options incorrect. When you see these words in your option choices, look very closely at them and carefully check your other option choices. Chances are the correct option will be one that does not contain these words.

- Another testing tip is to look for words in the option choices that are found up in the stem of the question. Often if you see an option that contains a word that is in the stem of the question, that option is the correct option.

- If you do not know the answer to a question, make your best educated guess. Try to eliminate as many of the options as possible. In a four (4) option multiple choice question, if you are able to eliminate one of the options you have a 25% chance of getting the question correct. If you are able to eliminate two (2) of the options as being incorrect you now have a 50% chance of getting the question correct!

- With the computerized testing format you are not able to go back and review questions as you have been able to do on paper/pencil exam. Throughout your nursing preparation you have taken many nursing examinations. Most of these examinations have been paper and pencil tests. With a paper and pencil test you have the opportunity to go back to previously answered questions, re-read the question and potentially change your answer to the question an unlimited number of times throughout the examination. Oftentimes this may have resulted in changing an incorrect response to a correct response . . . although probably equally as often a correct response was changed to an incorrect response! With the computer testing that is used in the NCLEX-RN® examination once you have confirmed your answer to a question and the computer has moved to the next question in your test, you cannot go back and review and question and change your answer to a question. It is this type of format for answering questions that you need to become comfortable with as you begin your NCLEX-RN® review. So from this time on when you are answering review questions, do not go back to a question that you have already selected and confirmed (selected and written an answer for). By practicing answering questions in this manner (answering a question and moving on to the next question) you will become comfortable with this format of testing used on the NCLEX-RN® exam. From this point on as you complete your practice questions you should: (1) read the question, (2) select an answer to the question, and (3) move to the next question since there is no going back.

Strategies to Manage Test Anxiety

It is normal to feel some anxiety as you prepare for this examination. In fact, you want to have a small amount of anxiety. As you study and prepare for the examination a mild to moderate level of anxiety about the exam will keep you committed, focused, and help you to better adhere to your study plan. With this same mild to moderate level of anxiety on the day of the exam you will have increased concentration during the exam itself. This increased ability to concentrate will help to improve your critical thinking and problem solving ability as you answer questions on the exam. In addition, it will also help you to better focus on the exam itself and you will not be distracted by things going on around you in the testing room. We have established that some anxiety is beneficial prior to and on the day of the exam. But what if at some point a mild to moderate level of anxiety begins to increase to a higher level or a sense of panic develops? For example, what if you come upon a few questions in a sequence that you do not feel comfortable with your answer and you feel your anxiety level increasing. The key to allowing anxiety to work for you is the ability to control anxiety when you need to. This ability to control your level of anxiety is what you will learn in this section of the book.

The following are some anxiety management strategies or relaxation techniques that can be used to effectively decrease and manage levels of anxiety. Review the various types of strategies identified, practice each of them and find the one that is most effective for you. Some individuals routinely practice relaxation or anxiety management techniques (yoga is a great example) so if you already have identified a strategy that works for you, this is not the time to make a change. Use the anxiety management or relaxation strategy that works best for you. It is important as with any skill that you practice this strategy or technique regularly as you begin your preparation for the exam in order to be able to use it effectively. On the day of the exam you want to be able to quickly and effectively manage your anxiety and relax. You will only be able to do this if you have a technique that works for you and are effectively able to employ the technique.

Guided Imagery

Guided imagery is a relaxation technique that can be used to develop a sense of calmness or tranquility in an individual experiencing stress. The mind creates a mental picture of something or somewhere the individual finds relaxing and tranquil. You will employ sight, sound, and sensation in a guided imagery experience. The following steps will guide you through a guided imagery relaxation exercise:

1. Sit comfortably in your chair with your eyes closed, feet flat on the floor, and hands in your lap or at your side. Let your breathing be slow and relaxed.
2. Imagine yourself somewhere you find relaxing (the beach, in a hammock, in the woods); identify the sights (sun, shade, trees, sky, water), sounds (waves lapping the shore, birds chirping, wind in the trees, and sensations (warm sand, cool breeze, warm sun, cool shade, relaxing swaying motion of the hammock) associated with that location.
3. Focus on your area, the sights, the sounds, and the sensations. Repeat the words associated with your sensation over to yourself as you imagine yourself in your area.
4. Continue feeling the sights, sounds, sensations until you feel more relaxed and calm.
5. Focus on how you feel right now and slowly open your eyes.

Progressive Muscle Relaxation

Progressive muscle relaxation works on the premise that tension is incompatible with relaxation so, when we relax our body and our mind, we eliminate the tension that tightens our muscles. And when we eliminate the tension that tightens our muscles we relax our body and mind. This is how we reduce stress and anxiety and thereby produce a sense of well being. The technique involves slowly tensing and releasing each muscle group starting slowly in the toes and finishing up at the head. The following steps will guide you through a progressive muscle relaxation exercise:

1. Sit comfortably in your chair with your eyes closed, feet flat on the floor, and hands in your lap or at your side. Let your breathing be slow and relaxed.
2. Begin by stretching your legs out in front of you.
3. Tighten your feet by curling your toes toward the sole of your foot. Visualize your feet and toes becoming tighter and tighter. Hold this tension for five (5) seconds then relax. Relax all the muscles in your feet.
4. Tighten the muscles in your calves and those in your thighs. Visualize your calves and thighs becoming tighter and tighter. Hold the tension for five (5) seconds and then relax. Relax all the muscles in your feet, in your calves, and in your thighs.
5. Focus on your toes, feet, calves, and thighs and feel the relaxation.
6. Tighten your hands by clenching your fists and tensing the muscles. Visualize the muscles in your hands becoming tighter and tighter. Hold this tension for five (5) seconds then relax. Relax all the muscles in your hands.
7. Tighten the muscles in your arms. Visualize the muscles in your arms becoming tighter and tighter. Hold the tension for five (5) seconds and then relax. Relax all the muscles in your arms and hands.
8. Focus on your toes, feet, calves, thighs, hands, and arms and feel the relaxation.
9. Tighten the muscles in your shoulders by shrugging your shoulders and tensing the muscles. Visualize the muscles in your shoulders becoming tighter and tighter. Hold this tension for five (5) seconds then relax. Relax all the muscles in your shoulders.
10. Tighten the muscles in your face by tightening your facial muscles. Visualize the muscles in your face becoming tighter and tighter. Hold the tension for five (5) seconds and then relax. Relax all the muscles in your face.
11. Focus on your toes, feet, calves, thighs, hands, arms, shoulders, and face and feel the relaxation.
12. Focus on how you feel right now and slowly open your eyes.

Deep Breathing

Deep breathing slowly increases the oxygen flow from your lungs to your brain. This exercise will help to decrease your anxiety level because by concentrating on counting and breathing you will not be focusing on the event that is causing you stress and/or anxiety.

The following steps will guide you through a deep breathing relaxation exercise:

1. Sit comfortably in your chair with your eyes closed, feet flat on the floor, and hands in your lap or at your side. Let your breathing be slow and relaxed.
2. Take deep measured breaths by inhaling slowly while counting to five (5) and then exhaling slowly while counting to ten (10).
3. Repeat the deep breathing sequence for ten (10) to fifteen (15) times.
4. Continue the breathing sequences until you begin to feel more calm and relaxed.
5. Focus on how you feel right now and slowly open your eyes.

Mind Clearing/Blanking Your Mind

Mental clearing or blanking is a relaxation technique that can be used to develop a sense of calmness or tranquility in an individual experiencing stress. This technique is very similar to that of visual imagery. The difference between the two is that in mind clearing or blanking, rather than creating a mental picture of something, the mind creates a mental picture of a blank black screen or blank black wall. While creating this blank mental picture repeat the phrase blank screen or blank blackboard to yourself. While doing this try not to let any other thoughts or feelings enter your mind. If they do, just return your attention to your blank screen or blank blackboard. At the end of this exercise you will feel more relaxed and calm. The following steps will guide you through a mind clearing/blanking relaxation exercise:

1. Sit comfortably in your chair with your eyes closed, feet flat on the floor, and hands in your lap or at your side. Let your breathing be slow and relaxed.
2. Remove all thoughts from your mind. Clear your mind by imagining a blank black screen or a blank black wall. Focus only on the blank screen or wall. Keep repeating the words blank screen or blank wall to yourself.
3. Remain focused on your blank screen or wall and keep repeating your phrase until you begin to feel more relaxed or calm.
4. Focus on how you feel right now and slowly open your eyes.

It is important to find the anxiety management strategy or relaxation technique you are most comfortable using and the one that is most effective for you. Take time as you are preparing for the examination to practice your technique of choice daily until you are very comfortable using the technique. If during the NCLEX-RN® examination you find yourself becoming anxious, you will easily and effectively be able to lower your anxiety level and continue on with your questions.

Tips from NCLEX-RN® Survivors

It is good to remember that you are not the first person to have ever taken the NCLEX-RN® examination. Included below are some insights from students who successfully prepared for and completed the examination.

"I found that completing a self-assessment prior to taking the exam really helped me to focus my study efforts . . ."

"For me, it was very useful to work on practice questions before taking the exam. I took some with me wherever I went and if I had some down time I just took them out and answered some . . ."

"I am not very good at budgeting my time. I found that creating a study plan for the weeks leading up to the test and sticking to it really allowed me to feel like I had prepared to the best of my ability . . ."

"There is nothing to compare the feeling of confidence you experience when you sit down for the exam and know that you have prepared yourself to the best of your ability . . ."

"Working on practice questions caused me to realize that I actually remembered what I had learned in all those nursing courses I had taken . . ."

"Being familiar with the types of questions and using a computerized test bank of questions to review helped when it was time to sit down for the actual exam. It was not like this was something I was seeing for the first time . . ."

"Throughout nursing school I always got very anxious when taking tests. I found that the stress relieving techniques I learned and practiced helped me to really reduce my anxiety before and during the test . . ."

"I can't stress enough the importance of knowing what my strengths and weaknesses were to me. It allowed me to really focus on areas I did not realize I needed work in. My suggestion for success is: Self-assessment, self-assessment, self-assessment . . ."

"I have always been a last-minute studier. For the NCLEX® exam I made myself a study plan and followed it for five weeks before taking the test. The difference it made in my comfort and confidence level was amazing . . ."

"I had answered so many practice questions by the time I took the exam, I felt like I had seen the test ahead of time!"

"Multiple response questions have always given me problems on tests. So when preparing for the NCLEX® exam I practiced them a lot. By the time I took the test I had become very comfortable with them . . ."

"My best friend and I decided to be study partners for the exam. We were able to help each other in areas we did not feel strong in . . ."

Conclusion

In conclusion, after completing this unit you should be well on your way to NCLEX-RN® success. To begin with, you have learned how to use this review book and the accompanying CD-ROM to prepare for your NCLEX-RN® examination. In addition to this you should be familiar with licensure requirements for registered nurses. The NCLEX-RN® Test Plan has been explored along with identification of the format of the examination and content areas found on the exam. Also, you now know the format of the types of questions you can expect to encounter on the exam. The comprehensive self-assessment of your learning needs you have completed is designed to help begin your study preparation and developed a plan for preparing for the exam. After prioritizing your content areas for study you have created a timeline and study plan to organize your preparation for the exam. Finally, you have learned how to psychologically prepare yourself for this very important test and have learned some effective strategies to use in order to manage any test anxiety you may experience prior to or during the examination. Now the rest is up to you. The fact that you have completed or are near completion of a Registered Nursing program means that you possess a significant amount of nursing skills and knowledge. All that is left to do is believe in yourself and follow the preparation plan you have developed for yourself. Once again, congratulations: you are well on your way to NCLEX-RN® success!

References

Bloom, B. (1956). *Taxonomy of educational objectives. Handbook I: Cognitive domain.* New York: David McKay.

Chitty, K. (2001). *Professional nursing: Concepts & challenges* (3rd ed.). Philadelphia: Saunders.

Crutchlow, E., Dudac, P., MacAvoy, S., & Madara, B. (2002). *Quick look nursing: Pathophysiology.* Thorofare, NJ: Slack.

Eddy, L. & Epeneter, B. (2002). The NCLEX-RN experience: Qualitative interviews with graduates of a baccalaureate nursing program. *Journal of Nursing Education. 41*(6), 273–278.

Lewis, S., Heitkemper, M., & Dirkson, S. (2004). *Medical-surgical nursing: Assessment and management of clinical problems* (6th ed.). St. Louis, MO: Mosby.

National Council of State Boards of Nursing (NCSBN). (2006). *2007 NCLEX-RN examination: Test plan for the national council licensure examination for registered nurses.* New York: Pearson Vue.

National Council of State Boards of Nursing (NCSBN). (2006). *2006 NCLEX-RN examination: Candidate bulletin.* New York: Pearson Vue.

Nuget, P. & Vitale, B. (2004). *Test success: Test taking techniques for beginning nursing students.* (4th ed.). Philadelphia: FA Davis.

Thies, K. & Travers, J. (2001). *Quick look nursing: Growth & development.* Thorofare, NJ: Slack.

Individualized Study Plan

Self-Assessment

Content Knowledge Assessment

Pretest Score—Identify areas of strength and areas needing more review.

_____

_____

_____

Historical Review—From your educational program identify content areas of strength and areas needing more review.

_____

_____

_____

_____

_____

_____

_____

_____

Data Prioritization—Prioritize your areas of content knowledge with #1 being the content area in which you feel most comfortable/confident of your knowledge. After you have your list, reverse the numbering order so that you begin your study with area #1 being the area in which you feel you need the most study and/or review (use additional pages as needed).

_____

_____

_____

_____

_____

_____

_____

_____

_____

Individualized Study Plan

Study Methods/Skills, Locations, Timeline

Study Methods—Methods I have used successfully in the past and will use now:

_____
_____
_____
_____
_____
_____
_____
_____
_____
_____

Study Location—Where I plan to study:

_____
_____
_____

My Study Timeline—Assessment of the time I will need to completely review my content areas:

(On the next page is a calendar to schedule appointments for study sessions and other important events occurring during your NCLEX-RN® preparation timeline.)

_____
_____
_____
_____
_____
_____
_____
_____
_____
_____
_____
_____

Month: _____

Sunday	Monday	Tuesday	Wednesday	Thursday	Friday	Saturday

Pretest

The questions in the Pretest are taken from the various sections within the book. You will see these questions again later in the book. The purpose of the Pretest is to test your knowledge across the various topic areas in the book at this moment. Answers to the Pretest questions appear on page 446.

1. The nurse must transfer a dependent client from a bed to a gurney. Which measure taken by the nurse will be safest for both the nurse and the client?
   1. Adjust the height of the client's bed.
   2. Avoid movements that twist the spine.
   3. Keep the client close to her body when lifting.
   4. Use a mechanical lift device appropriate for this client.

2. The nurse is teaching a client with a history of falls about home safety. Which of the following statements indicates that the client understands the instructions?
   1. "I will keep my walker at the end of my bed."
   2. "I will keep the ceiling light on in my room at all times."
   3. "I will put a nonskid floor mat on the side of the bed that I exit."
   4. "I will wear treaded slipper socks on my carpeted floors."

3. The nurse is training a group of certified nursing assistants (CNAs) about hand hygiene. Which of the following statements indicate that the CNAs need further instruction from the nurse?
   1. "As long as I am changing gloves between clients, it is not necessary to wash my hands."
   2. "I should wash my hands when my hands are visibly soiled."
   3. "I will not wear artificial nails when providing client care."
   4. "It is ok to use alcohol-based hand products after client contact."

4. The nurse is caring for a client with Hepatitis A. What action puts the nurse at highest risk for being exposed to Hepatitis A?
   1. Standing one foot away when the client coughs.
   2. Suctioning the client.
   3. Testing the client's stool for occult blood.
   4. Touching the client's arm when providing comfort.

5. When assessing a client's strength in preparation for ambulating out of bed, the nurse should do which of the following?
   1. Ask the client how strong they feel today.
   2. Ask the client if they have been up before.
   3. Check the pedal pulses and feet for edema.
   4. Instruct the client to push the soles of the feet against the nurse's palms.

6. To ensure accuracy when checking bowel sounds, how should the nurse auscultate the abdomen?
   1. After palpation and percussion.
   2. Before palpation and percussion.
   3. For at least five minutes in each quadrant.
   4. Start listening at the left lower quadrant.

7. A client's pulse oximetry to determine hemoglobin saturation is 85%. What should the nurse do first?
   1. Administer oxygen at four liters per minute.
   2. Call the client's doctor.
   3. Encourage coughing and deep breathing.
   4. Raise the head of the bed.

8. **The nurse instructs her elderly client not to strain when defecating because it could cause which of the following?**
   1. Dizziness.
   2. Dysrhythmias.
   3. Fecal incontinence.
   4. Rectal bleeding from hemorrhoids.

9. **Men tend to display which of the following traits when communicating with other workers?**
   1. They are more goal-oriented than process-orientated.
   2. They build and maintain personal relationships.
   3. They tell people what to do indirectly.
   4. They value the process aspect of decision-making.

10. **A client with post-traumatic stress disorder says to you, "They think you should be able to put it out of your mind. It happened so long ago—just get over it!" The nurse responds, "It must be very frustrating to encounter that kind of an attitude." The response is an example of which of the following?**
    1. Clarifying.
    2. Focusing.
    3. Paraphrasing.
    4. Reflection.

11. **At the immunization clinic, a father says to his six-year-old son who is fighting back tears, "Children who cry when they get needles are crybabies." The nurse assesses this communication to be which of the following?**
    1. Clear.
    2. Circular.
    3. Emotional.
    4. Masked.

12. **A nurse approaches a male patient and asks how he is feeling. The client states, "I'm feeling a bit nervous today." Which of the following is the nurse's best reply?**
    1. "Please explain what you mean by the word nervous."
    2. "What is making you feel nervous?"
    3. "Would a backrub ease your nervousness?"
    4. "You do look like you're nervous."

13. **To convert 0.8 grams to milligrams, the nurse should do which of the following?**
    1. Move the decimal point 3 places to the right.
    2. Move the decimal point 3 places to the left.
    3. Move the decimal point 2 places to the right.
    4. Move the decimal point 2 places to the left.

14. **When administering a flu vaccine, how does the nurse locate the deltoid muscle?**
    1. By locating the center of the arm between the elbow and the shoulder.
    2. By locating the midpoint of the lateral aspect of the upper arm.
    3. By palpating the lower edge of the acromion process and measuring four inches below to the center of the lateral aspect of the upper arm.
    4. By palpating the lower edge of the acromion process and measuring four finger-widths below to the midpoint and center of the lateral aspect of the upper arm.

15. **The nurse is preparing an injection using a single dose glass ampule. The nurse will do which of the following?**

1. Wear sterile gloves and break off the neck of the glass ampule with a single snap to the right side.
2. Wear sterile gloves and break off the neck of the glass ampule with a single snap in a forward motion.
3. Tap the top of the ampule, place a gauze pad or alcohol swab around the ampule neck, and break off the top with a forward motion away from the hands.
4. Tap the top of the ampule, place a gauze pad or unwrapped alcohol swab around the ampule neck, and break off the top with a forward motion away from the hands.

For the following question, fill in the blank with the correct route (intravenous, intramuscular, oral, rectal, subcutaneous, topical) of administration.

16. _____

Drugs that are safest and most convenient; most drugs are administered by this route.

17. Which of the following tasks, as defined in your state practice acts, cannot be delegated to the LPN/LVN?
    1. Tracheotomy care.
    2. Ostomy care.
    3. Testing a stool specimen for guaiac blood.
    4. Shift head to toe physical assessment

18. The nurse has just completed her shift report. Which client will she assign to the unlicensed personnel (UAP)?
    1. A stable three-hour postoperative thyroidectomy client.
    2. A stable one-day postoperative abdominal hysterectomy client.
    3. A stable three-day postoperative gastric bypass client.
    4. A stable two-hour postoperative cholestectomy client.

19. What nursing diagnosis takes priority in a client with borderline personality disorder (BPD)?
    1. Chronic low self esteem.
    2. Impaired social interaction.
    3. Risk for impulsive aggressive behavior.
    4. Risk for suicide.

20. The registered nurse checks with individuals throughout the day to see if they are completing tasks. What right of delegation is the nurse demonstrating?
    1. Right circumstances.
    2. Right communication.
    3. Right person.
    4. Right supervision.

21. Who is used as a triage officer during the time of a disaster?
    1. Members of the Federal Medical Emergency Agency (FEMA).
    2. The emergency room physician who directs all care.
    3. Representatives from the American Red Cross.
    4. Nurses and other emergency personnel.

22. According to the American Red Cross, a major disaster is classified as which of the following?
    1. A disaster that affects more than one family, occurs within the jurisdiction of one American Red Cross chapter, and requires limited human and material resources.
    2. A disaster that affects multiple families in a single state and may require disaster help from more than one Red Cross chapter.
    3. A disaster that requires the help of multiple Red Cross units, affects more than a single state, and may be expected to be declared an emergency by the President of the United States.
    4. A disaster that requires full or partial implementation of the Federal Response Plan. This disaster exceeds the ability of the state and local government capabilities to meet the needs of the situation.

23. **In disaster preparedness planning for a bioterrorism event that may involve anthrax, the nurse should know which of the following?**
    1. Anthrax vaccine is recommended for all hospital staff who deliver care to clients.
    2. Anthrax is typically contracted through ingestion of raw meat.
    3. Children are less likely to be effected by the exposure.
    4. Anthrax is not spread person to person.

24. **With the potential use of smallpox as a bioterrorism threat, a nurse must prepare to respond to a disaster event with this agent. The nurse's preparation is based on which of the following facts about smallpox? Select all that apply.**
    1. Smallpox is transmitted person to person through direct contact or droplet inhalation.
    2. Infection is characterized by severe respiratory distress, septicemia, and hemorrhagic meningitis.
    3. A vaccination for smallpox is available.
    4. Naturally occurring smallpox has been eradicated from the world.
    5. Smallpox is a bacterium that produces spores that can remain viable in the environment for long periods of time.
    6. There is no proven treatment.

25. **A client has been diagnosed with pulmonary tuberculosis. The client exhibits signs and symptoms that include which of the following?**
    1. Cough, decreased blood pressure, and decreased urinary output.
    2. Cough, chills, and leucocytosis.
    3. Fever, pain, and abdominal distention.
    4. A negative chest X-ray and weight gain.

26. **The nurse is caring for a client who has a chest tube with water seal drainage. Guidelines for care include which of the following?**
    1. Do not encourage the client to cough until the chest tube is removed.
    2. Elevate the drainage system to the level of the patient's chest.
    3. Keep the water seal and suction control chamber at the appropriate water levels by adding sterile water as needed.
    4. Strip or milk the tubing to promote drainage.

27. **What is a normal tidal volume (Vt) for a client on a ventilator?**
    1. 5–7 ml/kg.
    2. 7–9 ml/kg.
    3. 9–11 ml/kg.
    4. 11–13 ml/kg.

28. **Which population has a higher incidence of acquiring tuberculosis (TB)? Select all that apply.**
    1. Children 2 years and younger.
    2. Clients who are HIV positive.
    3. Adolescents.
    4. Pregnant women.
    5. African American males.

29. **What should the nurse have available if the patient receives an overdose of heparin?**
    1. Iron.
    2. Platelets.
    3. Protamine Sulfate.
    4. Vitamin K.

30. **Which of the following is a manifestation of chronic venous insufficiency?**
    1. Dry, necrotic ulcers in the feet.
    2. Edema.
    3. Hair loss.
    4. Thick, deformed toenails.

31. **Which is the antidote for a severe warfarin (Coumadin) overdose?**
    1. Protamine zinc.
    2. Protamine sulfate.
    3. Vitamin E.
    4. Vitamin K.

32. The nurse is giving warfarin (Coumadin) to a client with atrial fibrillation. What does the nurse understand the implications of this medication to be?
    1. Coumadin is helpful in converting atrial fibrillation to sinus rhythm.
    2. Coumadin is used to dissolve clots.
    3. Coumadin is used to prevent heart attacks in clients with atrial fibrillation.
    4. Coumadin is used to prevent strokes in clients with atrial fibrillation.

33. Which of the following is a common link between Crohn's disease and ulcerative colitis?
    1. Both are inflammatory.
    2. Both have the same degree of mucosal penetration.
    3. Both occur in the same population.
    4. Both share a similar distribution pattern.

34. Your client is scheduled for a barium enema. He asks why a laxative is necessary the evening before the test. How would the nurse best respond in order to help the client understand the procedure?
    1. "Because the doctor ordered it."
    2. "It assists with emptying the bowel for the best visualization."
    3. "It is our procedure at this facility."
    4. "It makes the X-ray more clear."

35. Which of the following represents the best evaluation criteria for monitoring the effectiveness of treatment aimed at reducing aggravating factors with the diagnosis of cholecystitis?
    1. The client displays no improvement on ultrasonography.
    2. The client maintains a serum albumin level within normal limits.
    3. The client maintains intake and output within normal limits.
    4. The client reports no pain following a low-fat meal.

36. A client with advanced liver disease presents with vomiting blood, tachycardia, cool, clammy skin, restlessness, and lethargy. All signs indicate a complication of portal hypertension. Based on the findings, the nurse determines the client is experiencing which complication of portal hypertension?
    1. Cirrhosis of the liver
    2. Bleeding esophageal varices
    3. Hepatomegaly
    4. Duodenal ulcer

37. According to the following lab results, which one indicates renal failure?
    1. BUN 10, serum creatinine 0.3.
    2. BUN 45, serum creatinine 1.0.
    3. BUN 11, serum creatinine 10.
    4. BUN 35, serum creatinine 8.

38. In teaching a new client with chronic renal failure about the process of peritoneal dialysis (PD), the nurse would explain which of the following to the client?
    1. PD occurs when blood is filtered through an artificial device called a dialyzer.
    2. PD is the dialysis of choice for clients with abdominal trauma.
    3. PD has fewer dietary and fluid restrictions than hemodialysis.
    4. PD is the treatment of choice with acute conditions.

39. The nurse is discharging a client from the hospital. The nurse knows that client has knowledge of their new prescription of furosemide (Lasix) when the client states which of the following?
    1. "I have to eat a diet low in potassium."
    2. "I have to limit my fluid intake."
    3. "My blood pressure will increase while I am on this medication."
    4. "I need to limit my sun exposure and wear sunscreen while on this medication."

40. A nurse would educate a client who was recovering from shock that their kidney function was altered from the trauma. The nurse would state that the client was in acute renal failure and that their kidneys were going to go through phases of recovery. List the phases of acute renal failure in order from the initial injury to the stabilization of kidney function.
    1. Diuretic phase.
    2. Onset phase.
    3. Oliguric phase.
    4. Recovery phase.

41. Following a hypophysectomy, the client complains of clear nasal drainage. What is the most appropriate initial action for the nurse?
    1. Notify the surgeon immediately.
    2. Encourage the client to blow his nose to clear the sinuses.
    3. Check the nasal drainage for glucose.
    4. Place the client in Trendelenberg position

42. Which of the following lab results would be typical of the client with Addison's disease?
    1. Blood urine nitrogen (BUN) of 3.5 mg/dl.
    2. Sodium (NA) of 185 mEq/L.
    3. Fasting blood glucose (FBS) of 55 mg/dl.
    4. Potassium (K) of 2.7 mEq/L.

43. The nurse is teaching a patient newly diagnosed with Type 1 diabetes mellitus how to administer insulin injections. Place the following steps in the correct order for drawing up and administering a dose of 25 units of NPH insulin.
    1. Wash hands.
    2. Draw back 25 units of air into the syringe and inject air into the insulin vial.
    3. Inject insulin.
    4. Withdraw 25 units of NPH insulin.
    5. Gently roll vial of NPH insulin.
    6. Inspect for and remove air bubbles.
    7. Choose and cleanse the site.
    8. Cleanse the top of the insulin vial with alcohol.

44. The nurse administers a dose of six units of regular insulin (Humulin R) to a patient. Knowing the action of regular insulin, when would the nurse anticipate that a hypoglycemia reaction could occur?
    1. Between 8:00AM and 10:00AM.
    2. Between 10:00AM and 12:00PM.
    3. Between 2:00PM and 10:00PM.
    4. Between 10:00PM and 8:00AM the next day.

45. In the following list, identify items to be included in a teaching plan for a thrombocytopenic client requiring bleeding precautions. Select all that apply.
    1. Avoid intramuscular injections.
    2. Brush teeth with a soft toothbrush.
    3. Avoid rectal temperatures, suppositories, and examinations.
    4. Avoid flossing your teeth.
    5. Blow your nose gently.
    6. Avoid fresh fruits and vegetables.
    7. Avoid contact sports and activities potentially causing trauma.
    8. Use a straight razor instead of an electric shaver.

46. A client with a white blood cell disorder asks how such a condition develops. The nurse begins by stating that all blood cells are produced in which of the following?
    1. Thymus.
    2. Central nervous system.
    3. Bone marrow.
    4. Spleen.

47. The nurse receives a unit of packed red blood cells (PRBCs) from the blood bank and notes that the time on the clock reads 4:10 PM. By what time must the blood begin infusing?
    1. 4:50 PM.
    2. 4:40 PM.
    3. 5:00 PM.
    4. 5:10 PM.

48. **During a client's routine physical examination, leukocytosis is detected. The nurse receiving this result knows that leukocytosis can indicate which of the following?**
    1. Anemia.
    2. Coagulation disorders.
    3. Infection and inflammation.
    4. Renal or hepatic disorders.

49. **Which of the following would indicate that a biopsy be recommended for skin lesions?**
    1. A health history can not be obtained.
    2. A more definitive diagnosis is needed.
    3. Palpation reveals abnormal findings.
    4. Topical medications have not worked.

50. **While working in a community clinic, a 10-year-old client complains of dandruff and a rash on the back of her neck. On examination, the nurse notices the dandruff flakes don't brush off the hair. The nurse suspects which of the following disorders?**
    1. Pediculosis capitus.
    2. Psoriasis.
    3. Seborrheic dermatitis.
    4. Tinea capitis.

51. **A client has just been admitted to your unit with psoriasis. The nurse needs to prepare the client for which of the following therapies to be initiated?**
    1. Laser treatments.
    2. Phototherapy.
    3. Radiation therapy.
    4. Topical fluorouracil (5-FU)

52. **Which statement best indicates an understanding of skin cancer risk factors?**
    1. "Because I'm dark-complected, I won't have to worry about skin cancer."
    2. "I really need to use sunscreen—even in winter."
    3. "I used to lie in the sun all the time but now I just go to the tanning bed."
    4. "My father was treated for melanoma, but my mother says not to worry."

53. **A client was informed that radiation therapy will be initiated for several weeks prior to surgery. The client and family are angry and state they believe the delay in surgical removal will delay eradication of the tumor. What would be the nurse's most appropriate initial topic of discussion to have with this client and family?**
    1. If radiation is effective, surgery will not be necessary.
    2. If you disagree with the doctor, you may seek a second opinion.
    3. Radiation will shrink the tumor before surgery.
    4. You have the right to refuse radiation so surgery can be done.

54. **A family noticed that after opiate pain management was initiated, the client was sedated and resting comfortably but sleeping continuously. After three days, the client is no longer sedated, and the family questions if pain control is lost. The nurse realizes that which of the following occurs after two to three days?**
    1. An alternate method of pain management must be employed.
    2. Most clients develop a tolerance to the sedative effects of opioids.
    3. The dose will have to be adjusted.
    4. The client will probably require combination pain control.

55. **The firmest recognized risk factor for pancreatic cancer is which of the following?**
    1. A high-fat diet.
    2. Cigarette smoking.
    3. Diabetes.
    4. Exposure to benzidine.

56. **The symptoms of gastric cancer are often identical to those of which of the following?**
    1. Esophagus cancer.
    2. Liver cancer.
    3. Myocardial infarction.
    4. Peptic ulcer disease.

57. The nurse is giving instructions to a patient with Parkinson's disease. Which instruction should the nurse include in the discharge teaching?
1. Many side effects are dose related and can be controlled by a dosage adjustment.
2. All drugs have side effects and most clients will get used to them.
3. Skipping a dose now and then is okay if the side effects are too annoying.
4. It is important to keep a list of all the side effects and bring it to your next doctor's visit.

58. Differentiate between bowel training for clients with upper motor neuron (UMN) spinal cord injury and lower motor neuron (LMN) spinal cord injury.

_____

_____

_____

_____

_____

_____

_____

59. A client has undergone a craniotomy to clip a cerebral aneurysm. Which postoperative complication is the client *least* likely to develop as a result of the surgery?
1. Hydrocephalus.
2. Diabetes insipidus.
3. Diabetes mellitus.
4. Syndrome of inappropriate ADH.

60. Motor function response in an unconscious client is purposeful when the nurse applies a painful stimulus and the client does which of the following?
1. Pushes the painful stimulus away.
2. Extends the body part toward the stimuli.
3. Shows no reaction to the painful stimuli.
4. Flexes the upper extremities and extends the lower extremities.

61. What portion of the bone contains pain receptors?
1. Endosteum.
2. Haversian system.
3. Marrow.
4. Periosteum.

62. The nurse, when assessing a client with systemic lupus erythematosus, can be expected to find which of the following? Select all that apply.
1. Neuropathies.
2. Pleural effusion.
3. Photosensitivity.
4. Thrombocytopenia.

63. A nurse is giving instructions to a client who had surgical correction of bilateral hallux valgus (bunion). What should the nurse's instructions include?
1. Expect the feet to be numb for several days postoperatively.
2. Rest frequently with the feet elevated.
3. Soak the feet in warm water several times a day.
4. Walk primarily on the heels to relieve pressure on the toes.

64. A client with a fracture has developed compartment syndrome. Which of the following are characteristic of impending compartment syndrome? Select all that apply.
1. Pain proximal to the injury.
2. Pallor.
3. Paresthesia.
4. Pulselessness.

65. In the preoperative area, the nurse notices that the surgical permit has not been signed; however, the client has been medicated with Ativan (lorazepam) and Demerol (meperidine). What should the nurse do?

1. Have the client sign the permit.
2. Have the client's friend sign the permit.
3. Notify the doctor.
4. Sign the permit for the client.

66. The client is unconscious on admission to the postanesthesia care unit (PACU). How should the nurse position the client?

1. In a lateral position.
2. In a prone position.
3. In a supine position.
4. With the head elevated.

67. Identify the client who is a high risk for developing respiratory problems in the postoperative course.

1. The client is ambulatory.
2. The client has no history of respiratory problems.
3. The client has undergone genitourinary surgery.
4. The client is obese.

68. The circulating nurse is preparing the surgical suite for a procedure. The nurse notices that a sterile package has become wet with sterile normal saline. Select the most appropriate action.

1. Discard the package.
2. Include it in the sterile field.
3. Let the package dry and use it in the procedure.
4. Save it for the next procedure.

69. Place the steps for inserting an IV in the proper order.

1. Catheter stabilization and application of dressing.
2. Check physician's order.
3. Insertion into vein.
4. Assemble equipment.
5. Don gloves.
6. Documentation of procedure.
7. Site preparation.
8. Site selection and vein dilation.

70. While preparing to administer a new container of TPN as a total nutrient admixture (TNA) or a 3:1 solution at 84 ml/hr, the nurse checks the order with another nurse. The client has a patent designated central line and an electronic infusion device (EID) at the bedside. The nurse gathers tubing for the new container. What is the appropriate size final filter for this infusion?

1. 0.22 micron.
2. 0.45 micron.
3. 1.2 micron.
4. 170–260 micron.

71. The nurse enters the client's room and realizes that due to a shortage of EIDs on the unit, a client is receiving an IV that is infusing at 28 drops/min with 20 drop factor (drop/ml) tubing. How many ml of solution will this client receive at the end of a 12-hour shift?

1. 84 ml.
2. 672 ml.
3. 1008 ml.
4. 1680 ml.

72. A client is admitted with a HCO_3 of 18 mEq (22–26), CO_2 of 28 mmHg (35–45). What pH value and acid base imbalance would most likely accompany these values?

1. Decreased pH and metabolic acidosis.
2. Decreased pH and respiratory acidosis.
3. Elevated pH and metabolic alkalosis.
4. Elevated pH and respiratory alkalosis.

73. A client with severe hepatic failure is ordered a high calorie, low protein diet. Which selection is most appropriate for the client?

1. Scrambled eggs, bacon, pancakes, orange slices.
2. Grilled cheese sandwich, potato chips, chocolate pudding.
3. Steak, french fries, corn, salad.
4. Chicken breast, mashed potatoes, spinach.

74. A client with a CVA is admitted to the rehab unit. At supper time, the nurse notices that the client experiences severe dysphagia and reports this to the physician. What form of nutritional support is most essential for this client?
1. NPO until dysphagia subsides.
2. Nasogastric tube feeding.
3. Total parenteral nutrition (TPN).
4. Soft residue diet.

75. The student nurse discusses the risk of aspiration with the parents of an 18-month-old. Which foods should be avoided?
1. Apples, crackers, and applesauce.
2. Cherries, peanuts, and hard candy.
3. Cheerios, fruit juice, and raisins.
4. Orange juice, toast, bananas.

76. The nurse reviews the monthly dietary recall journal of a geriatric client who has been recently been diagnosed with anemia. Which foods *best* identify essential nutrients that promote erthropoiesis?
1. Roast beef, broccoli, and whole grain bread.
2. Lasagna, garlic toast, and creamed corn.
3. Tacos, spanish rice, and cherry cobbler.
4. French toast, sausage, and figs.

77. When teaching a class of pregnant women about fetal development, the nurse should include which of the following?
1. "The baby's heart beat is audible by doppler at 12 weeks of pregnancy."
2. "The sex of the baby is determined by week 8 of pregnancy."
3. "Very fine hairs, called lanugo, cover your baby's entire body by week 36 of pregnancy."
4. "You will first feel your baby move by week 24 of pregnancy."

78. A laboring client delivers two hours after receiving meperidine (Demerol) IV. Which of the following medications should be available to counteract the effects of meperidine (Demerol) in the newborn?
1. Beractant (Survanta).
2. Betamethasone.
3. Fentanyl (Sublimaze).
4. Naloxone (Narcan).

79. A sudden loud noise produced the following response in a newborn: symmetric abduction and extension of the arms with the fingers fanning out and forming a "C" with the thumb and forefinger. A slight tremor was also noted. The nurse would document this finding as a positive

_____ reflex.
1. Babinski.
2. Moro.
3. Rooting.
4. Tonic neck.

80. A postpartum client delivered a healthy baby girl two days ago. Document the expected type of lochia at this time.

_____

81. The client states, "I'm a little nervous because I have never had a pelvic examination before." The nurse recognizes the client is anxious and explains which of the following about the exam?

1. The examiner will use a plastic speculum to visualize and inspect the woman's vulva, vagina, and cervix.

2. The woman's cervix will be inspected using a speculum.

3. The examiner will perform both a bimanual examination and an inspection that will include palpation of the cervix, uterus, and ovaries.

4. The exam will include an inspection of the vulva, vagina, and cervix using a speculum.

82. **Which of the following medications are used to prevent osteoporosis in menopausal women?**
    1. Levothyroxine (Snythroid).
    2. Vitamin E.
    3. Raloxiphine (Evista).
    4. Alendronate sodium (Fosamax).

83. **When rounding, the nurse observes that a six-hour postoperative hysterectomy client's Foley catheter drainage is becoming increasingly bloody in appearance. Which of the following could cause this?**
    1. The bladder may have been nicked during the surgical procedure.
    2. This is a normal response for this type of surgery.
    3. The client is probably dehydrated.
    4. The client may have a urinary tract infection.

84. **Effective techniques for sexually transmitted infection counseling include which of the following?**
    1. Asking closed-ended questions when obtaining the health history.
    2. Obtaining a reproductive health history on all women.
    3. Assuming that women in higher socially economic classes are not a risk for sexually transmitted infections.
    4. Assuming that women are aware of the consequences of sexually transmitted infections.

85. **An infant born to an HBsAg-positive mother should receive which of the following?**
    1. HBIG.
    2. Hepatitis B vaccine at day 0, 1–2 months, and 6 months.
    3. Hepatitis B vaccine within 12 hours of birth, plus HBIG.
    4. Hepatitis B vaccine within 24 hours of birth.

86. **You are sending a child home on an oral medication. Appropriate discharge instructions on giving a medication would include which of the following? Select all that apply.**
    1. How to store the drug.
    2. The name of the medication.
    3. The reason the child is taking the medication.
    4. To stop taking the medication when the child feels better.
    5. Side-effects of the medication.
    6. Use a kitchen spoon to administer the medication.
    7. When to return for the next set of vaccinations.
    8. Written instructions.

87. **Most children begin to speak their first words at which of the following ages?**
    1. 6 months.
    2. 12 months.
    3. 18 months.
    4. 24 months.

88. **Which of the following is an example of a 4-year-old's concept of self?**
    1. "I am a better swimmer than my brother."
    2. "I am better at drawing than at coloring."
    3. "I like to swim."
    4. "People like me because I play fair."

89. **When assessing a client taking clozapine (Clozaril) for side effects, what side effects does the nurse see most commonly?**
    1. Agranulocytosis and blood dyscrasias.
    2. Anticholinergic symptoms and increased serum prolactin levels.
    3. Dystonias and akasthesia.
    4. Weight gain and sedation.

90. **When assessing a client for presence of alcohol withdrawal delirium, the nurse watches for which of the following? Select all that apply.**
    1. Disorientation.
    2. Distractibility.
    3. Grandiosity.
    4. Paranoid delusions.
    5. Pressure of speech.
    6. Tremors.

91. **Confidential information can be released without the client's written consent in which of the following situations?**
    1. Commitment proceedings request.
    2. Insurance company request.
    3. Police request.
    4. Previous therapist request.

92. **When planning nursing care for a client on a monoamine oxidase inhibitor (MAOI), which of the following should the nurse realize?**
    1. MAOIs ar e fairly safe in overdose.
    2. The client may have problems with addiction.
    3. The client will have a decreased ability to use vitamin B_6.
    4. Tolerance to therapeutic effect may occur.

Unit 2 • Specific Aspects of Care

Safety and Infection Control

1. **While ambulating with the nurse, the client begins to fall. The nurse should do which of the following to stabilize the client?**
   1. Instruct the client to stand against the wall.
   2. Lean the client forward while lowering the client to the floor.
   3. Slide the client against the nurse's leg while lowering the client to the floor.
   4. Use a narrow base of support.

2. **The nurse is positioning a client for a urinary catheterization. Which action would best prevent musculoskeletal injury to the nurse while performing this procedure?**
   1. Narrowing the base of support.
   2. Positioning the client using a draw sheet.
   3. Raising the bed to a comfortable height.
   4. Using the nondominant hand to insert the catheter.

3. **During meal time, the nurse notices a client with his hands holding his throat area. Which situation would most require immediate action by the nurse?**
   1. The client has a high-pitched inspiratory stridor.
   2. The client is coughing and talking.
   3. The client is coughing only.
   4. The client is not making any sounds.

4. **The nurse must transfer a dependent client from a bed to a gurney. Which measure taken by the nurse will be safest for both the nurse and the client?**
   1. Adjust the height of the client's bed.
   2. Avoid movements that twist the spine.
   3. Keep the client close to her body when lifting.
   4. Use a mechanical lift device appropriate for this client.

5. **A nurse is caring for a hospitalized client in a continuous mitten restraint. Which of the following interventions should be included in the client's care plan? Select all that apply.**
   1. Document restraint checks and patient status every two hours.
   2. Educate the client's family about restraint use.
   3. Obtain the physician's order renewal every 72 hours.
   4. Provide 10 minutes of release and repositioning.
   5. Release the restraint and reposition the client every four hours.

6. **The nurse is instructing the client about the prevention of carbon monoxide poisoning. Which of the following statements from the client indicates that more teaching is needed?**
   1. "A high concentration of carbon monoxide can cause death."
   2. "I can detect the presence of carbon monoxide by a strong odor."
   3. "I can purchase a carbon monoxide detector for my home."
   4. "I should inspect my carbon monoxide detector annually."

7. A nurse is preparing a presentation about bicycle safety for a health fair. For which target audience would this presentation be most appropriate?
   1. Adolescents
   2. Infants, toddlers, and preschool children
   3. Middle-aged adults
   4. School-aged children

8. A nurse working the night shift is caring for a client who is at high risk for falls. Which of the following does the nurse need to consider when caring for this client? Select all that apply.
   1. Keep the client's room dark by keeping the door closed.
   2. Monitor the client at least every four hours to ensure safety.
   3. Move the client's room away from the nurses' station.
   4. Place fall risk indicators on the client's door.
   5. Teach the client to use the call light.
   6. Turn off the client's bed alarm so the client is not disturbed.

9. A quadriplegic client is sliding down in bed. Which of the following is the best method to reposition this client?
   1. One nurse lifting the client's legs while the client uses a trapeze.
   2. Two nurses lifting the client under the shoulders.
   3. Two nurses using a draw sheet.
   4. Two nurses using a friction reducing device.

10. The nurse looks into a client's room and notices a fire. What action should the nurse take first?
   1. Activate the fire alarm.
   2. Close all the doors and windows.
   3. Evacuate the client from the room.
   4. Extinguish the fire.

11. The nurse is teaching a client with a history of falls about home safety. Which of the following statements indicates that the client understands the instructions?
   1. "I will keep my walker at the end of my bed."
   2. "I will keep the ceiling light on in my room at all times."
   3. "I will put a nonskid floor mat on the side of the bed that I exit."
   4. "I will wear treaded slipper socks on my carpeted floors."

12. The nurse is providing discharge teaching to a client going home on oxygen therapy. The nurse recognizes further teaching is needed when the client states which of the following?
   1. "I can tell how much oxygen is being delivered by looking at the flowmeter."
   2. "I should call my doctor if I experience an increased pulse, increased respiratory rate, increased fatigue, or decreased ability to concentrate."
   3. "I will post a 'No smoking' sign on my door."
   4. "I should see a frosty buildup on the tank when I am refilling my portable oxygen."

13. The nurse is conducting a home safety risk appraisal for an elderly client. The client is attempting to eliminate the safety hazards in the home. Which findings would indicate the client is successful? Select all that apply.
   1. The home includes a bath tub with rails.
   2. Electric cords are behind the furniture.
   3. There is a seat located in the shower stall.
   4. Space heaters are present to ensure adequate heating.
   5. Throw rugs are used in the home.

14. The nurse must select the proper safe patient handling equipment to use when transferring a client from a sit to stand position. Which of the following is most important when determining how to transfer this client?
  1. The client's ability to communicate.
  2. The client's current weight-bearing status.
  3. The client's height.
  4. The type of equipment used in the past.

15. The nurse is supervising a certified nurse assistant (CNA) taking care of a client with a restraint. The nurse knows that the CNA understands the use of restraints when the CNA states which of the following?
  1. "I tied the restraint in a double knot."
  2. "I made sure the restraint was tight."
  3. "I tied the restraint to the moving part of the bed frame."
  4. "I put the bedrails up on all of the clients on the unit."

16. When caring for a client who is having a seizure, which of the following actions should be performed by the nurse? Select all that apply.
  1. Assess the client's airway patency.
  2. Place a tongue depressor in the client's mouth.
  3. Place the bed in a low position.
  4. Place the client in prone position.
  5. Restrain the client.
  6. Surround the client with furniture.

17. The nurse is conducting a home visit when the client starts to experience convulsions after accidentally ingesting a poisonous substance. What action by the nurse would be a priority for this client?
  1. Assess the client for airway patency.
  2. Identify the poison.
  3. Induce vomiting.
  4. Position the client with her head to the side.

18. The nurse is transferring a patient from a chair to a toilet 50 feet down the hall. The patient can bear weight and has upper extremity strength, but gets short of breath with prolonged ambulation. What is the most appropriate device for transferring this patient?
  1. A gait belt without handles.
  2. A lateral friction reducing device.
  3. A sit to stand lift.
  4. An overhead lift with a full body sling.

19. When planning care of the elderly client, the nurse knows that falls are common in the elderly. Falling can be prevented by which of the following? Select all that apply.
  1. Balance and strength exercises.
  2. Home safety evaluations.
  3. Locking beds and wheelchairs during transfers.
  4. Placing a bedside table within the client's reach.
  5. Use of sedatives.

20. When using ergonomics in preventing musculoskeletal injuries as it pertains to safe patient handling, the nurse should do which of the following?
  1. Fit the task of lifting a client to the nurse.
  2. Fit the nurse to the task of lifting a client.
  3. Find the strongest person to perform the task of lifting a client.
  4. Manually lift clients whenever possible.

21. Which of the following would the nurse observe in a client who is suffering ill effects from a wrist restraint?
  1. The client has a capillary refill of less than two seconds.
  2. The client has full range of motion in her wrist.
  3. The client is attempting to remove the restraint.
  4. The client's hand is cool and pale.

22. **A client has an infection that is spread through droplets. Which of the following is essential for the nurse to use when taking this client's temperature?**
    1. Gloves.
    2. Goggles.
    3. A gown.
    4. A mask.

23. **While working in a hospital, a coworker is splashed in the face with a cleaning solution. Where can the nurse quickly find detailed information about this chemical?**

    _____

24. **The nurse is training a group of Certified Nursing Assistants (CNAs) about hand hygiene. Which of the following statements indicate that the CNAs need further instruction from the nurse?**
    1. "As long as I am changing gloves between clients, it is not necessary to wash my hands."
    2. "I should wash my hands when my hands are visibly soiled."
    3. "I will not wear artificial nails when providing client care."
    4. "It is OK to use alcohol-based hand products after client contact."

25. **What action by the nurse is most important when performing a dressing change using surgical aseptic technique?**
    1. Comforting the client.
    2. Maintaining sterility.
    3. Obtaining extra gloves.
    4. Organizing supplies.

26. **The nurse must assign a room to a client with scabies. Which of the following options would be the best choice for this client?**
    1. A negative-pressure isolation room.
    2. A private room.
    3. A semi-private room with any client.
    4. A room with another client with scabies.

27. **When caring for a client with bronchitis, what is the best way the nurse can prevent the spread of infection?**

    _____

28. **A nurse is caring for a client with a respiratory infection. Which of the following is the most important action by the nurse to prevent the transmission of infection?**
    1. Using nonsterile gloves when in contact with body fluid.
    2. Washing hands after donning sterile gloves.
    3. Wearing a gown to protect skin and clothing.
    4. Washing hands after the removal of soiled gloves.

29. **When preparing a sterile field, which of the following conditions indicates to the nurse that the field is contaminated?**
    1. A dressing is laying two inches away from the border of the sterile field.
    2. A sterile item is being held just above waist level.
    3. A sterile package is opened over and placed into the middle of the sterile field.
    4. Sterile normal saline is poured onto the waterproof field.

30. **After establishing a sterile field to insert a Foley catheter, the nurse must don sterile gloves. Place these actions in the proper sequence:**
    1. Interlock fingers to fit the gloves into each finger.
    2. Pull the glove over the dominant hand.
    3. Slip the glove onto the nondominant hand.
    4. Slip the fingers of the dominant hand under the nondominant hand on the sterile glove side of the cuff.
    5. With the nondominant hand, grasp the inside of the dominant hand glove by the cuff.

31. **The nurse is caring for a client with Hepatitis A. What action puts the nurse at highest risk for being exposed to Hepatitis A?**
    1. Standing one foot away when the client coughs.
    2. Suctioning the client.
    3. Testing the client's stool for occult blood.
    4. Touching the client's arm when providing comfort.

32. **The nurse must auscultate the lungs of a client in isolation. Which of the following is the best way to prevent the spread of microorganisms to other clients?**
    1. Detach a contaminated needle from its syringe before disposal.
    2. Double-bag soiled equipment with impervious bags before removing it from the client's room.
    3. Keep the stethoscope used for that client in the room.
    4. Remove personal protective equipment just outside the client's door.

33. **The nurse is evaluating the need for the use of a wrist restraint for a client pulling out a peripheral IV. Which of the following should be considered before using the restraint?**
    1. The convenience of the staff.
    2. The need for use of a chemical restraint.
    3. The reason the client is pulling out the IV.
    4. The staffing level on that shift.

34. **The nurse teaches a client's daughter to perform a dressing change using sterile technique. Which of the following actions by the daughter should indicate to the nurse that the daughter understands prevention of infection?**
    1. The daughter placing herself between the sterile field and the client.
    2. The daughter putting on sterile gloves before opening dressing packages.
    3. The daughter putting on sterile gloves to remove the old dressing.
    4. The daughter washing hands before applying gloves.

35. **Which measure used by the nurse would be most effective in preventing exposure when caring for a client with Hepatitis B?**
    1. Applying a mask before entering the client's room.
    2. Placing a contaminated needle in a sharps container.
    3. Wearing a gown when changing an IV bag.
    4. Wearing gloves when taking the client's pulse.

36. **The nurse is finished caring for a client in an isolation room. The nurse begins to remove personal protective equipment. Put the following items in order beginning with what the nurse would remove first.**
    1. Gloves.
    2. Goggles.
    3. Gown.
    4. Mask.

37. **When teaching a client's spouse about wheelchair safety, the nurse recognizes further teaching is needed when the spouse makes which of the following statements?**
    1. "I should back in to and out of elevators."
    2. "I should push the wheelchair ahead of me when I go up a ramp."
    3. "I should slowly back down wheelchair ramps."
    4. "I should use the wheelchair to help push doors open."

38. A client with neutropenia is in protective, or reverse, isolation. The family asks why the client is in this type of isolation. Which of the following explanations by the nurse is the best response?

1. To protect other clients on the unit from infection.
2. To protect the client from environmental sources of infection.
3. To protect the client from his own bacteria.
4. To protect the staff from infection from the client.

39. A nurse who has a right dominant hand is going to don sterile gloves. Place an X in the spot on the gloves where the nurse will begin donning.

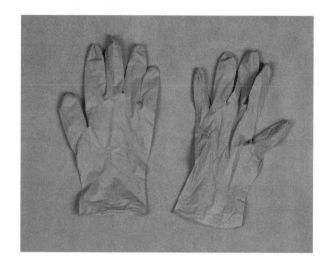

Fundamental Skills and Principles

1. Which best describes the nursing role of protecting the client and supporting a client's decisions?
   1. Advocate.
   2. Caregiver.
   3. Case Manager.
   4. Teacher.

2. According to Erikson, reminiscence of life events occurs in which stage of psychosocial development?
   1. Autonomy versus Shame and Doubt.
   2. Generativity versus Stagnation.
   3. Identity versus Role Diffusion.
   4. Ego Integrity versus Despair.

3. When leaving a client's room after providing care, it is most important to evaluate the client's ability to do which of the following?
   1. Ambulate to the bathroom.
   2. Push the call light to see if the client is able to activate it when needed.
   3. Turn the television on and off.
   4. Use the telephone to call family.

4. When assessing a client's strength in preparation for ambulating out of bed, the nurse should do which of the following?
   1. Ask the client how strong they feel today.
   2. Ask the client if they have been up before.
   3. Check the pedal pulses and feet for edema.
   4. Instruct the client to push the soles of the feet against the nurse's palms.

5. Using numbers, place the following steps of the nursing process in the correct sequence.
   ____ Compare actual outcomes of care to expected outcomes.
   ____ Critically analyze data to determine the significance and priorities.
   ____ Collect and organize data about the client.
   ____ Take corrective action and modify plan if goals are not met.
   ____ Determine the appropriateness of nursing diagnosis.
   ____ Deliver nursing care with individualized interventions.
   ____ Determine the response to interventions.
   ____ Set client-centered, measurable, and realistic goals.

6. What is the priority nursing intervention when feeding a confused client?
   1. Check that the client's dentures fit properly.
   2. Check the mouth to make sure it is empty between bites.
   3. Instruct the client what foods are present on the tray.
   4. Thicken all liquids to make swallowing easier.

7. The nurse should perform which of the following actions when providing fingernail care for a confused client who is incontinent of stool?
   1. Clean under the nail with an orange stick.
   2. File the nails in a rounded shape.
   3. Push the cuticles back with a metal nail file or scissors.
   4. Soak the hands in hot water.

8. **Which pulse rate should not be assessed on both sides of the body at the same time?**
   1. Brachial.
   2. Carotid.
   3. Femoral.
   4. Temporal.

9. **Which of the following are important concepts in providing bed and bath hygiene care for a client? Select all that apply.**
   1. Check the soiled bed linen for personal items such as eyeglasses.
   2. Finish care with a back rub using rubbing alcohol.
   3. Put a clean gown on the strongest arm first, then the weak arm.
   4. Ensure that the temperature of the bath water is 110–115°F.
   5. Shave the client in the direction of the hair growth.
   6. Use standard precautions for exposed body fluids.
   7. Wash the client's extremities from proximal to distal.
   8. Wash hands after disposing of client's linen in the soiled hamper.

10. **When the client has an irregular radial pulse on assessment, the nurse should first check which of the following?**
    1. The apical pulse for a full minute.
    2. The apical pulse with a Doppler.
    3. The pulse at two other sites.
    4. The radial pulse on the other arm.

11. **To ensure accuracy when checking bowel sounds, how should the nurse auscultate the abdomen?**
    1. After palpation and percussion.
    2. Before palpation and percussion.
    3. For at least five minutes in each quadrant.
    4. Start listening at the left lower quadrant.

12. **Which of the following statements best describes the application of the nursing process?**
    1. Assists in determining the length of stay determined by the insurance company.
    2. Determines the role of the healthcare team.
    3. Is individualized and changes to meet the needs of the client.
    4. Establishes the client's medical problem.

13. **The nurse should first do which of the following to determine the appropriateness of a nursing diagnosis?**
    1. Assess the patient again.
    2. Compare the defining characteristics to the client data.
    3. Establish goals and interventions.
    4. Review the "related to" etiologies.

14. **Which nursing intervention will interrupt the transmission of infection?**
    1. Changing linen for the client each day.
    2. Encouraging a healthy and increased protein diet.
    3. Hand washing before and after providing care to a client.
    4. Putting the client in a private room.

15. **Which of the following elevated diagnostic laboratory values would suggest that the client is attempting to fight an infection?**
    1. Blood urea nitrogen level (BUN).
    2. Potassium level (K⁺).
    3. Red blood cell count (RBC).
    4. White blood cell count (WBC).

16. **When is the best time to toilet a patient to encourage bowel training?**
    1. As soon as the client has the urge to defecate.
    2. Every hour while the patient is awake.
    3. Immediately before meals.
    4. When the patient feels abdominal cramping.

17. Which fluid could the nurse give to a client on a clear liquid diet?

1. Ginger ale.
2. Lemon sherbet.
3. Milkshake.
4. Vanilla ice cream.

18. The physician should be notified when the client's hourly urine output falls below which of the following?

1. 20 cc.
2. 30 cc.
3. 50 cc.
4. 100 cc.

19. What assessment data would be of greatest concern to the nurse who suspects a client is hypovolemic?

1. Decreased heart rate.
2. Dyspnea.
3. Increased blood pressure.
4. Thready pulse.

20. What should the nurse do immediately to evaluate a client's tolerance to a change in position when transferring a patient from a bed to a chair?

1. Allow the client to sit quietly to adjust to the change in position.
2. Ask the client if they feel dizzy or lightheaded.
3. Assess the client for bradycardia.
4. Check the client's blood pressure.

21. Which of the following are possible complications of a client on bedrest? Select all that apply.

1. Contractures of extremities.
2. Decreased pain.
3. Decreased dependency.
4. Diarrhea.
5. Pneumonia.
6. Pressure ulcers.
7. Thrombi.
8. Urinary calculi.

22. Which of the following statements by a client would alert the nurse that further teaching on the idea of a restful sleep is indicated?

1. "I don't take naps throughout the day."
2. "I go to bed and get up routinely at the same time each day."
3. "I have a small snack and take a bath before going to bed each day."
4. "I went to bed earlier than usual and I rested and watched television until I fell asleep."

23. What can the nurse do to support all clients' ability to sleep in the hospital setting?

1. Assess the client towards the end of the shift, closer to a normal awakening time.
2. Darken the room as much as possible by keeping the lights off.
3. Limit the noise and distractions on the unit.
4. Provide a bath or shower before bedtime.

24. A client's pulse oximetry to determine hemoglobin saturation is 85%. What should the nurse do first?

1. Administer oxygen at four liters per minute.
2. Call the client's doctor.
3. Encourage coughing and deep breathing.
4. Raise the head of the bed.

25. When attempting to apply a pulse oximeter probe to a client's finger, the nurse notes edema of both of the client's hands and thickened toe nails. The nurse should do which of the following?

1. Attach the probe softly and carefully to a finger to prevent discomfort.
2. Attach the probe to one earlobe.
3. Attach the probe to one of the client's toes.
4. Elevate the client's hand and check the pulse oximetry later.

26. **Which of the following are signs of infection in a patient? Select all that apply.**
    1. Bradycardia.
    2. Hypothermia.
    3. Increased body temperature.
    4. Increased neutrophils.
    5. Increased red blood cells.
    6. Increased white blood cells.
    7. Localized edema.
    8. Localized pain.

27. **Which of the following should the nurse do to be most effective in helping to liquefy or thin a client's respiratory secretions?**
    1. Assist the client to ambulate more frequently.
    2. Encourage coughing and deep breathing.
    3. Instruct the client to increase fluid intake.
    4. Teach the correct use of the incentive spirometer.

28. **What step is the most important when discontinuing a urinary catheter for a client?**
    1. Deflate the balloon completely before removing the catheter.
    2. Have the client take a deep breath as the catheter is removed.
    3. Provide perineal care before and after removing the catheter.
    4. Wear sterile gloves to remove the catheter.

29. **The nurse is emptying a client's urinal when she notices the urine is dark amber, cloudy, and has an unpleasant odor. The nurse would suspect the client has what condition?**
    1. A urinary tract infection.
    2. Urinary incontinence.
    3. Urinary frequency.
    4. Urinary retention.

30. **The nurse will first need to do which of the following before she obtains a wound drainage specimen for culture?**
    1. Irrigate the wound with normal saline prior to culturing.
    2. Irrigate the wound with the ordered antiseptic before culturing.
    3. Realize she cannot irrigate the wound until after the culture is obtained.
    4. Wipe the wound with sterile gauze with no solution prior to culturing.

31. **The nurse instructs her elderly client not to strain when defecating because it could cause which of the following?**
    1. Dizziness.
    2. Dysrhythmias.
    3. Fecal incontinence.
    4. Rectal bleeding from hemorrhoids.

32. **Identify what factors hinder defecation in a hospitalized client that the nurse should be aware of when planning teaching for a patient who is constipated. Select all that apply.**
    1. Discomfort with defecation.
    2. Excessive laxative use.
    3. Ignoring the urge to defecate when it occurs.
    4. Inadequate fluid intake.
    5. Increased fiber in the diet.
    6. Increased activity.

33. **According to Erikson, establishing relationships based on commitment mainly occurs in which state of psychosocial development?**
    1. Generativity versus Stagnation.
    2. Identity versus Role Diffusion.
    3. Intimacy versus Isolation.
    4. Trust versus Mistrust.

34. **What is the most important concept the nurse must consider in observing nonverbal behavior in her client?**

1. The client's behavior has less truth than what the client states.
2. The client's behavior does not have the same meaning in all sociocultural groups.
3. The client's behavior is usually a poor reflection of what the patient feels.
4. It is common that nonverbal communication is consciously motivated.

35. **Which of the following is an example of the working phase of a therapeutic relationship?**

1. Asking the client what brought them to the hospital today.
2. Beginning the client on progressive ambulation.
3. Discussing the achievement of self ambulation with the client and family before discharge.
4. Reviewing the medical and nursing history on the emergency department records.

36. **Which teaching method has been evaluated as most effective in a new diabetic client?**

1. Utilizing breaks after each unit of the teaching session.
2. Having the client repeat the steps of insulin administration.
3. Encouraging the client to ask many questions.
4. Confirming that the client is able to give his own insulin.

37. **Which of the following does the nurse need to realize when assessing for pain? Select all that apply.**

1. Administering medication for pain will eventually lead to addiction.
2. Each person's expression of pain may be different and individualized.
3. Intravenous narcotics are the longest acting pain relief method.
4. Pain level and pain tolerance can be assessed using a scale from 1 to 10.
5. The client needs to know the nurse believes what they are saying about their pain.
6. The client should show nonverbal signs as well as stating that he is in pain.

38. **Which source would be most helpful in aiding the nurse to provide psychological care to the client?**

1. Client concerns.
2. Family information.
3. Medical history.
4. Progress note.

39. **Mark an X on the picture below where the nurse is most likely to locate the dorsalis pedis pulse.**

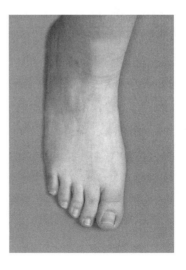

Communication

1. **Which of the following is the traditional view of the nurse-patient relationship (NPR)?**
   1. Building trust is essential in the early phases of the relationship.
   2. Each nurse-client contact is an opportunity for goal achievement.
   3. The nurse approaches the relationship with a sense of client autonomy.
   4. The relationship is equitable with equal participation by the nurse and the client.

2. **Which of the following indicates to the nurse that a client's passive-aggressive communication is improving?**
   1. The client's nonverbal message is less aggressive.
   2. The client sticks up for herself.
   3. The message is more in keeping with the client's actual feelings.
   4. The verbal and nonverbal messages are congruent.

3. **What communication skill would be used primarily in the orientation phase of the nurse-client relationship?**
   1. Eliciting information.
   2. Displaying patience with regression.
   3. Praising accomplishments.
   4. Summarizing gains.

4. **Men tend to display which of the following traits when communicating with other workers?**
   1. They are more goal-oriented than process-orientated.
   2. They build and maintain personal relationships.
   3. They tell people what to do indirectly.
   4. They value the process aspect of decision-making.

5. **The nurse, who is learning how to knit, discovers that a client on the unit is an expert knitter. The nurse asks the client for help with a difficult sequence of stitches. The nurse's supervisor evaluates this behavior to be which of the following?**
   1. Goal-directed.
   2. Professional.
   3. Therapeutic.
   4. Social.

6. **The nurse becomes overly involved with a client by disclosing excessive personal information. The nurse's supervisor evaluates this behavior as failing to honor nurse-client**
   _____.

7. **When planning to communicate with a client, the following activity takes priority.**
   1. Empathy.
   2. Giving information.
   3. Listening.
   4. Reflection.

8. A stable schizophrenic client asks the nurse, "I do not have to pay attention to the voices so much. Why is that?" The nurse replies, "Your body has an imbalance in the neurotransmitters dopamine and norepinephrine, which are responsible for you hearing the voices. Your medication has relieved these symptoms but you may develop extrapyramidal side effects that you will need to report." What criterion for successful communication has been violated?
   1. Appropriateness.
   2. Efficiency.
   3. Feedback.
   4. Flexibility.

9. The client says, "I have got to get out of this hospital! They have found out my address and are coming for my family!" The nurse responds, "Don't worry, no one will harm your family." What type of communication breakdown does this response represent?
   1. A failure to recognize the level of meaning.
   2. A failure to see individual uniqueness.
   3. Giving false reassurance to the client.
   4. Using value statements and clichés.

10. The client states, "When I found out about my husband cheating on me, it triggered a whole range of feelings. I need to talk with him but do not know how to do it right. I don't want to make him mad by crying and screaming." What response by the nurse would best help the client in this situation?
   1. Do you mean you have a hard time controlling your emotions?
   2. I hear you. That must be very frustrating.
   3. It sounds like you feel that you are to blame.
   4. So what are some alternatives?

11. A client with post-traumatic stress disorder says to you, "They think you should be able to put it out of your mind. It happened so long ago—just get over it!" The nurse responds, "It must be very frustrating to encounter that kind of an attitude." The response is an example of which of the following?
   1. Clarifying.
   2. Focusing.
   3. Paraphrasing.
   4. Reflection.

12. The nurse has become critical and defensive when communicating with a client. The team leader evaluates this behavior as a possible indicator of

   _____.

13. The nurse is describing the physical effects of chemotherapy to a newly diagnosed patient. During this explanation by the nurse, the patient is exhibiting which of the following steps in the communication process?
   1. Channeling.
   2. Decoding.
   3. Encoding.
   4. Feedback.

14. When using electronic communication (e-mail) with clients, what concerns might the nurse have? Select all that apply.
   1. Communication time may be increased.
   2. Instructions may not be understood.
   3. Messages may seem cold.
   4. Privacy might be breached.

15. The nurse has joined a project team. Team members are clarifying goals, adopting new roles, and defining tasks and standards for work to be done. The nurse assesses that the group is in what stage of development?
    1. Forming.
    2. Storming.
    3. Norming.
    4. Performing.

16. The nurse is planning a team meeting. What tools can the nurse use to promote an effective meeting? Select all that apply.
    1. An agenda.
    2. An encourager.
    3. An evaluator.
    4. A facilitator.
    5. An initiator.
    6. A recorder.

17. When planning communication with clients, the nurse realizes that the following are areas where cultural differences may be found. Select all that apply.
    1. Eye contact.
    2. Degree of closeness.
    3. Greeting.
    4. Sharing feelings.
    5. Touch.
    6. Valuing family.
    7. Valuing health.

18. When intervening with a client, the nurse recognizes that confrontational skills are most closely related to which of the following?
    1. Aggressive behavior.
    2. Assertive behavior.
    3. Controlling behavior.
    4. Nonassertive behavior.

19. The nurse is working to help a client learn to say "no" effectively. What statement by the client indicates that more teaching is necessary?
    1. "I cannot do that."
    2. "I have never done that before and I do not want to start now."
    3. "I have to work this week, write a paper for school, and my husband is out of town, so I'd rather not."
    4. "No, thank you, I do not care to do that."

20. A colleague apologizes to the nurse for snapping at her earlier in the day, explaining that he just found out some upsetting news. What response by the nurse is both assertive and appropriate?
    1. "Apology accepted. Things will turn out OK."
    2. "I forgive you. I can see you are upset by the unexpected news."
    3. "It's OK this time, but do not let it happen again."
    4. "It's OK. We all get upset at times."

21. When interviewing a client, the nurse verbally reflects the client's feelings and the reasons for them. This response is

   _____.

22. What response by the nurse indicates a positive perspective on criticism?
    1. "Criticism makes me feel like a stupid person."
    2. "I ask for specific facts about the behavior being criticized."
    3. "I feel obliged to agree with most criticism sent my way."
    4. "I usually do not reply to aggressive behavior."

23. When assessing a team for potential teamwork success, what communication-related criteria would be included?

1. Areas of expertise.
2. Good documentation.
3. Knowing one's own limits.
4. Recognition of common goals.

24. At the immunization clinic, a father says to his six-year-old son who is fighting back tears, "Children who cry when they get needles are crybabies." The nurse assesses this communication to be which of the following?

1. Clear.
2. Circular.
3. Emotional.
4. Masked.

25. When assessing a client, what statement would indicate negative self-talk?

1. "Everyone has to learn something new sometime."
2. "I am looking forward to making home visits, but I am also nervous."
3. "This is going to be difficult, but I know I can do it."
4. "Who can ever have enough experience to prepare for that job?"

26. The client is in conflict with her husband about methods to achieve the goal of "not talking back to adults" for their four-year-old son. The client decides the husband's position of power in the family will result in him winning and decides not to press her suggestions. The nurse assesses this behavior to be which of the following?

1. Lose-lose
2. Lose-win
3. Win-lose
4. Win-win

27. The nurse is discussing a client's goals with a physician colleague. The colleague leans back in the chair with both hands behind her head supporting the head. The nurse assesses that this nonverbal behavior indicates which of the following?

1. Confidence and superiority.
2. Doubt.
3. Powerful negative evaluation.
4. Thoughtful evaluation.

28. The nurse is using the communication principle of presence when establishing a collaborative relationship with a client. What intervention behaviors would you expect to see?

1. Calling the client by name and introducing himself.
2. Communicating to the client an understanding of how the client feels.
3. Displaying real thoughts and beliefs to the client.
4. Making eye contact, leaning forward, and listening attentively to the client.

29. Using Peplau's framework for phases in the nurse–client relationship, what phase involves a goal of "to clearly understand each other's preconceptions and expectations"?

1. Orientation phase.
2. Identification phase.
3. Exploitation phase.
4. Resolution phase.

30. In which of the following situations would a closed question be most appropriate?

1. Assessing a client for a well-balanced diet.
2. Assessing a client's receptiveness to a transfer to an extended care facility.
3. Assessing a client's reaction to a barium enema.
4. Assessing if the client took his antihypertensive medication this morning.

31. **A nurse approaches a male patient and asks how he is feeling. The client states, "I'm feeling a bit nervous today." Which of the following is the nurse's best reply?**
    1. "Please explain what you mean by the word nervous."
    2. "What is making you feel nervous?"
    3. "Would a backrub ease your nervousness?"
    4. "You do look like you're nervous."

32. **The introductory phase of communication involves the nurse acquainting herself with the patient and includes which of the following?**
    1. Beginning preparing the client for the interview.
    2. Identifying applicable goals and objectives.
    3. Providing advice to the client.
    4. Suggesting a referral to other care providers.

33. **Which of the following statements during shift report provides the most useful information related to priority-setting for the nurse?**
    1. A client admitted with hypertension has a blood pressure reading of 138/84.
    2. A client had a catheter removed six hours ago and has not voided.
    3. A client is only alert and oriented to person and place.
    4. A client three days postoperative is still complaining of incisional discomfort.

34. **A client expresses anxiety over an impending surgery. Which of the following is the nurse's best approach to this situation?**
    1. Acknowledge the client's anxiety and explore their feelings.
    2. Discuss the competency of the surgeon with the client.
    3. Discuss another individual's similar surgical experience with the client.
    4. Provide written information outlining the surgical procedure.

35. **A nurse is made aware of a client with partial hearing impairment during the admission assessment. Which of the following is the best way to communicate with the client?**
    1. Conduct only the physical portion of the assessment at this time.
    2. Face the client directly while addressing them and speak slowly in a low-pitched voice.
    3. Have a family member present during the assessment.
    4. Provide the assessment questions in a written format.

36. **A client expresses to the nurse that her husband is an alcoholic and has trouble keeping a job for longer than three months. Which of the following is the nurse's best response?**
    1. "Have you tried to contact Al-Anon?"
    2. "I'm so sorry to hear that."
    3. "This seems to worry you. I suggest you talk with the hospital chaplain."
    4. "What have you done in the past to help cope with this problem?"

37. **The client states, "I am so nervous about what to expect after my colonoscopy." The nurse's reply of "Are you feeling anxious about the results of your colonoscopy?" is an example of which of the following therapeutic communication techniques?**
    1. Clarification.
    2. Paraphrasing.
    3. Reflection.
    4. Restatement.

38. **The use of cues is involved in nonverbal communication. Which of the following is an example of a nonverbal cue?**
    1. Physical appearance.
    2. Reading.
    3. Symbols.
    4. Written words.

39. **When communicating with a client with expressive aphasia, the nurse should be aware of the importance of which of the following?**

    1. Allow a short time for the client to respond.
    2. Ask open-ended questions.
    3. Ask questions with yes or no answers, or questions that can be answered by blinking the eyes.
    4. Refer to the family members for client information.

Medication Administration

1. **Before administration of intramuscular meperidine (Demerol), which assessment is most important for the nurse to make?**
   1. Apical pulse rate.
   2. Blood pressure.
   3. Level of consciousness.
   4. Respiratory rate.

2. **The nurse is having difficulty reading the physician's order for a medication. The nurse knows the physician is very busy and does not like to be called. What should the nurse do?**
   1. Ask the ward clerk to interpret the physician's handwriting.
   2. Call the pharmacist to interpret the order.
   3. Call the physician to have the order clarified.
   4. Consult the unit manager to help interpret the order.

3. **When a nurse is preparing medication for the client and the nurse is called away for an emergency situation, which of the following should the nurse do?**
   1. Have another nurse guard the medication preparations until the nurse returns.
   2. Have another nurse finish preparing and administering the medications.
   3. Lock the medicines in a room and finish when the nurse returns from the emergency situation.
   4. Discard the prepared medications and begin again upon return.

4. **To convert 0.8 grams to milligrams, the nurse should do which of the following?**
   1. Move the decimal point 3 places to the right.
   2. Move the decimal point 3 places to the left.
   3. Move the decimal point 2 places to the right.
   4. Move the decimal point 2 places to the left.

5. **The nurse is instilling ear drops to a very young child and must straighten the ear canal by pulling the auricle of the ear. The nurse will pull the auricle in which directions?**
   1. Down and backward.
   2. Down and outward.
   3. Upward and backward.
   4. Upward and outward.

6. **The nurse administers a wrong medicine to a client. Which of the following actions should the nurse take?**
   1. Do nothing.
   2. Immediately report the error to the nurse manager and the client's physician.
   3. Monitor the client for adverse effects.
   4. Tell the client that a wrong medicine was given.

7. The nurse arrives for work and is asked to count narcotics with the nurse finishing her shift duty. The arriving nurse should be the nurse who does which of the following?

   1. Visually counts the actual number of the narcotics that remain in the locked narcotic cabinet after the previous nurse leaves the unit.
   2. Visually counts the actual number of narcotics that remain in the locked narcotic cabinet before the previous nurse leaves the unit.
   3. Visually counts the actual sign-out sheet for the balance of narcotics administered by nurses before the previous nurse leaves the unit.
   4. Visually counts the actual sign-out sheets for the balance of narcotics administered by nurses after the nurse leaves the unit.

8. Before administering a medication to a client, the nurse needs to identify the client. Which of the following methods of identification should the nurse perform?

   1. Ask the client's first name.
   2. Check the client's ID bracelet.
   3. Check the client's name on the medication administration record.
   4. Check the client's name with family or a significant other.

9. Identify the "rights of medication administration." Select all that apply.

   1. Right drug.
   2. Right dose.
   3. Right client.
   4. Right route.
   5. Right time.
   6. Right documentation.

10. The adult client has an order for penicillin to be given intramuscularly. Which of the following angles would be the correct one to use for injection into the ventrogluteal muscle site?

    1. A 45° angle
    2. A 60° angle
    3. A 75° angle
    4. A 90° angle

11. When administering a flu vaccine, how does the nurse locate the deltoid muscle?

    1. By locating the center of the arm between the elbow and the shoulder.
    2. By locating the midpoint of the lateral aspect of the upper arm.
    3. By palpating the lower edge of the acromion process and measuring four inches below to the center of the lateral aspect of the upper arm.
    4. By palpating the lower edge of the acromion process and measuring four finger-widths below to the midpoint and center of the lateral aspect of the upper arm.

12. The nurse needs to prepare and administer medication. The order reads 250 mg is to be given, and the label on the vial of medication reads 0.2 grams/2 ml. What is the correct amount of medication to be administered?

    1. 1.5 ml.
    2. 2.0 ml.
    3. 2.5 ml.
    4. 3.0 ml.

13. The medication order is for potassium chloride (KCL) 20 mEq. The bottle is labeled KCL elixir, 10 mEq/ml. How many milliliters will be given?

    1. 1 ml.
    2. 1.5 ml.
    3. 2 ml.
    4. 2.5 ml.

14. The medicine order is penicillin 750,000 units. The vial reads 300,000 units/2 ml. How many milliliters will be given?
1. 1.2 ml.
2. 3.5 ml.
3. 4 ml.
4. 5 ml.

15. The physician orders amoxicillin 250 mg every eight hours. On hand are 125 mg chewable amoxicillin tablets. The nurse will administer how many tablets?
1. ½ tablet.
2. 1 tablet.
3. 2 tablets.
4. 4 tablets.

Fill in the blank with the correct type of medication.

16. A gelatinous container to hold a drug in powder, liquid, or oil form is called a(n)

_____.

17. A powdered drug is compressed into a hard small disc. Some are scored, some have coatings to prevent them from dissolving in the stomach. This is called a(n)

_____.

18. A sweetened and aromatic solution of alcohol that is used as a vehicle for medicinal agents is called a(n)

_____.

19. The physician orders 14 units of regular insulin and 28 units of long-acting insulin to be given subcutaneously at the breakfast hour. What is the total number of units of insulin that the nurse will prepare in the insulin syringe?
1. 14 units.
2. 28 units.
3. 32 units.
4. 42 units.

20. The nurse hands the oral medication to the client and the client states that the medication is the wrong color. The nurse will take which of the following actions?
1. Return to the medicine room and check the medicine administration sheet with the physician's order.
2. Reassure the client that the medicine is same other than the fact that it comes from a different pharmacy company.
3. Explain that the medicine comes in different colors but that it is the correct medicine.
4. Tell the client that the correct medicine has been ordered by the physician and the client should take it.

21. The nurse enters an elderly client's room to administer oral medication. The nursing assistant is making the client's bed and states the client is in the bathroom. What should the nurse do?
1. Go into the bathroom and instruct the client to take the medicine at this time.
2. Leave the medicine on the bedside table and tell the client to take it when she's finished in the bathroom.
3. Leave and return later when the client is out of the bathroom.
4. Give the medicine to the nursing assistant to give to the client when she's finished in the bathroom.

22. **The nurse is to administer nitroglycerin paste, ½ inch, topically every 6 hours to the client. Why will the nurse wear disposable gloves?**

   1. The ointment causes discoloration when in contact with the skin.
   2. Application of the paste needs exact measurements to be effective.
   3. The ointment can cause a drop in blood pressure and headaches when in contact with the nurse's skin.
   4. The ointment causes blistering of the skin if it is in contact with the nurse's skin.

23. **After administering a vaginal medication requiring an applicator, the nurse will take which of the following actions?**

   1. Place the used applicator into the dispensing carton and place the carton in the client's medication cassette.
   2. Place the used applicator in the dispensing carton and place the carton in the client's top drawer of the bedside cabinet.
   3. Wash, rinse, and dry the applicator, then wrap it in a paper towel and place it in the client's top drawer of the bedside cabinet.
   4. Wash, rinse, and dry the applicator, then place it in the dispensing carton with the medicine and place the carton in the client's medicine cassette.

24. **The nurse is preparing an injection using a single dose glass ampule. The nurse will do which of the following?**

   1. Wear sterile gloves and break off the neck of the glass ampule with a single snap to the right side.
   2. Wear sterile gloves and break off the neck of the glass ampule with a single snap in a forward motion.
   3. Tap the top of the ampule, place a gauze pad or alcohol swab around the ampule neck, and break off the top with a forward motion away from the hands.
   4. Tap the top of the ampule, place a gauze pad or unwrapped alcohol swab around the ampule neck, and break off the top with a forward motion away from the hands.

25. **The nurse prepares a medication for injection from an opened multi-dose vial from the stock floor medication cabinet. The nurse will do which of the following?**

   1. Check the multi-dose vial for date, time, and initials when first opened and withdraw the needed amount into the syringe.
   2. Check the multi-dose vial for date, time, and initials when first opened, clean the rubber top with an alcohol swab, and withdraw the needed amount into the syringe.
   3. Check the multi-dose vial for date, time, and initials when first opened, inject an equal amount of air into the vial, and withdraw the same amount of medication as ordered.
   4. Check the multi-dose vial for date, time, and initials when first opened, clean the rubber top with an alcohol swab, inject an equal amount of air into the vial, and withdraw the same amount of medication as ordered.

26. **The nurse is to administer subcutaneous short-acting insulin combined with long acting insulin to the client before he eats breakfast at 8:00 AM. Which of the following should the nurse do?**

   1. Give the insulin at 7:30 AM.
   2. Give the insulin when the breakfast tray arrives.
   3. Give the insulin one half hour after breakfast with other routine medicines.
   4. Give the insulin at 7:30 AM after checking the blood glucose level results.

27. **The nurse is to administer a rectal suppository to the client. The nurse will instruct the client to lie in which position on the bed?**

   1. Sim's position.
   2. Prone.
   3. Lying on the right side.
   4. Lying on the left side.

28. **The client is prescribed antibiotic eye drops, 1 gtt, O.U., t.i.d. Where and when will the nurse place the eye medication?**
    1. In the right eye, twice per day.
    2. In both eyes, twice per day.
    3. In the left eye, three times a day.
    4. In both eyes, three times a day.

29. **The nurse at the beginning of the shift is checking for a medication to be given to a client in the client's medication drawer. The medication is missing. What should the nurse do?**
    1. Call the pharmacy, tell them the medication is missing, and document that the medication was available.
    2. Borrow the medication from another client's medication drawer and administer.
    3. Go to the pharmacy, obtain the missing dose, and administer the medication.
    4. Omit the dose and prepare other medications for the client and then administer.

For each of the following, fill in the blank with the correct route (intravenous, intramuscular, oral, rectal, subcutaneous, topical) of administration.

30. _____
    Drugs that are absorbed through the epidermal layer of the skin into the dermis.

31. _____
    Drugs that are safest and most convenient; most drugs are administered by this route.

32. _____
    Drugs that are inserted to stimulate peristalsis, to relieve nausea, and decrease local irritation.

33. _____
    Drugs that are injected into adipose (fatty) tissue, and enter the blood stream slower than IM and IV drugs.

34. **How should the nurse administer heparin subcutaneously?**
    1. Cleanse the skin with an alcohol swab, insert the needle, and aspirate and inject the heparin.
    2. Cleanse the skin with an alcohol swab, insert the needle, aspirate and inject the heparin, and massage the site.
    3. Cleanse the skin with an alcohol swab, insert the needle, inject the heparin, and observe for bleeding.
    4. Cleanse the skin with an alcohol swab, insert the needle, inject the heparin, and aspirate and observe for bleeding.

35. **The nurse is to administer potassium chloride (KCL). The nurse reviews the client's serum potassium level results and discovers the client's potassium level is 5.2 mEq/L. What should the nurse do?**
    1. Give the ordered KCL as prescribed and document.
    2. Omit the KCL dose and document it was not given.
    3. Call the prescribing physician and inform her of the client's serum potassium level results.
    4. Call the lab to verify the client's results.

36. **The nurse is preparing a medication for the client and observes the date of expiration occurred two months ago. Which action should the nurse perform?**
    1. Give the medication.
    2. Discard the medication.
    3. Omit the medication.
    4. Return the medication to the pharmacy.

37. **What will the nurse do when the client refuses to take the prescribed medication that the nurse has prepared?**

1. Tell the client the physician wants the client to take the medicine.
2. Ask the client to tell the nurse why the client refuses the medication.
3. Explain what the medication is and the action of the medication.
4. Document that the client refuses the medication.

38. **What steps will the nurse take to administer antitussive cough syrup to the client?**

1. Check the client's ID bracelet, administer the cough syrup, and encourage the client to drink plenty of liquids.
2. Check the client's ID bracelet, administer the cough medicine, and encourage the client to remain upright for 30 minutes.
3. Check the client's ID bracelet, administer the cough medicine, and encourage the client to take sips of water for the next 30 minutes.
4. Check the client's ID bracelet, administer the cough medicine, and ask the client not to drink liquids for 30 minutes.

39. **The nurse is preparing an injectable pain medication for the client from the narcotic supply cabinet. How will the nurse discard half of one milliliter from the medication cartridge to dispense the correct dose ordered?**

1. The nurse will discard the leftover medicine in the medicine room drain and document that one half milliliter was wasted, then sign his signature on the narcotics control sign-out document.
2. Ask a second nurse to witness the discarded one half milliliter of medicine and have the first nurse sign the signature on the narcotics control sign-out document.
3. Both nurses will witness the discarded one half milliliter of medicine and both will sign the narcotics control sign-out document.
4. The second nurse witnessing the discarded one half milliliter of medicine will sign out the narcotics control sign-out document.

Unit 2 Answers and Rationales

Test 1 Answers and Rationales

1. **Answer: 3**
   Rationale: To ensure the safety of the client, the client's weight should be against the nurse's leg. The client would not have enough time to seek out a wall for support. If leaned forward, the client moves away from the center of gravity. The nurse should establish a wide base of support.
   Cognitive Level: Application
   Nursing Process: Intervention
   NCLEX-RN Test Plan: SECE
   Reference: Potter, P., & Perry, A. (2005). *Fundamentals of nursing* (6th ed.). St. Louis, MO: Elsevier Mosby.

2. **Answer: 3**
   Rationale: Working with the bed at a comfortable height provides the proper position for the nurse to prevent musculoskeletal injury. The nurse should use a wide base of support. Although the nurse may need to position the client, positioning using a draw sheet may cause musculoskeletal injury. The nurse should use the dominant hand to insert the catheter to ensure better control and to avoid awkward postures.
   Cognitive Level: Analysis
   Nursing Process: Planning
   NCLEX-RN Test Plan: SECE
   Reference: DeLaune, S. C., & Ladner, P. K. (2006). *Fundamentals of nursing: Standards and practice* (3rd ed.). Clifton Park, NY: Thomson Delmar Learning.

3. **Answer: 4**
   Rationale: When the airway is totally blocked, the client is not able to make any sound. This requires immediate action. A high-pitched stridor indicates that the airway is partially obstructed. If the client is talking or coughing, the airway is partially obstructed.
   Cognitive Level: Application
   Nursing Process: Assessment
   NCLEX-RN Test Plan: SECE
   Reference: DeLaune, S. C., & Ladner, P. K. (2006). *Fundamentals of nursing: Standards and practice* (3rd ed.). Clifton Park, NY: Thomson Delmar Learning.

4. **Answer: 4**
   Rationale: The safest method for transferring this client is through use of a mechanical lifting device. The other answers refer to use of body mechanics. Body mechanics alone will not protect the nurse from injury or provide the safest transfer for the client.
   Cognitive Level: Analysis
   Nursing Process: Implementation
   NCLEX-RN Test Plan: SECE
   References: Patient Safety Center of Inquiry & Department of Defense. (2005). *Patient care ergonomics resource guide: Safe patient handling and movement.* Retrieved March 31, 2006, from http://www.visn8.med.va.gov/patientsafetycenter/resguide/ErgoGuidePtOne.pdf

   Potter, P., & Perry, A. (2005). *Fundamentals of nursing* (6th ed.). St. Louis, MO: Elsevier Mosby.

5. **Answers: 1, 2, and 4**
   Rationale: JCAHO's restraint standard states that documentation must occur at least every two hours. It is important for the client's family to understand the purpose of the restraint. JCAHO's standard states that restraint orders are to be renewed every 24 hours when a restraint is used continuously. Release and repositioning should be provided for a minimum of 10 minutes at least every two hours.
   Cognitive Level: Application
   Nursing Process: Planning
   NCLEX-RN Test Plan: SECE
   Reference: DeLaune, S. C., & Ladner, P. K. (2006). *Fundamentals of nursing: Standards and practice* (3rd ed.). Clifton Park, NY: Thomson Delmar Learning.

6. **Answer: 2**
   Rationale: Carbon monoxide is odorless. All other options are correct.
   Cognitive Level: Analysis
   Nursing Process: Evaluation
   NCLEX-RN Test Plan: HPM
   Reference: Potter, P., & Perry, A. (2005). *Fundamentals of nursing* (6th ed.). St. Louis, MO: Elsevier Mosby.

7. **Answer: 4**

    Rationale: Bicycle-related injuries are a major cause of injuries in school-aged children. Children 5 to 14 years old account for almost one third of bicyclist deaths from traffic accidents. Bicycle safety is not a primary risk at the other developmental stages.

    Cognitive Level: Application

    Nursing Process: Planning

    NCLEX-RN Test Plan: HPM

    Reference: Potter, P., & Perry, A. (2005). *Fundamentals of nursing* (6th ed.). St. Louis, MO: Elsevier Mosby.

8. **Answers: 4 and 5**

    Rationale: Fall risk indicators are used to alert staff of the client's fall risk status. Teaching the client about the call light will help ensure the client has a way to call for assistance. The client should be placed near the nurses' station for close monitoring and response to client's needs. The purpose of the bed alarm is to alert the staff when the client gets out of bed unassisted.

    Cognitive Level: Application

    Nursing Process: Implementation

    NCLEX-RN Test Plan: SECE

    Reference: DeLaune, S. C., & Ladner, P. K. (2006). *Fundamentals of nursing: Standards and practice* (3rd ed.). Clifton Park, NY: Thomson Delmar Learning.

9. **Answer: 4**

    Rationale: A friction-reducing device is the most effective method in moving the client up in bed. This client is not able to use the trapeze. Lifting the client under the shoulders places musculoskeletal strain on the nurse and could cause injury to the client's shoulders. A draw sheet does little to reduce friction.

    Cognitive Level: Application

    Nursing Process: Planning

    NCLEX-RN Test Plan: SECE

    Reference: Patient Safety Center of Inquiry & Department of Defense. (2005). *Patient care ergonomics resource guide: Safe patient handling and movement.* Retrieved March 31, 2006, from http://www.visn8.med.va.gov/patientsafetycenter/resguide/ErgoGuidePtOne.pdf

10. **Answer: 3**

    Rationale: In the event of a fire, first remove persons in the room. Close the doors and windows and activate the alarm only after everyone is removed from the room. Extinguishing the fire would be the last step.

    Cognitive Level: Application

    Nursing Process: Implementation

    NCLEX-RN Test Plan: SECE

    Reference: Potter, P., & Perry, A. (2005). *Fundamentals of nursing* (6th ed.). St. Louis, MO: Elsevier Mosby.

11. **Answer: 3**

    Rationale: The use of a nonskid floor mat beside the bed is effective in fall prevention. Assistive devices should be located on the exit side of the bed. A light on at all times is not necessary. A night light can be sufficient. Treaded slipper socks could increase the likelihood of falling, especially if client shuffles feet while walking.

    Cognitive Level: Analysis

    Nursing Process: Evaluation

    NCLEX-RN Test Plan: SECE

    Reference: Stalhandske, E. (2004). *National center for patient safety 2004 falls toolkit.* Retrieved March 31, 2006, from http://www.patientsafety.gov/SafetyTopics/fallstoolkit/notebook/06_interventions.pdf

12. **Answer: 4**

    Rationale: A snow-like precipitate indicates a leakage of oxygen. The flowmeter will show the amount of oxygen being delivered. An increase in pulse, respirations, and fatigue and a decrease in ability to concentrate are all signs of hypoxia. Smoking should not be permitted where oxygen, which is flammable, is in use.

    Cognitive Level: Application

    Nursing Process: Evaluation

    NCLEX-RN Test Plan: SECE

    Reference: Potter, P., & Perry, A. (2005). *Fundamentals of nursing* (6th ed.). St. Louis, MO: Elsevier Mosby.

13. **Answers: 1, 2, and 3**

    Rationale: The correct findings, when seen in a home, can help to decrease the risk for injury. Space heaters are a fire hazard. Throw rugs are slippery and can cause a fall.

Cognitive Level: Application

Nursing Process: Evaluation

NCLEX-RN Test Plan: SECE

Reference: DeLaune, S. C., & Ladner, P. K. (2006). *Fundamentals of nursing: Standards and practice* (3rd ed.). Clifton Park, NY: Thomson Delmar Learning.

14. **Answer: 2**

Rationale: While all of this information is important to know, it is most important to know the client's weight-bearing status. This is the key assessment criteria when determining how this client will be transferred. From this information, the nurse can determine the ability of the client to assist with the transfer.

Cognitive Level: Application

Nursing Process: Analysis

NCLEX-RN Test Plan: SECE

Reference: Patient Safety Center of Inquiry & Department of Defense. (2005). *Patient care ergonomics resource guide: Safe patient handling and movement.* Retrieved March 31, 2006, from http://www.visn8.med.va.gov/patientsafetycenter/ resguide/ErgoGuidePtOne.pdf

15. **Answer: 3**

Rationale: The restraint should be tied to a part of the bed that moves when the head is elevated or lowered. The restraint should be tied in a quick release knot that does not tighten when pulled to ensure that the restraint can be removed quickly. Restraints should be secure but not tight so they do not impede circulation. Not all clients necessarily need the bedrails up. Each client should be assessed individually for a need for bedrails.

Cognitive Level: Application

Nursing Process: Evaluation

NCLEX-RN Test Plan: SECE

Reference: Kozier, B., Erb, G., Berman, A., & Snyder, S. (2004). *Fundamentals of nursing: Concepts, process and practice* (7th ed.). Upper Saddle River, NJ: Pearson Education, Inc.

16. **Answers: 1 and 3**

Rationale: Continuously assessing the client's airway patency during a seizure is the priority. Placing the bed in a low position minimizes the risk for injury. Placing an item in the client's mouth or restraining the client can cause injury. The client should be placed in a side-lying position. Furniture should be removed from the area to protect the client from injury.

Cognitive Level: Application

Nursing Process: Implementation

NCLEX-RN Test Plan: SECE

Reference: Potter, P., & Perry, A. (2005). *Fundamentals of nursing* (6th ed.). St. Louis, MO: Elsevier Mosby.

17. **Answer: 1**

Rationale: Although identifying the poison and properly positioning the client are important, checking for a patent airway is the priority for this client. Inducing vomiting may cause aspiration or internal burns.

Cognitive Level: Application

Nursing Process: Assessment

NCLEX-RN Test Plan: SECE

Reference: Potter, P., & Perry, A. (2005). *Fundamentals of nursing* (6th ed.). St. Louis, MO: Elsevier Mosby.

18. **Answer: 3**

Rationale: A sit-to-stand lift is the most appropriate device to transfer this client. This device will allow the client to maintain mobility while ensuring that the client does not become short of breath. The gait belt should have handles. The gait belt with handles may be used, but the nurse may end up bearing the client's weight if the client becomes too short of breath. An overhead lift or a lateral friction-reducing device would not promote independence.

Cognitive Level: Analysis

Nursing Process: Analysis

NCLEX-RN Test Plan: SECE

Reference: Patient Safety Center of Inquiry & Department of Defense. (2005). *Patient care ergonomics resource guide: Safe patient handling and movement.* Retrieved March 31, 2006, from http://www.visn8.med.va.gov/patientsafetycenter/ resguide/ErgoGuidePtOne.pdf

19. **Answers: 1, 2, 3, and 4**

    Rationale: Exercises that increase balance and strength can help prevent falls. Home safety evaluations should be done to identify fall risk hazards in the home. Using the locks provides stability and prevents the bed or wheelchair from rolling. Placing items within reach prevents the client from searching or overreaching for needed items. Use of sedatives can be a fall risk factor.

    Cognitive Level: Application

    Nursing Process: Planning

    NCLEX-RN Test Plan: SECE

    Reference: Potter, P., & Perry, A. (2005). *Fundamentals of nursing* (6th ed.). St. Louis, MO: Elsevier Mosby.

20. **Answer: 1**

    Rationale: To best prevent musculoskeletal injuries, the task should be adjusted so that it fits the nurse. If the nurse has to adjust to the task, this may increase the risk of injury. Having the strongest person performing the lifting isn't appropriate. Manual lifting is not the safest way to prevent injury. Body mechanics alone is not adequate protection from musculoskeletal injury.

    Cognitive Level: Application

    Nursing Process: Implementation

    NCLEX-RN Test Plan: SECE

    Reference: Patient Safety Center of Inquiry & Department of Defense. (2005). *Patient care ergonomics resource guide: Safe patient handling and movement.* Retrieved March 31, 2006, from http://www.visn8.med.va.gov/patientsafetycenter/resguide/ErgoGuidePtOne.pdf

21. **Answer: 4**

    Rationale: An extremity that is cool and pale may indicate impaired circulation caused by a tight restraint. A quick capillary refill indicates that circulation is not impaired. The client should have full range of motion of the wrist. Attempting to remove the restraint may be a response from being restrained.

    Cognitive Level: Application

    Nursing Process: Assessment

    NCLEX-RN Test Plan: SECE

    Reference: Potter, P., & Perry, A. (2005). *Fundamentals of nursing* (6th ed.). St. Louis, MO: Elsevier Mosby.

22. **Answer: 4**

    Rationale: Because droplet precautions are needed with this client, a mask is a necessary barrier when the nurse is within three feet of the client. Wearing gloves, goggles, or a mask may not be necessary for this client.

    Cognitive Level: Application

    Nursing Process: Planning

    NCLEX-RN Test Plan: SECE

    Reference: Potter, P., & Perry, A. (2005). *Fundamentals of nursing* (6th ed.). St. Louis, MO: Elsevier Mosby.

23. **Answer: Material safety data sheets**

    Rationale: Material safety data sheets provide detailed information about chemicals found in the workplace. Information about what to do in case of an exposure can be found in these sheets.

    Cognitive Level: Application

    Nursing Process: Implementation

    NCLEX-RN Test Plan: SECE

    Reference: Potter, P., & Perry, A. (2005). *Fundamentals of nursing* (6th ed.). St. Louis, MO: Elsevier Mosby.

24. **Answer: 1**

    Rationale: Although gloves reduce hand contamination, hand hygiene is still required. Centers for Disease Control (CDC) guidelines, which are evidence-based, state that alcohol-based hand rubs can be used before and after each client. These guidelines also recommend to wash hands when they are visibly soiled and to avoid wearing artificial nails when caring for clients.

    Cognitive Level: Application

    Nursing Process: Evaluation

    NCLEX-RN Test Plan: SECE

    Reference: DeLaune, S. C., & Ladner, P. K. (2006). *Fundamentals of nursing: Standards and practice* (3rd ed.). Clifton Park, NY: Thomson Delmar Learning.

25. **Answer: 2**

    Rationale: Maintaining sterility takes precedence over the other actions. While the other actions would be helpful in this procedure, the most harm would come from breaking sterility.

    Cognitive Level: Analysis

Nursing Process: Planning
NCLEX-RN Test Plan: SECE
Reference: Potter, P., & Perry, A. (2005).
Fundamentals of nursing (6th ed.). St. Louis,
MO: Elsevier Mosby.

26. **Answer: 4**
Rationale: Contact precautions are necessary for this client. Clients infected with the same organism may share a room but should not be placed in a room with any other client. A private room may isolate the client and is not necessary. A negative-pressure isolation room is not necessary for this client.
Cognitive Level: Analysis
Nursing Process: Planning
NCLEX-RN Test Plan: SECE
Reference: Potter, P., & Perry, A. (2005).
Fundamentals of nursing (6th ed.). St. Louis,
MO: Elsevier Mosby.

27. **Answer: Handwashing**
Rationale: Handwashing is the best way to prevent the spread of infection. Contaminated hands are a main cause of cross contamination.
Cognitive Level: Application
Nursing Process: Planning
NCLEX-RN Test Plan: SECE
Reference: Potter, P., & Perry, A. (2005).
Fundamentals of nursing (6th ed.). St. Louis,
MO: Elsevier Mosby.

28. **Answer: 4**
Rationale: Handwashing is the single best way to prevent the spread of infection. Although the nurse may need to use personal protective equipment when caring for clients, handwashing is most important in breaking the chain of infection.
Cognitive Level: Application
Nursing Process: Implementation
NCLEX-RN Test Plan: SECE
Reference: Lewis, S., Heitkemper, M., & Dirksen, S. (2004). *Medical-surgical nursing: Assessment and management of clinical problems* (6th ed.). St. Louis, MO: Elsevier Mosby.

29. **Answer: 3**
Rationale: Opening a package over a sterile field can cause contamination to the sterile field. Placing the

item into the middle of the field requires reaching into the field, which can contaminate its surface. A one-inch border barrier from the edge of the field is considered contaminated. Objects should be held above the waist to maintain sterility. When the sterile field is waterproof, bacteria will not cross from the nonsterile to the sterile side if it becomes wet.
Cognitive Level: Application
Nursing Process: Evaluation
NCLEX-RN Test Plan: SECE
Reference: Potter, P., & Perry, A. (2005).
Fundamentals of nursing (6th ed.). St. Louis,
MO: Elsevier Mosby.

30. **Answer: 5, 2, 4, 3, 1**
Rationale: Gloving the dominant hand facilitates dexterity. Grasping by the cuff maintains sterility of the outer surface of the glove. The nondominant hand is gloved second. When interlocking fingers, contact is made with two sterile gloves. This will protect the gloved fingers.
Cognitive Level: Application
Nursing Process: Planning
NCLEX-RN Test Plan: SECE
Reference: Potter, P., & Perry, A. (2005).
Fundamentals of nursing (6th ed.). St. Louis,
MO: Elsevier Mosby.

31. **Answer: 3**
Rationale: Because Hepatitis A is transmitted through the fecal route, handling the client's feces is the highest risk activity. The modes of transmission described in the first two answers would be more applicable for a client with a respiratory infection. Touching this client would not be a high risk activity.
Cognitive Level: Application
Nursing Process: Implementation
NCLEX-RN Test Plan: SECE
Reference: Potter, P., & Perry, A. (2005).
Fundamentals of nursing (6th ed.). St. Louis,
MO: Elsevier Mosby.

32. **Answer: 3**
Rationale: To prevent the spread of infection, all equipment used for a client in isolation should be kept in the client's room and used only for that client. A needle should not be detached from the syringe before disposal. It is not necessary to double

bag items if impervious bags are used. Personal protective equipment should be removed inside the client's door.
Cognitive Level: Application
Nursing Process: Analysis
NCLEX-RN Test Plan: SECE
Reference: Potter, P., & Perry, A. (2005). *Fundamentals of nursing* (6th ed.). St. Louis, MO: Elsevier Mosby.

33. **Answer: 3**
Rationale: Determining the reason for the client pulling out the IV may help to determine an alternative to the restraint. Using restraints should not be based on staffing level or staff convenience. A chemical restraint should be used after other alternatives are exhausted.
Cognitive Level: Application
Nursing Process: Evaluation
NCLEX-RN Test Plan: SECE
Reference: Potter, P., & Perry, A. (2005). *Fundamentals of nursing* (6th ed.). St. Louis, MO: Elsevier Mosby.

34. **Answer: 1**
Rationale: Washing hands before applying gloves best shows that the daughter understands preventing infection. If the sterile field is placed between the daughter and client, the daughter would have to turn her back on the sterile field. It is not necessary to wear sterile gloves to open packages or to remove an old dressing.
Cognitive Level: Analysis
Nursing Process: Evaluation
NCLEX-RN Test Plan: SECE
Reference: Potter, P., & Perry, A. (2005). *Fundamentals of nursing* (6th ed.). St. Louis, MO: Elsevier Mosby.

35. **Answer: 2**
Rationale: Because Hepatitis B can be spread through blood, the nurse can best prevent exposure by properly disposing of a contaminated needle. The other measures are not necessary unless there is a potential for the nurse to be exposed to the client's blood.
Cognitive Level: Application
Nursing Process: Planning
NCLEX-RN Test Plan: SECE

Reference: DeLaune, S. C., & Ladner, P. K. (2006). *Fundamentals of nursing: Standards and practice* (3rd ed.). Clifton Park, NY: Thomson Delmar Learning.

36. **Answer: 1, 3, 4, 2**
Rationale: The nurse removes personal protective equipment in this order to discard from the most contaminated item to the least contaminated item. The mask is discarded after the gown to minimize contamination from the gown. The gown is a greater source of contaminant than the mask. Goggles are removed last as they are considered the least contaminated item.
Cognitive Level: Application
Nursing Process: Planning
NCLEX-RN Test Plan: SECE
Reference: DeLaune, S. C., & Ladner, P. K. (2006). *Fundamentals of nursing: Standards and practice* (3rd ed.). Clifton Park, NY: Thomson Delmar Learning.

37. **Answer: 4**
Rationale: When going through self-closing doors, the wheelchair should be backed out of the room. The spouse should keep the door open by backing against the door and guiding the wheelchair out of the room. All of the other options are correct.
Cognitive Level: Application
Nursing Process: Evaluation
NCLEX-RN Test Plan: SECE
Reference: DeLaune, S. C., & Ladner, P. K. (2006). *Fundamentals of nursing: Standards and practice* (3rd ed.). Clifton Park, NY: Thomson Delmar Learning.

38. **Answer: 2**
Rationale: In a client with a depressed immune response, protective isolation will provide protection from environmental sources of infection. Since the other options do not relate to protecting this vulnerable client, they do not apply.
Cognitive Level: Application
Nursing Process: Implementation
NCLEX-RN Test Plan: SECE
Reference: Lewis, S., Heitkemper, M., & Dirksen, S. (2004). *Medical-surgical nursing: Assessment and management of clinical problems* (6th ed.). St. Louis, MO: Elsevier Mosby.

39. Answer:

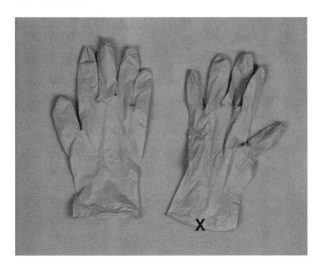

Rationale: Gloving the dominant hand facilitates dexterity. Grasping by the cuff maintains sterility of the outer surface of the glove.
Cognitive Level: Application
Nursing Process: Planning
NCLEX-RN Test Plan: SECE
Reference: Potter, P., & Perry, A. (2005). *Fundamentals of nursing* (6th ed.). St. Louis, MO: Elsevier Mosby.

Unit 2 Answers and Rationales

Test 2 Answers and Rationales

1. **Answer: 1**

   Rationale: The advocate protects the client, provides explanations in the client's language, acts as a change agent, and supports the client's decisions. She supports the client's rights and assists in asserting those rights when clients are unable to do so themselves.

   Cognitive Level: Application

   Nursing Process: Implementation

   NCLEX-RN Test Plan: SECE

   Reference: DeLaune, S. C., & Ladner, P. K. (2006). *Fundamentals of nursing: Standards and practice* (3rd ed.). Clifton Park, NY: Thomson Delmar Learning.

2. **Answer: 4**

   Rationale: In this stage of development, a person views his life as meaningful and fulfilling. This stage occurs when a person is older than age 45.

   Cognitive Level: Application

   Nursing Process: Implementation

   NCLEX-RN Test Plan: HMP

   Reference: DeLaune, S. C., & Ladner, P. K. (2006). *Fundamentals of nursing: Standards and practice* (3rd ed.). Clifton Park, NY: Thomson Delmar Learning.

3. **Answer: 2**

   Rationale: This meets safety and security needs so that the nurse will come as needed and prevent falls. The risk for falls can be reduced by orienting clients to the environment and providing ambulatory aids, placing personal belongings on tables near the bed, keeping beds in the lowest position with the side rails up, and illuminating the environment.

   Cognitive Level: Application

   Nursing Process: Evaluation

   NCLEX-RN Test Plan: SECE

   Reference: DeLaune, S. C., & Ladner, P. K. (2006). *Fundamentals of nursing: Standards and practice* (3rd ed.). Clifton Park, NY: Thomson Delmar Learning.

4. **Answer: 4**

   Rationale: It's necessary to assess the client for muscle strength (legs and upper arms) as immobile clients have decreased muscle strength, tone, and mass, which affects the ability to bear weight and raise the body.

   Cognition Level: Application

   Nursing Process: Assessment

   NCLEX-RN Test Plan: HPM

   Reference: Potter, P. A., & Perry, A. G. (2005). *Fundamentals of nursing* (6th ed.). St. Louis, MO: Elsevier Mosby.

5. **Answer: 7, 2, 1, 8, 3, 5, 6, 4**

   Rationale: The ANA's *Scope and Standards of Nursing Practice* describe the steps of the nursing process for the registered nurse as:

   Assessment—collects comprehensive data pertinent to the patient's health or the situation.

   Diagnosis—analyzes the assessment data to determine the diagnoses or issues.

   Outcome identification—expected outcomes for a plan individualized to the patient or the situation.

   Planning—develops a plan that prescribes strategies and alternatives to attain expected outcomes.

   Implementation—implements the identified plan including coordinating care delivery and health teaching and promotion.

   Evaluation—evaluates progress towards attainment of outcomes.

   Cognitive Level: Application

   Nursing Process: Assessment, Analysis, Planning, Implementation, and Evaluation

   NCLEX-RN Test Plan: PHYS

   Reference: Potter, P. A., & Perry, A. G. (2005). *Fundamentals of nursing* (6th ed.). St. Louis, MO: Elsevier Mosby.

6. **Answer: 2**

Rationale: The nurse should ensure that food is not pocketed or left in the mouth where it can be aspirated and obstruct the client's airway. Clients at high risk for aspiration are those clients with decreased level of alertness, decreased gag or cough reflexes, and clients who have difficulty managing saliva.

Cognition Level: Application

Nursing Process: Planning

NCLEX-RN Test Plan: PHYS

Reference: Potter, P. A., & Perry, A. G. (2005). *Fundamentals of nursing* (6th ed.). St. Louis, MO: Elsevier Mosby.

7. **Answer: 1**

Rationale: Removal of dirt decreases the risk for infection and the orange stick is shaped to not cause injury.

Cognitive Level: Application

Nursing Process: Implementation

NCLEX-RN Test Plan: PHYS

Reference: DeLaune, S. C., & Ladner, P. K. (2006). *Fundamentals of nursing: Standards and practice* (3rd ed.). Clifton Park, NY: Thomson Delmar Learning.

8. **Answer: 2**

Rationale: Never press both carotids at the same time. This may decrease blood flow to the brain and induce syncope.

Cognitive Level: Application

Nursing Process: Assessment

NCLEX-RN Test Plan: HPM

Reference: Bickley, L. S., & Szilagyi, P. G. (2003). *Bates' guide to physical examination and history taking* (8th ed.). Philadelphia: Lippincott Williams & Wilkins.

9. **Answers: 1, 4, 5, 6, and 8**

Rationale: Rubbing alcohol is drying and may cause skin breakdown. The weak arm should be gowned first to prevent stretching and discomfort of the arm. Washing extremities distal to proximal stimulates venous return.

Cognitive Level: Application

Nursing Process: Implementation

NCLEX-RN Test Plan: PHYS

Reference: DeLaune, S. C., & Ladner, P. K. (2006). *Fundamentals of nursing: Standards*

and practice (3rd ed.). Clifton Park, NY: Thomson Delmar Learning.

10. **Answer: 1**

Rationale: An irregular pulse is taken for a full minute for an accurate count. When the heart rhythm is irregular, the rate should be evaluated by cardiac auscultation because beats that occur earlier than others may not be detected peripherally, and the heart rate can be seriously underestimated. A doppler is not necessary as the pulse can be heard with a stethoscope.

Cognitive Level: Application

Nursing Process: Assessment

NCLEX-RN Test Plan: PHYS

Reference: Bickley, L. S., & Szilagyi, P. G. (2003). *Bates' guide to physical examination and history taking* (8th ed.). Philadelphia: Lippincott Williams and Wilkins.

11. **Answer: 2**

Rationale: Listen to the abdomen before performing percussion or palpation, since these maneuvers may alter the frequency of bowel sounds.

Cognitive Level: Application

Nursing Process: Assessment

NCLEX-RN Test Plan: HPM

Reference: Bickley, L. S., & Szilagyi, P. G. (2003). *Bates' guide to physical examination and history taking* (8th ed.). Philadelphia: Lippincott Williams & Wilkins.

12. **Answer: 3**

Rationale: The nursing process is dynamic and requires creativity for its application. The steps remain the same but the application and results will be different in each client situation.

Cognitive Level: Application

Nursing Process: Planning

NCLEX-RN Test Plan: PHYS

Reference: DeLaune, S. C., & Ladner, P. K. (2006). *Fundamentals of nursing: Standards and practice* (8th ed.). Clifton Park, NY: Thomson Delmar Learning.

13. **Answer: 2**

Rationale: Compare the data collected to the major and minor defining characteristics of each of the nursing diagnoses being considered to determine which meets the criteria.

Cognitive Level: Application
Nursing Process: Planning
NCLEX-RN Test Plan: PHYS
Reference: Potter, P. A., & Perry, A. G. (2005).
   Fundamentals of nursing (6th ed.). St. Louis,
   MO: Elsevier Mosby.

14. **Answer: 3**
   Rationale: Transmission of microorganisms from
   one client to another is prevented when microorgan-
   isms are removed from the hands. Handwashing is
   the most important intervention in preventing and
   controlling the transmission of infection.
   Cognitive Level: Application
   Nursing Process: Implementation
   NCLEX-RN Test Plan: SECE
   Reference: DeLaune, S. C., & Ladner, P. K.
      (2006). *Fundamentals of nursing: Standards
      and practice* (3rd ed.). Clifton Park, NY:
      Thomson Delmar Learning.

15. **Answer: 4**
   Rationale: When the white blood cell count is ele-
   vated (leukocytosis), it suggests the client is defend-
   ing against the pathogen causing an infection.
   Other options, if elevated, are not directly related
   to infection.
   Cognitive Level: Application
   Nursing Process: Analysis
   NCLEX-RN Test Plan: PHYS
   Reference: Potter, P. A., & Perry, A. G. (2005).
      Fundamentals of nursing (6th ed.). St. Louis,
      MO: Elsevier Mosby.

16. **Answer: 1**
   Rationale: Failure to heed the call to defecate may
   lead to overdistention of the rectum with hardening
   of the stool and subsequent constipation.
   Cognitive Level: Application
   Nursing Process: Implementation
   NCLEX-RN Test Plan: PHYS
   Reference: DeLaune, S. C., & Ladner, P. K.
      (2006). *Fundamentals of nursing: Standards
      and practice* (3rd ed.). Clifton Park, NY:
      Thomson Delmar Learning.

17. **Answer: 1**
   Rationale: Clear liquids are given to relieve thirst,
   prevent dehydration, and minimize irritation to the
   gastrointestinal tract.
   Cognitive Level: Application
   Nursing Process: Implementation
   NCLEX-RN Test Plan: PHYS
   Reference: Potter, P. A., & Perry, A. G. (2003).
      Fundamentals of nursing (6th ed.). St. Louis,
      MO: Elsevier Mosby.

18. **Answer: 2**
   Rationale: Document and report output less than
   30 ml/hour. This alerts the nurse to severe fluid
   imbalance and means the client has a decreased cir-
   culating fluid volume, inadequate renal perfusion,
   and/or kidney disease.
   Cognitive Level: Analysis
   Nursing Process: Assessment
   NCLEX-RN Test Plan: PHYS
   Reference: DeLaune, S. C., & Ladner, P. K.
      (2006). *Fundamentals of nursing: Standards
      and practice* (3rd ed.). Clifton Park, NY:
      Thomson Delmar Learning.

19. **Answer: 4**
   Rationale: A decreased volume of circulating
   blood and less pressure within the vessels gives the
   client weak thready peripheral pulses and flattened
   neck veins.
   Cognitive Level: Analysis
   Nursing Process: Assessment
   NCLEX-RN Test Plan: PHYS
   Reference: DeLaune, S. C., & Ladner, P. K.
      (2006). *Fundamentals of nursing: Standards
      and practice* (3rd ed.). Clifton Park, NY:
      Thomson Delmar Learning.

20. **Answer: 2**
   Rationale: As ambulation activities are initiated, it is
   important to assess the client's blood pressure, respiratory rate, pulse, skin color, and moisture as well as
   subjective responses. Feeling dizzy is a subjective
   response and asking the client about dizziness gives a
   quick evaluation for safety.
   Cognitive Level: Application
   Nursing Process: Evaluation

NCLEX-RN Test Plan: SECE

Reference: DeLaune, S. C., & Ladner, P. K. (2006). *Fundamentals of nursing: Standards and practice* (3rd ed.). Clifton Park, NY: Thomson Delmar Learning.

21. **Answers: 1, 5, 6, 7, and 8**
    Rationale: Urinary calculi due to stasis or urine, contractures of the extremities because of disuse of the muscles and joints, pneumonia due to pulmonary stasis, pressure ulcers due to increased pressure on bony prominences, and thrombi due to venous stasis are all possible complications of immobility.
    Cognition Level: Analysis
    Nursing Process: Evaluation
    NCLEX-RN Test Plan: PHYS
    Reference: DeLaune, S. C., & Ladner, P. K. (2006). *Fundamentals of nursing: Standards and practice* (3rd ed.). Clifton Park, NY: Thomson Delmar Learning.

22. **Answer: 4**
    Rationale: Lying down earlier may not help and may only lead to frustration. When activities other than sleeping, like watching TV, are done in bed, they are not correlated to the expectation of sleep like simply lying down to sleep. The nurse should facilitate maintenance of the client's usual bedtime routines as appropriate.
    Cognitive Level: Application
    Nursing Process: Evaluation
    NCLEX-RN Test Plan: PHYS
    Reference: DeLaune, S. C., & Ladner, P. K. (2006). *Fundamentals of nursing: Standards and practice* (3rd ed.). Clifton Park, NY: Thomson Delmar Learning.

23. **Answer: 3**
    Rationale: Limit environmental and procedural activities as well as staff communication noise as these are major deterrents to sleep in the hospital.
    Cognitive Level: Application
    Nursing Process: Implementation
    NCLEX-RN Test Plan: PHYS
    Reference: DeLaune, S. C., & Ladner, P. K. (2006). *Fundamentals of nursing: Standards and practice* (3rd ed.). Clifton Park, NY: Thomson Delmar Learning.

24. **Answer: 4**
    Rationale: Supporting the client with elevation of the head of the bed or with pillows can reduce the client's workload and minimize fatigue. Raising the head of the bed uses gravity to drop the abdominal organs away from the diaphragm, which provides increased expansion of the lungs.
    Cognitive Level: Application
    Nursing Process: Implementation
    NCLEX-RN Test Plan: PHYS
    Reference: DeLaune, S. C., & Ladner, P. K. (2006). *Fundamentals of nursing: Standards and practice* (3rd ed.). Clifton Park, NY: Thomson Delmar Learning.

25. **Answer: 2**
    Rationale: The earlobe is rarely edematous, is the least affected by decreased blood flow, and has better accuracy when saturations decrease. Assess and move the sensor to an alternate site. Assess the capillary refill and proximal pulse and if the client has poor circulation, use the earlobe, forehead, or a nasal sensor instead.
    Cognitive Level: Application
    Nursing Process: Assessment
    NCLEX-RN Test Plan: HPM
    Reference: DeLaune, S. C., & Ladner, P. K. (2006). *Fundamentals of nursing:Standards and practice* (3rd ed.). Clifton Park, NY: Thomson Delmar Learning.

26. **Answers: 3, 4, 6, 7, and 8**
    Rationales: 3—Increased body temperature. The inflammatory process has begun to fight infection. Fever is caused by phagocytic release of pyrogens from bacterial cells that cause a rise in the hypothalamic set point or temperature-regulating center of the brain.

    4—Increased neutrophils. Through the process of phagocytosis, these specialized white blood cells, called neutrophils and monocytes, ingest and destroy microorganisms.

    6—Increased white blood cells or leukocytosis. This is the body's response to white blood cells leaving blood vessels as inflammation becomes systemic.

    7—Localized edema. Edema occurs as injury causes tissue necrosis. The body releases histamine, bradykinin, prostaglandin, and serotonin, which increases the permeability of small blood vessels. Fluid, protein, and cells enter interstitial spaces and the accumulated fluid appears as localized swelling or edema.

8—Localized pain. This occurs because the swelling of inflamed tissue increases the pressure on nerve endings, causing pain.

Cognitive Level: Analysis
Nursing Process: Analysis
NCLEX-RN Test Plan: PHYS
Reference: Potter, P. A., & Perry, A. G. (2005). *Fundamentals of nursing* (6th ed.). St. Louis, MO: Elsevier Mosby.

27. **Answer: 3**
Rationale: Increasing fluids promotes liquefaction of pulmonary secretions, which facilitate expectoration to clear the lungs.
Cognitive Level: Application
Nursing Process: Implementation
NCLEX-RN Test Plan: PHYS
Reference: DeLaune, S. C., & Ladner, P. K. (2006). *Fundamentals of nursing: Standards and practice* (3rd ed.). Clifton Park, NY: Thomson Delmar Learning.

28. **Answer: 1**
Rationale: Complete deflation of the balloon holding the catheter in place with a syringe prevents trauma to the urethra as the catheter is removed.
Cognitive Level: Application
Nursing Process: Implementation
NCLEX-RN Test Plan: PHYS
Reference: Potter, P. A., & Perry, A. G. (2005). *Fundamentals of nursing* (6th ed.). St. Louis, MO: Elsevier Mosby.

29. **Answer: 1**
Rationale: The urine appears cloudy and concentrated because of the presence of white blood cells, red blood cells, and bacteria. Pus and bacteria can cause the unpleasant smell.
Cognitive Level: Analysis
Nursing Process: Analysis
NCLEX-RN Test Plan: PHYS

Reference: DeLaune, S. C., & Ladner, P. K. (2006). *Fundamentals of nursing: Standards and practice* (3rd ed.). Clifton Park, NY: Thomas Delmar Learning.

30. **Answer: 1**
Rationale: Irrigation decreases the risk of culturing normal flora and other exudates such as protein. Irrigating with an antiseptic prior to obtaining the specimen may destroy the bacteria.
Cognitive Level: Application
Nursing Process: Implementation
NCLEX-RN Test Plan: PHYS
Reference: Potter, P. A., & Perry, A. G. (2005). *Fundamentals of nursing* (6th ed.). St. Louis, MO: Elsevier Mosby.

31. **Answer: 2**
Rationale: Pressure can be exerted to expel feces through a voluntary straining (Valsalva Maneuver) in which client contracts the abdominal muscles and holds their breath while bearing down. Clients with cardiovascular disease, glaucoma, increased intracranial pressure, or a new surgical wound can be placed at further risk, such as cardiac irregularities and elevated blood pressure.
Cognitive Level: Application
Nursing Process: Implementation
NCLEX-RN Test Plan: PHYS
Reference: Potter, P. A., & Perry, A. G. (2005). *Fundamentals of nursing* (6th ed.). St. Louis, MO: Elsevier Mosby.

32. **Answer: Options 1–4 should be selected.**
Rationale: Each client is unique with their bowel habits and specific information should be reviewed to determine which areas to emphasize with the client during teaching to prevent constipation. Lack of privacy should also be considered in the hospitalized client.

A number of conditions, including hemorrhoids, rectal surgery, rectal fistulas, and abdominal surgery, can result in discomfort, which often causes the client to suppress the urge to defecate to avoid pain and constipation may develop.

Chronic use of laxatives causes the large intestine to lose muscle tone and become less responsive to stimulation by laxatives.

Anything that prevents the client from responding to the urge to defecate and disrupts regular habits can cause possible alterations such as constipation.

Reduced fluid intake slows the passage of food through the intestine and can result in hardening of stool contents.

Cognitive Level: Application.

Nursing Process: Implementation

NCLEX-RN Test Plan: HPM

Reference: Potter, P. A., & Perry, A. G. (2005). *Fundamentals of nursing* (6th ed.). St. Louis, MO: Elsevier Mosby.

33. **Answer: 3**

Rationale: In the Intimacy versus Isolation psychosocial state, young adults age 18–25 develop commitments to others and to a life work (career). In the Generativity versus Stagnation state, people of middle age (25–65) fulfill life goals dealing with family, career, and society, and give to and care for others. In the Identity versus Role Diffusion state, adolescents (age 12–20) transition from childhood to adulthood. In the Trust versus Mistrust state, newborn infants to children age 18 months strive to have needs met by others and develop trust in caregivers.

Cognitive Level: Application

Nursing Process: Planning

NCLEX-RN Test Plan: HPM

Reference: DeLaune, S. C., & Ladner, P. K. (2006). *Fundamentals of nursing: Standards and practice* (3rd ed.). Clifton Park, NY: Thomson Delmar Learning.

34. **Answer: 2**

Rationale: Sociocultural background is a major influence on the meaning of nonverbal behavior. In the United States, with its diverse cultural communities, nonverbal messages between people can be easily misinterpreted. Options 1 and 4 are incorrect because unconsciously motivated nonverbal behavior may more accurately indicate a person's intended meaning than the verbal words. Nonverbal carries more weight than verbal because nonverbal is influenced by the unconscious. Option 3 is incorrect because it is more likely that the nonverbal behavior reflects the client's true feelings.

Cognitive Level: Application

Nursing Process: Assessment

NCLEX-RN Test Plan: PSYC

Reference: Potter, P. A., & Perry, A. G. (2005). *Fundamentals of nursing* (6th ed.). St. Louis, MO: Elsevier Mosby.

35. **Answer: 2**

Rationale: The working phase (Option 2) is when the nurse and client work together to solve problems and accomplish goals. The orientation phase (Option 1) is when the nurse and client meet to get to know one another. The termination phase (Option 3) is what the nurse does during the end of the relationship. The preinteraction phase (Option 4) is what the nurse does before meeting the client.

Cognitive Level: Analysis

Nursing Process: Assessment

NCLEX-RN Test Plan: PSYC

Reference: Potter, P. A., & Perry, A. G. (2005). *Fundamentals of nursing* (6th ed.). St. Louis, MO: Elsevier Mosby.

36. **Answer: 4**

Rationale: Positive behavior changes are seen and documented. The client sees the value of being able to give his own insulin and is incorporating it into his life style. The other answer options give less effective methods. In Option 1, rewards are being utilized to increase motivation for learning. Option 2 indicates learning is taking place but not a behavior change yet. Option 3 indicates readiness to learn.

Cognitive Level: Analysis

Nursing Process: Evaluation

NCLEX-RN Test Plan: HPM

Reference: Potter, P. A., & Perry, A. G. (2005). *Fundamentals of nursing* (6th ed.). St. Louis, MO: Elsevier Mosby.

37. **Answers: 2, 4, and 5**

Rationale: 2—Each person's expression of pain may be different and individualized. In some cultures it is unacceptable to complain about pain or tolerance to pain signifies strength and courage.

4—Pain level and pain tolerance can be assessed using a scale of 1–10. To assess a client's pain level, ask the client how much pain they are having on a scale of 1–10. For pain tolerance, the nurse can ask the client at what point on a scale of 1–10 they feel that they must have pain medication.

5—The client needs to know the nurse believes what they are saying about their pain. The client's self report of the existence and intensity of pain is the most accurate and reliable evidence of the nature of the pain.

Cognitive Level: Application
Nursing Process: Assessment
NCLEX-RN Test Plan: PHYS
Reference: DeLaune, S. C., & Ladner, P. K. (2006). *Fundamentals of nursing: Standards and practice* (3rd ed.). Clifton Park, NY: Thomson Delmar Learning.

38. **Answer: 1**
Rationale: Information obtained directly from the client (client concern) is the most accurate and provides the best information available to the nurse. The client is considered to be a primary source of information. The other options (family information, medical history, and progress notes) are considered to be secondary sources of information. Although these secondary sources may provide information to the nurse, they are not as helpful to the nurse as information directly from the client.
Cognitive Level: Application
Nursing Process: Planning
NCLEX-RN Test Plan: PSYC
Reference: Chitty, K., & Black, B. (2007). *Professional nursing: Concepts & challenges* (5th ed.). Philadelphia: Elsevier Saunders.

39. **Answer:**

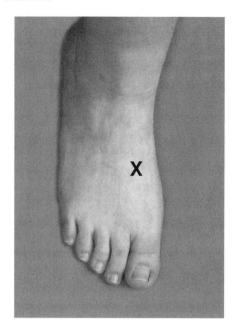

Rationale: With the client's foot relaxed, the nurse locates the dorsalis pedis pulse. The artery runs along the top of the foot in line with the groove between the extensor tendons of the great toe and first toe. Often an examiner finds the pulse by placing the fingertips between the great and first toe and slowly inching up the foot.
Cognitive Level: Application
Nursing Process: Assessment
NCLEX-RN Test Plan: PHYS
Reference: Potter, P. A., & Perry, A. G. (2005). *Fundamentals of nursing* (6th ed.). St. Louis, MO: Elsevier Mosby.

Unit 2 Answers and Rationales

Test 3 Answers and Rationales

1. **Answer: 1**
   Rationale: This is characteristic of the traditional NPR where nurses had time to build the three phase NPR. Today clients are more acutely ill, nurses' workloads have increased, and clients spend fewer days in the hospital than in the past. The result is that the nurse's time with a client may be limited to one or two contacts. This has led to reconceptualizing the NPR using the theory of human relatedness as a framework.
   Cognitive Level: Analysis
   Nursing Process: Analysis
   NCLEX-RN Test Plan: PSYC
   Reference: Chitty, K. K. (2005). *Professional nursing: Concepts & challenges* (4th ed.). St. Louis, MO: Elsevier Saunders.

2. **Answer: 4**
   Rationale: In passive-aggressive communication, the verbal message is aggressive while the nonverbal message is passive. Improvement is demonstrated when there is congruence between the two modes of communication.
   Cognitive Level: Analysis
   Nursing Process: Evaluation
   NCLEX-RN Test Plan: PSYC
   Reference: Chitty, K. K. (2005). *Professional nursing: Concepts & challenges* (4th ed.). St. Louis, MO: Elsevier Saunders.

3. **Answer: 1**
   Rationale: One of the main tasks of the orientation phase is the nurse and client getting to know each other. This requires that the nurse elicit information.
   Cognitive Level: Application
   Nursing Process: Implementation
   NCLEX-RN Test Plan: PSYC
   Reference: Chitty, K. K. (2005). *Professional nursing: Concepts & challenges* (4th ed.). St. Louis, MO: Elsevier Saunders.

4. **Answer: 1**
   Rationale: Responses 2, 3, and 4 are more characteristic of female communication with coworkers.
   Cognitive Level: Analysis
   Nursing Process: Analysis
   NCLEX-RN Test Plan: PSYC
   Reference: Chitty, K. K. (2005). *Professional nursing: Concepts & challenges* (4th ed.). St. Louis, MO: Elsevier Saunders.

5. **Answer: 4**
   Rationale: The social relationship meets the needs of both parties. It is not necessarily goal-directed, professional, or therapeutic.
   Cognitive Level: Application
   Nursing Process: Evaluation
   NCLEX-RN Test Plan: PSYC
   Reference: Chitty, K. K. (2005). *Professional nursing: Concepts & challenges* (4th ed.). St. Louis, MO: Elsevier Saunders.

6. **Answer: Professional boundaries**
   Rationale: The nurse is responsible for maintaining professional boundaries with clients. Actions overstepping these boundaries to meet the needs of the nurse are boundary violations. The nurse should avoid personal relationships with clients.
   Cognitive Level: Analysis
   Nursing Process: Evaluation
   NCLEX-RN Test Plan: PSYC
   Reference: Chitty, K. K. (2005). *Professional nursing: Concepts & challenges* (4th ed.). St. Louis, MO: Elsevier Saunders.

7. **Answer: 3**
   Rationale: No verbal message can be received if the receiver is not listening. The other responses are helpful techniques for responding to a client's communication.
   Cognitive Level: Application
   Nursing Process: Planning
   NCLEX-RN Test Plan: PSYC
   Reference: Chitty, K. K. (2005). *Professional nursing: Concepts & challenges* (4th ed.). St. Louis, MO: Elsevier Saunders.

8. **Answer: 2**
   Rationale: Efficiency requires the use of clear, simple, paced words suitable to the client's understanding.
   Cognitive Level: Analysis
   Nursing Process: Intervention
   NCLEX-RN Test Plan: PSYC
   Reference: Chitty, K. K. (2005). *Professional nursing: Concepts & challenges* (4th ed.). St. Louis, MO: Elsevier Saunders.

9. **Answer: 3**
   Rationale: The nurse has not clarified, and thus has no way of knowing, what the client's actual concerns are and who the client fears.
   Cognitive Level: Analysis
   Nursing Process: Intervention
   NCLEX-RN Test Plan: PSYC
   Reference: Chitty, K. K. (2005). *Professional nursing: Concepts & challenges* (4th ed.). St. Louis, MO: Elsevier Saunders.

10. **Answer: 4**
    Rationale: Response 4 is the only problem-solving response.
    Cognitive Level: Analysis
    Nursing Process: Intervention
    NCLEX-RN Test Plan: PSYC
    References: Stuart, G. W., & Laraia, M. T. (2005). *Principles and practices of psychiatric nursing* (8th ed.). St. Louis, MO: Elsevier Mosby.

    Mohr, W. K. (2003). *Psychiatric-mental health nursing* (5th ed.). Philadelphia: Lippincott Williams & Wilkins.

11. **Answer: 4**
    Rationale: The nurse's response reflects the emotion underlying the client's message.
    Cognitive Level: Analysis
    Nursing Process: Intervention
    NCLEX-RN Test Plan: PSYC
    Reference: Mohr, W. K. (2003). *Psychiatric-mental health nursing* (5th ed.). Philadelphia: Lippincott Williams & Wilkins.

12. **Answer: Countertransference**
    Rationale: Countertransference is the development of an emotional relationship with the patient by the nurse. When this occurs, the nurse may lose objectivity in the interaction with the patient.

   Cognitive Level: Analysis
   Nursing Process: Analysis
   NCLEX-RN Test Plan: PSYC
   Reference: Mohr, W. K. (2003). *Psychiatric-mental health nursing* (5th ed.). Philadelphia: Lippincott Williams & Wilkins.

13. **Answer: 3**
    Rationale: Encoding occurs when the receiver of the communication listens, processes, and develops an understanding of the information.
    Cognitive Level: Analysis
    Nursing Process: Analysis
    NCLEX-RN Test Plan: PSYC
    Reference: Catalano, J. T. (2006). *Nursing now! Today's issues, tomorrow's trends* (4th ed.). Philadelphia: F.A. Davis.

14. **Answers: 2, 3, and 4**
    Rationale: Without feedback, it is difficult to know if the client understood the directions. Some people do not read well and are reluctant to admit it. E-mail messages are often short and can be perceived as cold. Nurses need to remember that they are talking to a person, not a computer. Family members often share an e-mail account. Thus, privacy may be breached.
    Cognitive Level: Application
    Nursing Process: Implementation
    NCLEX-RN Test Plan: PSYC
    Reference: Riley, J. B. (2004). *Communication in nursing* (5th ed.). St. Louis, MO: Elsevier Mosby.

15. **Answer: 3**
    Rationale: In order to communicate effectively in groups, the nurse must have knowledge of group development and dynamics. This particular group is in the norming stage, which is characterized by defining rules and standards needed to getting the work done.
    Cognitive Level: Analyzing
    Nursing Process: Assessment
    NCLEX-RN Test Plan: PSYC
    Reference: Riley, J. B. (2004). *Communication in nursing* (5th ed.). St. Louis, MO: Elsevier Mosby.

16. **Answers: 1, 4, and 6**
    Rationale: An agenda, a recorder (secretary), and someone to keep the group moving (facilitator) are tools for effective group functioning.

Cognitive Level: Application
Nursing Process: Planning
NCLEX-RN Test Plan: PSYC
Reference: Riley, J. B. (2004). *Communication in nursing* (5th ed.). St. Louis, MO: Elsevier Mosby.

17. **Answers: 1, 2, 3, 4, and 5**
    Rationale: Responses 1, 2, 3, 4, and 5 are areas where cultural differences can be found.
    Cognitive Level: Application
    Nursing Process: Planning
    NCLEX-RN Test Plan: PSYC
    Reference: Riley, J. B. (2004). *Communication in nursing* (5th ed.). St. Louis, MO: Elsevier Mosby.

18. **Answer: 2**
    Rationale: Confrontation skills allow one to take calm, controlled, assertive action.
    Cognitive Level: Analysis
    Nursing Process: Intervention
    NCLEX-RN Test Plan: PSYC
    Reference: Riley, J. B. (2004). *Communication in nursing* (5th ed.). St. Louis, MO: Elsevier Mosby.

19. **Answer: 3**
    Rationale: Things "Not to Do" include beginning your refusal with a list of excuses (response 3).
    Cognitive Level: Analysis
    Nursing Process: Evaluation
    NCLEX-RN Test Plan: PSYC
    Reference: Riley, J. B. (2004). *Communication in nursing* (5th ed.). St. Louis, MO: Elsevier Mosby.

20. **Answer: 2**
    Rationale: Response 2 is appropriate and assertive and recognizes the colleague's feelings.
    Cognitive Level: Analysis
    Nursing Process: Implementation
    NCLEX-RN Test Plan: PSYC
    Reference: Riley, J. B. (2004). *Communication in nursing* (5th ed.). St. Louis, MO: Elsevier Mosby.

21. **Answer: Empathetic**
    Rationale: Empathy is a way of communicating to clients that we understand how they feel and why they feel that way.
    Cognitive Level: Application
    Nursing Process: Implementation
    NCLEX-RN Test Plan: PSYC

Reference: Riley, J. B. (2004). *Communication in nursing* (5th ed.). St. Louis, MO: Elsevier Mosby.

22. **Answer: 2**
    Rationale: Response 2 represents a positive and helpful perception of criticism.
    Cognitive Level: Analysis
    Nursing Process: Evaluation
    NCLEX-RN Test Plan: PSYC
    Reference: Riley, J. B. (2004). *Communication in nursing* (5th ed.). St. Louis, MO: Elsevier Mosby.

23. **Answer: 2**
    Rationale: Response 2 is the only communication related criteria.
    Cognitive Level: Application
    Nursing Process: Assessment
    NCLEX-RN Test Plan: PSYC
    Reference: Rankin, S. H., Stallings, K. D., & London, F. (2005). *Patient education in health and illness* (5th ed.). Philadelphia: Lippincott Williams & Wilkins.

24. **Answer: 4**
    Rationale: Response 4 provides a distorted message and masks criticism of the child.
    Cognitive Level: Analysis
    Nursing Process: Assessment
    NCLEX-RN Test Plan: PSYC
    Reference: Wright, L. M., & Leahey, M. (2005). *Nurses and families* (4th ed.). Philadelphia: F.A. Davis.

25. **Answer: 4**
    Rationale: Response 4 is the only example of negative self-talk.
    Cognitive Level: Analysis
    Nursing Process: Assessment
    NCLEX-RN Test Plan: PSYC
    Reference: Riley, J. B. (2004). *Communication in nursing* (5th ed.). St. Louis, MO: Elsevier Mosby.

26. **Answer: 2**
    Rationale: In a lose-win situation, the conflict is resolved at the expense of the client.
    Cognitive Level: Application
    Nursing Process: Assessment
    NCLEX-RN Test Plan: PSYC
    Reference: Riley, J. B. (2004). *Communication in nursing* (5th ed.). St. Louis, MO: Elsevier Mosby.

27. **Answer:** 1

    Rationale: The nonverbal communication of the physician communicates confidence and superiority.

    Cognitive Level: Analysis

    Nursing Process: Assessment

    NCLEX-RN Test Plan: PSYC

    Reference: Hood, L. J., & Leedy, S. K. (2006). *Conceptual basis of professional nursing* (6th ed.). Philadelphia: Lippincott Williams & Wilkins.

28. **Answer:** 4

    Rationale: The principle of presence involves being in the moment with the client and you would expect to see the behaviors listed in Response 4.

    Cognitive Level: Analysis

    Nursing Process: Intervention

    NCLEX-RN Test Plan: PSYC

    Reference: Hood, L. J., & Leedy, S. K. (2006). *Conceptual basis of professional nursing* (6th ed.). Philadelphia: Lippincott Williams & Wilkins.

29. **Answer:** 2

    Rationale: In the Identification Phase, the nurse and the client decide how best to meet the client's goals.

    Cognitive Level: Analysis

    Nursing Process: Planning

    NCLEX-RN Test Plan: PSYC

    Reference: Hood, L. J., & Leedy, S. K. (2006). *Conceptual basis of professional nursing* (6th ed.). Philadelphia: Lippincott Williams & Wilkins.

30. **Answer:** 4

    Rationale: A "yes" or "no" answer is all that is required of the client for the nurse to make the determination called for in Response 4.

    Cognitive Level: Application

    Nursing Process: Assessment

    NCLEX-RN Test Plan: PSYC

    Reference: Riley, J. B. (2004). *Communication in nursing* (5th ed.). St. Louis, MO: Elsevier Mosby.

31. **Answer:** 1

    Rationale: Asking the client to describe his feelings seeks more information and demonstrates that the nurse is attentive.

    Cognitive Level: Application

    Nursing Process: Implementation

    NCLEX-RN Test Plan: PSYC

    Reference: Hogan, M. A., Bowles, D., & White, J. E. (2003). *Nursing fundamentals: Reviews & rationales.* Upper Saddle River, NJ: Pearson Prentice Hall.

32. **Answer:** 2

    Rationale: The introductory phase is the time when the nurse and client identify goals and objectives.

    Cognitive Level: Knowledge

    Nursing Process: Planning

    NCLEX-RN Test Plan: HPM

    Reference: Hogan, M. A., Bowles, D., & White, J. E. (2003). *Nursing fundamentals: Reviews & rationales.* Upper Saddle River, NJ: Pearson Prentice Hall.

33. **Answer:** 2

    Rationale: Not urinating following a catheter removal requires nursing intervention, a thorough assessment for abdominal distension, monitoring intake and output, and possibly notifying the physician to obtain a straight catheterization order.

    Cognitive Level: Application

    Nursing Process: Planning

    NCLEX-RN Test Plan: SECE

    Reference: Hogan, M. A., Bowles, D., & White, J. E. (2003). *Nursing fundamentals: Reviews & rationales.* Upper Saddle River, NJ: Pearson Prentice Hall.

34. **Answer:** 1

    Rationale: Exploring the client's feelings is a way of expressing the importance of client feelings.

    Cognitive Level: Application

    Nursing Process: Planning

    NCLEX-RN Test Plan: PSYC

    Reference: Hogan, M. A., Bowles, D., & White, J. E. (2003). *Nursing fundamentals: Reviews & rationales.* Upper Saddle River, NJ: Pearson Prentice Hall.

35. **Answer:** 2

    Rationale: Speaking slowly in a low-pitched voice and facing the client promotes understanding for client with hearing impairment.

    Cognitive Level: Application

    Nursing Process: Analysis

    NCLEX-RN Test Plan: PSYC

Reference: Hogan, M. A., Bowles, D., & White, J. E. (2003). *Nursing fundamentals: Reviews & rationales.* Upper Saddle River, NJ: Pearson Prentice Hall.

36. **Answer: 4**

    Rationale: Asking what the client has done previously stimulates problem-solving for the client and allows the nurse to assess coping mechanisms.

    Cognitive Level: Application

    Nursing Process: Implementation

    NCLEX-RN Test Plan: PSYC

    Reference: Hogan, M. A., Bowles, D., & White, J. E. (2003). *Nursing fundamentals: Reviews & rationales.* Upper Saddle River, NJ: Pearson Prentice Hall.

37. **Answer: 1**

    Rationale: Clarification is a manner in which the client is asked to verify that the received message is accurate.

    Cognitive Level: Application

    Nursing Process: Assessment

    NCLEX-RN Test Plan: PSYC

    Reference: Christensen, B. L., & Kockrow, E. O. (2003). *Foundations of nursing.* St. Louis, MO: Elsevier Mosby.

38. **Answer: 1**

    Rationale: Physical appearance is a nonverbal cue that can influence the client's perceptions during an interaction. Other nonverbal cues are tone and rate of voice, volume of speech, eye contact, and use of touch.

    Cognitive Level: Application

    Nursing Process: Assessment

    NCLEX-RN Test Plan: PSYC

    Reference: Christensen, B. L., & Kockrow, E. O. (2003). *Foundations of nursing.* St. Louis, MO: Elsevier Mosby.

39. **Answer: 3**

    Rationale: Clients with expressive aphasia are able to communicate best when asked questions that require simple one or two word commands, such as yes/no or blinking the eyes.

    Cognitive Level: Application

    Nursing Process: Assessment

    NCLEX-RN Test Plan: PSYC

    Reference: Christensen, B. L., & Kockrow, E. O. (2003). *Foundations of nursing.* St. Louis, MO: Elsevier Mosby.

Unit 2 Answers and Rationales

Test 4 Answers and Rationales

1. **Answer: 4**
   Rationale: The respiratory rate needs to be assessed before giving the client a narcotic because a narcotic may cause severe respiratory depression that can be life threatening.
   Cognitive Level: Application
   Nursing Process: Assessment
   NCLEX-RN Test Plan: SECE
   Reference: Potter, P., & Perry, A. (2005). *Fundamentals of nursing* (6th ed.). St. Louis, MO: Elsevier Mosby.

2. **Answer: 3**
   Rationale: The nurse should validate the order with the prescriber to ensure that all the elements are correct. The order should include the right drug, dose, time, route and patient for correct medication administration.
   Cognitive Level: Application
   Nursing Process: Assessment
   NCLEX-RN Test Plan: SECE
   Reference: Potter, P., & Perry, A. (2005). *Fundamentals of nursing* (6th ed.). St. Louis, MO: Elsevier Mosby.

3. **Answer: 3**
   Rationale: The nurse administers only medicines that the nurse prepares.
   Cognitive Level: Application
   Nursing Process: Planning
   NCLEX-RN Test Plan: SECE
   Reference: Potter, P., & Perry, A. (2005). *Fundamentals of nursing* (6th ed.). St. Louis, MO: Elsevier Mosby.

4. **Answer: 1**
   Rationale: Conversions between grams and milligrams requires moving the decimal point three places to the right.
   Cognitive Level: Application
   Nursing Process: Assessment

NCLEX-RN Test Plan: SECE
Reference: Curren, A., & Munday, L. (1998). *Dimensional analysis for meds.* San Diego, CA: W I Publications.

5. **Answer: 1**
   Rationale: In infants and young children, the nurse straightens the cartilaginous canal by grasping the auricle of the ear and pulling it gently down and backward.
   Cognitive Level: Application
   Nursing Process: Implementation
   NCLEX-RN Test Plan: SECE
   Reference: Potter, P., & Perry, A. (2005). *Fundamentals of nursing* (6th ed.). St. Louis, MO: Elsevier Mosby.

6. **Answer: 2**
   Rationale: The nurse should acknowledge the error in practice and report it to the immediate supervisor. The nurse should also complete an incident report according to hospital policy.
   Cognitive Level: Application
   Nursing Process: Implementation
   NCLEX-RN Test Plan: SECE
   Reference: Potter, P., & Perry, A. (2005). *Fundamentals of nursing* (6th ed.). St. Louis, MO: Elsevier Mosby.

7. **Answer: 2**
   Rationale: Physically checking the actual supply of narcotic drugs and comparing the number to the written sign-out documents protects the nurse at the beginning of the tour of duty. Discrepancies can then be rectified before the previous nursing staff leave the hospital, all according to the controlled substance laws.
   Cognitive Level: Application
   Nursing Process: Implementation
   NCLEX-RN Test Plan: SECE
   Reference: Potter, P., & Perry, A. (2005). *Fundamentals of nursing* (6th ed.). St. Louis, MO: Elsevier Mosby.

8. **Answer: 2**

   Rationale: Safe medication administration depends on the nurse following the six rights for medication administration, specifically the right client.

   Cognitive Level: Application

   Nursing Process: Implementation

   NCLEX-RN Test Plan: SECE

   Reference: Potter, P., & Perry, A. (2005). *Fundamentals of nursing* (6th ed.). St. Louis, MO: Elsevier Mosby.

9. **Answers: 1, 2, 3, 4, 5, and 6**

   Rationale: All nurses must adhere to the process of medication administration because these basic skills protect each client from medication errors.

   Cognitive Level: Application

   Nursing Process: Implementation

   NCLEX-RN Test Plan: SECE

   Reference: DeLaune, S. C., & Ladner, P. K. (2006). *Fundamentals of nursing: Standards and practice* (3rd ed.). New York: Thomson Delmar Learning.

10. **Answer: 4**

    Rationale: Intramuscular injections require deep muscle penetration at a 90° angle at the insertion point.

    Cognitive Level: Application

    Nursing Process: Evaluation

    NCLEX-RN Test Plan: SECE

    Reference: Potter, P., & Perry, A. (2005). *Fundamentals of nursing* (6th ed.). St. Louis, MO: Elsevier Mosby.

11. **Answer: 4**

    Rationale: The nurse palpates the lower edge of the acromion process, which forms the base of a triangle in line with the midpoint of the lateral aspect of the upper arm. The injection site is the center of the triangle 3–5 cm below the acromion process.

    Cognitive Level: Application

    Nursing Process: Implementation

    NCLEX-RN Test Plan: SECE

    Reference: Potter, P., & Perry, A. (2005). *Fundamentals of nursing* (6th ed.). St. Louis, MO: Elsevier Mosby.

12. **Answer: 3**

    Rationale:

    Initially convert grams to milligrams:

    $$0.2 \text{ gm} = 200 \text{ mg}$$

    Utilize the formula:

    $$\frac{\text{Amount Desired}}{\text{Amount Available}} \times \text{Quantity}$$

    $$\frac{250 \text{ mg}}{200 \text{ mg}} \times 2 \text{ ml}$$

    $$\frac{250 \text{ mg}}{\underset{100}{\cancel{200}} \text{ mg}} \times \frac{\cancel{2}^{1}}{1}$$

    $$\frac{250 \text{ mg}}{100 \text{ mg}} = 2.5 \text{ ml}$$

    Cognitive Level: Application

    Nursing Process: Evaluation

    NCLEX-RN Test Plan: SECE

    Reference: Potter, P., & Perry, A. (2005). *Fundamentals of nursing* (6th ed.). St. Louis, MO: Elsevier Mosby.

13. **Answer: 3**

    Rationale:

    Utilize the formula:

    $$\frac{\text{Amount Desired}}{\text{Amount Available}} \times \text{Quantity}$$

    $$\frac{20 \text{ mEq}}{10 \text{ mEq}} \times 1 \text{ ml}$$

    $$\frac{20}{10} \times 1$$

    $$\frac{20}{10} = 2 \text{ ml}$$

    Cognitive Level: Application

    Nursing Process: Evaluation

    NCLEX-RN Test Plan: SECE

    Reference: Potter, P., & Perry, A. (2005). *Fundamentals of nursing* (6th ed.). St. Louis, MO: Elsevier Mosby.

14. **Answer: 4**
    Rationale:
    Utilize the formula:

    $$\frac{\text{Amount Desired}}{\text{Amount Available}} \times \text{Quantity}$$

    $$\frac{750,000 \text{ u}}{300,000 \text{ u}} \times 2 \text{ ml}$$

    $$\frac{750,000}{\underset{150,000}{300,000}} \times \frac{\overset{1}{2}}{1}$$

    $$\frac{750,000}{150,000} = 5.0 \text{ ml}$$

    Cognitive Level: Application
    Nursing Process: Evaluation
    NCLEX-RN Test Plan: SECE
    Reference: Potter, P., & Perry, A. (2005).
    Fundamentals of nursing (6th ed.). St. Louis,
    MO: Elsevier Mosby.

15. **Answer: 3**
    Rationale:
    Utilize the formula:

    $$\frac{\text{Amount Desired}}{\text{Amount Available}} \times \text{Quantity}$$

    $$\frac{250 \text{ mg}}{125 \text{ mg}} \times 1 \text{ tab}$$

    $$\frac{250}{125} \times 1$$

    $$\frac{250}{125} = 2 \text{ tablets}$$

    Cognitive Level: Application
    Nursing Process: Evaluation
    NCLEX-RN Test Plan: SECE
    Reference: Potter, P., & Perry, A. (2005).
    Fundamentals of nursing (6th ed.). St. Louis,
    MO: Elsevier Mosby.

16. **Answer: Capsule**

17. **Answer: Tablet**

18. **Answer: Elixir**
    Rationale for questions 16–18: The nurse needs to
    understand the components of manufactured medi-
    cines to teach the client about prescribed medicines,
    their effects, storage, and benefits.
    Cognitive Level: Application
    Nursing Process: Implementation
    NCLEX-RN Test Plan: SECE
    Reference: Kozier, B., Erb, G., Berman, A., &
    Snyder, S. (2004). *Techniques in clinical nursing*
    (5th ed.). Upper Saddle River, NJ: Pearson
    Prentice Hall.

19. **Answer: 4**
    Rationale: Each order for units of insulin is com-
    bined in the same syringe and added together for a
    total amount in the insulin syringe.
    Cognitive Level: Application
    Nursing Process: Evaluation
    NCLEX-RN Test Plan: SECE
    Reference: Potter, P., & Perry, A. (2005).
    Fundamentals of nursing (6th ed.). St. Louis,
    MO: Elsevier Mosby.

20. **Answer: 1**
    Rationale: Advise the client to always question the
    nurse if the medicine delivered to the client looks
    different (color, shape, size).
    Cognitive Level: Application
    Nursing Process: Implementation
    NCLEX-RN Test Plan: SECE
    Reference: Adams, M., Josephson, D., & Holland, L.
    (2004). *Pharmacology for nurses.* Upper Saddle
    River, NJ: Pearson Prentice Hall.

21. **Answer: 3**
    Rationale: The skill of medicine administration is
    not delegated to ancillary personnel.
    Cognitive Level: Application
    Nursing Process: Implementation
    NCLEX-RN Test Plan: SECE
    Reference: Altman, G. (2004). *Delmar's fundamental
    and advanced nursing skills* (2nd ed.). New York:
    Thompson Learning.

22. **Answer: 3**
    Rationale: Nitroglycerine paste (NTP) can have side effects of headache and a drop in blood pressure. The nurse needs to be careful not to have contact with the paste while applying this topical medication.
    Cognitive Level: Application
    Nursing Process: Implementation
    NCLEX-RN Test Plan: SECE
    Reference: Altman, G. (2004). *Delmar's fundamental and advanced nursing skills* (2nd ed.). New York: Thomson Learning.

23. **Answer: 3**
    Rationale: The vaginal area is not sterile. The applicator will contain bacteria and residual medication and should be washed in warm soapy water, rinsed and dried, and placed in a secure place in the client's room for future use.
    Cognitive Level: Application
    Nursing Process: Implementation
    NCLEX-RN Test Plan: SECE
    Reference: Potter, P., & Perry, A. (2005). *Fundamentals of nursing* (6th ed.). St. Louis, MO: Elsevier Mosby.

24. **Answer: 4**
    Rationale: Placing a protective pad around the ampule protects the nurse's fingers and face from shattered glass when breaking the ampoule, while not contaminating the medication with alcohol.
    Cognitive Level: Application
    Nursing Process: Implementation
    NCLEX-RN Test Plan: SECE
    Reference: Potter, P., & Perry, A. (2005). *Fundamentals of nursing* (6th ed.). St. Louis, MO: Elsevier Mosby.

25. **Answer: 4**
    Rationale: For multidose vials, the nurse who opens the vial will write her initials, the date, and time on the vial itself to ensure that future doses will be prepared correctly and the vial will be discarded beyond a certain numbers of days. Rubber seals must be swabbed with alcohol and allowed to dry before inserting the needle to prevent microorganisms from entering the vial. Air must be injected in an equal amount to the medicine withdrawn to prevent a buildup of negative pressure when aspirating the medication.
    Cognitive Level: Application
    Nursing Process: Implementation
    NCLEX-RN Test Plan: SECE
    Reference: Potter, P., & Perry, A. (2005). *Fundamentals of nursing* (6th ed.). St. Louis, MO: Elsevier Mosby.

26. **Answer: 4**
    Rationale: Short-acting insulin has an onset of 30 minutes. Insulin should be given at a specific time before meals, usually one half hour. The nurse should always check the blood glucose levels prior to administering short-acting insulin.
    Cognitive Level: Application
    Nursing Process: Implementation
    NCLEX-RN Test Plan: SECE
    Reference: DeLaune, S. C., & Ladner, P. K. (2006). *Fundamentals of nursing: Standards and practice* (3rd ed.). New York: Thomson Delmar Learning.

27. **Answer: 1**
    Rationale: The SIM's position exposes the anus and helps the client relax the external anal sphincter muscle for easier insertion of the suppository.
    Cognitive Level: Application
    Nursing Process: Implementation
    NCLEX-RN Test Plan: SECE
    Reference: Potter, P., & Perry, A. (2005). *Fundamentals of nursing* (6th ed.). St. Louis, MO: Elsevier Mosby.

28. **Answer: 4**
    Rationale: Common abbreviations found in medication orders use Latin abbreviations. The abbreviation gtt means guttal, from the Latin word *gutta*, which means "drop." The abbreviation O.U. refers to the Latin phrase *oculi unitas*, meaning "both eyes." The abbreviation t.i.d. refers to the Latin phrase *ter in die*, which means "three times per day."
    Cognitive Level: Application
    Nursing Process: Implementation
    NCLEX-RN Test Plan: SECE
    Reference: DeLaune, S. C., & Ladner, P. K. (2006). *Fundamentals of nursing: Standards and practice* (3rd ed.). Clifton Park, NY: Thomson Delmar Learning.

29. **Answer: 3**
    Rationale: Medications are dispensed by the pharmacy to the nursing units according to physician's orders. Drugs should not be borrowed from one client's supply to administer to another client.

Cognitive Level: Application
Nursing Process: Implementation
NCLEX-RN Test Plan: Implementation
Reference: DeLaune, S. C. & Ladner, P. K. (2006). *Fundamentals of nursing: Standards and practice* (3rd ed.). Clifton Park, NY: Thomson Delmar Learning.

30. **Answer: Topical**

31. **Answer: Oral**

32. **Answer: Rectal**

33. **Answer: Subcutaneous**
    Rationale for questions 30–33: The nurse needs to know the correct route for drug administration for the most effective mode of absorption.
    Cognitive Level: Application
    Nursing Process: Implementation
    NCLEX-RN Test Plan: SECE
    Reference: Mills, E. (2004). *Nursing procedures* (4th ed.). Philadelphia: Lippincott Williams and Wilkins.

34. **Answer: 3**
    Rationale: The nurse does not aspirate on the plunger when giving heparin subcutaneously; doing so may cause tissue damage.
    Cognitive Level: Application
    Nursing Process: Implementation
    NCLEX-RN Test Plan: SECE
    Reference: DeLaune, S. C., & Ladner, P. K. (2006). *Fundamentals of nursing: Standards and practice* (3rd ed.). Clifton Park, NY: Thomson Delmar Learning.

35. **Answer: 3**
    Rationale: Some medications require monitoring of blood levels to determine effectiveness. If levels are higher or lower than the therapeutic range, adjustments must be made by the prescribing practitioner.
    Cognitive Level: Analysis
    Nursing Process: Implementation
    NCLEX-RN Test Plan: SECE
    Reference: DeLaune, S. C., & Ladner, P. K. (2006). *Fundamentals of nursing: Standards and practice* (3rd ed.). Clifton Park, NY: Thomson Delmar Learning.

36. **Answer: 4**
    Rationale: Laws require all medication to have an expiration date. Outdated medication should be returned to pharmacy for proper disposal.
    Cognitive Level: Application
    Nursing Process: Implementation
    NCLEX-RN Test Plan: SECE
    Reference: DeLaune, S. C., & Ladner, P. K. (2006). *Fundamentals of nursing: Standards and practice* (3rd ed.). Clifton Park, NY: Thomson Delmar Learning.

37. **Answer: 4**
    Rationale: The client has the right to refuse medications; however, if the client understands the action of the medication, they may be willing to take it.
    Cognitive Level: Analysis
    Nursing Process: Implementation
    NCLEX-RN Test Plan: SECE
    Reference: DeLaune, S. C., & Ladner, P. K. (2006). *Fundamentals of nursing: Standards and practice* (3rd ed.). Clifton Park, NY: Thomson Delmar Learning.

38. **Answer: 4**
    Rationale: Soothing cough medications coat the throat for the most beneficial effect. Fluids taken after the dose of cough medications dilute the effect of the cough syrup.
    Cognitive Level: Application
    Nursing Process: Implementation
    NCLEX-RN Test Plan: SECE
    Reference: Mills, E. (2004). *Nursing procedures* (4th ed.). Philadelphia: Lippincott Williams and Wilkins, p. 229.

39. **Answer: 3**
    Rationale: The disposal of any narcotic drug must be cosigned by another nurse as mandated by law.
    Cognitive Level: Application
    Nursing Process: Implementation
    NCLEX-RN Test Plan: SECE
    Reference: Mills, E. (2004). *Nursing procedures* (4th ed.). Philadelphia: Lippincott Williams and Wilkins, p. 229.

Unit 3 • Managing Client Care

Delegation and Prioritization

1. **The process of assignment making does not include which of the following?**
   1. Delegation of duties and all aspects of care for a client to individual personnel.
   2. Clear concise direction.
   3. Delegation of responsibility and authority for the performance of care.
   4. Intimidation.

2. **When determining whether unlicensed assistive personnel (UAP) understand how to do a procedure safely and correctly, which rights of delegation must the nurse assess? Select all that apply.**
   1. The task.
   2. The circumstance.
   3. The person.
   4. The environment.

3. **The nurse has 10 clients on her module. The clients have multiple required treatments. She delegates ostomy/wound care to the unlicensed assistive personnel (UAP). Which of the following describes this example?**
   1. Overdelegation.
   2. Indirect delegation.
   3. Underdelegation.
   4. Supervisory rights.

4. **Which of the following tasks, as defined in your state practice acts, cannot be delegated to the LPN/LVN?**
   1. Tracheotomy care.
   2. Ostomy care.
   3. Testing a stool specimen for guaiac blood.
   4. Shift head to toe physical assessment.

5. **A storm has resulted in the nurse being the only RN on a medical-surgical unit with one UAP. When considering the resources available to her, she might elect to focus on which of the following?**
   1. Interventions that prevent life-threatening emergencies.
   2. Reinforcement of patient teaching plans.
   3. Review of home environments for patients scheduled to be discharged in the morning.
   4. Stocking of the unit supplies.

6. **The nurse is assigned to a group of clients on the evening shift, and a UAP is working with the nurse. Which of the following interventions can be assigned to the UAP?**
   1. Administration of an antibiotic cream to the client's arm after the UAP gives the client a bath.
   2. Completion of a health history and admission assessment on a client that is not in acute distress.
   3. Obtain vital signs on a client who is four hours postoperative.
   4. Monitor and adjust the client's IV drip rate after the nurse instructs the UAP to perform this task properly.

7. The nurse is working with unlicensed assistive personnel (UAP) today. She has experienced conflict with a particular UAP during previous encounters. She is responsible for the care of 20 clients today. She assigns the UAP to stock supplies and transport clients for the shift. She plans on assigning herself vital signs, baths, treatments, and medication passes on the 20 clients on her module. Which of the following priority traps is this nurse using?

   1. Doing whatever hits first.
   2. Taking the path of least resistance.
   3. Completing tasks by default.
   4. Relying on misguided inspiration.

8. The nurse has determined that a client has a dressing that needs to be changed before it saturates the client's clothing and bed. She delegates this task to the LPN/LVN. Several hours later, the client's family requests that the client's dressing and soiled bed are changed. What should the nurse do at this time?

   1. Change the dressing herself.
   2. Disregard the family's request.
   3. Find the LPN/LVN and explore the family's complaint to determine what happened.
   4. Check to see if the LPN/LVN completed care on her other assigned patients.

9. The nurse takes into consideration which of the following elements when delegating a task to the LPN/LVN?

   1. The state nurse practice act.
   2. The LPN/LVN competency level and number of years in nursing.
   3. The willingness of the LPN/LVN to perform the task.
   4. The temperament and mood of the LPN/LVN.

10. The new graduate nurse asks the experienced nurse why she must delegate nursing tasks. Which of the following is the primary reason for delegating tasks?

   1. To provide appropriate resources for the client.
   2. To simplify the nurse's work day.
   3. To provide for the immediate needs of the clients.
   4. To decrease health care costs.

11. The nurse has just completed her shift report. Which client will she assign to the unlicensed personnel (UAP)?

   1. A stable three-hour postoperative thyroidectomy client.
   2. A stable one-day postoperative abdominal hysterectomy client.
   3. A stable three-day postoperative gastric bypass client.
   4. A stable two-hour postoperative cholestectomy client.

12. A new graduate nurse delegates the following activities to the unlicensed assistive personnel (UAP). Which activity should she perform herself?

   1. Administration of a fleet enema.
   2. Repositioning of a stable client.
   3. Intravenous pain medication administration.
   4. Bathing of a stable client.

13. The nurse is beginning her 7–3 PM shift. Which client activity will take priority when delegating to the UAP?

   1. A diabetic client who is ordered a morning dose of Humulin insulin to cover his blood sugar before breakfast.
   2. A client requesting a fresh cup of coffee.
   3. Distributing water to the clients under her care.
   4. Collecting and delivering a clean voided urine specimen to the lab.

14. **The unlicensed assistive personnel (UAP) reports that the newly admitted abdominal hysterectomy client's dressing is saturated with blood. What task could be delegated to the UAP at this time?**
    1. An abdominal dressing change.
    2. Vital signs.
    3. Assessment of bladder distention in this client.
    4. Assessment of the incisional site.

15. **What is the most important goal for a client experiencing anorexia nervosa?**
    1. The client will reach a weight of 90% average for height and weight.
    2. The client shows an accurate perception of body image.
    3. The client feels in control of behavior.
    4. The client's sense of autonomy with the family unit improves.

16. **The severest stage of depression for a hospitalized client has been alleviated. What nursing diagnosis takes priority at this time?**
    1. Hopelessness.
    2. Risk for self-directed violence.
    3. Self-esteem disturbance.
    4. Social isolation.

17. **You are a team leader for 10 clients and have an inexperienced licensed practical nurse (LPN) and an experienced unlicensed assistive personnel (UAP) on your team. Several times you have found the LPN chatting sociably at the front desk. You follow up on tasks delegated to the LPN and find them not completed. The LPN has left the unit for a break without telling you or the aide. What assessment of the LPN's behavior is most warranted at this time?**
    1. The LPN has inherent resistance to authority and needs counseling.
    2. The LPN believes herself incapable of completing the delegated tasks and needs education.
    3. The delegated tasks are inappropriate and need to be reassigned.
    4. The LPN may be overwhelmed and further assessment is needed.

18. **The registered nurse is planning a large project involving a community diabetic foot-care education and management program. The registered nurse breaks the project down into short-term, intermediate, and long-term goals. What is an example of a short-term goal?**
    1. Contact area physicians to see if there is interest and if there are any subject recruitment possibilities.
    2. Develop a general program plan including time-frame and content to be covered.
    3. Reserve a facility for the event.
    4. Secure identified handouts and teaching materials.

19. **When prioritizing care by developing a "do later" list of items, the registered nurse puts off most items that involve interacting with others over the telephone. The registered nurse recognizes this behavior as**

    _____.

20. **Which of the following managerial policies will lead to effective and safe delegation?**
    1. The manager expects the delegate to perform the task with outstanding skill.
    2. The manager continuously oversees the delegated work to ensure compliance.
    3. The manager directly observes a performance of the delegated task.
    4. The manager reassumes the task when the delegate is having difficulty.

21. The new graduate nurse is trying to be fair in making staff assignments. There are several patients that need IV medications and high-level assessment skills. The nurse takes the total assignment for all these patients and leaves total responsibility for the remaining client to the other personnel. What error of delegation has the nurse made?

1. Adopting old patterns.
2. Failure to release control.
3. Overloading himself.
4. Unclear communication.

22. When teaching (for the purpose of delegation) the unlicensed assistive personnel (UAP) to set limits on manipulative behavior, which response by the UAP indicates more teaching is needed?

1. "Consistency among all staff is important."
2. "I will set limits each time I see a dysfunctional behavior."
3. "I understand that limit-setting counteracts resistance."
4. "A goal is for the client to ask directly for what is wanted."

23. When delegating to a licensed practical nurse (LPN), the registered nurse (RN) is best guided by which of the following?

1. Agency policies for the LPN.
2. The documented experience level of the LPN.
3. The documented skill level of the LPN.
4. State LPN scope of practice guidelines.

24. What nursing diagnosis takes priority in a client with borderline personality disorder (BPD)?

1. Chronic low self esteem.
2. Impaired social interaction.
3. Risk for impulsive aggressive behavior.
4. Risk for suicide.

25. What activities below would be appropriate for a registered nurse to assign to the unlicensed assistive personnel (UAP)? Select all that apply.

1. Accompanying a depressed client to occupational therapy.
2. Assessing a hypomanic client for exhaustion.
3. Checking a client in soft wrist restraints.
4. Setting limits with a manic client.
5. Monitoring a newly admitted alcoholic whose last drink was two days ago.
6. Monitoring a client who has been on a tricyclic antidepressant (TCA) for two weeks.
7. Recording intake and output on a manic client.

26. What assessment would indicate to the registered nurse that an activity should not be delegated to the unlicensed assistive personnel (UAP)?

1. Family members are with the client most of the day.
2. The client's condition is unstable.
3. There is some potential for harm to the client.
4. The UAP is in close contact with the nurse.

27. Which statement by the unlicensed assistive personnel (UAP) indicates that the UAP needs help setting priorities?

1. "I have my assignment and will start with room 1, then work my way to room 10."
2. "I will give Mr. J his meal tray first as he is going early to physical therapy."
3. "After breakfast, I will help pack belongings of the clients to be discharged this morning."
4. "I will start with partial baths before breakfast."

28. **When making an assignment, the registered nurse recognizes that the unlicensed assistive personnel (UAP) has which of the following responsibilities?**
    1. Accountability for providing nursing care.
    2. A legal scope of practice.
    3. Responsibility for comprehensive care of assigned clients.
    4. No accountability for nursing care.

29. **When the registered nurse delegates tasks, the nurse is freed of the time it would take to carry out delegated responsibilities. However, for the tasks, the nurse remains**

    _____.

30. **The nurse needs to ensure that the licensed practical nurse (LPN) is legally allowed to perform a task. The nurse assesses the LPN's**

    _____.

31. **The registered nurse checks with individuals throughout the day to see if they are completing tasks. What right of delegation is the nurse demonstrating?**
    1. Right circumstances.
    2. Right communication.
    3. Right person.
    4. Right supervision.

32. **What item takes priority in client care?**
    1. Bathing.
    2. Contacting referrals.
    3. Pain management.
    4. Teaching.

33. **Which of the following interventions does the registered nurse feel takes priority for a heroin-addicted client who is pregnant?**
    1. Education to maintain status quo until delivery.
    2. Provide immediate total drug freedom.
    3. Provide methadone maintenance.
    4. Provide appropriate detoxification.

34. **The RN is preparing the assignment for the day shift. Which patient is appropriate for the RN to assign the LPN?**
    1. Mrs. Smith, age 44, chronic renal failure, admitted for peritoneal dialysis this afternoon.
    2. Mrs. Anderson, age 37, newly admitted for angina, cardiac enzymes pending.
    3. Mrs. Johnson, age 66, pleural effusion, bilateral chest tubes to Pleurovac.
    4. Miss Andrews, age 48, total right hip replacement, two days postoperative.

35. **The PACU calls the RN to admit a 13-year-old female with an appendectomy on the general pediatric unit. Which roommate would be most appropriate?**
    1. Room 203A, 14-year-old male with sickle cell crisis.
    2. Room 204B, 13-year-old female with tonsillitis.
    3. Room 206A, 15-year-old male with head injury.
    4. Room 208B, 12-year-old female with diabetes mellitus.

36. **An RN from the labor and delivery unit is pulled to work on a medical-surgical unit. Which patient is appropriate for the charge nurse to assign the pulled RN to care for?**
    1. Mrs. Simon, a 66-year-old with terminal end renal disease.
    2. Ms. Beck, a 45-year-old with acute pancreatitis.
    3. Mrs. Newton, a 37-year-old with a total abdominal hysterectomy, one day postoperative.
    4. Mr. Quinn, a 72-year-old with a cerebral vascular accident, newly admitted.

37. **The RN listens to the report from the previous shift. Which patient should the nurse see first?**
    1. Room 7201, a 6-year-old with diabetes, blood sugar ordered this morning.
    2. Room 7202, a 2-month-old with pertussis, O_2 at 3 L/min mask.
    3. Room 7203, a 4-month-old with gastro-enteritis, three stools during the past shift.
    4. Room 7204, a 6-month-old with dehydration, IV decreased to 42 cc/hr last shift.

38. **The UAP refuses to take a specimen to the lab. What should the RN do?**
    1. Take the specimen to the lab.
    2. Report the UAP to the charge nurse.
    3. Complete an incident report and submit it to the supervisor.
    4. Discuss the incident with the UAP.

39. **The UAP reports to work the afternoon shift. Identify what is NOT appropriate to assign the UAP.**
    1. Vital signs for patients on this unit.
    2. Application of antiembolic stockings.
    3. Administer acetaminophen for a client with a headache.
    4. Tally I&O for the end of shift.

Disasters Nursing/Bioterrorism

1. **Place the following phases of the disaster cycle in appropriate order.**
   1. Nondisaster or interdisaster phase.
   2. Impact phase.
   3. Reconstruction or rehabilitation phase.
   4. Predisaster or warning phase.
   5. Emergency phase.

2. **There has been a major school bus accident in the community with many injured children seen on the ground. A 10-year-old boy is found lying in the road. His respiratory rate is 10 breaths per minute. He has good distal pulses and groans to painful stimuli. After this quick assessment, what would be your first intervention?**
   1. Try to find his parents' home phone number in his book bag.
   2. Place a red tag on his upper body and yell for help.
   3. Place a yellow tag on him since he's breathing and has no apparent wounds.
   4. Continue to assess his neurological status using the Glasgow Coma Scale.

3. **A multiple car accident has occurred on the local expressway. Among the many casualties is an adult male, found trapped under the car. Upon examination, you find that he is apneic, but has a weak pulse at 120 beats per minute. After repositioning his upper airway, he remains apneic. As a nurse in the field, how do you proceed?**
   1. Start CPR and continue until EMS arrives.
   2. Place a red tag on the man's upper body and yell for help.
   3. Place a black tag on the man's upper body and attempt to help the next accident victim.
   4. Reposition his upper airway again before assessing his respirations.

4. **Who is used as a triage officer during the time of a disaster?**
   1. Members of the Federal Emergency Management Agency (FEMA).
   2. The emergency room physician who directs all care.
   3. Representatives from the American Red Cross.
   4. Nurses and other emergency personnel.

5. **According to the Joint Commission on Accreditation of Healthcare Organizations, all hospitals must perform which of the following tasks?**
   1. Develop a disaster plan and send it to all nurse managers in the building.
   2. Develop a disaster plan and hold a disaster drill twice each year.
   3. Select a disaster representative from the emergency room department who is responsible for all internal disaster activities.
   4. Develop a disaster plan, hold disaster drills twice a year, and regularly evaluate these plans and activities.

6. **A tornado has ripped through a community leaving demolished homes and extensive damage. As a nurse arriving at the site, you find many people who need medical attention, among them, a man walking aimlessly around mumbling to himself. Another neighbor tells you that he is a diabetic. What would be included in your assessment and action?**

    1. Assess his level of consciousness. If he obeys commands, place a yellow tag on his upper body.
    2. Diabetics are treated differently. Place a red tag on his upper body and yell for help.
    3. Attempt to find diabetic supplies and test his blood sugar immediately.
    4. Ask him what he has lost.

7. **An adult arrives at the emergency department after being injured in a work-related explosion. His leg is wrapped in a blanket. As you unwrap the blanket, you note that the skin is torn with torn tissue underneath. You note that this is what type of wound?**

    1. An abrasion.
    2. An avulsion.
    3. A laceration.
    4. A puncture.

8. **Identify an appropriate nursing diagnosis for a patient who is physically uninjured but who is stressed after being involved in a flood disaster.**

    _____

9. **A nurse is the triage officer in the emergency department when four patients arrive at the same time by ambulance after a factory explosion. Which patient does she prioritize as needing immediate care?**

    1. An adult complaining of shortness of breath; respiratory rate is < 30/min; capillary refill is < 2 seconds. The patient is conscious.
    2. An unconscious adult with a sucking chest wound; respirations are > 30/min; capillary refill is < 2 seconds.
    3. A conscious adult with a dislocated right shoulder; respirations are < 30/min; capillary refill is < 2 seconds.
    4. An unconscious adult with no respirations; capillary refill is > 2 seconds. Paramedics have already tried to reposition airway without results.

10. **The nurse is working with community members in order to aid them in preparation for any disaster. She helps them compile a list of emergency supplies needed in case of a disaster. Which of the following would be included in the list? Select all that apply.**

    1. A three day supply of water and food that will not spoil.
    2. One change of clothing and protective footwear.
    3. Passport and birth certificate.
    4. Candles and matches.
    5. Sanitation supplies, including toilet paper, soap, feminine hygiene products, and plastic garbage bags.

11. **According to the American Red Cross, a major disaster is classified as which of the following?**
    1. A disaster that affects more than one family, occurs within the jurisdiction of one American Red Cross chapter, and requires limited human and material resources.
    2. A disaster that affects multiple families in a single state and may require disaster help from more than one Red Cross chapter.
    3. A disaster that requires the help of multiple Red Cross units, affects more than a single state, and may be expected to be declared an emergency by the President of the United States.
    4. A disaster that requires full or partial implementation of the Federal Response Plan. This disaster exceeds the ability of the state and local government capabilities to meet the needs of the situation.

12. **A bomb has exploded in the bus station. You are a nurse assisting in this disaster triage. After an initial assessment, you have to prioritize the needs of the patients. Which patient needs to be sent to the emergency department on the next emergency vehicle?**
    1. An unconscious adult who has a large head wound with gray matter exposed; absent respirations; capillary refill > 2 seconds.
    2. A conscious adult with second degree burns on both lower legs; respiratory rate is > 30/min; capillary refill is < 2 seconds.
    3. An unconscious 6-month-old infant with no respirations; no visible injuries; no pulse.
    4. A conscious adult wearing a medic-alert diabetic bracelet; respirations are < 30/min; capillary refill is < 2 seconds, but patient is complaining of feeling clammy and shaky.

13. **After a recent flooding disaster where homes were destroyed and families were displaced, the teacher in the elementary school is expected to observe which of the following behaviors? Select all that apply.**
    1. Students want to return to school to maintain their previous schedule.
    2. Students exhibit regressive behaviors such as bed wetting, thumb sucking, crying, and clinging to parents.
    3. Students have fantasies that the disaster never happened.
    4. Students have an inability to concentrate and refuse to go back to school.

14. **One of the initial assessments required for victims of disaster, especially a mass trauma, is a complete head to toe examination of the person affected. What physical assessment techniques should the nurse be taught in order to perform this skill?**
    1. Look, feel, listen, and smell.
    2. Assessment and percussion.
    3. Auscultation of abnormal heart sounds.
    4. Assessment and palpation of the abdomen.

15. **Which of the following is a hospital-based system that is used as a framework for reporting and communicating during a disaster? The plan also assigns specific roles to individuals to create a chain of command during a stressful time.**
    1. Red Cross disaster plan.
    2. New York City disaster plan.
    3. Hospital Emergency Incident Command System (HEICS).
    4. Bureau for Health and Human Services Disaster Plan.

16. An adult is found in a building four days after an explosion occurred. It is winter and the temperature in the building is 10°F. The patient presents with pain, loss of sensation, edema, and red, blistered areas on both legs. The skin on both legs is hard and cold to the touch. Additionally, he states that both legs are "stinging and burning." The nurse suspects that this patient is experiencing frostbite of both legs. What nursing interventions are appropriate?

1. Immerse the legs in cold water, gently circulating the water around the extremity.
2. After thawing, gently wrap the extremity and elevate it to prevent further edema.
3. Rub the area vigorously to promote the warming process.
4. Debride the blisters and then call the physician.

17. The nurse in the emergency department has just been notified that there has been a gang riot in the community with four injured victims arriving within ten minutes. In preparing the trauma rooms for their imminent arrival, this nurse anticipates which of the following?

1. If low velocity missiles were used as the weapons, such as knives, the tissue damage may be only along the path of the weapon because of the low energy force of the weapon. It is not life threatening.
2. If high velocity missiles were used as the weapons, such as guns, rifles, or paint guns, there could be tissue damage but the nurse is not concerned about toxins of chemicals injected.
3. It is not necessary to know the caliber of the gun since all gunshot wounds are similar.
4. The assessment of possible injuries must take into consideration the possibility of more extensive internal injuries.

18. Victim of a suspected terror event involving inhalation anthrax, a client is brought to the emergency room. The nurse will observe for major symptoms associated with a possible exposure including which of the following?

1. Respiratory distress would be expected almost immediately upon exposure.
2. Fever, malaise, headache, and a cough present within hours of inhalation exposure.
3. Skin lesions progressing from pruritic papules to necrotic ulcers begin appearing within one hour of exposure.
4. Severe dyspnea, hypoxia, and septic shock follow a prodromal period of malaise, headache, fever, and chills.

19. Police inform the emergency room that a bioterrorism event is suspected and to prepare for casualties. The emergency room nurse first notifies which outside agency?

1. The local health department.
2. The CDC (Centers for Disease Control and Prevention).
3. FEMA (Federal Emergency Management Agency).
4. Local safety forces.

20. In evaluating the effects of an acute radiation exposure, the nurse would monitor the results of which laboratory blood test?

1. Potassium.
2. Blood cell count.
3. Creatinine.
4. Ammonia.

21. **Four days following an acute radiation exposure, which of the following complaints would indicate to the nurse that the client is experiencing a complication of the radiation exposure?**
    1. Fever and chills.
    2. Leg restlessness.
    3. An inability to sleep through the night.
    4. Itchy, dry skin.

22. **A client exposed to the nerve agent sarin has atropine prescribed. The nurse knows that the main purpose for administering this medication is which of the following?**
    1. To loosen respiratory secretions.
    2. To slow the gastrointestinal tract.
    3. To improve cerebral blood flow.
    4. To act as an antidote.

23. **Upon admission, the nurse should give highest priority to meeting which need of a client who has inhalation anthrax?**
    1. Respiratory support.
    2. Infection control.
    3. Fluid balance.
    4. Neurological desensitization.

24. **In disaster preparedness planning for a bioterrorism event that may involve anthrax, the nurse should know which of the following?**
    1. Anthrax vaccine is recommended for all hospital staff who deliver care to clients.
    2. Anthrax is typically contracted through ingestion of raw meat.
    3. Children are less likely to be affected by the exposure.
    4. Anthrax is not spread person to person.

25. **In disaster preparedness planning for a bioterrorism event that may involve smallpox, the nurse should know which of the following?**
    1. Health care providers will need to become familiar with the clinical presentation of smallpox and how it differs from chickenpox.
    2. Smallpox is not a communicable disease risk.
    3. The majority of the American population under 50 years of age is vaccinated for the disease.
    4. Fatality rates for smallpox would be expected to be less than one percent of those infected.

26. **In disaster preparedness planning for a bioterrorism event that may involve chemical agents, the nurse should know which of the following?**
    1. Health care workers will need training regarding antidotes.
    2. Communicability of the agents will be a big concern.
    3. Decontamination procedures are only needed for radiological and nuclear terrorism.
    4. Anthrax is one of the most likely chemical agents to be used as a weapon.

27. **As part of a nurse's responsibility in preplanning for a response to a bioterrorism disaster, which of the following is necessary for her to know?**
    1. Know in advance community medical and social services that will be available.
    2. Evaluate the impact of a disaster on the community.
    3. Assess survivors of a disaster for levels of psychological stress.
    4. Link victims with support agencies to help with food, clothing, shelter, and counseling needs.

28. Victim of a disaster, a client is prescribed ciprofloxacin. The nurse knows this medication is part of the treatment regime for a bioterrorism disaster involving which of the following?
    1. Smallpox.
    2. Sarin gas.
    3. Ebola virus.
    4. Anthrax.

29. The nurse understands that disaster management of a bioterrorism event will involve mitigation. Which of the following are included in mitigation activities for a health care delivery system?
    1. Having infection control policies and procedures in place.
    2. Identifying a spokesperson for media communication.
    3. Triage for casualties.
    4. Having a personal disaster plan.

30. A client consults the nurse in the immunization clinic for overseas travelers regarding their need for anthrax vaccine because they will be traveling with an international aid organization to Eastern Europe. The nurse's response is based on the following:
    1. No vaccine exists for anthrax.
    2. Anthrax is not endemic to Eastern Europe.
    3. Anthrax vaccine is under Defense Department control, and is primarily for military use.
    4. Anthrax vaccine is highly recommended by the Centers for Disease Control and Prevention (CDC) for travelers to Eastern Europe.

31. With the potential use of smallpox as a bioterrorism threat, a nurse must prepare to respond to a disaster event with this agent. The nurse's preparation is based on which of the following facts about smallpox? Select all that apply.

    1. Smallpox is transmitted person to person through direct contact or droplet inhalation.
    2. Infection is characterized by severe respiratory distress, septicemia, and hemorrhagic meningitis.
    3. A vaccination for smallpox is available.
    4. Naturally occurring smallpox has been eradicated from the world.
    5. Smallpox is a bacterium that produces spores that can remain viable in the environment for long periods of time.
    6. There is no proven treatment.

32. With the potential use of ricin as a terrorism threat, a nurse must prepare to respond to a disaster event with this agent. The nurse's preparation is based on which of the following facts about ricin? Select all that apply.
    1. Ricin is a spore producing bacterium.
    2. Ricin causes injury by inhibiting protein synthesis.
    3. Ricin can be inhaled or ingested.
    4. Ricin treatment is supportive; there is no antidote.
    5. Ricin is a toxin found in castor beans.
    6. A vaccination is available, though it is not routine.

33. Upon arrival at the hospital, the nurse should give highest priority to meeting which need of a client who has inhalation sulfur mustard (mustard gas)?
    1. Neurological desensitization.
    2. Infection control.
    3. Fluid balance.
    4. Decontamination.

34. A child weighing 25 kg and who has been exposed to anthrax is ordered to receive "doxycycline 2.2 mg per kg Q 12 hours IV." Calculate the correct dose for the nurse to administer.

35. A nurse understands weapons of terror are of different classifications requiring specific medical responses. Match the following potential weapons of terrorism with their correct category.

A. Bacteria and viruses   1. Mustard gas
                                     2. Botulinum
B. Biotoxins   3. A dirty bomb
                                     4. Pneumonic plague
C. Chemical weapons   5. Anthrax
                                     6. Smallpox
D. Radiologic weapons   7. Ricin
                                     8. Tularemia

36. In disaster preparedness planning for a bioterrorism event that may involve tularemia, the nurse should know which of the following?

1. Vaccination would be recommended for all hospital staff that deliver care to clients.
2. Tularemia is transmitted person to person.
3. Tularemia responds well to antibiotics.
4. Exposure would require decontamination procedures.

37. As part of disaster preparedness planning for a bioterrorism event, the emergency room nurse is checking on the supply of personal protective equipment for the health care staff. Knowing that there are several levels of protection, the availability of full face shields, water repellent gowns, and rubber boots would be considered which of the following?

1. The minimum protection needed.
2. The preferred protection to have available.
3. Components of specialized protection equipment.
4. Unnecessary for most responses to a bioterrorism event.

38. A school nurse preparing supplies and equipment as part of the school's disaster plan assembles a "To Go" bag. Essential elements in this bag include all of the following EXCEPT:

1. A list of students and staff.
2. A blueprint of school property.
3. A portable automatic external defibrillator (AED).
4. Walkie-talkies.

39. Following a bioterrorism event with a chemical agent, the nurse chooses to secure an inpatient unit of 24 infants before securing the inpatient psychiatric unit of 32 adults, knowing that infants are at increased risk to chemical agents that are absorbed through the skin. Why are the infants more susceptible to these agents?

1. Infants have a slower metabolic rate.
2. Infants have a larger body surface area relative to weight.
3. Infants have an immature nervous system.
4. Infants are obligatory nose breathers.

Unit 3 Answers and Rationales

Test 5 Answers and Rationales

1. **Answer: 4**
   Rationale: Intimidation has no place in delegation. Delegation means transferring to a competent individual the authority to perform a selected nursing task in a specific selected situation.
   Cognitive Level: Analysis
   Nursing Process: Planning
   NCLEX-RN Test Plan: SECE
   Reference: Kelly-Heidenthal, P. (2003). *Nursing leadership and management.* Clifton Park, NY: Thomson Delmar Learning.

2. **Answers: 1, 2, and 3**
   Rationale: The nurse must consider the job description of the UAP and determine whether the UAP understands how to do a procedure correctly and safely and whether the task requires UAP competency.
   Cognitive Level: Analysis
   Nursing Process: Planning
   NCLEX-RN Test Plan: SECE
   Reference: Kelly-Heidenthal, P. (2003). *Nursing leadership and management.* Clifton Park, NY: Thomson Delmar Learning.

3. **Answer: 1**
   Rationale: Overdelegation puts the client at risk. Delegating duties inappropriately to personnel to perform is inappropriate when the personnel are inadequately educated because it places the client at risk.
   Cognitive Level: Application
   Nursing Process: Planning
   NCLEX-RN Test Plan: SECE
   Reference: Kelly-Heidenthal, P. (2003). *Nursing leadership and management.* Clifton Park, NY: Thomson Delmar Learning.

4. **Answer: 4**
   Rationale: LPN/LVNs are able to perform and function at a higher level than UAPs. The LPN/LVN education includes standardized training and competency evaluation. Duties include reinforcing teaching from a standardized plan of care and

updating initial assessments made by an RN. The role of the LPN/LVN is determined by the State Nurse Practice act.
   Cognitive Level: Application
   Nursing Process: Planning
   NCLEX-RN Test Plan: SECE
   Reference: Kelly-Heidenthal, P., & Marthaler, M. T. (2005). *Delegation of nursing care.* Clifton Park, NY: Thomson Delmar Learning.

5. **Answer: 1**
   Rationale: Once nurses have decided on client priorities, they must consider what can be achieved with available resources. Life-threatening emergencies or saving a life when a life-threatening event occurs are priorities and must be completed no matter how short the staffing. Nurses must protect their clients and maintain both patient and staff safety as well as perform important nursing activities.
   Cognitive Level: Analysis
   Nursing Process: Planning
   NCLEX-RN Test Plan: SECE
   Reference: Kelly-Heidenthal, P., & Marthaler, M. T. (2005). *Delegation of nursing care.* Clifton Park, NY: Thomson Delmar Learning.

6. **Answer: 3**
   Rationale: Unlicensed assistive personnel (UAP) generally can be assigned routine tasks on a stable client. Obtaining vital signs is within the job description of the UAP. UAPs cannot administer medications (including topical medications and adjustment of IV drip rates) as this action requires nursing judgment and assessment.
   Cognitive Level: Analysis
   Nursing Process: Planning
   NCLEX-RN Test Plan: SECE
   Reference: Killion, S. W., & Dempski, K. M. (2000). *Quick look nursing: Legal and ethical issues.* Thorofare, NJ: Slack, Inc.

7. **Answer: 2**
   Rationale: The nurse is taking the path of least resistance. She is under the assumption it is easier to

do the task herself rather than risk confrontation with the UAP.

Cognitive Level: Application

Nursing Process: Planning

NCLEX-RN Test Plan: SECE

Reference: Kelly-Heidenthal, P., & Marthaler, M. T. (2005). *Delegation of nursing care.* Clifton Park, NY: Thomson Delmar Learning.

8. **Answer: 3**

Rationale: The RN is directly responsible for the care of the client. This includes ensuring that nursing orders are carried out, such as the LPN/LVN completing their assignment of care and treatments. It is the responsibility of the RN to determine why the dressing change was not completed as requested.

Cognitive Level: Application

Nursing Process: Evaluation

NCLEX-RN Test Plan: SECE

Reference: Kelly-Heidenthal, P., & Marthaler, M. T. (2005). *Delegation of nursing care.* Clifton Park, NY: Thomson Delmar Learning.

9. **Answer: 1**

Rationale: Elements to be considered when delegating a task to the LPN/LVN are the state nurse practice act, nursing professional standards, knowledge and skill of the LPN/LVN, and the individual's strengths and weaknesses.

Cognitive Level: Application

Nursing Process: Planning

NCLEX-RN Test Plan: SECE

Reference: Kelly-Heidenthal, P. (2003). *Nursing leadership and management.* Clifton Park, NY: Thomson Delmar Learning.

10. **Answer: 1**

Rationale: The primary reason for delegation is to complete a job in the most effective and efficient way using the most appropriate resources. Tasks are delegated to personnel who are educated and skilled in the assigned task.

Cognitive Level: Application

Nursing Process: Evaluation

NCLEX-RN Test Plan: SECE

Reference: Kelly-Heidenthal, P., & Marthaler, M. T. (2005). *Delegation of nursing care.* Clifton Park, NY: Thomson Delmar Learning.

11. **Answer: 3**

Rationale: Two factors to consider when assigning and delegating clients to the UAP are complexity of client needs and the skill, education, and competency of the UAP. The gastric bypass client is three days postoperative and, if stable, will require the least amount of skill and monitoring.

Cognitive Level: Analysis

Nursing Process: Planning

NCLEX-RN Test Plan: SECE

Reference: Kelly-Heidenthal, P., & Marthaler, M. T. (2005). *Delegation of nursing care.* Clifton Park, NY: Thomson Delmar Learning.

12. **Answer: 3**

Rationale: According to the patient safety act of 1996, UAPs may perform duties for which they have been appropriately trained and educated. UAPs can provide supportive care. Intravenous pain administration is an RN duty that should not be delegated to a UAP.

Cognitive Level: Application

Nursing Process: Planning

NCLEX-RN Test Plan: SECE

Reference: Kelly-Heidenthal, P., & Marthaler, M. T. (2005). *Delegation of nursing care.* Clifton Park, NY: Thomson Delmar Learning.

13. **Answer: 1**

Rationale: Maslow's hierarchy of human needs provides the nurse with a base for establishing priorities. However, Covey and Merrill have classified activities as urgent or not urgent, important or not important. An activity that is both urgent and important takes precedence over lower priority activities. As nurses begin their shifts, they must give priority to those activities that will impact and make the most difference in patient outcome. Timely insulin administration is required to maintain the blood sugar level in diabetic clients.

Cognitive Level: Application

Nursing Process: Planning

NCLEX-RN Test Plan: SECE

Reference: Kelly-Heidenthal, P., & Marthaler, M. T. (2005). *Delegation of nursing care.* Clifton Park, NY: Thomson Delmar Learning.

14. **Answer: 2**

    Rationale: UAPs are trained and educated to take vital signs, but are not competent, educated, or permitted to assess clients. The nurse is responsible for assessing clients. Postoperative bleeding may be due to hemorrhage. The nurse is responsible for assessing and evaluating the client's status, especially when there is a reported change in status. High priority, unstable clients require nursing assessment, evaluation, and stabilization.

    Cognitive Level: Analysis

    Nursing Process: Planning

    NCLEX-RN Test Plan: SECE

    Reference: Kelly-Heidenthal, P., & Marthaler, M. T. (2005). *Delegation of nursing care.* Clifton Park, NY: Thomson Delmar Learning.

15. **Answer: 1**

    Rationale: Physiologic parameters take precedence over body image, self-esteem, and autonomy.

    Cognitive Level: Application

    Nursing Process: Planning

    NCLEX-RN Test Plan: SECE

    Reference: Kneisl, C. R., Wilson, H. S., & Trigoboff, E. (2004). *Contemporary psychiatric-mental health nursing.* Upper Saddle River, NJ: Pearson Prentice Hall.

16. **Answer: 2**

    Rationale: There is an increased risk of suicide at this time as the client now has the energy and cognitive ability to plan suicide and implement the plan. Other responses are appropriate diagnoses for a depressed client. However, they do not take priority at this time.

    Cognitive Level: Application

    Nursing Process: Analysis

    NCLEX-RN Test Plan: SECE

    Reference: Kneisl, C. R., Wilson, H. S., & Trigoboff, E. (2004). *Contemporary psychiatric-mental health nursing.* Upper Saddle River, NJ: Pearson Prentice Hall.

17. **Answer: 4**

    Rationale: All responses represent reasons for subordinate resistance to delegation. However, before considering the basis for the resistance, more assessment is needed.

    Cognitive Level: Analysis

    Nursing Process: Assessment

    NCLEX-RN Test Plan: SECE

    Reference: Marquis, B. L., & Huston, C. J. (2006). *Leadership roles and management functions in nursing: Theory and application* (5th ed.). Philadelphia: Lippincott Williams & Wilkins.

18. **Answer: 2**

    Rationale: Long-term goals have later deadlines. Responses 3 and 4 are longer term goals. However, before they can be achieved, the nurse needs to know if there is interest from area physicians and how many clients to expect. Before the physicians are contacted, the registered nurse needs to have a program plan to present to them.

    Cognitive Level: Analysis

    Nursing Process: Planning

    NCLEX-RN Test Plan: SECE

    Reference: Marquis, B. L., & Huston, C. J. (2006). *Leadership roles and management functions in nursing: Theory and application* (5th ed.). Philadelphia: Lippincott Williams & Wilkins.

19. **Answer: Procrastination**

    Rationale: Procrastination involves delaying needlessly. It shrinks productivity. It rarely results from a single cause and can be related to performance anxiety, escapism, and low frustration tolerance.

    Cognitive Level: Analysis

    Nursing Process: Planning

    NCLEX-RN Test Plan: SECE

    Reference: Marquis, B. L., & Huston, C. J. (2006). *Leadership roles and management functions in nursing: Theory and application* (5th ed.). Philadelphia: Lippincott Williams & Wilkins.

20. **Answer: 3**

    Rationale: Managers should validate the delegate's skills by directly observing a performance of the task. Not every delegated task needs to be handled with outstanding skill—satisfactory may be adequate when one is learning the skill.

    Cognitive Level: Application

    Nursing Process: Implementation

    NCLEX-RN Test Level: SECE

    Reference: Marquis, B. L., & Huston, C. J. (2006). *Leadership roles and management functions in nursing: Theory and application* (5th ed.). Philadelphia: Lippincott Williams & Wilkins.

21. **Answer: 3**
Rationale: A common delegation error of a new graduate nurse is overloading herself. In this case, the nurse needs to work in partnership with the other personnel who can provide routine care.
Cognitive Level: Analysis
Nursing Process: Planning
NCLEX-RN Test Plan: SECE
Reference: Ellis, J. R., & Hartley, C. L. (2005). *Managing and coordinating nursing care* (4th ed.). Philadelphia: Lippincott Williams & Wilkins.

22. **Answer: 2**
Rationale: When limits are globally set, the client is more likely to rebel. All other responses are appropriate.
Cognitive Level: Analysis
Nursing Process: Evaluation
NCLEX-RN Test Plan: SECE
Reference: Kneisl, C. R., Wilson, H. S., & Trigoboff, E. (2004). *Contemporary psychiatric-mental health nursing.* Upper Saddle River, NJ: Pearson Prentice Hall.

23. **Answer: 4**
Rationale: Agency policies operate within the state scope of practice laws.
Cognitive Level: Application
Nursing Process: Planning
NCLEX-RN Test Plan: SECE
Reference: Ellis, J. R., & Hartley, C. L. (2005). *Managing and coordinating nursing care* (4th ed.). Philadelphia: Lippincott Williams & Wilkins.

24. **Answer: 4**
Rationale: Clients with BPD have one of the highest suicide rates of all of the personality disorders (3–10%). This is related to their impulsiveness, profound mood swings, and unstable yet impulsive relationships. All other responses are appropriate nursing diagnoses. However, number 4 takes priority.
Cognitive Level: Analysis
Nursing Process: Analysis
NCLEX-RN Test Plan: SECE
Reference: Stuart, G. W., & Laraia, M. T. (2005). *Principles and practices of psychiatric nursing* (8th ed.). St. Louis, MO: Elsevier Mosby.

25. **Answers: 1, 4, and 7**
Rationale: Non-nursing activities, such as those listed in Responses 1, 4, and 7, are safe to delegate to the UAP as long as there has been prior education. All data collected by the UAP are analyzed by the registered nurse. The nurse cannot delegate any activity that uses the nursing process or involves client teaching.
Cognitive Level: Application
Nursing Process: Planning
NCLEX-RN Test Plan: SECE
References: Kneisl, C. R., Wilson, H. S., & Trigoboff, E. (2004). *Contemporary psychiatric-mental health nursing.* Upper Saddle River, NJ: Pearson Prentice Hall.

Marquis, B. L., & Huston, C. J. (2006). *Leadership roles and management functions in nursing: Theory and application* (5th ed.). Philadelphia: Lippincott Williams & Wilkins.

Stuart, G. W., & Laraia, M. T. (2005). *Principles and practices of psychiatric nursing* (8th ed.). St. Louis, MO: Elsevier Mosby.

26. **Answer: 2**
Rationale: Responses 1, 3, and 4 are strategic assessments that indicate that delegation to a properly educated UAP can be carried out in a safe manner. In Responses 1 and 4, assistance is readily available to the UAP. There would need to be more than "some" potential for danger to the client to rule out delegation. Delegation nursing care of a highly unstable client to the UAP is inappropriate.
Cognitive Level: Analysis
Nursing Process: Assessment
NCLEX-RN Test Plan: SECE
References: Marquis, B. L., & Huston, C. J. (2006). *Leadership roles and management functions in nursing: Theory and application* (5th ed.). Philadelphia: Lippincott Williams & Wilkins.
Ellis, J. R., & Hartley, C. L. (2005). *Managing and coordinating nursing care* (4th ed.). Philadelphia: Lippincott Williams & Wilkins.

27. **Answer: 1**
Rationale: Response 1 indicates that the UAP does not have a prioritized timeline for task completion. All other responses indicate a priority.
Cognitive Level: Analysis

Nursing Process: Evaluation
NCLEX-RN Test Plan: SECE
Reference: Marquis, B. L., & Huston, C. J. (2006).
*Leadership roles and management functions in
nursing: Theory and application* (5th ed.).
Philadelphia: Lippincott Williams & Wilkins.

28. **Answer: 4**
Rationale: UAPs have no legal scope of practice
(although they may have an agency job description)
and, thus, no accountability for nursing care. The
registered nurse is accountable and responsible for
client care. UAPs are delegated specific tasks of
client care, not comprehensive care of clients.
Cognitive Level: Application
Nursing Process: Planning
NCLEX-RN Test Plan: SECE
Reference: Ellis, J. R., & Hartley, C. L. (2005).
Managing and coordinating nursing care (4th ed.).
Philadelphia: Lippincott Williams & Wilkins.

29. **Answer: Accountable**
Rationale: There is legal responsibility (accountabil-
ity) in delegation. The nurse is accountable for dele-
gating according to the five rights.
Cognitive Level: Application
Nursing Process: Implementation
NCLEX-RN Test Plan: SECE
Reference: Ellis, J. R., & Hartley, C. L. (2005).
Managing and coordinating nursing care (4th ed.).
Philadelphia: Lippincott Williams & Wilkins.

30. **Answer: Scope of practice**
Rationale: Scope of practice is a description of what
each person's license or job description allows them
to do.
Cognitive Level: Analysis
Nursing Process: Implementation
NCLEX-RN Test Plan: SECE
Reference: Ellis, J. R., & Hartley, C. L. (2005).
Managing and coordinating nursing care (4th ed.).
Philadelphia: Lippincott Williams & Wilkins.

31. **Answer: 4**
Rationale: Supervision involves determining that the
delegated tasks are being completed. The nurse needs
to determine if care is progressing according to
schedule, and if not, why progress has not occurred.

Cognitive Level: Application
Nursing Process: Implementation
NCLEX-RN Test Level: SECE
Reference: Ellis, J. R., & Hartley, C. L. (2005).
Managing and coordinating nursing care (4th ed.).
Philadelphia: Lippincott Williams & Wilkins.

32. **Answer: 3**
Rationale: Items essential to maintaining life and
critical symptom management (pain management)
take priority over items related to moving towards
self-care (teaching and contacting referrals) and cre-
ating comfort (bathing).
Cognitive Level: Analysis
Nursing Process: Planning
NCLEX-RN Test Level: SECE
Reference: Ellis, J. R., & Hartley, C. L. (2005).
Managing and coordinating nursing care (4th ed.).
Philadelphia: Lippincott Williams & Wilkins.

33. **Answer: 3**
Rationale: Most abused drugs pass through the placental membrane. During pregnancy, the safest situation is drug free, with one exception. For pregnant
women addicted to heroin, methadone maintenance
is safer for the fetus than acute detoxification
(Responses 2 and 4). Continued use of heroin is
not appropriate (Response 1).
Cognitive Level: Application
Nursing Process: Intervention
NCLEX-RN Test Plan: SECE
Reference: Stuart, G. (2005). *Handbook of psychiatric
nursing* (6th ed.). St. Louis, MO: Elsevier Mosby.

34. **Answer: 4**
Rationale: The patient with total hip replacement is
the most stable. The other choices are less stable
and would require frequent assessment. The LPN
can perform dressing changes if required, and assist
with ambulation.
Cognitive Level: Analysis
Nursing Process: Planning
NCLEX-RN Test Plan: SECE
Reference: Kelly-Heidenthal, P., & Marthaler, M. T.
(2005). *Delegation of nursing care.* Clifton Park,
NY: Thomson Delmar Learning.

35. **Answer: 4**

    Rationale: The RN is responsible for deciding the room assignments for clients. The RN must be cognizant of the client's diagnosis and the presence or absence of infectious disease. Clients with similar diagnoses or infections should be placed together. Clients with a bacteria, viral, fungal, or other infection are considered "dirty". Clients who are postoperative are considered "clean" and must be assigned a room with other patients free of infectious disease. Therefore, the postoperative appendectomy (clean) patient should be assigned to the room with the client admitted with diabetes mellitus. Other options are incorrect.

    Cognitive Level: Analysis

    Nursing Process: Planning

    NCLEX-RN Test Plan: SECE

    Reference: Kelly-Heidenthal, P., & Marthaler, M. T. (2005). *Delegation of nursing care.* Clifton Park, NY: Thomson Delmar Learning.

36. **Answer: 3**

    Rationale: The pulled RN from labor and delivery will have a strong knowledge base to assess for vaginal drainage or active bleeding and other complications for the postoperative client who had a total abdominal hysterectomy.

    Cognitive Level: Analysis

    Nursing Process: Planning

    NCLEX-RN Test Plan: SECE

    Reference: Catalano, J. T. (2006). *Nursing now!* (4th ed.). Philadelphia: F.A. Davis Company.

37. **Answer: 2**

    Rationale: The patient with a severe respiratory infection, such as pertussis, is at risk of respiratory distress and requires frequent monitoring and assessment. The young age of 2 months places this patient at risk for complications, such as airway obstruction. Airway takes priority over other options.

    Cognitive Level: Analysis

    Nursing Process: Planning

    NCLEX-RN Test Plan: SECE

    Reference: Kelly-Heidenthal, P., & Marthaler, M. T. (2005). *Delegation of nursing care.* Clifton Park, NY: Thomson Delmar Learning.

38. **Answer: 4**

    Rationale: In the event that the UAP refuses to perform a task, the RN should attempt to open communication and discuss the matter in order to obtain more information. Further intervention should be sought only after the RN attempts to discuss the matter with the UAP. Should the UAP continue to refuse and becomes insubordinate, the RN must delegate the task to other available personnel, document the incident, and report the incident to the clinical nurse manager.

    Cognitive Level: Analysis

    Nursing Process: Planning

    NCLEX-RN Test Plan: SECE

    Reference: Catalano, J. T. (2006). *Nursing now!* (4th ed.). Philadelphia: F.A. Davis Company.

39. **Answer: 3**

    Rationale: The RN can assign tasks related to feeding, basic hygiene, or ambulation, provided that essential training and supplies are available. The UAP is not permitted to administer any medication to clients. Administration of medication is within the RN or LPN scope of practice.

    Cognitive Level: Analysis

    Nursing Process: Planning

    NCLEX-RN Test Plan: SECE

    Reference: Catalano, J. T. (2006). *Nursing now!* (4th ed.). Philadelphia: F.A. Davis Company.

Unit 3 Answers and Rationales

Test 6 Answers and Rationales

1. **Answer:** 1, 4, 2, 5, 3
   Rationale: The nondisaster stage is the time for early planning and preparation, prior to the event occurring. The predisaster phase follows when there is knowledge of an impending disaster. The impact stage occurs after the disaster has occurred and the community is experiencing the immediate effects. This is followed by the emergency phase when there is an immediate response of aid and assistance by the community resources. Reconstruction or rehabilitation is the last phase.
   Cognitive Level: Application
   Nursing Process: Implementation
   NCLEX-RN Test Plan: SECE
   Reference: Langan, J. C., & James, D. C. (2005). *Preparing nurses for disaster management.* Upper Saddle River, NJ: Pearson Prentice Hall.

2. **Answer:** 2
   Rationale: Any child who has a respiratory rate of less than 10 or greater than 45 should be tagged with red, indicating immediate care should be given. During a multiple casualty accident, there is not time to perform a complete neurological assessment.
   Cognitive Level: Analysis
   Nursing Process: Analysis
   NCLEX-RN Test Plan: SECE
   References: Beachley, M. L. (2005). Nursing in a disaster. In F. Maurer & C. Smith, (Eds.), *Community/public health nursing practice: Health for families and populations* (pp. 496–516). Philadelphia: Elsevier.

   Romig, L. E. (n.d.). *Jumpstart pediatric multiple casualty incident triage.* Retrieved April 26, 2005 from http://www.jumpstarttriage.com

3. **Answer:** 3
   Rationale: When assessing an apneic adult casualty in a disaster situation, attempt to reposition the upper airway once. If the person still does not breathe, a black tag (dying or death) should be placed on the upper body and the rescuer should attempt to aid the next person.

   Cognitive Level: Analysis
   Nursing Process: Implementation
   NCLEX-RN Test Plan: SECE
   Reference: Romig, L. E. (n.d.). *Combined start/jumpstart triage algorithm.* Retrieved April 26, 2005 from http://www.jumpstarttriage.com/ JumpSTART_and_MCI_Triage.php

4. **Answer:** 4
   Rationale: Nurses and other emergency personnel are used as triage officers because physicians are administering emergency care to the more critical victims.
   Cognitive Level: Application
   Nursing Process: Implementation
   NCLEX-RN Test Plan: SECE
   Reference: Beachley, M. L. (2005). Nursing in a disaster. In F. Maurer & C. Smith, (Eds.), *Community/public health nursing practice: Health for families and populations* (pp. 496–516). Philadelphia: Elsevier.

5. **Answer:** 4
   Rationale: Hospital disaster plans should be developed for both internal and external disasters. In order for the hospital to be prepared, these plans should be practiced at least twice per year and evaluated for accuracy and efficiency.
   Cognitive Level: Application
   Nursing Process: Implementation
   NCLEX-RN Test Plan: SECE
   Reference: Beachley, M. L. (2005). Nursing in a disaster. In F. Maurer & C. Smith (Eds.), *Community/public health nursing practice: Health for families and populations* (pp. 496–516). Philadelphia: Elsevier.

6. **Answer:** 1
   Rationale: In a disaster situation, if an adult can obey a command, his coding for triage is yellow (urgent; second priority). If he cannot obey a command, he has a decreased level of consciousness and is placed in the most urgent (red) category. Having diabetes does not automatically place that person in the most urgent (red) category.
   Cognitive Level: Analysis

Nursing Process: Assessment

NCLEX-RN Test Plan: SECE

Reference: Beachley, M. L. (2005). Nursing in a disaster. In F. Maurer & C. Smith (Eds.), *Community/public health nursing practice: Health for families and populations* (pp. 496–516). Philadelphia: Elsevier.

7. **Answer: 3**

Rationale: Lacerations are torn wounds with torn tissue underneath. An abrasion occurs when the skin is scraped or rubbed off. An avulsion is the tearing away of tissue from a body part, and a puncture is seen when an object penetrates the skin leaving a small surface opening.

Cognitive Level: Application

Nursing Process: Assessment

NCLEX-RN Test Plan: SECE

Reference: Langan, J. C., & James, D. C. (2005). *Preparing nurses for disaster management.* Upper Saddle River, NJ: Pearson Prentice Hall.

8. **Answer: Ineffective coping related to lack of available resources.**

Rationale: This is an acceptable nursing diagnosis as defined in the NANDA classification system.

Cognitive Level: Application

Nursing Process: Planning

NCLEX-RN Test Plan: PSYC

Reference: Lewis, S. M., Heitkemper, M. M., & Dirksen, S. R. (2004). *Medical-surgical nursing* (6th ed.). St. Louis, MO: Elsevier Mosby.

9. **Answer: 2**

Rationale: Any adult with a respiratory rate of over 30 breaths per minute needs immediate attention. Additionally, this patient is unconscious, which constitutes altered mental status. Patients #1 and #3 are both conscious and have normal respiratory rates and capillary refill. In a disaster situation, patient #4 is apneic after repositioning of his airway so that patient is considered dead.

Cognitive Level: Analysis

Nursing Process: Assessment

NCLEX-RN Test Plan: PHY

Reference: Romig, L. E. (n.d.). *Combined start/jumpstart triage algorithm.*

Retrieved April 26, 2005, from http://www.jumpstarttriage.com/JumpSTART_ and_MCI_Triage.php

10. **Answers: 1, 2, 4, and 5**

Rationale: All of the items, except a passport and birth certificate, listed are needed in case of a disaster. A passport or birth certificate would only be needed if the community member was going to travel out of the country. That is not an issue during a disaster.

Cognitive Level: Application

Nursing Process: Implementation

NCLEX-RN Test Plan: SECE

Reference: Hassmiller, S. B. (2003). Disaster management. In M. Stanhope & J. Lancaster (Eds.), *Community & public health nursing* (6th ed., pp. 470–489). St. Louis, MO: Elsevier Mosby.

11. **Answer: 3**

Rationale: This is the definition of the scope of a major disaster. #1 is a local disaster, #2 is a state disaster and #4 is the definition of a Presidentially Declared Disaster.

Cognitive Level: Comprehension

Nursing Process: Assessment

NCLEX-RN Test Plan: SECE

Reference: Hassmiller, S. B. (2003). Disaster management. In M. Stanhope & J. Lancaster (Eds.), *Community & public health nursing* (6th ed., pp. 470–489). St. Louis, MO: Elsevier Mosby.

12. **Answer: 2**

Rationale: This patient has a respiratory rate that is greater than 30 breaths per minute, which is indicative of needing immediate help. In a disaster, #1 and #3 are considered dead and would receive a black tag in the field. The patient who is a diabetic should be watched but does not need immediate assistance. This patient would receive a yellow tag.

Cognitive Level: Analysis

Nursing Process: Analysis

NCLEX-RN Test Plan: SECE

Reference: Romig, L. E. (n.d.). *Combined start/jumpstart triage algorithm.* Retrieved April 26, 2005, from http://www.jumpstarttriage.com/ JumpSTART_and_MCI_Triage.php

13. **Answers: 2, 3, and 4**
    Rationale: Exhibiting regressive behaviors, having fantasies that nothing occurred, and the inability to concentrate are common behaviors after a disaster trauma.
    Cognitive Level: Analysis
    Nursing Process: Assessment
    NCLEX-RN Test Plan: SECE
    Reference: Hassmiller, S. B. (2003). Disaster management. In M. Stanhope & J. Lancaster (Eds.), *Community & public health nursing* (6th ed., pp. 470–489). St. Louis, MO: Elsevier Mosby.

14. **Answer: 1**
    Rationale: The nurse needs the simple techniques of overall observation of looking; feeling, which includes palpation of deformities, tenderness, pulsations, and temperature; listening, which includes assessment of breath sounds; and smelling, which includes a fruity breath smell of someone in diabetic ketoacidosis.
    Cognitive Level: Application
    Nursing Process: Assessment
    NCLEX-RN Test Plan: PHY
    Reference: Langan, J. C., & James, D. C. (2005). *Preparing nurses for disaster management.* Upper Saddle River, NJ: Pearson Prentice Hall.

15. **Answer: 3**
    Rationale: The Hospital Emergency Incident Command System (HEICS) is a hospital-based incident command system used throughout the country as a framework for reporting and communication, which entails assignment of specific roles to members of the health care team.
    Cognitive Level: Comprehension
    Nursing Process: Assessment
    NCLEX-RN Test Plan: SECE
    Reference: Langan, J. C., & James, D. C. (2005). *Preparing nurses for disaster management.* Upper Saddle River, NJ: Pearson Prentice Hall.

16. **Answer: 2**
    Rationale: Gently wrapping the extremity will not cause vasoconstriction. Elevation will decrease the progression of the edema. Frostbite care includes immersion of the site in warm water (100°–106°F). Rubbing the area during the warming process may cause increased tissue damage, and debriding blisters should only be done by physician's order.

Cognitive Level: Application
Nursing Process: Implementation
NCLEX-RN Test Plan: PHY
Reference: Schwytzer, D. (2004). Common problems encountered in emergency and critical care nursing. In M. A. Hogan & T. Madayag (Eds.), *Medical-surgical nursing: Reviews and rationales* (pp. 1–44). Upper Saddle River, NJ: Pearson Prentice Hall.

17. **Answer: 4**
    Rationale: There can be more significant internal injuries than what is observed at the entrance wound due to patient movement. Low velocity missile weapons, such as a knife, usually cause damage along a path. However, it can be life threatening if it strikes a vital or highly vascular organ. A nurse should always be concerned about chemical toxins due to any gunshot wound.
    Cognitive Level: Application
    Nursing Process: Assessment
    NCLEX-RN Test Plan: SECE
    Reference: Schwytzer, D. (2004). Common problems encountered in emergency and critical care nursing. In M. A. Hogan & T. Madayag (Eds.), *Medical-surgical nursing: Reviews and rationales* (pp. 1–44). Upper Saddle River, NJ: Pearson Prentice Hall.

18. **Answer: 4**
    Rationale: The incubation period for inhaled anthrax is approximately 7–10 days.
    Cognitive Level: Application
    Nursing Process: Assessment
    NCLEX-RN Test Plan: SECE
    Reference: Department of Health and Human Services Centers for Disease Control and Prevention. (2002). *Fact sheet: Anthrax information for health care providers.* Retrieved April 15, 2006, from http://www.bt.cdc.gov/agent/anthrax/anthrax-hcp-factsheet.asp

19. **Answer: 1**
    Rationale: After the hospital emergency department and administration, the next agency in the chain of command to be notified is the local health department.
    Cognitive Level: Comprehension

Nursing Process: Implementation
NCLEX-RN Test Plan: SECE
Reference: Langan, J. C., & James, D. C. (2005).
 Preparing nurses for disaster management. Upper
 Saddle River, NJ: Pearson Prentice Hall.

20. **Answer: 2**
 Rationale: The effect of acute radiation exposure is
 the depression of red and white blood cell counts.
 Cognitive Level: Application
 Nursing Process: Evaluation
 NCLEX-RN Test Plan: PHYS
 Reference: Veenema, T. G. (2003). *Disaster nursing
  and emergency preparedness for chemical,
  biological, and radiological terrorism and other
  hazards.* New York: Springer.

21. **Answer: 1**
 Rationale: The client is at risk for infection due to
 damaged white blood cells.
 Cognitive Level: Application
 Nursing Process: Evaluation
 NCLEX-RN Test Plan: PHYS
 Reference: Veenema, T. G. (2003). *Disaster nursing
  and emergency preparedness for chemical,
  biological, and radiological terrorism and other
  hazards.* New York: Springer.

22. **Answer: 4**
 Rationale: Atropine is the known first line antidote
 to be administered in a sarin nerve gas exposure.
 Cognitive Level: Analysis
 Nursing Process: Analysis
 NCLEX-RN Test Plan: PHYS
 Reference: Langan, J. C., & James, D. C. (2005).
  Preparing nurses for disaster management. Upper
  Saddle River, NJ: Pearson Prentice Hall.

23. **Answer: 1**
 Rationale: Signs and symptoms of inhalation anthrax
 exposure quickly progress to respiratory failure.
 Cognitive Level: Analysis
 Nursing Process: Planning
 NCLEX-RN Test Plan: PHYS
 Reference: Veenema, T. G. (2003). *Disaster nursing
  and emergency preparedness for chemical,
  biological, and radiological terrorism and other
  hazards.* New York: Springer.

24. **Answer: 4**
 Rationale: Anthrax predominately occurs as a cutaneous infection, but the use of anthrax as a biological weapon typically involves inhalational anthrax.
 Human to human transmission of anthrax has not
 been reported.
 Cognitive Level: Analysis
 Nursing Process: Planning
 NCLEX-RN Test Plan: SECE
 Reference: Veenema, T. G. (2003). *Disaster nursing
  and emergency preparedness for chemical,
  biological, and radiological terrorism and other
  hazards.* New York: Springer.

25. **Answer: 1**
 Rationale: Because of the potential for bioterrorism
 and the fact that many health care providers have
 never seen this disease, it is important to become
 familiar with the clinical and epidemiologic features of
 smallpox and how it is differentiated from chickenpox.
 Cognitive Level: Analysis
 Nursing Process: Planning
 NCLEX-RN Test Plan: SECE
 Reference: Stanhope, M., & Lancaster, J. (2005).
  Community and public health nursing (6th ed.).
  St. Louis, MO: Elsevier Mosby.

26. **Answer: 1**
 Rationale: Public health responsibilities for pre-
 paredness planning regarding chemical attacks
 include developing capabilities for the education of
 first responders and health care personnel about
 chemical antidotes.
 Cognitive Level: Analysis
 Nursing Process: Planning
 NCLEX-RN Test Plan: SECE
 Reference: Langan, J. C., & James, D. C. (2005).
  Preparing nurses for disaster management. Upper
  Saddle River, NJ: Pearson Prentice Hall.

27. **Answer: 1**
 Rationale: The preplanning phase of disaster pre-
 paredness involves developing a response plan; key
 to developing this plan is knowing the resources that
 will be available in the community.
 Cognitive Level: Analysis
 Nursing Process: Planning
 NCLEX-RN Test Plan: SECE

Reference: Mauer, F. A., & Smith, C. M. (2005). *Community and public health nursing practice: Health for families and populations.* St. Louis, MO: Elsevier Saunders.

28. **Answer: 4**
    Rationale: Anthrax is the only bacterial infection choice. Ciprofloxacin is an antimicrobial drug, effective against bacterial infections, and the drug of choice for an anthrax exposure.
    Cognitive Level: Application
    Nursing Process: Analysis
    NCLEX-RN Test Plan: PHYS
    Reference: Veenema, T. G. (2003). *Disaster nursing and emergency preparedness for chemical, biological, and radiological terrorism and other hazards.* New York: Springer.

29. **Answer: 1**
    Rationale: Mitigation is action taken to prevent or reduce the harmful effects of a disaster, and involves future-oriented activities. Infection control policies and procedures will prevent or minimize the severity of a biological bioterrorism event.
    Cognitive Level: Application
    Nursing Process: Planning
    NCLEX-RN Test Plan: SECE
    Reference: Langan, J. C., & James, D. C. (2005). *Preparing nurses for disaster management.* Upper Saddle River, NJ: Pearson Prentice Hall.

30. **Answer: 3**
    Rationale: Anthrax vaccine is produced exclusively under contracts to the Department of Defense. Virtually all vaccine produced in the United States is primarily for military use and a small number of other official government uses.
    Cognitive Level: Analysis
    Nursing Process: Analysis
    NCLEX-RN Test Plan: SECE
    Reference: Langan, J. C., & James, D. C. (2005). *Preparing nurses for disaster management.* Upper Saddle River, NJ: Pearson Prentice Hall.

31. **Answers: 1, 3, 4, and 6**
    Rationale: Smallpox is a virus that had been eliminated worldwide in the 1970s; consequently immunization is no longer required. This successful public health achievement has made smallpox a biologic weapon.
    Cognitive Level: Application
    Nursing Process: Planning
    NCLEX-RN Test Plan: SECE
    Reference: Lehne, R. A. (2004). *Pharmacology for nursing care* (5th ed.). St. Louis, MO: Elsevier Saunders.

32. **Answers: 2, 3, 4, and 5**
    Rationale: Ricin is a toxin derived from castor beans. It can be ingested or inhaled and there is no known antidote. Vaccination is not available; this is not a microbiologic agent.
    Cognitive Level: Application
    Nursing Process: Planning
    NCLEX-RN Test Plan: SECE
    Reference: Lehne, R. A. (2004). *Pharmacology for nursing care* (5th ed.). St. Louis, MO: Elsevier Saunders.

33. **Answer: 4**
    Rationale: Mustard gas is an alkylating agent and vesicant. Management centers on rapid decontamination, supportive care, and drug therapy.
    Cognitive Level: Analysis
    Nursing Process: Planning
    NCLEX-RN Test Plan: PHYS
    Reference: Lehne, R. A. (2004). *Pharmacology for nursing care* (5th ed.). St. Louis, MO: Elsevier Saunders.

34. **Answer: 55 mg Q 12 hours**
    Rationale: The math calculation to determine this answer requires the nurse to multiply 2.2 (drug) by 25 (child's body weight in kg) to obtain the correct dose.
    Cognitive Level: Analysis
    Nursing Process: Analysis
    NCLEX-RN Test Plan: PHYS
    Reference: Lehne, R. A. (2004). *Pharmacology for nursing care* (5th ed.). St. Louis, MO: Elsevier Saunders.

35. **Answers: 1-C, 2-B, 3-D, 4-A, 5-A, 6-A, 7-B, 8-A**
    Rationale: Weapons of terrorism can be of different categories, each requiring different disaster preparedness directed toward their unique characteristic ability to do harm.

Cognitive Level: Comprehension
Nursing Process: Planning
NCLEX-RN Test Plan: SECE
Reference: Lehne, R. A. (2004). *Pharmacology for nursing care* (5th ed.). St. Louis, MO: Elsevier Saunders.

36. **Answer: 3**
    Rationale: Tularemia is very infectious, but is not spread person to person. It responds very well to antibiotic therapy, in particular streptomycin. There is no vaccine for this microbe. Decontamination procedures are not necessary for bacterial and viral agents, with a possible exception of cutaneous anthrax.
    Cognitive Level: Analysis
    Nursing Process: Planning
    NCLEX-RN Test Plan: SECE
    References: Lehne, R. A. (2004). *Pharmacology for nursing care* (5th ed.). St. Louis, MO: Elsevier Saunders.

    Langan, J. C., & James, D. C. (2005). *Preparing nurses for disaster management.* Upper Saddle River, NJ: Pearson Prentice Hall.

37. **Answer: 1**
    Rationale: Adequate supplies of protective gear are essential for health care providers in the event of a bioterrorism event. Levels of protection include minimum, preferred, and specialized, each requiring more sophisticated gear. The items in this question are all minimum protection items needed to keep staff from harm.
    Cognitive Level: Application
    Nursing Process: Planning
    NCLEX-RN Test Plan: SECE
    Reference: Langan, J. C., & James, D. C. (2005). *Preparing nurses for disaster management.* Upper Saddle River, NJ: Pearson Prentice Hall.

38. **Answer: 3**
    Rationale: An AED is unlikely to be needed with a well child population. Communication capability, accountability of children and staff, and an understanding of the school environment layout are essential.
    Cognitive Level: Application
    Nursing Process: Planning
    NCLEX-RN Test Plan: SECE
    Reference: Langan, J. C., & James, D. C. (2005). *Preparing nurses for disaster management.* Upper Saddle River, NJ: Pearson Prentice Hall.

39. **Answer: 2**
    Rationale: An infant's larger body surface area in proportion to their weight allows for more rapid absorption of noxious substances. Infants are obligatory nose breathers, but this does not increase their risk for cutaneous absorption. They have higher metabolic rates than adults.
    Cognitive Level: Application
    Nursing Process: Implementation
    NCLEX-RN Test Plan: PHYS
    Reference: Langan, J. C., & James, D. C. (2005). *Preparing nurses for disaster management.* Upper Saddle River, NJ: Pearson Prentice Hall.

Unit 4 • Adult Nursing

Respiratory

1. **A client with pulmonary edema is started on furosemide (Lasix). What would the nurse include in the discharge teaching?**
   1. A decrease in urine output is to be expected.
   2. The client should eat foods with plenty of potassium.
   3. The client should expect an increase in swelling in the hands and feet.
   4. The client should take the medication at bedtime.

2. **If airflow is obstructed while attempting to ventilate a victim during CPR, what should the rescuer do?**
   1. Give two slow breaths followed by 15 chest compressions.
   2. Perform a finger sweep.
   3. Perform five chest compressions.
   4. Reposition the victim's head and reattempt to ventilate.

3. **A client is wearing a nasal cannula. The flow rate is set at 2 L/min. The nurse understands the O_2 concentration that the client is receiving is:**
   1. 28%.
   2. 45%.
   3. 50%.
   4. 60%.

4. **A client has been diagnosed with pulmonary tuberculosis. The client exhibits signs and symptoms that include which of the following?**
   1. Cough, decreased blood pressure, and decreased urinary output.
   2. Cough, chills, and leucocytosis.
   3. Fever, pain, and abdominal distention.
   4. A negative chest X-ray and weight gain.

5. **Analysis of arterial blood gasses (ABGs) and oxymetry are the best methods to assess which of the following?**
   1. Acid-base balance.
   2. Adequate oxygenation.
   3. The efficiency of gas transfer in the lungs.
   4. Mixed venous gas sample.

6. ***Early* signs and symptoms of inadequate oxygenation include which of the following?**
   1. Arrhythmias, diaphoresis, and hypotension.
   2. Combativeness, dyspnea at rest, and use of accessory muscles.
   3. Cool, clammy skin, decreased urinary output, and unexplained fatigue.
   4. Unexplained restlessness, irritability, and tachypnea.

7. **A nurse is auscultating the breath sounds of a client who has been diagnosed with asthma. On expiration, the nurse hears continuous high-pitched squeaking sounds. The nurse knows that this respiratory abnormality can be described as which of the following?**
   1. Crackles.
   2. Rhonchi.
   3. Stridor.
   4. Wheezes.

8. **Select all of the options that apply to the description and purpose of hematocrit.**

   1. The test reflects the amount of hemoglobin available for combination with oxygen.
   2. The test reflects the ratio of blood cells to plasma.
   3. The normal range for an adult female is 12–16 g/dl (120–160 g/L).
   4. The normal value for an adult male is 40–54%.
   5. Venous blood is used.

9. **Target groups for influenza immunization include which of the following? Select all that apply.**

   1. Adults of any age with chronic cardiac or pulmonary disease.
   2. Anyone 50 years old or older.
   3. Healthcare workers.
   4. Immunocompromised adults.
   5. Residents in long term care facilities.
   6. Women who will be in the second or third trimester of pregnancy during influenza season.

10. **A 16-year-old comes into the ER following a motor vehicle accident. The client is dyspnic and has severe pain. The left chest is sucked in during inspiration and it bulges out during expiration. The nurse understands these are symptoms most suggestive of which of the following?**

    1. Atelectesis.
    2. Flail chest.
    3. Fractured ribs.
    4. Pneuomothorax.

11. **The nurse is caring for a client who has a chest tube with water seal drainage. Guidelines for care include which of the following?**

    1. Do not encourage the client to cough until the chest tube is removed.
    2. Elevate the drainage system to the level of the patient's chest.
    3. Keep the water seal and suction control chamber at the appropriate water levels by adding sterile water as needed.
    4. Strip or milk the tubing to promote drainage.

12. **A client is complaining of pleuritic pain on the right side. The nurse notices that the client has dyspnea, a decreased movement of the chest wall, and absent breath sounds on the client's right chest. These symptoms are most suggestive of which of the following?**

    1. Pleural effusion.
    2. Pulmonary embolism.
    3. Pulmonary infection.
    4. Empyema.

13. **A client is ordered oxygen therapy via a nasal cannula. The nurse understands that this method of oxygen delivery does which of the following?**

    1. Delivers a constant concentration of oxygen.
    2. Delivers a high concentration of oxygen.
    3. Mixes room air with oxygen.
    4. Restricts the client from coughing and talking while wearing the device.

14. **A client in the hospital has a productive cough and has been diagnosed with tuberculosis. While in the hospital, prevention of disease transmission should include which of the following?**

    1. Contact isolation.
    2. Respiratory isolation.
    3. Standard isolation.
    4. Ultraviolet lights.

15. **A client is being sent home with the need for home oxygen. Client and family teaching will include which of the following statements? Select all that apply.**
    1. Cleanse the mask or collar with water every other day.
    2. Ensure that the straps on the mask are secure but not too tight.
    3. Observe the client's lips and chin for skin breakdown from pressure points.
    4. Post "no smoking" warning signs at home where they can be seen.

16. **A client has been diagnosed with emphysema and has dyspnea with minimal exertion. The nurse understands that this client is at risk for developing which of the following?**
    1. Respiratory acidosis.
    2. Respiratory alkalosis.
    3. Metabolic acidosis.
    4. Metabolic alkalosis.

17. **A client has been brought into the ER with a head injury. He is not breathing. Which of the following is causing this absent ventilation?**
    1. Pon's apneustic center.
    2. Serum bicarbonate level.
    3. Sympathetic nervous system.
    4. Trauma to the brainstem.

18. **A client in the hospital with pulmonary edema has developed tachypnia, dyspnea, crackles, and hypoxemia, which are not relieved by O_2 therapy. This client is now diagnosed with acute respiratory distress syndrome (ARDS). This client will develop which of the following acid-base imbalances?**
    1. Respiratory acidosis.
    2. Respiratory alkalosis.
    3. Metabolic acidosis.
    4. Metabolic alkalosis.

19. **Which of the following statements concerning ARDS is true?**
    1. One of the causes of ARDS is CHF.
    2. Pulmonary capillary wedge pressure is elevated in ARDS.
    3. Surfactant production is reduced in ARDS.
    4. ARDS has a low mortality rate.

20. **The nurse auscultates bilateral breath sounds on a client two days postoperative. She notices absent breath sounds in the bases. The nurse recognizes this is most likely due to which of the following?**
    1. Atelectesis.
    2. Rales.
    3. Rhonchi.
    4. Wheezes.

21. **A client, newly diagnosed with asthma, is started on theophylline (Theo-Dur, Slo-Bid) and is going to be discharged to home. In the discharge teaching, the nurse instructs the client that this medication will cause which of the following?**
    1. Hemolytic anemia.
    2. Increased appetite.
    3. Increased ocular pressure.
    4. Tachycardia.

22. **Which of the following is a common cause of acute respiratory acidosis?**
    1. Alveolar hyperventilation.
    2. Alveolar hypoventilation.
    3. Anxiety and fear.
    4. Pain.

23. **A client comes into the ER complaining of chest pain. The chest pain is described as a sharp, knife-like pain, and the client is able to point to the pain focal area with one finger. The nurse understands that which of the following conditions describes this chest pain?**
    1. Angina.
    2. Cardiogenic pain.
    3. Myocardial infarction.
    4. Pleuritic pain.

24. **What is a normal tidal volume (Vt) for a client on a ventilator?**
    1. 5–7 ml/kg.
    2. 7–9 ml/kg.
    3. 9–11 ml/kg.
    4. 11–13 ml/kg.

25. **Place an X over the anatomical location that the nurse would hear bronchial breath sounds.**

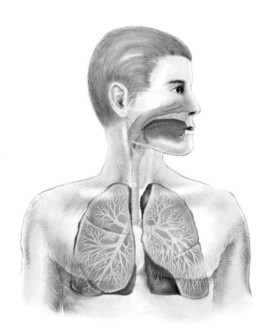

26. **Place these common signs and symptoms of pulmonary embolism in order of *frequency*.**
    1. Cough.
    2. Crackles.
    3. Dyspnea.
    4. Pleural pain.
    5. Tachycardia.
    6. Tachypnea.
    7. Unilateral leg swelling and pain.

27. **A seven-year-old client is brought into the ER. Her parents report that she is a healthy child who awoke with a temp of 102.2°F, complaints of an extreme sore throat, and drooling with difficulty swallowing. What would be a *priority* for the nurse assigned to this client?**
    1. Start an IV to provide hydration and medication.
    2. Obtain a throat and blood culture stat.
    3. Administer an antipyretic to manage fever and pain.
    4. Place the child in an upright position leaning forward.

28. **The nurse prepares to teach a child the proper MDI technique with spacer. Identify the correct sequence.**
    1. Hold breath for 5–10 seconds, then breathe normally.
    2. Shake to increase the pressure in the canister.
    3. Place the mouthpiece in the mouth and make a seal with the lips.
    4. Attach the MDI canister to the mouthpiece.
    5. Inspire slowly to the total lung capacity.
    6. Expire to the functional residual capacity.

29. **Which response indicates that the parent of a child with a streptococcal infection understands instructions for prevention of the disease?**
    1. "I will continue to push oral fluids for my son."
    2. "I will take his temperature every four hours."
    3. "He has frequent sore throats in the winter months."
    4. "I will discard his toothbrush and buy another."

30. **Identify signs of impending airway obstruction. Select all that apply.**
    1. Increased temperature.
    2. Increased pulse and respirations.
    3. Vomiting.
    4. Retractions.
    5. Muscle tremors.
    6. Restlessness.

31. **Which population has a higher incidence of acquiring tuberculosis (TB)? Select all that apply:**
    1. Children 2 years and younger.
    2. Clients who are HIV positive.
    3. Adolescents.
    4. Pregnant women.
    5. African American males.

32. **The school nurse interprets the peak expiratory flow rate for a client with asthma. Which zone signals a *medical alert* and indicates that the client may need their inhaler?**
    1. Green.
    2. Red.
    3. Yellow.
    4. Blue.

33. **When administering drugs during CPR (or a "code"), what would be a *priority* for the nurse?**
    1. Flush with saline between medications to prevent drug interactions.
    2. Check the expiration dates of emergency drugs.
    3. Identify potential adverse reactions of emergency drugs.
    4. Audit the emergency drugs that will be replaced on the medication cart.

34. **What is the *expected outcome* for a client with a nursing diagnosis of ineffective airway clearance related to inflammation?**
    1. Closely monitor blood pH less than 7.25.
    2. Client will experience reduction of anxiety.
    3. Client will breathe easily and without dyspnea.
    4. Teach percussion, postural drainage, and encourage coughing.

35. **The nurse receives a lab value indicating a theophylline level of 23 ug/ml for a client. What is the nurse's expected action?**
    1. Hold the client's morning dose of theophylline.
    2. Inform the physician that the blood level is below the desired therapeutic range.
    3. Have the lab redraw the blood level for verification.
    4. Increase the dose of theophylline for effectiveness.

36. **For a client with a pulmonary embolism, an order is received for a 5000 unit IV Heparin (heparin sodium) bolus followed by a drip at 1800 units per hour. A premixed bag of 25,000 units in 500 ml of dextrose in water is available for the drip. With 20 drop factor tubing, what is the rate of this IV?**

    _____

37. **While a client is receiving a heparin drip, the nurse receives an aPTT (activated partial thromboplastin time) result of 100 seconds. The nurse would anticipate doing which of the following? Select all that apply.**
    1. Assess the client.
    2. Call the physician.
    3. Continue the infusion.
    4. Decrease the drip per nomogram.
    5. Increase the drip per nomogram.
    6. Prepare to administer protamine sulfate.
    7. Prepare to administer vitamin K.
    8. Reassess the aPTT in six hours.
    9. Reassess the aPTT in the morning.
    10. Reassess the aPTT in three hours.
    11. Stop the infusion for one hour.
    12. Stop the infusion for six hours.

38. **Determine if the following are "early" or "late" signs and symptoms of inadequate oxygenation.**

1. ＿＿ Combativeness and/or coma.
2. ＿＿ Cool, clammy skin or cyanosis.
3. ＿＿ Dyspnea on exertion and mild hypertension.
4. ＿＿ Pausing for breath between sentences and words, and dyspnea at rest.
5. ＿＿ Hypotension.
6. ＿＿ Retraction of interspaces on inspiration and use of accessory muscles.
7. ＿＿ Tachycardia and tachypnea.
8. ＿＿ Unexplained apprehension, restlessness, or irritability.

39. **Differentiate which of these is seen with respiratory acidosis (ac) and which is seen with respiratory alkalosis (al).**

1. ＿＿ Apathy, lethargy, and disorientation.
2. ＿＿ CO_2 deficit.
3. ＿＿ Flushing and tachycardia.
4. ＿＿ Hyperactive reflexes and symptoms of tetany.
5. ＿＿ Irritability.
6. ＿＿ Rapid shallow respirations.

Cardiovascular

1. **Before administering digoxin (Lanoxin), what is the most important action for the nurse to take?**
   1. Provide foods high in potassium (K⁺).
   2. Take the client's blood pressure.
   3. Take an apical pulse.
   4. Weigh the client daily.

2. **The client is complaining of a headache after administration of nitroglycerine. What should the nurse instruct the client to do?**
   1. Decrease the nitroglycerine dose.
   2. Do not take the next scheduled dose of nitroglycerine.
   3. Lie down in a cool environment and rest.
   4. Tell a healthcare worker immediately.

3. **The client is diagnosed with angina. What should the nurse teach the client about taking Nitroglycerine SL?**
   1. After taking one SL NTG without a relief of symptoms, the client should call his doctor.
   2. Carry NTG in your pocket when you leave the house.
   3. Replace the NTG every year.
   4. Take NTG before exercising to prevent angina from occurring.

4. **What should the nurse have available if the patient receives an overdose of heparin?**
   1. Iron.
   2. Platelets.
   3. Protamine Sulfate.
   4. Vitamin K.

5. **A client has just been diagnosed with mitral valve stenosis. The nurse is teaching the client about the disease. Place an X on the mitral valve to illustrate its position to the client. Where would the nurse place the X?**

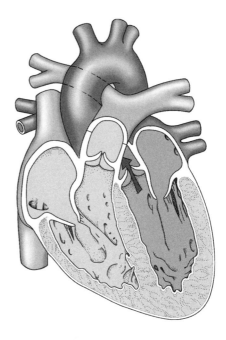

6. **A client has just returned from a cardiac catheterization. Nursing care for this client would include which of the following options?**
   1. Check the extremity, distal to catheterization site for color, temperature, pulse, and capillary refill.
   2. Keep the extremity bent at a 45° angle immediately postoperative.
   3. Keep the head of the bed elevated to 45°.
   4. Place a loose dressing over the catheterization site.

7. The nurse is reading an EKG strip. There are 9 QRS complexes in a six-second strip. What is the client's heart rate?

_____.

8. Modifiable risk factors for atherosclerosis include which of the following? Select all that apply.
   1. Age.
   2. Diet.
   3. Hypercholesterolemia.
   4. Hypertension.
   5. Obesity.
   6. Smoking.
   7. Weight loss.

9. Dyspnea, edema, fatigue, and tachycardia are clinical manifestations of which of the following?
   1. Asthma.
   2. Aortic valve regurgitation.
   3. Heart failure.
   4. Pneumonia.

10. A client with hypotension is being treated with dopamine hydrochloride (Inotropin). Dopamine 400 mg in 250 ml D_5W is ordered at 300 mcg/kg/hr. The client weighs 80 kg. How many cc/hr will the client receive?

_____

11. Which of the following is a manifestation of chronic venous insufficiency?
   1. Dry, necrotic ulcers in the feet.
   2. Edema.
   3. Hair loss.
   4. Thick, deformed toenails.

12. Which of the following may contribute to deep vein thrombosis?
   1. Dehydration, immobility, and oral contraceptives.
   2. Dehydration, oral contraceptives, and a high intake of calcium.
   3. Hypertension, immobility, and dehydration.
   4. Immobility, diabetes, and digoxin (Lanoxin).

13. A client diagnosed with deep vein thrombosis (DVT) has an IV infusion of heparin sodium ordered at 800 units/hour. The concentration in the bag is 10,000 units/100 ml. What should the nurse set the infusion pump at to deliver 800 units/hour?

_____

14. How would the nurse interpret this cardiac rhythm?

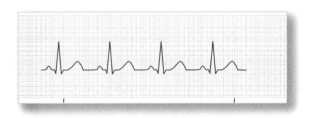

_____

15. When auscultating a client's heart sounds, the nurse hears turbulence occurring between the S1 and S2 heart sounds. The nurse recognizes this finding as indicative of which of the following?
   1. Cardiac murmurs.
   2. Fourth heart sound (S4).
   3. Normal heart sounds.
   4. Third heart sound (S3).

16. **A P wave on an ECG represents an impulse that begins in which of the following?**
    1. In the AV node and depolarizes the atria.
    2. In the AV node and repolarizes the atria.
    3. In the SA node and depolarizes the atria.
    4. In the SA node and repolarizes the atria.

17. **Unmodifiable risk factors for a client with coronary artery disease include which of the following?**
    1. Age.
    2. Cigarette smoking.
    3. Hypertension.
    4. Physical inactivity.

18. **A client in the hospital with angina tells his nurse that he is having chest pain. What does the nurse understand this to mean?**
    1. The client's symptoms are associated with irreversible cardiac muscle damage.
    2. The client is experiencing a heart attack.
    3. The client will have pain relief with rest, nitroglycerine, or both.
    4. The client will have ST changes on the ECG.

19. **Antiplatelet aggregation therapy is a first line of treatment for which of the following?**
    1. Angina.
    2. Arrhythmia.
    3. Pulmonary embolus.
    4. Valve disease.

20. **A client in the CCU is complaining of chest pain. He categorizes his chest pain as a 6 (on a 1 to 10 scale). His BP is 108/72. The nurse gives the client NTG 1/150 sublingual. After 5 minutes, the client states that his chest pain is now a 2. What should the nurse do next?**
    1. Administer another NTG.
    2. Check the blood pressure.
    3. Check the pulse rate.
    4. Obtain an EKG.

21. **A client is experiencing shortness of breath in the supine position, fatigue, jugular vein distention, and a third heart sound (S3). The nurse concludes that these are signs and symptoms of which of the following?**
    1. Coronary artery disease.
    2. Heart failure.
    3. Hypertension.
    4. Valvular heart disease.

22. **Which diuretic is a potassium sparing diuretic?**
    1. Furosemide (Lasix).
    2. Hydrochlorothiazide (Esidrix).
    3. Mannitol (Osmitrol).
    4. Spironolactone (Aldactone).

23. **Which anticoagulant requires less laboratory monitoring and is often used to prevent deep vein thrombosis (DVT) following total knee or hip surgery?**
    1. Aspirin.
    2. Enoxaparin (Lovonox).
    3. Heparin.
    4. Warfarin sodium (Coumadin).

24. **Which is the antidote for a severe warfarin (Coumadin) overdose?**
    1. Protamine zinc.
    2. Protamine sulfate.
    3. Vitamin E.
    4. Vitamin K.

25. **Nursing considerations when administering digoxin (Lanoxin) to an adult include which of the following?**
    1. Holding the medication if the heart rate is above 100 beats per minute.
    2. Instructing the client to eat foods that are low in potassium.
    3. Taking an apical pulse for 15 seconds before administration.
    4. Understanding that signs and symptoms of nausea, vomiting, and anorexia need to be reported to the physician.

26. The nurse interprets this rhythm as:

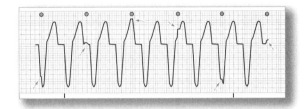

   1. Sinus tachycardia.
   2. Supraventricular tachycardia.
   3. Ventricular fibrillation.
   4. Ventricular tachycardia.

27. The client has the following rhythm, which the nurse interprets as which of the following?

   1. Sinus tachycardia.
   2. Supraventricular tachycardia.
   3. Ventricular fibrillation.
   4. Ventricular tachycardia.

28. A client comes to the ER and states that she has had chest pain lasting for 10 minutes after walking up the steps. After resting, her pain subsided. Which of the following is the client experiencing?

   1. Acute myocardial infarction.
   2. Angina.
   3. Heart failure.
   4. Pneumothorax.

29. Which of the following assessment findings by the nurse indicates right ventricular failure?

   1. A dry hacking cough.
   2. Jugular vein distention.
   3. Nocturia.
   4. Pulmonary edema.

30. When checking capillary refill on a client, the color returns to normal in 10 seconds. The nurse understands that this finding is indicative of which of the following?

   1. Impaired arterial blood flow to the extremities.
   2. Impaired venous blood flow to the extremities.
   3. Normal capillary refill time.
   4. Thrombus formation in the vein.

31. The nurse is giving warfarin (Coumadin) to a client with atrial fibrillation. What does the nurse understand the implications of this medication to be?

   1. Coumadin is helpful in converting atrial fibrillation to sinus rhythm.
   2. Coumadin is used to dissolve clots.
   3. Coumadin is used to prevent heart attacks in clients with atrial fibrillation.
   4. Coumadin is used to prevent strokes in clients with atrial fibrillation.

32. The client is being discharged after his treatment for atrial fibrillation. He will take warfarin (Coumadin) at home. Which of the following statements indicates that the client understands the effects of Coumadin?

   1. "I will begin an exercise program."
   2. "I will get routine PTT levels drawn."
   3. "I will take aspirin instead of Tylenol for my headaches."
   4. "I will use my electric razor for shaving instead of using my razor blades."

33. Place in order the proper sequencing of steps for one-rescuer cardiopulmonary resuscitation (CPR).

   1. Activate Emergency Medical Services (EMS).
   2. Airway.
   3. Assess.
   4. Breathing.
   5. Circulation.
   6. Compression/ventilation.
   7. Continuation of CPR.
   8. Reassessment.

34. **Which of the following is important to teach the client who has received an implantable cardiac defibrillator?**
    1. The client will no longer be allowed to travel by air due to security screening.
    2. Family members should learn CPR.
    3. Routine ICD checks are needed every year.
    4. The ICD is small enough to fit into the client's pockets.

35. **The client who is at risk for infective endocarditis must understand the significance of prophylactic antibiotic therapy before which of the following occurs?**
    1. All chest X-rays.
    2. All dental procedures.
    3. Beginning an exercise program.
    4. Becoming pregnant.

36. **The nurse suspects the presence of a deep vein thrombosis (DVT) based on which of the following findings?**
    1. Coolness of the leg.
    2. Decreased pedal pulses.
    3. Pain in the ankle and foot.
    4. Unilateral leg edema.

37. **Prior to caring for a client who is being treated with enoxaparin (Lovenox) for the treatment of deep vein thrombosis (DVT), the nurse understands which of the following about this medication?**
    1. Routine coagulation tests are required daily.
    2. The nurse must expel air bubbles before administering it subcutaneously.
    3. There is less risk for bleeding complication than with heparin.
    4. Vitamin K partially reverses the effects.

38. **A client is preparing for an exercise stress test. The nurse understands that the client needs additional teaching if he makes which of the following comments?**
    1. "I will not smoke prior to my test."
    2. "I will take my medications the morning of my test."
    3. "I will allow for eight hours of sleep the night prior to the test."
    4. "I will only have coffee the morning of my exam."

39. **An adult client is experiencing cardiac arrest and the nurse is performing CPR. Which of the following is the correct hand position on the client's chest?**
    1. The middle of the sternum.
    2. Over the upper half on the client's chest.
    3. Over the xyphoid process.
    4. Two finger widths above the xyphoid process.

Gastrointestinal

1. **Your client is being treated for chronic cholecystitis. Client education has been ordered. What dietary instructions should the nurse include in the teaching plan?**
   1. An acid-ash diet.
   2. A high fiber diet.
   3. A low fat diet.
   4. A low sodium diet.

2. **The nurse is interviewing a client with acute pancreatitis. What factor is most likely to be present in the client's history?**
   1. Alcohol abuse.
   2. Congestive heart failure.
   3. COPD.
   4. Diabetes mellitus.

3. **Gastric ulcer disease can be managed with minimal medical intervention beyond the initial treatment. However, there is a risk for serious complications of this disease. Which of the following is the most concerning of these complications?**
   1. Anorexia.
   2. Esophagitis.
   3. Pulmonary embolism.
   4. Sudden hemorrhage.

4. **Which of the following is a common link between Crohn's disease and ulcerative colitis?**
   1. Both are inflammatory.
   2. Both have the same degree of mucosal penetration.
   3. Both occur in the same population.
   4. Both share a similar distribution pattern.

5. **A client with a nasogastric tube in place is ordered a sublingual medication. How would the nurse apply her knowledge of medication administration to this situation?**
   1. Change the form of the medication to a liquid, then administer it.
   2. Crush the medication and administer it through the nasogastric tube.
   3. Dissolve the medication in water and administer it through the nasogastric tube.
   4. Place the medication under the client's tongue as indicated.

6. **A client on the surgical unit has an extremely long horizontal incision held together with a continuous suture line. The oncoming nurse must implement the order to increase activity to walking in the hall three times every day. The nurse reviews the client history and considers the risk factors for wound dehiscence. What risk factors should the nurse recall? Select all that apply.**
   1. Abdominal distention.
   2. Altered mental status.
   3. Dehydration.
   4. Increased abdominal pressure.
   5. Low hemoglobin.
   6. Obesity.
   7. Pain medication administration.
   8. Wound infection.

7. The nurse is assessing the abdomen of a client who is admitted to the emergency department for treatment of multiple problems. Which finding would justify further investigation?
   1. Asymmetry of the lower quadrants.
   2. Concave umbilicus.
   3. Flat appearance below the umbilicus.
   4. Rounded abdominal contour.

8. The nurse is teaching a family member how to position a client to receive tube feedings in the home. Which of the following positions by the family reveals an understanding of the education given by the nurse?
   1. Allowing the client to assume their position of comfort.
   2. Elevating the head of the bed 10°.
   3. Placing the client in the left-side lying position.
   4. Positioning the client in a chair.

9. A client is 5'9" and weighs 98 lbs. She has tenting (delayed) skin turgor, pallored coloring, and admits to anorexia and diarrhea. Which of the following data would be consistent with her diagnosis of malabsorption?
   1. Calcium 17 mg/dl.
   2. Infiltrates bilaterally.
   3. Hgb 7.6 g/dl, Hct 24%.
   4. K+ 7.1 mEq/L.

10. A client with acute gastritis is admitted to the medical unit. Blood tests are drawn and reveal the following results:

Sodium	135 mEq/L
Potassium	2.3 mEq/L
Chloride	96 mEq/L
CO_2	32 mEq/L
Glucose	145 mg/dL

Which of these results should the nurse identify as critical and report immediately?

11. Your client is scheduled for a barium enema. He asks why a laxative is necessary the evening before the test. How would the nurse best respond in order to help the client understand the procedure?
   1. "Because the doctor ordered it."
   2. "It assists with emptying the bowel for the best visualization."
   3. "It is our procedure at this facility."
   4. "It makes the X-ray more clear."

12. Skin care is especially important for the client with an ileostomy. The nurse develops a plan of care for prevention of skin breakdown for such a client. This plan is constructed based on the understanding of which of the following?
   1. Ileostomy bags are not sterile.
   2. Ileostomy drainage contains enzymes.
   3. No skin barrier is applied with an ileostomy.
   4. The fecal content collected is firm.

13. A client was recently in an automobile accident and has multiple injuries requiring surgery. Postoperatively she is being treated for a paralytic ileus (adynamic ileus). The nurse determines which of the following would most likely be ordered for a client with a paralytic ileus?
   1. Antacids.
   2. Bulk-forming agent.
   3. Nasogastric tube insertion.
   4. Truss application.

14. **A client in critical condition is recovering after a major abdominal surgery lasting nine hours. The physician is requesting the total number of milliliters the client received in the operating room. The fluids administered include:**

Lactated ringers at 150 ml/hour
Cefazolin sodium (Ancef) 2 gm IV piggyback
    in 100 ml of normal saline
Two units of packed RBCs at 275 ml and
    250 ml
Bolus of 250 ml normal saline every four hours
Ranitidine (Zantac) 50 mg IV in 50 ml D_5W
    over 30 minutes

How many milliliters will the nurse report as the total amount of fluid intake during surgery?

_____

15. **A client comes to the ER with complaints of "stomach pains." What approach would the nurse use to conduct a physical examination of the abdomen?**
    1. Auscultation, percussion, palpation, and inspection.
    2. Inspection, auscultation, percussion, and palpation.
    3. Inspection, palpation, percussion, and auscultation.
    4. Palpation, percussion, auscultation, and inspection.

16. **A client returns to the unit after an endoscopy to investigate frequent throat burning. In order to implement the safest position postendoscopy, the nurse would select which of the following for the client?**
    1. High Fowler's.
    2. Prone.
    3. Reverse Trendelenberg.
    4. Side-lying.

17. **A 56-year-old client is admitted with cirrhosis of the liver. Which of the following should the nurse expect to be in the plan of care? Select all that apply.**
    1. Administration of furosemide (Lasix).
    2. Administration of warfarin (Coumadin).
    3. A calorie reduction diet.
    4. A chest X-ray everyday while the client is acute.
    5. A liver function blood test.
    6. The client should be up in hallway two times each shift.

18. **The nurse is assessing a client post abdominal laparoscopy. The client is complaining of shoulder discomfort and wants to know if this is normal? How should the nurse respond?**
    1. "I'm not sure, I'll check with your doctor."
    2. "No, this should not occur. I will call your doctor immediately."
    3. "No, you must have strained your shoulder in some way. Let me massage it out for you."
    4. "Yes, this may occur due to the filling of the abdominal cavity with carbon dioxide for better viewing."

19. **A 16-year-old male client reports to the nurse that he is experiencing nausea, anorexia, and vomiting. His mother reports a low-grade fever with tenderness over his right lower stomach area. Based on the above findings, the nurse determines the client is most likely experiencing what inflammatory disorder?**

_____

20. "My head, my head," yells a client being seen at a physician's office. The nurse practitioner reviews the client's history and discovers a new diagnosis of GERD with drug therapy initiated 10 days ago. What inference can be made based on this information?
   1. A diagnosis of GERD can lead to headaches.
   2. The client did not start the drug therapy as directed.
   3. The client is exhibiting a side effect that may occur with ranitidine (Zantac).
   4. There must be a brain tumor present.

21. An elderly client with a history of COPD presents to the emergency room with complaints of foul diarrhea, nausea, and abdominal tenderness. He was just discharged three days ago after receiving treatment for a severe urinary tract infection. Considering this data, what conclusion can the nurse come to?
   1. A bowel infection with *Clostridium difficile* has occurred.
   2. Dinner last evening did not agree with this client.
   3. The client has now caught the flu.
   4. The urinary tract infection is back.

22. During the assessment of a client with diverticular disease, where would the nurse anticipate abdominal pain?
   1. Lower left quadrant.
   2. Upper left quadrant.
   3. Lower right quadrant.
   4. Upper right quadrant.

23. Constipation is a problem in the elderly population. Identify an appropriate outcome for interventions aimed at preventing or minimizing constipation.
   1. The client should avoid physical exercise.
   2. The client should drink one or two glasses of water daily.
   3. The client should eat a high-fiber diet.
   4. The client should maintain a sedentary lifestyle.

24. Which of the following represents the best evaluation criteria for monitoring the effectiveness of treatment aimed at reducing aggravating factors with the diagnosis of cholecystitis?
   1. The client displays no improvement on ultrasonography.
   2. The client maintains a serum albumin level within normal limits.
   3. The client maintains intake and output within normal limits.
   4. The client reports no pain following a low-fat meal.

25. At 3:30 AM, a bowel section postoperative client has a new 1000 ml bag of IV fluid hung by the nurse. If the IV infuses at 120 ml/hour as ordered, how much fluid should infuse by 6 AM?

   _____

26. A client admitted with GERD is to be discharged this afternoon. Which of the following statements, if made by the client, reveals the understanding of the teaching on this disorder?
   1. "I can eat whatever I want."
   2. "I no longer need to use a pillow and will sleep on my side."
   3. "I will lie down after meals."
   4. "I will sleep with the head of my bed elevated."

27. A client has a new colostomy and is to start a teaching program based on the information needed for care in the home. The nurse understands the pathophysiology of the sigmoid colon when he or she educates the client that the stool from a colostomy at the sigmoid colon area will be in which of the following presentations?
   1. Formed.
   2. Liquid.
   3. Pastelike.
   4. Semisoft.

28. Following an open cholecystectomy, the plan of care includes measures to prevent postoperative complications. Which of the following are measures to prevent postoperative complications in clients with an open cholecystectomy? Select all that apply.

1. Educating the client on the use of an incentive spirometry.
2. Medicating the client with a stool softener at bedtime to ensure soft bowel movements the next day.
3. Medicating for pain reduction with opiates.
4. Monitoring the nasogastric tube for proper functioning.
5. Providing a mechanical soft diet only after return of the gag reflex.
6. Removing the T-Tube after the first ambulation.

29. A client has experienced an acute episode of gastritis but wishes to start eating again. The nurse understands that the protective barrier to the stomach has been penetrated, therefore, the nurse should recommend which of the following examples of food to start out with?

1. Broth, coffee, and juice.
2. Cream soup, diet cola, and ice cream.
3. Gelatin, water, and toast.
4. Milk, sherbet, and toast.

30. A client is suspected of having hepatitis A. The nurse understands that this client mostly likely contracted this type of hepatitis in which of the following ways?

1. The client was born of a mother who is hepatitis positive.
2. The client has received several blood transfusions in the past.
3. The client has been on recent missionary work to a third world country.
4. The client is using intravenous street drugs.

31. A client with advanced liver disease presents with vomiting blood, tachycardia, cool, clammy skin, restlessness, and lethargy. All signs indicate a complication of portal hypertension. Based on the findings, the nurse determines the client is experiencing which complication of portal hypertension?

1. Cirrhosis of the liver.
2. Bleeding esophageal varices.
3. Hepatomegaly.
4. Duodenal ulcer.

32. The client is admitted with a diagnosis of Hepatitis B. Which of the following orders would the nurse question if prescribed?

1. Administration of antiemetics for nausea and vomiting.
2. A low-fat, high calorie diet.
3. Strict intake and output monitoring.
4. Instructions for the client to be up in a chair three times a day.

33. The nurse is completing a medication review of a client newly diagnosed with elevated cholesterol levels. During the review, the nurse should pay close attention to which factor since the client is also taking an anticoagulant?

1. Attempting to follow a low-fat diet.
2. Family usage of a cholesterol lowering agent.
3. Sprinkling flax seeds on breakfast food every day.
4. Using garlic as a cholesterol lowering agent.

34. The nurse practitioner has prescribed lansoprazole (Prevacid) 15 mg PO to be given once a day. Which time would the nurse schedule the medication to be given?

1. After lunch.
2. Any time would produce the therapeutic effect.
3. Before breakfast.
4. With the evening meal.

35. A client was recently started on docusate sodium (Colace). Which statement from the client indicates that the therapeutic effect of this medication has been achieved?

1. "I am finally having regular bowel movements."
2. "My stomach pain is gone!"
3. "My stools are no longer green."
4. "There is no more blood in my bowel movements."

36. A client comes to the emergency room with suspected gastrointestional bleeding. In planning care, which of the following would be a nursing priority for this client?

1. Assessing vital signs.
2. Explaining the procedure for an upper GI series.
3. Investigating the client's pain history.
4. Testing emesis for blood.

37. A client has an order for a "high cleansing enema." Based on the nurse's knowledge, how will the enema be administered?

1. At a level of comfort for the client.
2. At eight inches above the anus.
3. Level with the upper, exposed hip.
4. Slowly raised above the recommended height of 12 inches.

38. Post hemicolectomy, a client asks why he has a nasogastric tube. The nurse's best response for the client would be:

1. "It will be out shortly, then you can eat."
2. "It will help with your belly pain."
3. "The tube decompresses your stomach of the gas and fluid contents so the surgical site can begin healing."
4. "Your doctor wants you to have it."

Renal and Genitourinary

1. A client comes to the emergency department with renal failure. Which of the following lab results would you expect to see from this client?
   1. pH 7.25, HCO_3 20, PCO_2 30.
   2. pH 7.30, HCO_3 22, PCO_2 50.
   3. pH 7.50, HCO_3 20, PCO_2 32.
   4. pH 7.55, HCO_3 28, PCO_2 31.

2. A patient presents to the hemodialysis unit for his first treatment since his diagnosis of end stage renal disease. He states to the dialysis nurse, "I decided to come today, but I am not sure if I will need to come back again this week. I am feeling much better since my discharge from the hospital and I think my kidneys are working again." This patient is demonstrating which stage of Kübler-Ross's stages of dying?
   1. Bargaining.
   2. Denial.
   3. Depression.
   4. Anger.

3. A client is admitted to the hospital with a serum potassium level of 6.8. Which one of the following meds would you administer to treat this electrolyte imbalance?
   1. Lactulose 15 ml PO.
   2. Renagel 800 mg PO.
   3. Kayexalate 30 grams PO.
   4. Aranesp 100 mcg/ml SQ.

4. According to the following lab results, which one indicates renal failure?
   1. BUN 10, serum creatinine 0.3.
   2. BUN 45, serum creatinine 1.0.
   3. BUN 11, serum creatinine 10.
   4. BUN 35, serum creatinine 8.

5. How would you classify the oliguric phase of acute renal failure (ARF)?
   1. Normal renal tubular function is reestablished during this phase.
   2. BUN and serum creatinine levels begin to decrease.
   3. Fluid output is less than 400 ml per 24 hours.
   4. Fluid output is greater than 1000 ml per 24 hours.

6. A client on hemodialysis with chronic renal failure (CRF) has been educated by the dietician on limiting foods high in potassium in his diet. The client would be taught about consumption of which of the following food selections that are high in potassium. Select all that apply.
   1. Orange juice.
   2. Tomatoes.
   3. Bananas.
   4. Corn flakes.
   5. Raisins.

7. A client being discharged to home with a new vascular access to the right forearm needs teaching about Steal syndrome. As the discharge nurse, which of the following signs and symptoms would you educate the client about?

   1. A raised red rash around the vascular access site.
   2. Bleeding profusely from the vascular access site.
   3. Cold and numb fingers of the right arm.
   4. Foul smelling drainage from vascular access site.

8. A client comes back to the floor after his first hemodialysis treatment. He displays symptoms of confusion, vomiting, and restlessness. By what name is this complication of hemodialysis known?

   1. Dialysis disequilibrium syndrome.
   2. Steal syndrome.
   3. Peritonitis.
   4. Septicemia.

9. After a client's hemodialysis treatment, a nurse would expect to find an improvement with which of the following blood values?

   1. Hgb/Hct.
   2. Calcium.
   3. Ammonia.
   4. Potassium.

10. A client on hemodialysis with chronic renal failure (CRF) has been educated by the dietician on limiting foods high in phosphorus in her diet. The client would be taught about consumption of which of the following food selections that are high in phosphorus? Select all that apply.

    1. Milk.
    2. Nuts.
    3. Orange juice.
    4. Bread.

11. In teaching a new client with chronic renal failure about the process of peritoneal dialysis (PD), the nurse would explain which of the following to the client?

    1. PD occurs when blood is filtered through an artificial device called a dialyzer.
    2. PD is the dialysis of choice for clients with abdominal trauma.
    3. PD has fewer dietary and fluid restrictions than hemodialysis.
    4. PD is the treatment of choice with acute conditions.

12. A client has a history of having renal calculi (stone) formation. What type of diet should this client avoid?

    1. A low protein diet.
    2. A low phosphorous diet.
    3. A high dietary intake of calcium.
    4. A high fluid intake.

13. Which of the following serum or urine lab values would a nurse expect to find in a client with dehydration?

    1. Decreased specific gravity.
    2. Decreased BUN.
    3. Increased BUN.
    4. Ketones.

14. Which of the following is the lab value that measures the end product of muscle and protein metabolism and is used to diagnosis renal disease?

    1. Bilirubin.
    2. Specific gravity.
    3. BUN (blood urea nitrogen).
    4. Creatinine.

15. A client with chronic renal failure (CRF) may display which of the following metabolic disturbances in relation to the disease's clinical manifestations? Select all that apply.

    1. Sleep disturbances.
    2. Restless leg syndrome.
    3. Pneumonia.
    4. Pruritus/dry skin.

16. **What is the most important serious complication that the nurse must monitor for after a client has a percutaneous renal biopsy?**
    1. Infection.
    2. Flank pain.
    3. Urinary retention.
    4. Bleeding.

17. **Which of the following is the most appropriate nursing intervention for a client who has had an intravenous pyelogram (IVP)?**
    1. Assess the client for hematuria in the urine.
    2. Check the insertion site for bleeding.
    3. Offer the client a warm sitz bath.
    4. Force fluids.

18. **Which condition would contraindicate a client from having a renal transplant?**
    1. Having hepatitis B.
    2. Having a pacemaker.
    3. Being 65-years-old.
    4. Having a chronic infection.

19. **A client is scheduled to have a renal biopsy. Prior to the procedure, what is the nurse's responsibility? Select all that apply.**
    1. Type and cross the client for blood.
    2. Ensure the consent form is signed.
    3. Administer prednisone and benadryl for a minor allergy to iodine.
    4. Make client NPO for four to six hours before the procedure.
    5. Obtain coagulation studies.
    6. Clamp the client's Foley before the procedure.
    7. Have the client hold Coumadin for three days before the procedure.
    8. Have the client remove all metal objects.

20. **Which of the following drugs is used to treat benign prostatic hypertrophy (BPH)?**
    1. Danazol (Danocrine).
    2. Finasteride (Proscar, Propecia).
    3. Fluoxymesterone (Halotestin).
    4. Methyltestosterone (Android).

21. **When a client has been ordered phenazopyridine (Pyridium), the nurse needs to educate the client about which of the following expected side effects of this drug?**
    1. Burning during urination.
    2. Reddish orange urine.
    3. Hematuria.
    4. Hypertension.

22. **A nurse assesses a client who was just newly diagnosed with chronic renal failure. The nurse forms a nursing diagnosis of "Anticipatory Grieving" due to which of the following statements?**
    1. "I know that I will get a kidney transplant; I am healthy."
    2. "I can now eat whatever I want. It will be dialyzed out of my system."
    3. "I can never have sex with my wife again because I might become impotent."
    4. "I know that renal failure runs in my family and I can prevent it."

23. **After a renal biopsy, the most appropriate nursing interventions are which of the following? Select all that apply.**
    1. Dipstick urine for hematuria.
    2. Assess for flank pain.
    3. Monitor for extravasation of tissue surrounding the site.
    4. Encourage ambulation.
    5. Administer aspirin for pain.
    6. Offer the client a warm sitz bath.
    7. Monitor the client's ketone level.
    8. Monitor the client's temperature.

24. The nurse is discharging a client from the hospital. The nurse knows that client has knowledge of their new prescription of furosemide (Lasix) when the client states which of the following?
1. "I have to eat a diet low in potassium."
2. "I have to limit my fluid intake."
3. "My blood pressure will increase while I am on this medication."
4. "I need to limit my sun exposure and wear sunscreen while on this medication."

25. The nurse caring for a client with benign prostatic hyperplasia (BPH) understands which of the following about the symptoms of this disease process?
1. Symptoms are acutely present with the onset of prostate enlargement.
2. Symptoms gradually lessen as the degree of obstruction increases.
3. Symptoms are experienced by the client as a result of urinary obstruction.
4. Symptoms are primarily urinary retention and infection.

26. The nurse caring for an adult client with polycystic kidney disease (PKD) knows that an early and commonly seen symptom of this disease process would be which of the following?
1. Steady, dull flank pain.
2. Hypotension.
3. Confusion.
4. Sharp back pain.

27. In planning nursing interventions to help relieve urinary symptoms in a patient with interstitial cystitis (IC), the nurse should include which of the following?
1. Informing the client that a urinary tract infection (UTI) is unlikely to develop.
2. Educating the client on dietary restrictions necessary to control painful symptoms.
3. Informing the client that high potency vitamins are recommended.
4. Educating the client to drink tea instead of coffee.

28. During an assessment of the renal system, the nurse uses the

_____

landmark for locating the kidneys, which is located between the lower portion of the twelfth rib and the vertebral column.

29. A client is admitted to the hospital with acute poststreptococcal glomerulonephritis (APSGN). Which of the following is the nurse's top priority in caring for this patient?
1. Encouraging a high protein diet.
2. Encouraging fluid intake.
3. Administering diuretics and antihypertensives.
4. Administering corticosteroids.

30. As compared to younger adults, older adults who experience urinary tract infections (UTIs) tend to exhibit the following primary clinical manifestations.
1. Fever and chills.
2. Dysuria and flank pain.
3. Suprapubic pain.
4. Cognitive impairment, fatigue, and anorexia.

31. A nurse would educate a client who was recovering from shock that their kidney function was altered from the trauma. The nurse would state that the client was in acute renal failure and that their kidneys were going to go through phases of recovery. List the phases of acute renal failure in order from the initial injury to the stabilization of kidney function.
1. Diuretic phase.
2. Onset phase.
3. Oliguric phase.
4. Recovery phase.

32. **For a patient with a recurrent urinary tract infection (UTI), which of the following statements describe the primary drug therapy regimen for this disease process?**

    1. A one- to three-day treatment regimen of antibiotic therapy.
    2. A three- to five-day treatment regimen of antibiotic therapy.
    3. Consideration of a 10-day trial of suppressive antibiotic therapy.
    4. Phenazopyridine (Pyridium) to relieve discomfort associated with a UTI.

33. **A client with recurrent urinary tract infections (UTIs) is educated by the nurse on the disease process and health promotion measures. The following statement from the client would indicate to the nurse the need for further instruction.**

    1. "I will need to wipe my perineal area from back to front after urination."
    2. "I will need to empty my bladder regularly and completely."
    3. "I will need to evacuate my bowels regularly."
    4. "I need to drink an adequate amount of liquid each day."

34. **A client with a new ileal conduit presents to your nursing unit. While planning her care, the nurse determines that the following nursing diagnoses would relate to this client's needs. Select all that apply.**

    1. Anxiety.
    2. Disturbed body image.
    3. Risk for impaired skin integrity.
    4. Risk for infection.

35. **The nurse identifies a risk factor for a urinary tract infection in a patient who relates a history of which of the following?**

    1. COPD.
    2. Diabetes mellitus.
    3. Anemia.
    4. Osteoporosis.

36. **Postoperative management of an ileal conduit should include which of the following? Select all that apply.**

    1. Planning care to prevent surgical complications such as atelectasis and shock.
    2. Encouraging the client to increase fluid intake to help flush the ileal conduit.
    3. Educating the client that shrinkage of the stoma site is a sign of poor healing.
    4. Educating the client about signs of infection and possible obstruction.

37. **A client with nephrotic syndrome is educated by the nurse on his disease and course of treatment. The following statement from the client would indicate a need for further instruction.**

    1. "I can expect to experience swelling in my hands and feet."
    2. "The protein in my blood will probably be low and my cholesterol may be high."
    3. "I will need to take medication to control the swelling and high cholesterol."
    4. "I may eat a diet that is not restricted in salt or protein."

38. **Indications for use of urinary catheterization include which of the following? Select all that apply.**

    1. Relief of urinary retention.
    2. Convenience for the nursing staff or client's family.
    3. Measurement of residual urine after urination.
    4. Routine acquisition of a urine specimen.

39. **A client presents with urinary incontinence after surgery. She experiences leakage of small amounts of urine frequently during the day and night, along with urinating frequently in small amounts. Her bladder has been distended and is usually palpable upon examination. The physician has ordered urinary catheterization to treat this urinary incontinence, which is known as which of the following?**

1. Stress incontinence.
2. Urge incontinence.
3. Overflow incontinence.
4. Reflex incontinence.

40. **A client develops urge incontinence. Methods of treatment that can be used with this type of urinary incontinence may include which of the following? Select all that apply.**

1. Use of anticholingergic drugs.
2. Use of vaginal estrogen creams.
3. Use of calcium channel blockers.
4. Use of urinary catheterization.

Endocrine

1. The nurse has just reviewed instructions for an oral glucose tolerance test (OGTT) with a client. Which of the following statements made by the client indicate a need for more teaching?
   1. "I will eat a light breakfast the morning of the test."
   2. "I will expect to take 100 mg of glucose at the start of the test."
   3. "I can expect to have my blood drawn at 30 and 60 minute intervals during the test."
   4. "I will report any symptoms of dizziness, sweating, and/or weakness if they occur during the test."

2. A client presents with a diagnosis of hypopituitarism. When performing the history and physical exam, which of the following findings should the nurse anticipate?
   1. Increased cardiac output.
   2. Truncal obesity.
   3. Increased blood pressure.
   4. Hyperactivity or increased energy levels.

3. A client presents to the clinic with a diagnosis of acromegaly. Which of the following should the nurse expect to see during the physical examination of the client? Select all that apply.
   1. Large hands and feet.
   2. Thickening and protruding of the jaw.
   3. Arthritic changes.
   4. Diaphoresis.
   5. Organomegaly.
   6. Hypotension.
   7. Dysphagia.
   8. Deepening of the voice.

4. Following a hypophysectomy, the client complains of clear nasal drainage. What is the most appropriate initial action for the nurse?
   1. Notify the surgeon immediately.
   2. Encourage the client to blow his nose to clear the sinuses.
   3. Check the nasal drainage for glucose.
   4. Place the client in Trendelenberg position.

5. The nurse would expect the client with Addison's crisis to exhibit which of the following signs and symptoms? Select all that apply.
   1. Generalized weakness.
   2. Cardiovascular collapse.
   3. Shock.
   4. Severe hypertension.
   5. Severe hypotension.
   6. Abdominal pain.

6. Following a hypophysectomy, the nurse teaches the client to report which of the following?
   1. Cushing's disease.
   2. Grave's disease.
   3. Diabetes mellitus.
   4. Hypopituitarism.

7. Vasopressin (Pitressin) is ordered for the client with diabetes insipidus in order to do which of the following?
   1. Stimulate the pancreas to secrete insulin.
   2. Slow the absorption of glucose in the intestine.
   3. Increase reabsorption of water in the tubules.
   4. Increase blood pressure.

8. A client presents at the clinic with a diagnosis of Cushing's syndrome. Which of the following symptoms would the nurse expect to find during the physical examination? Select all that apply.
   1. Fat deposits in the abdominal region (truncal obesity).
   2. Fat pads over the upper back (buffalo hump).
   3. Round (moon) face.
   4. Muscle weakness and wasting.
   5. Hypotension and brachycardia.
   6. Thinning and bruising of the skin.

9. Dietary management of the client with Addison's disease includes which of the following?
   1. High protein, high calcium, low calorie, high nutrition.
   2. Low protein, high calcium, low calorie, high nutrition.
   3. Low protein, high calcium, high calorie, high nutrition.
   4. Low protein, low calcium, high calorie, high nutrition.

10. The client with Addison's disease is ordered glucocorticoid therapy. Which of the following statements indicates that the client has a correct understanding of the medication regimen?
   1. "Dosage adjustments in my medication dosages may be needed."
   2. "On days I feel good, I will not need to take the medication."
   3. "I will adjust my dosages based on my home blood glucose test results."
   4. "I am on an every-other-day dosing regimen."

11. Which of the following lab results would be typical of the client with Addison's disease?
   1. Blood urine nitrogen (BUN) of 3.5 mg/dl.
   2. Sodium (NA) of 185 mEq/L.
   3. Fasting blood glucose (FBS) of 55 mg/dl.
   4. Potassiuim (K) of 2.7 mEq/L.

12. The client with Addison's disease may present with which of the following signs and symptoms?
   1. Muscle spasms.
   2. Hunger.
   3. Fatigue and emotional labiality.
   4. Weight gain.

13. A client has undergone surgery for removal of the adrenal gland (adrenalectomy). Postoperatively, it is important for the nurse to monitor which of the following? Select all that apply.
   1. Intake and output.
   2. Electrolytes.
   3. WBC levels.
   4. Temperature.

14. A client presents with a diagnosis of Cushing's disease. Physical assessment by the nurse reveals which of the following findings?
   1. Bruised areas on the skin.
   2. Postural hypotension.
   3. Weight loss.
   4. Decreased body hair.

15. After pituitary surgery, the nurse should carefully assess the client and report which of the following findings immediately?
   1. A urine test positive for glucose and ketones.
   2. A blood glucose level greater than 450 mg/dl.
   3. Urine output of 1–2 liters/day.
   4. Urine specific gravity less than 1.010.

16. **A patient presents to the outpatient clinic with a diagnosis of hyperthyroidism. During the physical assessment of this client, which of the following signs and symptoms would the nurse expect to find? Select all that apply.**
    1. Enlarged thyroid (goiter).
    2. Weight gain.
    3. Intolerance to cold.
    4. Generalized puffiness and edema around the eyes and face.
    5. Palpitations.
    6. Bradycardia.
    7. Hypertension.
    8. Nervousness and fine tremors of the hands.
    9. Protruding eyeballs (exophthalmos).
    10. Loss of body hair.

17. **Which of the following lab results are consistent with a diagnosis of Cushing's disease?**
    1. A two hour postprandial blood glucose of 40 mg/dl.
    2. A urinary calcium level of 6.2 mg/dl.
    3. A potassium (K) level of 2.7 mEq/L.
    4. A sodium (Na) level of 128 mEq/L.

18. **A client is undergoing thyroid tests (T_3, T_4, TSH) for hypothyroidism. Which of the following laboratory test results are indicative of hypothyroidism?**
    1. Elevated T_3 & T_4 levels and normal TSH.
    2. Normal T_3 & T_4 levels and elevated TSH.
    3. Elevated T_3 & T_4 levels and decreased TSH.
    4. Decreased T_3 & T_4 levels and elevated TSH.

19. **A patient is newly diagnosed with hypothyroidism. During the physical assessment of this client, the nurse would expect to identify which of the following signs and symptoms? Select all that apply.**
    1. Enlarged thyroid (goiter).
    2. Weight gain.
    3. Protruding eyeballs (exophthalmas).
    4. Hypertension.
    5. Nervousness and fine tremors of hands.

6. Intolerance to cold.
7. Palpitations.
8. Bradycardia.
9. Loss of body hair.
10. Generalized puffiness and edema around the eyes and face.

20. **A client is admitted with a diagnosis of hyperthyroidism rule out (r/o) Grave's disease. The nurse assessing the client would expect to find which of the following?**
    1. Weight gain.
    2. Anorexia.
    3. Cold skin.
    4. Tachycardia.

21. **In explaining the use of radioactive iodine (RAI) in the treatment of Grave's disease, which of the following statements made by the nurse best describes how the medication works?**
    1. The radioactive iodine decreases the levels of thyroid hormone by slowing the body's production.
    2. The radioactive iodine reduces the uptake of thyroxine.
    3. Radioactive iodine stabilizes the thyroid hormone levels preoperatively in preparation for a thyroidectomy.
    4. Radioactive iodine destroys thyroid tissue so the thyroid hormones are no longer produced.

22. **A client is taking levothyroxene sodium (Synthroid) for treatment of hypothyroidism. The client should verbalize which of the following regarding her medication regimen?**
    1. "The medication should be taken prn to alleviate symptoms."
    2. "The medication should be taken in divided doses to ensure therapeutic drug levels."
    3. "The medication should be taken in the morning to prevent sleeplessness."
    4. "The medication must be taken on an empty stomach."

23. **A client is taking methimazole (Tapazol) for treatment of hyperthyroidism. The client correctly verbalizes which of the following regarding her medication regimen?**
    1. "The medication should be taken on an empty stomach."
    2. "The medication should be taken in divided doses."
    3. "The medication should be taken at the same time each day."
    4. "The medication should be taken as needed when symptoms occur."

24. **The nurse is teaching a patient newly diagnosed with Type 1 diabetes mellitus how to administer insulin injections. Place the following steps in the correct order for drawing up and administering a dose of 25 units of NPH insulin.**
    1. Wash hands.
    2. Draw back 25 units of air into the syringe and inject air into the insulin vial.
    3. Inject insulin.
    4. Withdraw 25 units of NPH insulin.
    5. Gently roll vial of NPH insulin.
    6. Inspect for and remove air bubbles.
    7. Choose and cleanse the site.
    8. Cleanse the top of the insulin vial with alcohol.

25. **In explaining the use of levothyroxine sodium (Synthroid) in treating hypothyroidism, which of the following best explains how the medication works?**
    1. The medication works to decrease the levels of thyroid hormone by decreasing the body's production of the hormone.
    2. The medication reduces the uptake of thyroxin.
    3. The medication stimulates the thyroid gland to produce more thyroid hormone.
    4. The medication replaces the thyroid hormone that is not being produced in sufficient amounts.

26. **Which of the following is the most significant controllable risk factor in the development of Type 2 diabetes mellitus?**
    1. Hypertension.
    2. Family history of diabetes.
    3. Cigarette smoking.
    4. Obesity.

27. **A patient diagnosed with Type 2 diabetes mellitus is admitted to the hospital with a blood glucose level of 800 mg/dl and a diagnosis of hyperosmolar hyperglycemic nonketotic syndrome (HHNKS). Which of the following symptoms would the nurse expect to find?**
    1. Fruity breath odor.
    2. Dehydration.
    3. Urine posture for ketones.
    4. Hypertension.

28. **The nurse is teaching a client how to draw up their insulin. The client is taking 5 units Humulin R and 15 units of Humulin N insulin. Please place the following steps in the correct order for mixing these insulins in a single syringe for the injection.**
    1. Gently roll vial of NPH insulin.
    2. Draw back 5 units of air into the syringe and inject into the vial of Humulin R insulin.
    3. Wash hands.
    4. Draw up 15 units of air into the syringe and inject into the vial of Humulin N insulin.
    5. Cleanse the tops of both insulin vials with alcohol.
    6. Draw up 5 units of Humulin R insulin into the syringe.
    7. Check for and remove any bubbles from Humulin R insulin.
    8. Insert needle into skin at selected site and inject 20 units of insulin.
    9. Draw up 15 units of Humulin N insulin into the syringe.
    10. Choose and cleanse the site.

29. During a home visit, the visiting nurse finds a patient with Type 1 diabetes who has been experiencing flu-like symptoms for the last 14–16 hours. Which of the following statements made by the patient indicates a need for more teaching?
    1. "I am testing my blood glucose every 3–4 hours."
    2. "I am testing my urine for ketones every 3–4 hours."
    3. "I am holding my insulin until my appetite returns."
    4. "I am drinking liquids (water and broth) every hour."

30. The nurse administers 24 units of NPH insulin to a patient at 8:00 AM. When does the nurse feel that the client is most likely to develop a hypoglycemic reaction?
    1. Between 8:00 AM and 10:00 AM.
    2. Between 10:00 AM and 12:00 PM.
    3. Between 2:00 PM and 10:00 PM.
    4. Between 10:00 PM and 8:00 AM the next day.

31. The nurse administers a dose of six units of regular insulin (Humulin R) to a patient at 8:00 AM. Knowing the action of regular insulin, when would the nurse anticipate that a hypoglycemia reaction could occur?
    1. Between 8:00 AM and 10:00 AM.
    2. Between 10:00 AM and 12:00 PM.
    3. Between 2:00 PM and 10:00 PM.
    4. Between 10:00 PM and 8:00 AM the next day.

32. A second generation patient with Type 2 diabetes mellitus is prescribed the oral hypoglycemia agent glyburide (Micronase, DiaBeta, Glynase). How does the nurse explain the basic mechanism of action of this medication in lowering blood glucose?
    1. It stimulates the pancreas to release insulin.
    2. It potentates the action of insulin.
    3. It increases the renal threshold of glucose.
    4. It decreases the renal threshold of glucose.

33. The nurse checks the patient's finger stick blood glucose and identifies a test result of 40 mg/dl. Which of the following signs/symptoms might the client be experiencing with this blood glucose result? Select all that apply.
    1. Tachycardia.
    2. Palpitations.
    3. Diaphoresis.
    4. Tremors.
    5. Headache.
    6. Dizziness.
    7. Irritability.
    8. Confusion.
    9. Thirst.

34. The nurse is working with a patient who is just beginning to use their new external insulin pump. Which statement made by the client indicates a need for more teaching regarding the use of the pump?
    1. "I will change my tubing and site every three days."
    2. "I will use only regular insulin (buffered) in my pump."
    3. "My pump delivers a continuous (basal) rate of insulin and I will use it to deliver additional (bolus) insulin with meals."
    4. "When I disconnect the pump overnight, I will use the sterile cap to cover the end of the tubing."

35. A client presents with lipodystrophy on both upper thighs. It would be most important for the nurse to assess which of the following?
    1. Whether the client aspirates before administering the insulin.
    2. Whether the client administers the insulin at a 45° angle.
    3. Whether the client cleanses the site with alcohol before each injection.
    4. Whether the client rotates injection sites using sites other than the thighs.

36. **A client presents to the clinic with a blood glucose level of 600 mg/dl. Which of the following signs and symptoms would the nurse expect to find during the physical assessment? Select all that apply.**

   1. Increased hunger (polyphagia).
   2. Increased thirst (polydypsia).
   3. Increased urination (polyuria).
   4. Cold, clammy skin.
   5. Fatigue.

37. **A patient with Type 2 diabetes mellitus is admitted to the emergency room with a blood glucose of 846 mg/dl and is complaining of polyuria, polydypsia, polyphasia, weight loss, and weakness. The nurse reviews the physical documentation and would expect to see which of the following diagnoses?**

   1. Porphyria.
   2. Pheochromocytoma.
   3. Diabetic ketoacedosis (DKA).
   4. Hyperosmolar hyperglycemic nonketotic syndrome (HHNKS).

38. **A patient with Type 2 diabetes mellitus is being seen in the clinic for a follow-up visit. Which of the following laboratory results should the nurse report to the physician?**

   1. A blood cholesterol of 140 mg/dl.
   2. A fasting blood glucose (FBG) of 250 mg/dl.
   3. Glycosylated hemoglobin (HBA$_1$C) of 4%
   4. Blood triglyceride levels of 120 mg/dl.

39. **A patient in the outpatient clinic complains of blurry vision, increased thirst, and increased urination. Which of the following lab results would the nurse expect to find?**

   1. HBA$_1$C of 3.0%.
   2. HBA$_1$C of 4.0%.
   3. HBA$_1$C of 10.5%.
   4. HBA$_1$C of 7%.

40. **A client with diabetes is on a dose of 37 units of Humulin R insulin. On the following 1 cc (100 unit) syringe, identify the position on the syringe indicating 37 units of insulin.**

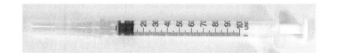

Hematology and Immunology

1. **A septic client develops disseminated intravascular coagulation (DIC). Which of the following describes DIC?**
   1. A chronic condition that is always controllable with lifelong heparin usage.
   2. A common bleeding disorder that is characterized by an elevated platelet count.
   3. A complex and serious blood disorder caused by abnormally activated coagulation.
   4. A disease triggered by a genetic disorder involving vitamin K deficiency.

2. **A client with disseminated intravascular coagulation (DIC) will experience simultaneous alterations in normal hemostatic mechanisms and clotting processes. The nurse knows this client will most likely develop which of the following?**
   1. Excessive thrombosis and bleeding.
   2. Decreased platelet production.
   3. Immediate sodium and fluid retention.
   4. Increased thromboplastin and fibrinogen levels.

3. **For a client experiencing an acute episode of disseminated intravascular coagulation (DIC), the nurse expects the initial laboratory values for partial thromboplastin time, prothrombin time, and thrombin time to be reported as which of the following?**
   1. Normal.
   2. Prolonged or elevated.
   3. Decreased or shortened.
   4. Elevated then decreased.

4. **In the following list, identify items to be included in a teaching plan for a thrombocytopenic client requiring bleeding precautions. Select all that apply.**
   1. Avoid intramuscular injections.
   2. Brush teeth with a soft toothbrush.
   3. Avoid rectal temperatures, suppositories, and examinations.
   4. Avoid flossing your teeth.
   5. Blow your nose gently.
   6. Avoid fresh fruits and vegetables.
   7. Avoid contact sports and activities potentially causing trauma.
   8. Use a straight razor instead of an electric shaver.

5. **The nurse knows that a client with immune or idiopathic thrombocytopenic purpura (ITP) is affected by an autoimmune disease that causes the destruction and reduction of which of the following?**
   1. Circulating white blood cells.
   2. Circulating red blood cells.
   3. Circulating granulocytes.
   4. Circulating platelets.

6. **Which of the following is important education for the nurse to provide a client with a thrombocytopenic disorder?**
   1. Use a rectal suppository for relief of constipation.
   2. Take medications by injection rather than the oral route whenever possible.
   3. Notify the dentist of underlying platelet problems prior to any invasive procedure.
   4. Take aspirin and ibuprofen for any headaches that may occur.

7. A unit of blood (500 ml) is started with a flow rate of 42 gtt/min and drop factor of 10 gtt/ml. Assuming no complications occur, how long will the transfusion run until it is complete?

_____

8. A client's platelet count is reported as 9,000/mm³. For which of the following is the client at risk?
   1. Spontaneous bleeding.
   2. Head trauma.
   3. Anemia.
   4. Increased susceptibility to infection.

9. A recently married female client is concerned with her family history of hemophilia A. The nurse knows this is a valid concern because hemophilia A can be described as which of the following?
   1. An X-linked genetic clotting disorder that results in asymptomatic Factor IX deficiency.
   2. A Y-linked genetic clotting disorder characterized by decreased platelet count with normal bleeding and coagulation times.
   3. A disorder almost always associated with a simultaneous diagnosis of HIV.
   4. An X-linked genetic clotting disorder that results in Factor VIII deficiency with potential hemorrhagic episodes.

10. A client with bleeding problems is diagnosed with vitamin K deficiency. The nurse knows that vitamin K is essential because it assists with normal blood clotting by performing which of the following?
   1. Regulating Factors VIII and IX utilization.
   2. Promoting prothrombin formation in the liver.
   3. Stimulating platelet proliferation and differentiation.
   4. Assisting with iron absorption.

11. A client with a white blood cell disorder asks how such a condition develops. The nurse begins by stating that all blood cells are produced in which of the following?
   1. Thymus.
   2. Central nervous system.
   3. Bone marrow.
   4. Spleen.

12. A student asks a nurse to explain how humoral immunity defends against invading antigens. The nurse's response should include which of the following choices?
   1. Humoral immunity is mediated by antibodies produced by B-lymphocytes.
   2. Humoral immunity is mediated by T-lymphocytes.
   3. Humoral immunity involves the utilization of phagocytic NK cells.
   4. Humoral immunity defends against only viral infections.

13. A client begins chilling and itching during a platelet transfusion reaction. Place the following nursing actions in the correct order of performance.
   1. Notify the physician and blood bank.
   2. Stop the infusion and maintain intravenous access and patency with saline solution.
   3. Treat symptoms per physician order.
   4. Assess vital signs and airway patency.
   5. Return the platelet bag and tubing with any unused product to the blood bank for analysis.

14. Following a kidney transplant, a client shows signs of transplant rejection. What causes this treatment response?
   1. A humoral immune response.
   2. An inflammatory response.
   3. An antiviral immune response.
   4. A cellular immune response.

15. A client states that he believes an infectious respiratory virus was acquired due to exposure to a sick colleague at work. The nurse is aware that this client is experiencing which type of immunity?
   1. Natural passive.
   2. Natural active.
   3. Artificial passive.
   4. Artificial active.

16. A nurse is preparing an in-service training about human immunodeficiency virus (HIV) for a church-based group. What information should the nurse include about HIV transmission?
   1. It is primarily transmitted through casual contact.
   2. It is primarily transmitted through accidental puncture wounds.
   3. It is primarily transmitted through contact with infected body fluids or needles.
   4. It is primarily transmitted through tears and saliva.

17. Client A shares a needle with HIV-positive Client B and Client A becomes infected. In the chain of infection, who/what was the reservoir for infection that led to Client A becoming infected?

   _____

18. While providing a community-based program about HIV and AIDS, a nurse is asked what symptoms a person may initially experience with HIV infection. The nurse explains that early manifestations of HIV during the primary infection stage include which of the following?
   1. Pneumocystis carinii pneumonia (PCP).
   2. Flu-like symptoms and night sweats.
   3. Wasting syndrome.
   4. Kaposi's sarcoma.

19. Which is *not* an appropriate nursing action for a client with acquired immunodeficiency syndrome (AIDS) who is experiencing fevers and night sweats?
   1. Encourage oral fluid intake.
   2. Change bed linens as needed.
   3. Use a pillow with a moisture resistant cover.
   4. Wake the client every four hours to administer prn acetaminophen (Tylenol).

20. Which of the following are potential nursing diagnoses for a client who is newly diagnosed with early stage HIV. Select all that apply.
   1. Fear.
   2. Spiritual distress.
   3. Risk for poisoning.
   4. Ineffective coping.
   5. Disturbed thought processes.
   6. Deficient knowledge.
   7. Ineffective protection.
   8. Anxiety.

21. A nurse who is caring for an adult female with a hemoglobin level of 10.1 g/dl can interpret this result to most likely be related to which of the following conditions noted in the health history?
   1. Emphysema.
   2. Peripheral vascular disease (PVD).
   3. Iron deficiency anemia.
   4. Gestational diabetes.

22. Prior to transfusing a unit of blood, the nurse should consider which of the following to be a qualified staff member to assist in ensuring that the blood label information matches that of the patient?
   1. A registered nurse.
   2. A radiology technician.
   3. A medical student.
   4. A phlebotomist.

23. **Which of the following assessment data are essential for the nurse to obtain immediately prior to initiating a blood transfusion?**
    1. Height and weight.
    2. Intake and output.
    3. Vital signs.
    4. Most recent hemoglobin and hematocrit levels.

24. **The nurse receives a unit of packed red blood cells (PRBCs) from the blood bank and notes that the time on the clock reads 4:10 PM. By what time must the blood begin infusing?**
    1. 4:50 PM.
    2. 4:40 PM.
    3. 5:00 PM.
    4. 5:10 PM.

25. **When caring for an immunosuppressed client, the nurse knows which of the following precautions are important? Select all that apply.**
    1. Wash hands thoroughly before entering the room.
    2. Wear a mask, gloves, and gown as appropriate.
    3. Restrict visitation by people with active infections.
    4. Discourage the client from bathing.
    5. Instruct the client to avoid crowds.
    6. Encourage the client to eat only fresh fruits and vegetables.
    7. Instruct the client to cook all foods thoroughly.
    8. Dispose of all linen in the trash after use.

26. **When planning care for a client requiring a blood transfusion, the nurse knows the total infusion time for a unit of packed red blood cells (PRBCs) should not exceed which of the following?**
    1. 2 hours.
    2. 6 hours.
    3. 8 hours.
    4. 4 hours.

27. **The nurse should remain in the room with the client during the most critical time of a blood transfusion, which is considered to be which of the following?**
    1. The first 2 minutes.
    2. The final 2 minutes.
    3. The first 15 minutes.
    4. The final 15 minutes.

28. **A client develops chills and back pain during a blood product transfusion. What should be the first action of the nurse?**
    1. Stop the transfusion immediately.
    2. Cover the client with a blanket.
    3. Notify the physician.
    4. Slow the rate of the blood transfusion.

29. **The nurse is preparing a handout about blood and its components for a unit in-service training. Which statements about blood and its components should be included in the handout? Select all that apply.**
    1. Blood is a type of connective tissue.
    2. Approximately 55% of blood is composed of formed elements (blood cells) and 45% is composed of plasma.
    3. Blood transports oxygen, hormones, and nutrients throughout the body.
    4. White blood cells are the only type of blood cell that develops from the stem cell within the bone marrow.
    5. Blood helps to maintain fluid and electrolyte balance.
    6. Blood protects against infection.

30. **A client arrives for initial evaluation following a diagnosis of systemic lupus erythematosus (SLE). The nurse knows that a classic cutaneous manifestation of SLE is which of the following?**
    1. Facial pallor.
    2. Brittle nails.
    3. Total body alopecia.
    4. Butterfly rash on the bridge of the nose.

31. **During a client's routine physical examination, leukocytosis is detected. The nurse receiving this result knows that leukocytosis can indicate which of the following?**

1. Anemia.
2. Coagulation disorders.
3. Infection and inflammation.
4. Renal or hepatic disorders.

32. **The nurse should report which of the following as a critical value for an adult?**

1. Total WBC 10,000/mm^3.
2. Total WBC 1,700/mm^3.
3. Hemoglobin 12.7 g/dl.
4. Platelet count 140,000/mm^3.

33. **A client with acute leukemia arrives for blood count assessment 10 days following treatment with aggressive chemotherapy. Which of the following hematologic laboratory abnormalities should the nurse expect to see? Select all that apply.**

1. Decreased platelet count.
2. Decreased BUN and creatinine.
3. Decreased white blood cell count.
4. Increased platelet count.
5. Decreased red blood cell count.
6. Increased red blood cell count.

34. **Which is an appropriate nursing goal for a client who has been battling AIDS for 10 years, has experienced advanced disease progression, and is at the end of life?**

1. The client will verbalize an understanding of the mode of disease transmission.
2. The client will experience a weight gain of one to two pounds per week.
3. The client will increase attendance at community social activities.
4. The client will maintain adequate comfort with minimal episodes of breakthrough pain.

35. **A client asks about the functions of various organs. The nurse's response should include that the thymus, spleen, and lymph nodes are organs that assist with which of the following?**

1. Immunity.
2. Digestion.
3. Electrolyte balance.
4. Vitamin absorption.

36. **Which of the following clinical conditions can the nurse suspect is most likely occurring when an immunosuppressed client develops disorientation, diminished urine output, and vital signs of T 102.1, P 124, R 24, BP 92/60?**

1. Acute renal failure.
2. Pneumothorax.
3. Septic shock.
4. Compartment syndrome.

37. **When caring for a client with iron-deficiency anemia, the nurse knows that regular assessment and analysis of various elements of the red blood cell (RBC) count are essential. Which important iron-containing and oxygen-carrying element of the RBC count is important to monitor?**

_____

38. **The nurse recognizes which of the following as a common treatment for a client diagnosed with pernicious anemia?**

1. Vitamin B$_{12}$ (cyanocobalamin) injections or supplements.
2. Iron supplements.
3. Frequent blood transfusions.
4. Vitamin B$_6$ (pyridoxine) supplements.

39. A client receiving an intravenous contrast agent in preparation for a CT scan develops facial flushing, peripheral tingling, fullness in the mouth and throat, periorbital swelling, and itching, which progresses to bronchospasm and dyspnea. What type of immunologic reaction is the client most likely experiencing?

_____

40. Why can splenomegaly affect blood cell counts in a client?
1. The spleen works directly with the bone marrow to produce blood cells.
2. When the spleen enlarges, its normal filtering capacity increases, often causing a decrease in the number of circulating blood cells.
3. When the spleen enlarges, its normal filtering capacity decreases, often causing an increase in the number of circulating blood cells.
4. Anemia is primarily caused by disorders of the spleen.

Integumentary

1. **When assessing a client with a new skin lesion, it is most important to ask the client about which of the following?**
   1. Allergies.
   2. Diet.
   3. Pets.
   4. Use of sunscreen products.

2. **When interviewing a client, which question would be *least* effective in obtaining important health history information regarding their skin disorder?**
   1. Does your skin condition keep you awake at night?
   2. Have you had any changes in your diet?
   3. How do you handle stress?
   4. How does your skin condition make you feel about yourself?

3. **The client with psoriasis needs to use several of the following treatments to control their disease. Select all that apply.**
   1. Coal tar preparations.
   2. Corticosteroids.
   3. Intralesional therapy.
   4. Laser therapy.
   5. Moisturizing creams.
   6. Phototherapy.

4. **Which of the following would indicate that a biopsy be recommended for skin lesions?**
   1. A health history can not be obtained.
   2. A more definitive diagnosis is needed.
   3. Palpation reveals abnormal findings.
   4. Topical medications have not worked.

5. **An elderly client comes to the clinic with a rash of their upper chest and back. What should the nurse do during the skin assessment?**
   1. Note dry, flaky skin as a normal finding.
   2. Perform a lesion-specific examination before the general inspection of the skin.
   3. Pinch up a fold of skin to check for turgor.
   4. Use a penlight to examine the lesions more closely.

6. **Why is turning a client every two hours while lying on a hypothermia blanket important?**
   1. It decreases the skin damage that may result from vasoconstriction.
   2. It decreases the amount of time that they will need the therapy.
   3. It prevents shivering.
   4. It promotes client comfort.

7. **The nurse working in a dermatologist's office is aware that skin cancer is a common diagnosis because there are several risk factors. Select all the risk factors that apply.**
   1. Dark skin, dark hair, and brown eyes.
   2. Light skin, light hair, and blue eyes.
   3. Blistering sunburns.
   4. Chronic skin irritations.
   5. Genetic predisposition.
   6. Regular use of sunscreen.

8. **While working in the emergency room, the nurse would be most concerned about a bee sting on a client who has which of the following?**
   1. Developed a large, reddened, swollen area with the last sting.
   2. Had hives and trouble breathing with the last sting.
   3. Had a rise in blood pressure when bitten.
   4. Has a history of fever and chills when bitten.

9. **A female client comes to the doctor's office with a pustular inflammation of her cheeks. Which of the following would the nurse include in her teaching plan for this client?**
   1. Apply moist compresses frequently throughout the day.
   2. Adhere to strict dietary changes.
   3. Squeeze the larger pustules periodically.
   4. Use a new cosmetic pad each time she applies makeup.

10. **While working in a community clinic, the nurse would include which of the following in the health teaching plan for a client with warts?**
    1. They are viral and may reappear.
    2. They cannot be transmitted.
    3. They only appear in childhood.
    4. They will spread if not treated.

11. **While working in a community clinic, a ten-year-old client complains of dandruff and a rash on the back of her neck. On examination, the nurse notices the dandruff flakes don't brush off the hair. The nurse suspects which of the following disorders?**
    1. Pediculosis capitus.
    2. Psoriasis.
    3. Seborrheic dermatitis.
    4. Tinea capitis.

12. **After a recent camping trip, a client comes to the doctor's office with complaints of pruritus and reddened, fluid-filled vesicles on her lower leg. The nurse suspects which of the following disorders?**
    1. Cellulitis.
    2. Contact dermatitis.
    3. Folliculitis.
    4. Seborrheic dermatitis.

13. **Arrange these types of skin cancers from least to most severe.**
    1. Basal cell carcinoma.
    2. Malignant melanoma.
    3. Squamous cell carcinoma.

14. **You are caring for a client that developed poison ivy after a recent camping trip. Which statement demonstrates that they understand how to keep from getting this form of contact dermatitis again?**
    1. "If I'm careful not to touch the leaves of the plant I can still go camping in that area."
    2. "I'll have to scrub myself with soap and hot water after camping in this area."
    3. "I'll have to wash my shoes, clothes, and gear so that I won't get sores from touching them."
    4. "I'm glad our dog didn't get poison ivy so he can stay with us in the tent."

15. **A client comes to the office with complaints of a "bump" in front of his right ear that has become bigger over the last six months. On examination the nurse notes a pink, one centimeter nodule without drainage. The client has no complaints of pain or pruritus. The nurse suspects**

   _____.

16. A client has been diagnosed with atopic dermatitis. She has severe pruritus. She has found several therapies on the Internet. Which of the following therapies would be least effective?
    1. Cool, moist compresses.
    2. Cornstarch baths.
    3. Oatmeal preparations.
    4. Warm, moist compresses.

17. A client at the clinic is diagnosed with contact dermatitis of the neck and upper chest. Which of the following is an important first step in managing this disease?
    1. Identify the causative agent.
    2. Obtain allergy testing.
    3. Take antihistamines to control itching.
    4. Try over-the-counter hydrocortisone cream first.

18. An elderly client is admitted with painful, open, weeping vesicles from herpes zoster or shingles. The nurse would expect their room environment to include which of the following?
    1. Isolation techniques.
    2. Semi-private room.
    3. Sharing of equipment between clients.
    4. Unrestricted visiting.

19. The nurse is caring for a client with newly diagnosed herpes zoster or shingles. They are aware that the most important priority of care is which of the following?
    1. Frequent dressing changes.
    2. Frequent wound assessment.
    3. Isolation precautions.
    4. Reposition the client every two hours.

20. The nurse is caring for a client with pruritus. Several nursing diagnoses need to be included in the plan of care. Select all that apply.
    1. Acute pain and itching.
    2. Disturbed body image.
    3. Disturbed personal identity.
    4. Disturbed sleep pattern.
    5. Ineffective protection.
    6. Impaired skin integrity.

21. When formulating a teaching plan for a client with herpes zoster, the nurse should include which of the following?
    1. Informing the client that people who have not had chickenpox will not develop them if exposed to the client.
    2. Informing the client that they are contagious only if the lesions are draining.
    3. Recurrence of infection can be triggered by stress and fatigue.
    4. With recurrence of infection, vesicles will appear before the pain begins.

22. A client is seen in the outpatient clinic for treatment of psoriasis. The nurse should anticipate which of the following findings?
    1. Abdominal lesions.
    2. Hyperpigmented skin.
    3. Intense pain.
    4. Silvery, white scales.

23. When formulating a teaching plan for the client with psoriasis, the nurse should encourage which of the following for his scaly lesions?
    1. Occlusive dressings on the lesions as much as possible throughout the day.
    2. Soaking in a warm bath for as long as can be tolerated.
    3. Soft brushing of scales while bathing.
    4. Warm, moist compresses at night.

24. **A client has just been admitted to your unit with psoriasis. The nurse needs to prepare the client for which of the following therapies to be initiated?**
    1. Laser treatments.
    2. Phototherapy.
    3. Radiation therapy.
    4. Topical fluorouracil (5-FU).

25. **A client has a lot of questions concerning the various treatment options for his newly diagnosed basal cell carcinoma. The nurse is aware that there are several treatments used in the management of this disease. Select all that apply.**
    1. Corticosteroids.
    2. Cryosurgery.
    3. Electrosurgery.
    4. Immunotherapy.
    5. Phototherapy.
    6. Surgical excision.

26. **A client with psoriasis tells the nurse that they are unable to work because of the horrible appearance of their lesions. The nurse includes which of the following nursing diagnoses in the plan of care that best describes this client's feelings?**
    1. Anxiety related to lack of knowledge of the disease process.
    2. Ineffective coping related to lack of social support.
    3. Self-esteem disturbance related to the lack of financial support.
    4. Social isolation related to decreased activities and fear of rejection.

27. **A client with psoriasis has a topical corticosteroid cream as one of their several treatments. In teaching this client about this medication, which of the following should the nurse tell them?**
    1. Creams should be applied in a thick layer to completely cover the lesions.
    2. Discontinuing the medication will cause an exacerbation of the psoriasis.
    3. Rubbing the medication completely into the lesions will increase absorption.
    4. Topical corticosteroids usually do not cause systemic side effects.

28. **What information would the nurse need to know when developing a teaching plan for a client with psoriasis?**
    1. Treatment includes liberal application of moisturizing creams, topical cortico-steroids, and medication for anxiety.
    2. Treatment focuses on colloidal baths, pain management, and assisting with their disturbed body image.
    3. Treatment includes teaching clients about UV light therapy, tar preparations, and assisting with altered self-concept.
    4. Treatment includes warm moist compresses, application of retinoid creams, and stress management.

29. **A client comes to the office with complaints of a mole that has increased in size and changed in color. On examination, the nurse notes an elevated two centimeter lesion that is dark brownish-black in color with irregular borders. The nurse suspects**

    _____.

30. **A client presents to the office for evaluation of multiple moles (nevi). Which of the following characteristics are important to note in the examination?**
    1. Color variation and irregular borders.
    2. Irregular borders and drainage.
    3. Location and color variation.
    4. Pruritus and location.

31. **Which statement best indicates an understanding of skin cancer risk factors?**
1. "Because I'm dark-complected, I won't have to worry about skin cancer."
2. "I really need to use sunscreen—even in winter."
3. "I used to lie in the sun all the time but now I just go to the tanning bed."
4. "My father was treated for melanoma, but my mother says not to worry."

32. **A client has just been admitted to your unit with a diagnosis of herpes zoster or shingles. They have had several complaints over the last two weeks. Place the following symptoms in order of their typical occurrence with this disease process.**
1. Crusted lesions.
2. Paresthesia.
3. Postneuralgia.
4. Redness and swelling.
5. Vesicles.
6. Weeping blisters.

33. **A client with suspected malignant melanoma will most often relate which of the following about their lesion?**
1. Pain.
2. Pruritus.
3. Purplish in color.
4. Purulent drainage.

34. **A client has just been admitted to your unit with malignant melanoma. The nurse needs to prepare the client for which of the following therapies?**
1. Cryosurgery.
2. Laser treatments.
3. Radiation therapy.
4. Surgical excision.

35. **A client comes to the outpatient clinic with recurrent herpes simplex 1 lesions that are uncontrolled by current medication. The nurse would expect to focus their assessment on which area of the body?**

_____

36. **Which action by a client would be least effective in preventing skin cancer?**
1. A high fiber diet.
2. Monthly skin examinations.
3. Stopping smoking.
4. Using a sunscreen.

37. **A client has just been admitted to your unit with basal cell carcinoma. The lesion would most likely be described as which of the following?**
1. A pearly, shiny nodule.
2. A red, edematous macule.
3. A rough, scaly tumor.
4. A weeping vesicle.

38. **One of your assigned clients, whose leg is severely infected, is complaining of soreness of his mouth and refuses to eat. Assessment of his mouth reveals a white, milky plaque that does not come off with rubbing. The nurse suspects which of the following conditions?**
1. Candidiasis from antibiotic therapy.
2. Dermatitis from immunosuppressive therapy.
3. Herpes simplex from corticosteroid therapy.
4. Squamous cell carcinoma from smoking abuse.

39. **A client comes to the outpatient clinic with recurrent tinea pedis or "athlete's foot." The nurse needs to be aware that this is what type of infection?**

_____

Oncology

1. **Select the seven signs of cancer.**
   1. A nonhealing sore.
   2. Bleeding or discharge from any body orifice.
   3. Bloating.
   4. Change in bowel or bladder habits.
   5. Change in moles or warts.
   6. Fatigue.
   7. Indigestion or swallowing problems.
   8. Lump in the breast or elsewhere.
   9. Nagging or persistent cough or hoarseness.

2. **A client who has been receiving chemotherapy as an outpatient is admitted with anorexia and dehydration secondary to candida esophagitis. Which of the following topics of instruction provided by the nurse in the outpatient setting may have averted this hospitalization?**
   1. Avoid persons with communicable disease.
   2. Daily assessments of oral mucosa.
   3. Obtain daily lab tests.
   4. Report nausea and vomiting.

3. **After chemotherapy, a client with myelosuppression is at risk for which of the following?**
   1. Anorexia and malnutrition.
   2. Bleeding from the gums.
   3. Diarrhea and dehydration.
   4. Full body alopecia.

4. **A client was informed that radiation therapy will be initiated for several weeks prior to surgery. The client and family are angry and state they believe the delay in surgical removal will delay eradication of the tumor. What would be the nurse's most appropriate initial topic of discussion to have with this client and family?**
   1. If radiation is effective, surgery will not be necessary.
   2. If you disagree with the doctor, you may seek a second opinion.
   3. Radiation will shrink the tumor before surgery.
   4. You have the right to refuse radiation so surgery can be done.

5. **A client that is neutropenic should do which of the following?**
   1. Eat plenty of fresh fruits and vegetables.
   2. Avoid crowds.
   3. Exercise mildly, like gardening.
   4. Take temperature weekly.

6. **In teaching a client about chemotherapy side effects, which of the following information should be included?**
   1. Side effects are expected.
   2. Side effects are not treatable.
   3. Side effects are unavoidable.
   4. Side effects will require hospitalization.

7. The physician progress notes state 'nadir in three weeks' on a client who has just received chemotherapy. In planning for discharge, the nurse would carefully determine the client's understanding of the need to return to the physician's office to obtain which of the following scheduled treatments?
   1. Hydration.
   2. Laboratory tests.
   3. Medications.
   4. Radiation treatments.

8. The nurse preparing a client for radiation treatment will tell them to expect which of the following?
   1. Alopecia.
   2. Diarrhea.
   3. Fatigue.
   4. Reproductive dysfunction.

9. On obtaining laboratory orders for a client admitted with a history of multiple myeloma, the nurse will note an increase in which of the following labs?
   1. Absolute neutropil count (ANC).
   2. Calcium.
   3. Platelets.
   4. White blood cells.

10. A client is scheduled for debulking. While preparing the client, the nurse is aware that debulking is which of the following?
    1. A conference with the physician and the family.
    2. A diagnostic procedure.
    3. A surgical procedure.
    4. A treatment for constipation.

11. A family noticed that after opiate pain management was initiated, the client was sedated and resting comfortably but sleeping continuously. After three days, the client is no longer sedated, and the family questions if pain control is lost. The nurse realizes that which of the following occurs after two to three days?

    1. An alternate method of pain management must be employed.
    2. Most clients develop a tolerance to the sedative effects of opiods.
    3. The dose will have to be adjusted.
    4. The client will probably require combination pain control.

12. After a course of chemotherapy, a client experiences severe nausea and vomiting. The nurse monitors the patient for signs and symptoms of which of the following?
    1. Metabolic acidosis.
    2. Metabolic alkalosis.
    3. Respiratory acidosis.
    4. Respiratory alkalosis.

13. After radiation treatment, the patient complains of dryness, redness, and scaling within the designated radiation treatment markings. What should the nurse instruct the client to do?
    1. Apply hydrating lotions.
    2. Apply moist heat.
    3. Sit in the sun for 10 minutes a day.
    4. Wash with plain soap and water.

14. In evaluating a series of lab tests for cancer markers, the nurse recognizes that AFP will be elevated in

    _____,

    CA 15-3 will increase with

    _____,

    CEA will be elevated with

    _____ and

    Free PSA will increase with

    _____.

    1. Breast cancer, colon cancer, liver cancer, prostatic cancer.
    2. Breast cancer, liver cancer, colon cancer, prostatic cancer.
    3. Liver cancer, breast cancer, colon cancer, prostatic cancer.
    4. Prostatic cancer, breast cancer, colon cancer, liver cancer.

15. A client is receiving treatment for Stage IV ovarian cancer and asks the nurse to discuss the prognosis. What would the prognosis be at this stage with aggressive surgical, radiation, and chemotherapy treatment?
    1. Good.
    2. Guarded.
    3. Poor.
    4. Very good.

16. A 32-year-old female tells the nurse that she was just informed that she tested positive for a mutant BRCA-1 gene. This female has up to an 85% risk of which of the following?
    1. Delivering a child with Down's syndrome.
    2. Developing Alzheimer's disease.
    3. Developing breast cancer.
    4. Developing ovarian cancer.

17. A client with advanced breast cancer is scheduled for an autologous stem cell transplant. Which of the following will the client receive immediately prior to the transplant?
    1. A unit of whole blood.
    2. Antibiotic therapy.
    3. Genetic counseling.
    4. High doses of chemotherapy.

18. In educating the public on diagnostic studies that will detect early colorectal cancer, the nurse knows that the American Cancer Society recommends that persons who are asymptomatic, have no risk factors, and are age 50 or older should have a rectal examine with fecal occult blood testing every

    _____,

    a flexible sigmoidoscopy every

    _____,

    and a barium enema every

    _____.

    1. Six months, five years, five years.
    2. Two years, five years, ten years.
    3. One year, five years, five years.
    4. One year, two years, five years.

19. After several courses of chemotherapy, a client has labs drawn. The nurse is aware that after massive cell destruction there is an elevation of what lab test?
    1. Ammonia.
    2. Hemoglobin A1C.
    3. Lactic acid.
    4. Uric acid.

20. A client's wife is distraught that even after three radiation treatments the client's prostate cancer does not seem to be responding. What test is done to differentiate benign disease from a malignancy of the prostate?
    1. PKU.
    2. Free PSA.
    3. PSA.
    4. PTH.

21. Other than by direct spread of prostatic cancer cells through the prostatic capsule, common sites of metastasis include which of the following?
    1. Bladder, kidneys, and seminal vesicles.
    2. Bladder, kidneys, and testes.
    3. Bones, brain, and lymph nodes.
    4. Bones, liver, and lungs.

22. A client with lung cancer is scheduled for a lobectomy. The nurse prepares the client to expect which of the following postoperatively?
    1. A sternal incision.
    2. Chest tubes.
    3. Moderate pain.
    4. Pulmonary function studies.

23. A client has just received a diagnosis of small cell lung cancer and questions the nurse regarding treatment. Which of the following does the nurse realize about this type of cancer?
    1. It can be treated with surgery.
    2. It is not associated with smoking.
    3. It is most treatable.
    4. It has the poorest prognosis.

24. The firmest recognized risk factor for pancreatic cancer is which of the following?
    1. A high-fat diet.
    2. Cigarette smoking.
    3. Diabetes.
    4. Exposure to benzidine.

25. A client with liver cancer develops dyspnea, tachypnea, tachycardia, cough, pleuritic chest pain, crackles, fever, and hemoptysis. These symptoms support what frequently observed complication of liver cancer?
    1. Advanced cirrhosis.
    2. Congestive heart failure.
    3. Pulmonary embolism.
    4. Spontaneous pneumothorax.

26. A client was just diagnosed with testicular cancer. Which of the following statements will the nurse include in a discussion with the client? Select all that apply.
    1. Incidence is greater in men than in women.
    2. Cigarette smoking is the greatest risk factor.
    3. Flank pain is an early symptom.
    4. Obesity is a risk factor.
    5. Hematuria is a risk factor.

27. Most cancers of the liver are the result of which of the following?
    1. Chronic liver disease.
    2. Hepatocellular carcinoma.
    3. Metastasis from remote sites.
    4. Primary hepatic carcinoma.

28. A nurse is caring for a client with colon cancer who is being evaluated for metastasis. What laboratory studies will the nurse examine in following diagnostic assessment of the initial disease progression?
    1. Bone marrow function tests.
    2. Liver function tests.
    3. Pulmonary function tests.
    4. Renal function tests.

29. A client who is two days postoperative for surgery to remove cancer of the colon is very depressed. After much discussion, the nurse learns that prior to surgery the physician discussed the need for a colostomy, but the client noticed there were two colostomies instead of one. Which of the following should the nurse explain to the client?
    1. One colostomy drains the small intestine, while the other drains the large intestine.
    2. One is the colostomy and one is for wound drainage.
    3. The colostomy is probably temporary.
    4. The tumor was larger than expected.

30. After a Billroth II (gastrojejunostomy) surgery, a client is at great risk for which of the following?
    1. Ascites.
    2. Bowel obstruction.
    3. Dumping syndrome.
    4. Esophageal varies.

31. The symptoms of gastric cancer are often identical to those of which of the following?
    1. Esophagus cancer.
    2. Liver cancer.
    3. Myocardial infarction.
    4. Peptic ulcer disease.

32. An important aspect of nursing care for the client with pancreatic cancer and their family is the management of which of the following?
    1. Chemotherapy side effects.
    2. Radiation side effects.
    3. Smoking cessation.
    4. The grieving process.

33. The nurse is vigilant that oncologic emergencies can suddenly occur and differ from *expected* adverse outcomes of treatment. Which of the following are categorized as oncologic emergencies? Select all that apply.
    1. Cardiac tamponade.
    2. Carotid blowout.
    3. Hypercalcemia.
    4. SIADH.
    5. Spinal cord compression.
    6. Superior vena cave syndrome.
    7. Third space syndrome.
    8. Tumor lysis syndrome.

34. The nurse will conduct a seminar and provide information on men's health to a community group of clients. What should the nurse include in preparing the program regarding a testicular self exam?
    1. Discuss monthly self exams.
    2. Explain that the testes can be examined together.
    3. Indicate the best time to examine the testes is after the morning void.
    4. No need to discuss anatomy if the group is all male.

35. A client who began chemotherapy two days prior presents with a complaint of oliguria, hematuria, cramps, and confusion. Laboratory studies show an increased blood urea nitrogen, creatinine, potassium, phosphorus, and uric acid. Calcium is decreased. This client is most likely suffering from which of the following?
    1. Acute renal failure.
    2. Metabolic alkalosis.
    3. Tumor lysis syndrome.
    4. Urinary tract infection.

36. The physician has reviewed a chemotherapy combination protocol consisting of four different medications with a client with early Hodgkin's disease and their family. The nurse finds the client and family crying and extremely emotional. They are barely able to express their understanding of the bleak outlook associated with such an aggressive treatment plan. What action should the nurse take?
    1. Allow them to verbalize their concerns.
    2. Notify the physician.
    3. Reinforce the treatment rationale.
    4. Request a hospice referral.

37. A client receiving treatment for leukemia is at risk for which of the following? Select all that apply.
    1. Aplastic anemia.
    2. Bleeding.
    3. Dyspnea on exertion.
    4. Edema.
    5. Fatigue.
    6. Fractures.
    7. Infections.
    8. Opportunistic infections.

38. The doctor has prescribed a treatment protocol for a client who has metastatic cancer. Which of the following are true for the treatment for metastatic tumors? Select all that apply.

1. Even with early intervention, tumors are difficult to treat.
2. Some metastatic tumors are resistant to chemotherapy.
3. Some metastatic tumors are resistant to radiation.
4. Surgical resection is best if tumors are small.

39. In regard to radiation and chemotherapy, select all that apply in recruiting malignant cells to start growing and dividing.

1. It is a good plan.
2. It will cause metastasis.
3. Larger tumors are easier to treat.
4. Both therapies are never done concurrently.

Neurology

1. **What instruction should the nurse include in the discharge-teaching plan of a client who has been diagnosed with multiple sclerosis?**
   1. It is very important to engage in a progressive exercise program to build strength and endurance.
   2. It is important with this disease to relax muscles; a hot tub spa is a good form of relaxation.
   3. It is important to engage in social activity, and volunteering to read to schoolchildren will keep you active.
   4. It is very important to develop a daily schedule that reduces fatigue and conserves energy.

2. **A client is admitted with a possible medical diagnosis of Guillain-Barre syndrome. Which question is most important for the nurse to ask the client?**
   1. Have you had an MMR immunization?
   2. Have you had a recent upper respiratory infection?
   3. Have you had any recent travel to Great Britain?
   4. Have you been to China in the last two weeks?

3. **In adults, pneumococcal meningitis is the most common bacterial meningitis. Which symptoms most clearly relate to meningitis?**
   1. Headache, fever, and stiff neck.
   2. Fever, chills, and malaise.
   3. Deterioration in level of consciousness.
   4. Seizures.

4. **The nurse is giving instructions to a patient with Parkinson's disease. Which instruction should the nurse include in the discharge teaching?**
   1. Many side effects are dose related and can be controlled by a dosage adjustment.
   2. All drugs have side effects and most clients will get used to them.
   3. Skipping a dose now and then is okay if the side effects are too annoying.
   4. It is important to keep a list of all the side effects and bring it to your next doctor's visit.

5. **To prevent accidents in Parkinson clients with bradykinesia, tremors, and rigidity, the nurse should advise the client to do which of the following?**
   1. Wear crepe-soled shoes for support and stability.
   2. Avoid incontinence by hurrying to get to the bathroom.
   3. Shuffle their feet when ambulating.
   4. Maintain a wide-based gait.

6. **The nurse is conducting an Alzheimer's class for a group of ancillary personnel. Which of the following would be most important for the nurse to explain to the personnel?**
   1. They need to provide supervision to protect clients from becoming injured, humiliated, or lost.
   2. They need to limit client activities and visitors to minimize emotional outbursts.
   3. They need to speak clearly and loudly to clients who are unable to form words or sentences.
   4. They need to explain all procedures in full detail to the client before initiating.

7. A conscious client is brought into the emergency room with a suspected cervical cord injury. Which of the following interventions should be done by the nurse in the emergency room? Select all that apply.
   1. Assess adequacy of respirations.
   2. Assess vital signs.
   3. Instruct the client not to move.
   4. Perform a complete neurological assessment.
   5. Assess for evidence of an associated head injury.
   6. Straighten the head and neck.
   7. Assess for visceral damage.

8. While caring for a client who has quadriplegia, which nursing measures are most essential for prevention of pulmonary emboli? Select all that apply.
   1. Assess the client's extremities for coolness, paleness, and decreased pulses.
   2. Assess the client's intravenous sites and legs for redness, swelling, and venous dilation.
   3. Apply elastic compression stockings or an intermittent compression device to improve blood return to the heart.
   4. Perform passive range of motion exercises to promote venous drainage.
   5. Measure the client's calves and thighs daily.
   6. Monitor PT and PTT results daily.
   7. Give all IM injections in the legs and massage the site to improve circulation.

9. Which interventions should the nurse plan to include in a client's care to prevent autonomic dysreflexia? Select all that apply.
   1. Monitor bowel movement regularity.
   2. Check for fecal impactions.
   3. Check the urinary drainage system for obstructions.
   4. Monitor blood pressure for hypertension.
   5. Instruct the client to wear a medic-alert bracelet at all times.

10. In developing a plan of care for a client with a spinal cord injury and paralysis, the nurse recognizes that it is essential to consider preventative skin care measures. Which of the following would be appropriate? Select all that apply.
    1. Systematically assess the client's skin for erythema and massage nonerythematous areas.
    2. Implement a positioning and turning schedule every 1–2 hours for clients confined to bed using the logrolling technique.
    3. Use pillows, foam wedges, or gel pads under bony prominences and keep heels off the bed surface.
    4. Keep the client's skin dry with powder.
    5. Massage over erythematous bony prominences.
    6. Use moisture barriers and disposable briefs as needed.

11. Differentiate between bowel training for clients with upper motor neuron (UMN) spinal cord injury and lower motor neuron (LMN) spinal cord injury.

    _____
    _____
    _____

12. Which best exemplifies the nurse's awareness of emotional and psychological needs of spinal cord injured clients and their families in the post acute rehabilitation phase of their care? Select all that apply.

1. Establish a therapeutic relationship.
2. Establish a trusting environment.
3. Allow the client to verbalize all concerns.
4. Judge the client's behavior and initiate behavior modification.
5. Answer questions honestly and refer those you are unable to answer to the appropriate source.
6. Use the multidisciplinary team meetings to discuss emotional-psychological status.
7. Recognize that clients may be going through a wide array of emotional responses and should be excluded from the decision making process.

13. **Complete the following: The most sensitive indicator of overall brain function is**

_____.

14. **When using the Glasgow Coma Scale to evaluate levels of consciousness, which of the following most accurately describes a score of 8?**
1. Indicates the need for nursing care to meet requirements of a comatose client.
2. Would reflect a fully alert, well-oriented person.
3. Is indicative of a deep coma.
4. Indicates stabilization of the neurological status.

15. **Clients with basal skull fractures require special consideration in nursing care. The nurse knows which intervention should not be performed with this type of fracture?**
1. Suctioning the client through the nasal passages.
2. Placing the client in semi-Fowler position.
3. Inserting an intravenous line in the lower extremities.
4. Suctioning the client for more than 15 seconds.

16. **A client is admitted with a diagnosis of epidural hematoma. This condition is most often manifested by which of the following?**
1. Momentary unconsciousness followed by a lucid period lasting a brief time followed by rapid deterioration in the level of consciousness.
2. An interval of about 48 hours before the client begins to experience headache, drowsiness, slowed mental processes, and confusion, which gradually worsens.
3. An interval from two days to two weeks before the client begins to show neurodeficits or the level of consciousness is not improved.
4. A time lapse of months between the injury and development of symptoms.

17. **Which occurrence, if present in a head injured client, would indicate the need for immediate intervention?**
1. Temperature 99° (axillary).
2. Pulse 100 RR (apical).
3. Respirations 24 regular with increased depth.
4. Blood pressure 140/84 in the right arm.

18. **While performing a neurological assessment on a client with a supratentorial lesion, the nurse observes that the client has difficulty looking upward, downward, and medially, and the pupil is dilated in the right eye. The client is experiencing diplopia. These symptoms most clearly relate to which of the following?**
1. Cranial Nerve II (optic) dysfunction due to possible pressure on the right optic nerve.
2. Cranial Nerve II (optic) dysfunction due to possible pressure on the left optic nerve.
3. Cranial Nerve III (oculomotor) dysfunction due to pressure on the right oculomotor nerve.
4. Cranial Nerve III (oculomotor) dysfunction due to pressure on the left oculomotor nerve.

19. The rupture of a cerebral aneurysm causes a sudden increase in intracranial pressure. Which of the following findings would *not* be associated with increased intracranial pressure?
    1. Violent headache and rapid loss of consciousness.
    2. Neck pain and stiffness.
    3. Hemiparesis or hemiplegia.
    4. Vomiting.

20. In assessing a client with meningitis, which of the following would indicate that the client has a positive Kernig's sign?
    1. Passive flexing of the neck causes involuntary flexion of both legs at the hip and knee.
    2. After flexing of the thigh to 90° at the hip, the client is unable to extend the leg completely without pain.
    3. When briskly rotating the head from side to side, the eyes move in the direction opposite the head.
    4. A painful stimulus causes the client to withdraw the stimulated body part.

21. The nurse caring for a client with a ruptured aneurysm observes the client for signs of a rebleed. The nurse knows the client is most at risk for rebleed in which of the following time frames?
    1. 3 days postbleed.
    2. 7 days postbleed.
    3. 11 days postbleed.
    4. 21 days postbleed.

22. A client has a cerebral aneurysm. Which nursing measure will be essential to his/her care?
    1. To provide a nonstimulating environment.
    2. To encourage self-care.
    3. To allow natural sunlight in room.
    4. To encourage family and friend visitation.

23. Explain the rationale for the following preventive measures for clients with a cerebral bleed.

Corticosteroids
Anticonvulsants
Antihypertensives
Low sodium, low cholesterol diet

_____

24. A client has undergone a craniotomy to clip a cerebral aneurysm. Which postoperative complication is the client *least* likely to develop as a result of the surgery?
    1. Hydrocephalus.
    2. Diabetes insipidus.
    3. Diabetes mellitus.
    4. Syndrome of inappropriate ADH.

25. An elderly right-handed female was admitted with a brain infarction. The following abnormal findings were noted on the neuro exam:

Inability to move her left arm and attempts to move left leg were poor
Left homonymous hemianopsia
Facial asymmetry
Oriented to person and place but not time

Identify nursing diagnoses for the above assessment findings.

_____

26. A client with a right cerebral vascular accident consistently asks for a fork when served meal trays. On further investigation, it is noted that the client does not eat food on the left side of the tray. The nurse identifies the problem and initiates which of the following interventions to help the client learn to compensate for the visual deficit?
    1. Provide for increased self-care by placing food and utensils on the right side of the tray.
    2. Encourage the client to use the right hand when feeding self.
    3. Provide for increased self-care by placing food and utensils on the left side of the tray.
    4. Encourage the client to use the left hand when feeding self.

27. **While caring for a client with a left-brain cerebral vascular accident, the nurse observes that the client shaved only the left side of his face during morning care. The nurse would interpret this behavior as which of the following?**
    1. The client is exhibiting signs of confusion and requires re-orienting by the nurse when performing morning care.
    2. The client is confused and will need to have morning care provided by a nursing assistant.
    3. The client is exhibiting signs of self-neglect and perceives only the left side of the body.
    4. The client is exhibiting signs of depression and is not interested in performing self-care.

28. **It is important to teach family members of a stroke victim interventions for safe swallowing and the prevention of aspiration. The most critical concept for the family to understand is which of the following?**
    1. Offer mouth care before meals to stimulate saliva and facilitate swallowing.
    2. Place food in the unaffected side of the mouth to facilitate chewing.
    3. Encourage the client to take small bites and chew food thoroughly.
    4. Place the client in the upright position to facilitate swallowing.

29. **The nurse assigned a client with global aphasia to the licensed practical nurse (LPN). The nurse validates that the LPN understands global aphasia. Which response best describes this problem?**
    1. It is the inability to use or comprehend language and symbols.
    2. It is a result of impaired hearing and speech.
    3. It is as if a foreign language is being spoken.
    4. It is the inability to express words or name objects.

30. **A client is admitted to the hospital after being involved in an automobile accident. The client is unresponsive, the pupils sluggishly react to light, and there is bilateral decorticate posturing. The corneal reflexes are diminished. The nurse assesses this reflex by performing which of the following?**
    1. Examining the eye with a penlight.
    2. Instilling drops of dye on the cornea.
    3. Visualizing the red reflex.
    4. Touching the cornea lightly with a wisp of cotton.

31. **Motor function response in an unconscious client is purposeful when the nurse applies a painful stimulus and the client does which of the following?**
    1. Pushes the painful stimulus away.
    2. Extends the body part toward the stimuli.
    3. Shows no reaction to the painful stimuli.
    4. Flexes the upper extremities and extends the lower extremities.

32. **In developing a plan of care for an unconscious client with a loss of the corneal reflex, the nurse recognizes that it is essential to consider which of the following?**
    1. Keep the room darkened with reduced lighting and the window covering closed.
    2. Apply an eye shield and keep the eye moist with lubricating eye drops.
    3. Alternate warm and cold saline compresses.
    4. Alternate an eye patch to each eye.

33. **When beginning a tube feeding in an unconscious client, the nurse recognizes that the client is not tolerant of the feeding if which of the following is true?**
    1. The client exhibits abdominal distention, vomiting, and diarrhea.
    2. The residual aspirate is 45 mL.
    3. The urine specific gravity is 1.003.
    4. The serum sodium is 136 and the potassium is 4.2.

34. **A client is receiving a continuous enteral tube feeding and is to receive phenytoin (Dilantin) via the tube. In developing a plan of care, the nurse recognizes that it is essential to consider which of the following?**
    1. The client may require larger doses of phenytoin to maintain a therapeutic level.
    2. The client may develop phenytoin toxicity.
    3. The client requires lower doses of phenytoin to maintain therapeutic levels.
    4. The client requires no dose adjustment because of a tube feeding.

35. **Proper administration of phenytoin (Dilantin) is very important. The nurse knows which of the following?**
    1. The drug can crystallize if given too slowly.
    2. The drug can depress the myocardium and cause dysrhythmias.
    3. The drug can cause phlebitis in peripheral veins.
    4. The drug can cause client discomfort.

36. **The nurse should institute which of the following seizure precautions with a client with tonic-clonic seizures? Select all that apply.**
    1. Keep the suction setup at the bedside.
    2. Keep the side rails up when in bed.
    3. Keep the bed in the lowest position.
    4. Keep the oxygen setup at the bedside.
    5. Keep the airway taped to the bed.
    6. Keep restraints to prevent injury.
    7. Keep the physician informed of seizure activity.

37. **Differentiate between the signs and symptoms of cholinergic crisis and myasthenic crisis.**

    _____

    _____

    _____

38. **A client is being discharged on pyridostigmine (Mestinon). Which information is most important for the nurse to teach the client about this medication?**
    1. The daily dosage and time interval must be carefully adjusted to their needs.
    2. The medication can be taken with crackers or milk to reduce nausea.
    3. Do not take this medication with any over-the-counter medications without checking with the physician.
    4. It is sometimes advisable to take this medication at night.

39. **A medication is being titrated to maintain the diastolic blood pressure of less than 80. The solution strength is 6 mg in 100 mL D$_5$W. The order is 2–4 mcg/min. Calculate the infusion rate for a controller.**

    _____

Musculoskeletal

1. **In assessing a client with carpal tunnel syndrome, a nurse would expect to find which of the following?**
   1. Decreased radial pulse.
   2. Numbness and tingling during the day.
   3. Pale, cool extremities.
   4. Positive Phalen's sign.

2. **Which of the following would the nurse assess when completing a health history and clinical examination of a client diagnosed with a rotator cuff injury?**
   1. Does the client golf?
   2. An inability to initiate or maintain abduction of the arm or shoulder.
   3. A negative Neer's test.
   4. A positive Tinel's sign.

3. **Which of the following treatments is appropriate for a client diagnosed with bursitis?**
   1. Exercise.
   2. Heat to the affected extremity.
   3. Immobilization of the affected part.
   4. Use of corticosteroids.

4. **What portion of the bone contains pain receptors?**
   1. Endosteum.
   2. Haversian system.
   3. Marrow.
   4. Periosteum.

5. **When assessing a client with a herniated intervertebral disc, what would some of the signs and symptoms be? Select all that apply.**
   1. Coughing, sneezing, or bending lessens the pain.
   2. Paresthesis.
   3. Sciatica.
   4. Severe back pain that worsens with motion.

6. **A client is diagnosed with Paget's disease. Which manifestations would the nurse include when teaching the client about the disease? Select all that apply.**
   1. Bladder and/or bowel dysfunction.
   2. Chalkstick-type fractures of the lower extremities.
   3. Symptoms of hypercalcemia in immobilized clients.
   4. Vertebral collapse.

7. **Degenerative disc disease commonly occurs in which of the following populations?**
   1. Athletes, particularly African-American males.
   2. People as they age.
   3. Those with a narrowing of the spinal canal.
   4. Those with a poor dietary calcium intake.

8. **A client is on cyclophosphamide (cytoxan) to treat SLE. The nurse should instruct the client to do which of the following?**
   1. Contact the physician if unusual bleeding occurs.
   2. Notify the physician of new symptoms of muscular weakness.
   3. Report any behavioral changes.
   4. Report signs of infection, such as chills, fever, or sore throat.

9. **When preparing a client with SLE for discharge from the hospital, which of the following factors should be included? Select all that apply.**
   1. Clothing options such as elastic waist pants without zippers.
   2. The importance of avoiding exposure to infection.
   3. The importance of skin care.
   4. Management of stiffness and pain.

10. **Ineffective protection is an appropriate nursing diagnosis for the client with SLE. What would be your most important intervention for the hospitalized client?**
    1. Administer prescribed medications.
    2. Monitor lab finding.
    3. Practice careful hand washing.
    4. Provide appropriate skin care.

11. **The nurse, when assessing a client with systemic lupus erythematosus, can be expected to find which of the following? Select all that apply.**
    1. Neuropathies.
    2. Pleural effusion.
    3. Photosensitivity.
    4. Thrombocytopenia.

12. **A nurse is teaching workers at an industrial park what to do if a traumatic amputation would occur at their workplace. Which of the following guidelines would help preserve the amputated part until it could surgically be attached? Select all that apply.**
    1. Don't worry about the amputated part, the important thing is to get the person to the hospital.
    2. Put the amputated part in a plastic bag and put the bag on ice.
    3. Put the amputated part in a storage bag with warm water.
    4. Wrap the amputated part in a clean cloth soaked in saline if possible.

13. **What would be the most important nursing intervention for the first 24 hours after surgery when caring for a client who had a limb amputation?**
    1. Abducting the limb on a scheduled basis.
    2. Applying traction to the limb.
    3. Elevating the limb on a pillow.
    4. Keeping the residual limb flat on the bed.

14. **A client with osteoarthritis is scheduled for an arthroplasty. The nurse explains that the purpose of the procedure is to do which of the following?**
    1. Assess the extent of joint damage.
    2. Fuse a joint and reduce pain.
    3. Prevent further joint damage.
    4. Replace the joint and improve function.

15. **When teaching a client recently diagnosed with osteoarthritis about the risk factors for the disease, which risk factors should be included? Select all that apply.**
    1. Decreased estrogen.
    2. Epstein Barr virus.
    3. Excessive weight.
    4. Inactivity.

16. **Which of the following classifications of medications is commonly used with osteoarthritis, rheumatoid arthritis, and gout?**
    1. Narcotics.
    2. NSAIDs.
    3. Steroids.
    4. Uricosurics.

17. **What is involved in the pathophysiology of gout?**
    1. A reduction of uric acid, which allows calcium to precipitate.
    2. The formation of tophi in the kidneys, which impairs excretion of uric acid.
    3. Inflammation resulting from intra-articular deposition of urate crystals.
    4. A thinning of articular cartilage, leading to splitting and fragmentation.

18. **Which statement is correct concerning antirheumatoid agents? Select all that apply.**
    1. They are given at high doses during maintenance therapy.
    2. They are indicated for short-term use.
    3. They have immunomodulating effects.
    4. They have minor adverse effects.

19. **Clients taking antigout medications should be instructed to do which of the following?**
    1. Continue to take the medication even if diarrhea occurs.
    2. Drink alcoholic beverages to increase absorption of the medication.
    3. Increase their fluid intake to at least 2000 mL per day.
    4. Increase their intake of turkey and organ meats.

20. **When teaching a patient about bisphosphonates for the treatment of gout, which of the following should be included? Select all that apply.**
    1. Increase the client's fluid intake to 3–4 L/day.
    2. Limit foods, such as milk, fruits, carbonated drinks, most vegetables, molasses, and baking soda, that will cause the urine to be more alkaline in order to decrease the chance of stone formation,
    3. Recognize signs of hypocalcemia, such as seizures, muscle spasms, facial twitching, and paresthesias.
    4. Take the medication on an empty stomach and wait at least 30 minutes before eating.

21. **Which of the following medications may contribute to iatrogenic osteoporosis?**
    1. Heparin.
    2. NSAIDs.
    3. Steroids.
    4. Thyroid hormones.

22. **What risk factors identified by the nurse would put a client at risk for developing osteoporosis?**
    1. Early menopause, low calcium intake, excessive alcohol or caffeine, a sedentary lifestyle, and smoking.
    2. A history of falls, a diet deficient in protein and/or or caffeine.
    3. Obesity, stress, family history, and smoking.
    4. Poor dietary intake of calcium, obesity, depression, and excess alcohol.

23. **A nurse is teaching a client newly diagnosed with fibromyalgia about the disorder. What should the nurse include in her teaching?**
    1. FMS is characterized by progression of worsening inflammation.
    2. Many symptoms are similar to chronic fatigue syndrome.
    3. More men than women are affected.
    4. Trigger points are a definitive diagnostic test.

24. **A nurse is giving instructions to a client who had surgical correction of bilateral hallux valgus (bunion). What should the nurse's instructions include?**
    1. Expect the feet to be numb for several days postoperatively.
    2. Rest frequently with the feet elevated.
    3. Soak the feet in warm water several times a day.
    4. Walk primarily on the heels to relieve pressure on the toes.

25. **A nurse is educating co-workers on how to minimize back pain and avoid repeat episodes of low back pain. Which of the following should be included? Select all that apply.**
    1. Maintain appropriate weight.
    2. Sleep in a prone position.
    3. Sleep in a side-lying position with knees flexed.
    4. Use a soft mattress for sleeping.

26. **Which of the following would suggest to the nurse at an urgent care center that a client may have an ankle sprain?**
    1. The client dropped a 10-pound weight on his lower leg at the health club.
    2. The client has ankle pain after running a 10-mile race.
    3. The client has a twisting injury while running bases during a baseball game.
    4. The client was hit by another soccer player on the field.

27. **A client is scheduled for an electromyogram. The nurse should explain that this diagnostic test involves which of the following?**
    1. Administration of a fixed dose of radiostope two hours before the procedure.
    2. Measurement of the heat of muscle contractions radiating from the skin surface.
    3. Placement of electrodes on the skin to record electrical activity of the muscles.
    4. Placement of thin needles into the muscles.

28. **Which of the following is a normal assessment finding of the musculoskeletal system when a nurse assesses a client?**
    1. Full range of motion of all joints without pain or laxity.
    2. Lateral curvature of the spine.
    3. Muscle atrophy.
    4. Muscle strength of 3.

29. **While caring for a client after a spinal fusion has been performed, the nurse should recognize that the interventions for this surgery differ from a simple laminectomy in which of the following ways?**
    1. Body alignment is maintained by the fusion procedure.
    2. Earlier ambulation is permitted because the spine is more stabilized.
    3. Teaching regarding body mechanics and prevention of further back injuries is not as important.
    4. The donor site for the bone graft may be more painful than the spinal incision.

30. **When a client is admitted to the hospital with a fractured extremity, the nurse would first focus the assessment on which of the following?**
    1. The actual fracture site.
    2. The area distal to the fracture.
    3. The area proximal to the fracture.
    4. The extremity not affected for comparison.

31. **A client with a fracture has developed compartment syndrome. Which of the following are characteristic of impending compartment syndrome? Select all that apply.**
    1. Pain proximal to the injury.
    2. Pallor.
    3. Paresthesia.
    4. Pulselessness.

32. **Which of the following would the nurse assess in a client with a fracture of the hip?**
    1. Absence of pain at fracture site.
    2. External rotation.
    3. Lengthening of the affected extremity.
    4. Muscle flaccidity.

33. **A client that has had a femoral head prosthesis inserted should be instructed by the nurse to avoid which of the following activities?**
    1. Placing a large pillow between legs when turning.
    2. Putting on shoes and socks.
    3. Using a lifted toilet seat.
    4. Using a walker.

34. **What information should a nurse include when performing discharge teaching for a client who had a hip replacement with a femoral head prosthesis? Select all that apply.**
    1. Cross your legs or feet while seated.
    2. Inform your dentist of the presence of the prosthesis before dental work.
    3. Use a pillow between your legs when lying on your "good side" or when supine.
    4. Use a toilet elevator on the toilet seat.

35. **A client is taking ibuprofen (Motrin) to treat hip pain. To minimize gastric mucosal irritation, the nurse should teach the client to take this medication at which of the following times?**
    1. At bedtime.
    2. Immediately after a meal.
    3. On arising.
    4. When the client's stomach is empty.

36. **A client with a fractured ulna has been taking cyclobenzoprine (Flexeril). Which of the following would the nurse identify as the drug's primary effect?**
    1. Killing of microorganisms caused by an open fracture.
    2. Reduction in itching caused by skin rash.
    3. Relief of muscle spasms.
    4. Relief of pain.

37. **A client is admitted to the hospital and diagnosed with a fractured tibia to which a cast is applied. Out of the following, which nursing action would be most important after the cast is in place?**
    1. Assessing capillary refill.
    2. Discussing proper cast care.
    3. Pain management.
    4. Performing ROM with the client.

38. **When teaching a client recently discharged from an emergency room with a cast on their arm from a fracture, which of the following would not be included with regard to cast care?**
    1. Apply ice directly over fracture site for first 24 hours.
    2. Dry cast thoroughly after exposure to water with a towel or hair dryer.
    3. Elevate extremity above level of heart for first 48 hours.
    4. Insert any foreign objects inside cast.

39. **Client teaching concerning the use of NSAIDs includes which of the following?**
    1. Avoid combining the use of NSAIDs with alcohol or aspirin.
    2. Avoid giving acetaminophen to children under age 18.
    3. Take enteric coated aspirin with an antacid to decrease GI side effects.
    4. Take NSAIDs on an empty stomach.

Unit 4 Answers and Rationales

Test 7 Answers and Rationales

1. **Answer: 2**
   Rationale: Furosemide (Lasix) is a loop diuretic that will increase urine output and decrease edema. Give furosemide early in the day so that the increased urination will not disturb the client's sleep. Arrange for a potassium rich diet or potassium supplements as needed due to the loss of potassium with the increased diuresis.
   Cognitive Level: Analysis
   Nursing Process: Planning
   NCLEX-RN Test Plan: PHYS
   Reference: Karch, A. M. (2005). *2005 Lippincott's nursing drug guide.* Philadelphia: Lippincott Williams & Wilkins.

2. **Answer: 4**
   Rationale: If the victim cannot be ventilated the first time, reposition the head and try to ventilate again. If the victim cannot be ventilated after repositioning the head, the rescuer should proceed with maneuvers to remove any foreign bodies that may be obstructing the airway.
   Cognitive Level: Analysis
   Nursing Process: Evaluation
   NCLEX-RN Test Plan: SECE
   Reference: Lewis, S. M., Heitkemper, M. M., & Dirksen, S. R. (2004). *Medical-surgical nursing: Assessment and management of clinical problems* (6th ed.). St. Louis, MO: Elsevier Mosby.

3. **Answer: 1**
   Rationale: A flow rate of 2 L/min gives an O_2 concentration of approximately 28%. Face masks will deliver O_2 concentrations of 35–50% with flow rates of 6–12 L/min. A nonrebreathing mask, which delivers high concentrations of O_2, can deliver O_2 concentrations of 60–90%.
   Cognitive Level: Analysis
   Nursing Process: Planning
   NCLEX-RN Test Plan: PHYS

   Reference: Lewis, S. M., Heitkemper, M. M., & Dirksen, S. R. (2004). *Medical-surgical nursing: Assessment and management of clinical problems* (6th ed.). St. Louis, MO: Elsevier Mosby.

4. **Answer: 2**
   Rationale: Acute pneumonia may result when large amounts of tubercle bacilli are discharged from the liquefied necrotic lesion into the lung or lymph nodes. The clinical manifestations are similar to those of bacterial pneumonia, including chills, fever, productive cough, pleuritic pain, and leucocytosis.
   Cognitive Level: Application
   Nursing Process: Assessment
   NCLEX-RN Test Plan: PHYS
   Reference: Lewis, S. M., Heitkemper, M. M., & Dirksen, S. R. (2004). *Medical-surgical nursing: Assessment and management of clinical problems* (6th ed.). St. Louis, MO: Elsevier Mosby.

5. **Answer: 3**
   Rationale: Two methods that are used to assess the efficiency of gas transfer in the lungs are analysis of ABGs and oxymetry. ABGs are used to measure acid-base balance, but oxymetry is not. An assessment of PaO_2 or SaO_2 is usually sufficient to determine adequate oxygenation. Blood drawn from a pulmonary artery catheter is termed a mixed venous blood gas sample because it consists of venous blood that has returned to the heart from tissue beds and "mixed" in the right ventricle.
   Cognitive Level: Analysis
   Nursing Process: Analysis
   NCLEX-RN Test Plan: PHYS
   Reference: Lewis, S. M., Heitkemper, M. M., & Dirksen, S. R. (2004). *Medical-surgical nursing: Assessment and management of clinical problems* (6th ed.). St. Louis, MO: Elsevier Mosby.

6. **Answer: 4**
   Rationale: Early signs include unexplained apprehension, restlessness or irritability, tachypnia,

tachycardia, dyspnea on exertion, and mild hypertension. The other responses are late symptoms of inadequate oxygenation.
Cognitive Level: Application
Nursing Process: Assessment
NCLEX-RN Test Plan: PHYS
Reference: Lewis, S. M., Heitkemper, M. M., & Dirksen, S. R. (2004). *Medical-surgical nursing, Assessment and management of clinical problems* (6th ed.). St. Louis, MO: Elsevier Mosby.

7. **Answer: 4**
Rationale: Crackles are a series of explosive, high-pitched sounds heard just before the end of inspiration; a crackle is a similar sound to that made by rolling hair between the fingers just behind the ear. Rhonchi are continuous rumbling, snoring, or rattling sounds. Stridor is a continuous musical sound of *constant* pitch. Wheezes are also continuous, but are a high-pitched squeaking sound, first evident on expiration, but possibly evident on inspiration as the obstruction worsens. At times, wheezes are audible without a stethoscope.
Cognitive Level: Application
Nursing Process: Assessment
NCLEX-RN Test Plan: PHYS
Reference: Lewis, S. M., Heitkemper, M. M., & Dirksen, S. R. (2004). *Medical-surgical nursing: Assessment and management of clinical problems* (6th ed.). St. Louis, MO: Elsevier Mosby.

8. **Answers: 2, 4, 5**
Rationale: Answers 2, 4, and 5 describe hematocrit. Answers 1 and 3 describe hemoglobin. Venous blood is used for both.
Cognitive Level: Analysis
Nursing Process: Analysis
NCLEX-RN Test Plan: PHYS
Reference: Lewis, S. M., Heitkemper, M. M., & Dirksen, S. R. (2004). *Medical-surgical nursing: Assessment and management of clinical problems* (6th ed.). St. Louis, MO: Elsevier Mosby.

9. **Answers: 1, 2, 3, 4, 5, and 6**
Rationale: All of the answers are target groups for influenza immunization.
Cognitive Level: Application
Nursing Process: Evaluation
NCLEX-RN Test Plan: SECE

Reference: Lewis, S. M., Heitkemper, M. M., & Dirksen, S. R. (2004). *Medical-surgical nursing: Assessment and management of clinical problems* (6th ed.). St. Louis, MO: Elsevier Mosby.

10. **Answer: 2**
Rationale: Atelectasis refers to collapsed, airless alveoli. Pneumothorax is air in the pleural space involving decreased movement of the involved chest wall. Fractured ribs include pain at the site of the injury. The client would splint the affected area and takes shallow breaths to decrease the pain. Flail chest results from multiple rib fractures causing instability. During inspiration, the affected portion is sucked in, and during expiration it bulges out. This paradoxic chest movement prevents adequate ventilation of the lung in the injured site.
Cognitive Level: Analysis
Nursing Process: Assessment
NCLEX-RN Test Plan: PHYS
Reference: Lewis, S. M., Heitkemper, M. M., & Dirksen, S. R. (2004). *Medical-surgical nursing: Assessment and management of clinical problems* (6th ed.). St. Louis, MO: Elsevier Mosby.

11. **Answer: 3**
Rationale: Keep the water seal and suction control chamber at the appropriate water levels by adding sterile water as needed because water loss by evaporation may occur. Never elevate the drainage system to the level of the client's chest because this will cause fluid to drain back into the lungs. Encourage the client to breathe deeply periodically to facilitate lung expansion. Do not strip or milk the chest tube routinely because this increases pleural pressures.
Cognitive Level: Application
Nursing Process: Implementation
NCLEX-RN Test Plan: PHYS
Reference: Lewis, S. M., Heitkemper, M. M., & Dirksen, S. R. (2004). *Medical-surgical nursing: Assessment and management of clinical problems* (6th ed.). St. Louis, MO: Elsevier Mosby.

12. **Answer: 1**
Rationale: Common clinical manifestations of pleural effusion are progressive dyspnea and decreased movement of the chest wall on the affected side. There may be pleuritic pain from the underlying disease and absent or decreased breath sounds over

the affected area. Pleural effusions occur secondary to conditions mentioned in responses 2, 3, and 4.
Cognitive Level: Analysis
Nursing Process: Assessment
NCLEX-RN Test Plan: PHYS
Reference: Lewis, S. M., Heitkemper, M. M., & Dirksen, S. R. (2004). *Medical-surgical nursing: Assessment and management of clinical problems* (6th ed.). St. Louis, MO: Elsevier Mosby.

13. **Answer: 3**
Rationale: The amount of O_2 inhaled depends on the room air and the client's breathing pattern. It is useful for a client who requires low O_2 concentrations. It allows clients to eat, cough, or talk while wearing the device.
Cognitive Level: Analysis
Nursing Process: Planning
NCLEX-RN Test Plan: PHYS
Reference: Lewis, S. M., Heitkemper, M. M., & Dirksen, S. R. (2004). *Medical-surgical nursing: Assessment and management of clinical problems* (6th ed.). St. Louis, MO: Elsevier Mosby.

14. **Answer: 2**
Rationale: If hospitalization is needed, it is usually for a brief period. Clients strongly suspected of having TB should be placed in respiratory isolation. A negative pressure isolation room may be used. The purpose of protective isolation is to protect the vulnerable patient from environmental sources of infection.
Cognitive Level: Analysis
Nursing Process: Implementation
NCLEX-RN Test Plan: PHYS
Reference: Lewis, S. M., Heitkemper, M. M., & Dirksen, S. R. (2004). *Medical-surgical nursing: Assessment and management of clinical problems* (6th ed.). St. Louis, MO: Elsevier Mosby.

15. **Answers: 2 and 4**
Rationale: Oxygen in the home increases the risk of fire injuries. Do not use electric razors, portable radios, open flames, wool blankets, or mineral oils in the area where the oxygen is in use. Do not allow smoking in the home. Remove the mask or collar and cleanse with water 2–3 times a day. Ensure that the straps are not too tight. Observe the tops of the ears for skin breakdown from pressure points.

Cognitive Level: Application
Nursing Process: Implementation
NCLEX-RN Test Plan: PHYS
Reference: Lewis, S. M., Heitkemper, M. M., & Dirksen, S. R. (2004). *Medical-surgical nursing: Assessment and management of clinical problems* (6th ed.). St. Louis, MO: Elsevier Mosby.

16. **Answer: 1**
Rationale: Hypoxemia (especially with activity) may be present. Decreased ventilation causes CO_2 retention resulting in an increase in carbonic acid and *respiratory acidosis*. The other choices are incorrect because respiratory alkalosis occurs with increased exhalation of CO_2, and metabolic acidosis and metabolic alkalosis both have metabolic etiologies.
Cognitive Level: Analysis
Nursing Process: Evaluation
NCLEX-RN Test Plan: PHYS
Reference: Crutchlow, E. M., Dudac, P. J., MacAvoy, S., & Madara, B. R. (2002). *Quick look Nursing: Pathophysiology.* Thorofare, NJ: Slack, Inc.

17. **Answer: 4**
Rationale: The medulla oblongata in the lower brainstem contains "pacemaker" cells that stimulate autonomic ventilation. This controls the rate and depth of respiration. Stimulation of the apneustic center in the pons triggers gasping ventilation when the higher respiratory center is damaged by trauma.
Cognitive Level: Application
Nursing Process: Assessment
NCLEX-RN Test Plan: PHYS
Reference: Crutchlow, E. M., Dudac, P. J., MacAvoy, S., & Madara, B. R. (2002). *Quick look Nursing: Pathophysiology.* Thorofare, NJ: Slack, Inc.

18. **Answer: 1**
Rationale: Alveoli damage results in a decreased ability to exchange carbon dioxide for oxygen. Decreased ventilation (hypoxemia) causes CO_2 retention resulting in respiratory acidosis. The other choices are incorrect because respiratory alkalosis occurs with increased exhalation of CO_2. The others have metabolic etiologies.
Cognitive Level: Analysis
Nursing Process: Evaluation
NCLEX-RN Test Plan: PHYS

Reference: Crutchlow, E. M., Dudac, P. J., MacAvoy, S., & Madara, B. R. (2002). *Quick look Nursing: Pathophysiology.* Thorofare, NJ: Slack, Inc.

19. **Answer: 3**

Rationale: Type II alveolar cells are damaged as part of the ARDS cascade, leading to a decrease in surfactant production and alveolar collapse. Risk factors for developing this noncardiogenic pulmonary edema include aspiration of gastric contents, all types of shock, oxygen toxicity, fat embolism, major trauma, smoke inhalation, multiple blood transfusions, viral pneumonia, and burns. The PCWP is elevated in pulmonary edema caused by CHF, but is normal in pulmonary edema caused by ARDS since the edema is not caused by a deficient heart muscle. ARDS has a high mortality rate.

Cognitive Level: Application

Nursing Process: Planning

NCLEX-RN Test Plan: PHYS

Reference: Crutchlow, E. M., Dudac, P. J., MacAvoy, S., & Madara, B. R. (2002). *Quick look Nursing: Pathophysiology.* Thorofare, NJ: Slack, Inc.

20. **Answer: 1**

Rationale: Atelectesis is an incomplete alveolar expansion or collapse. Areas of alveolar collapse will result in absent breath sounds. Rales, rhonchi and wheezes are all examples of adventitious breath sounds.

Cognitive Level: Analysis

Nursing Process: Assessment

NCLEX-RN Test Plan: PHYS

Reference: Crutchlow, E. M., Dudac, P. J., MacAvoy, S., & Madara, B. R. (2002). *Quick look Nursing: Pathophysiology.* Thorofare, NJ: Slack, Inc.

21. **Answer: 4**

Rationale: Tachycardia is a side effect of theophylline (Theo-Dur, Slo-Bid). It causes CNS stimulation. Increased intraocular pressure and hemolytic anemia are not side effects of theophylline. Anorexia is also a side effect of theophylline.

Cognitive Level: Application

Nursing Process: Planning

NCLEX-RN Test Plan: PHYS

Reference: Crutchlow, E. M., Dudac, P. J., MacAvoy, S., & Madara, B. R. (2002). *Quick look Nursing: Pathophysiology.* Thorofare, NJ: Slack, Inc.

22. **Answer: 2**

Rationale: Alveolar hypoventilation is a common cause for respiratory acidosis. Alveolar hyperventilation, including anxiety, pain and fear, causes acute respiratory alkalosis.

Cognitive Level: Application

Nursing Process: Evaluation

NCLEX-RN Test Plan: PHYS

Reference: Wagner, D. W., Johnson, K., & Kidd, P. S. (2006). *High acuity nursing* (4th ed.). Upper Saddle River, NJ: Pearson Prentice Hall.

23. **Answer: 4**

Rationale: The type of chest pain that a client describes can be helpful in differentiating cardiogenic (originating from the heart) from pleuritic (originating from the pleura) pain. Cardiogenic pain is generally described as dull, pressure-like discomfort often radiating to the jaw, back, or left arm. The client often uses the palm of the hand indicating a general area of pain. Pleuritic pain is frequently described as sharp and knife-like, and the client is able to point to the pain focal area with one finger.

Cognitive Level: Analysis

Nursing Process: Assessment

NCLEX-RN Test Plan: PHYS

Reference: Wagner, D. W., Johnson, K., & Kidd, P. S. (2006). *High acuity nursing* (4th ed.). Upper Saddle River, NJ: Pearson Prentice Hall.

24. **Answer: 2**

Rationale: Normal tidal volume is 7–9 ml/kg or about 500 ml for an average-sized man (approximately 75 kg).

Cognitive Level: Application

Nursing Process: Planning

NCLEX-RN Test Plan: PHYS

Reference: Wagner, D. W., Johnson, K., & Kidd, P. S. (2006). *High acuity nursing* (4th ed.). Upper Saddle River, NJ: Pearson Prentice Hall.

25. Answer:

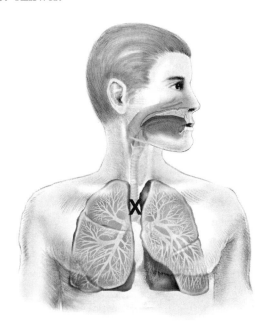

Rationale: These are all normal breath sounds. Bronchial (tubular) breath sounds are located over the trachea. Vesicular breath sounds are located over the lung fields. Bronchovesicular breath sounds are located in all lobes near major airways.
Cognitive Level: Application
Nursing Process: Assessment
NCLEX-RN Test Plan: PHYS
Reference: Wagner, D.W., Johnson, K., & Kidd, P.S. (2006). *High acuity nursing* (4th ed.). Upper Saddle River, NJ: Pearson Prentice Hall, p.107.

26. Answer: 3, 4, 5, 7, 6, 2, 1
Rationale: Although the presenting manifestations of PE are frequently described in general terms, not all episodes of PE present in the same way. The order of sequence of occurrence of signs and symptoms are as follows.
Dyspnea
Pleural pain
Tachycardia
Unilateral leg swelling and pain
Tachnypnea
Crackles (rales)
Cough
Cognitive Level: Application
Nursing Process: Assessment

NCLEX-RN Test Plan: PHYS
Reference: Wagner, D.W., Johnson, K., & Kidd, P.S. (2006). *High acuity nursing* (4th ed.). Upper Saddle River, NJ: Pearson Prentice Hall.

27. Answer: 4
Rationale: This client presents with symptoms of epiglottitis. The child is in respiratory distress. The nurse must keep the child in an upright position and prepare the parents that their child will be taken to the OR quickly. IV antibiotics will be given postoperatively. Examination of the throat is contraindicated, therefore, procedures such as intubation, blood and throat cultures, or IV starts will be done in the OR.
Cognitive Level: Analysis
Nursing Process: Implementation
NCLEX-RN Test Plan: SECE
Reference: Potts, N. L., & Mandleco, B. L. (2002). *Pediatric nursing: Caring for children and their families.* Clifton Park, NY: Delmar.

28. Answer: 4, 2, 6, 3, 5, 1
Rationale: Inhaled medications are administered via metered-dose inhaler (MDI). Children are taught to use a spacer with their MDIs. Spacers make the administration of inhaled medication easier and facilitate better distribution and inhalation of the medication. Spacers minimize large droplets from being deposited in the mouth, which in the case of corticosteroid MDIs, can cause candidal mouth infections. Mouth pieces require the child to be able to hold their breath for between 5 and 10 seconds once the medication is released from the MDI canister. The proper technique is important to adequate administration.
Cognitive Level: Application
Nursing Process: Implementation
NCLEX-RN Test Plan: PHYS
Reference: Potts, N. L., & Mandleco, B. L. (2002). *Pediatric nursing: Caring for children and their families.* Clifton Park, NY: Delmar.

29. Answer: 4
Rationale: Children who have positive throat cultures for streptococcal infection should be instructed to discard their toothbrush and replace it with a new one after they have been taking antibiotics for 24 hours.
Cognitive Level: Analysis
Nursing Process: Evaluation

192 • UNIT 4: ADULT NURSING

NCLEX-RN Test Plan: SECE
Reference: Hockenberry, M. J. (2005). *Wong's essentials of pediatric nursing.* St. Louis, MO: Elsevier Mosby.

30. **Answers: 2, 4, and 6**
    Rationale: Early signs of impending airway obstruction include an increase in pulse and respiratory rates; substernal, suprasternal, and intercostals retractions; flaring nares; and increased restlessness. It is important for the nurse to recognize impending respiratory failure so that intubation can be implemented without delay.
    Cognitive Level: Application
    Nursing Process: Assessment
    NCLEX-RN Test Plan: PHYS
    Reference: Hockenberry, M. J. (2005). *Wong's essentials of pediatric nursing.* St. Louis, MO: Elsevier Mosby.

31. **Answers: 1, 2, and 3**
    Rationale: Very young children have a higher incidence of disseminated disease. TB is a serious disease during the first two years of life, during adolescence, and for those who are HIV positive. Except in cases of tuberculous meningitis, death seldom occurs in treated children. The recommended drug therapy includes drugs such as INH, PZA, and rifampin, which has decreased the death rate and spread from primary lesions.
    Cognitive Level: Analysis
    Nursing Process: Assessment
    NCLEX-RN Test Plan: SECE
    Reference: Hockenberry, M. J. (2005). *Wong's essentials of pediatric nursing.* St. Louis, MO: Elsevier Mosby.

32. **Answer: 2**
    Rationale: The peak expiratory flow rate (PERF) measures the maximum flow rate that can be forcefully exhaled in one second. Three zones of measurement are used to interpret PERF. Green (80 to 100% personal best) signals good control of asthma. Yellow (50 to 79% of personal best) signals caution. Asthma is not well controlled, and an acute exacerbation may be present. Maintenance therapy may need to be increased. The nurse should call the practitioner if the client stays in this zone. Red (below

50% of personal best) indicates a medical alert. Severe airway narrowing may be occurring. A short-acting bronchodilator should be administered. Notify the practitioner if the PERF does not return immediately and stay in yellow or green zones.
    Cognitive Level: Analysis
    Nursing Process: Evaluation
    NCLEX-RN Test Plan: PHYS
    Reference: Hockenberry, M. J. (2005). *Wong's essentials of pediatric nursing.* St. Louis, MO: Elsevier Mosby.

33. **Answer: 1**
    Rationale: When administering drugs during CPR or a "Code," the nurse should use a saline flush between medications to prevent drug interactions. The nurse must also document all drugs, dosages, and the time and route of administration. Other options, although important, are not the highest priority during CPR or a "Code."
    Cognitive Level: Application
    Nursing Process: Implementation
    NCLEX-RN Test Plan: SECE
    Reference: Hockenberry, M. J. (2005). *Wong's essentials of pediatric nursing.* St. Louis, MO: Elsevier Mosby.

34. **Answer: 3**
    Rationale: Option 3 is the only correct answer. The desired outcome addresses the client's response. Options 1 and 4 are nursing interventions. Option 2 is a client goal not relevant to the nursing diagnosis.
    Cognitive Level: Application
    Nursing Process: Diagnosis
    NCLEX-RN Test Plan: PHYS
    Reference: Hockenberry, M. J. (2005). *Wong's essentials of pediatric nursing.* St. Louis, MO: Elsevier Mosby.

35. **Answer: 1**
    Rationale: Theophylline toxicity can occur with a serum level of 20 ug/ml or greater. Side effects from theophylline include nausea, vomiting, headache, irritability, and insomnia. Early signs of toxicity are nausea, tachycardia, and irritability; seizures and dysrhythmias occur at blood theophylline levels greater than 30 ug/ml.
    Cognitive Level: Analysis

Nursing Process: Implementation
NCLEX-RN Test Plan: SECE
Reference: Hockenberry, M. J. (2005). *Wong's essentials of pediatric nursing.* St. Louis, MO: Elsevier Mosby.

36. **Answer: 36 ml/hr**
    Rationale:

$$\frac{ml}{hr} = \frac{500\ ml}{25{,}000\ units} \times \frac{1800\ units}{hour}$$

    Cognitive Level: Knowledge
    Nursing Process: Planning
    NCLEX-RN Test Plan: SECE
    Reference: Phillips, L. D. (2005). *Manual of I.V. therapeutics* (4th ed.). Philadelphia: F.A. Davis.

37. **Answers: 1, 2, 4, 9, 10, and 11**
    Rationale: An optimal aPTT is achieved when it is 1.5–2.5 times the control value. If the control is 36, an aPTT of 90 indicates more than adequate coagulation. A clotting time of 100 seconds indicates the client is more than adequately anticoagulated. The client should be assessed for bleeding and neurological stability. The infusion is to be discontinued for one hour and restarted according to the nomogram. Heparin half-life is 30–180 minutes. Two hours after it is restarted (or three hours after it was initially stopped), an aPTT is drawn to determine therapeutic blood levels. The doctor should be notified since the client is at risk for a bleeding injury. Protamine sulfate is a heparin antagonist and is used for heparin overdose. This client has an increased aPTT but is not experiencing a heparin overdose. Vitamin K is the antidote for Coumadin overdose that is determined with PT results.
    Cognitive Level: Analysis
    Nursing Process: Evaluation
    NCLEX-RN Test Plan: SECE
    Reference: Karch, A. M. (2005). *Lippincott's nursing drug guide.* Philadelphia: Lippincott Williams and Wilkins.

38. **Answer: 1(late), 2(late), 3(early), 4(late), 5(late), 6(late), 7(early), 8(early)**
    Rationale: Brain tissue is highly sensitive to oxygen, and initial signs of deprivation are apprehension, restlessness, or irritability. As the demand for oxygen increases, cardiac output increases with an increase in the heart rate, blood pressure, and respiratory rate. Activities that increase oxygen demand will cause dyspnea. As the oxygen deprivation progresses, CNS symptoms become more pronounced, dyspnea occurs even at rest, and the patient begins to use accessory muscles. Oxygenated blood is shunted to vital organs causing hypotension, with cool, clammy skin or cyanosis.
    Cognitive Level: Analysis
    Nursing Process: Assessment
    NCLEX-RN Test Plan: PHYS
    Reference: Lewis, S. M., Heitkemper, M. M., & Dirksen, S. R. (2004). *Medical surgical nursing* (6th ed.). St. Louis, MO: Mosby.

39. **Answer: 1(ac), 2(al), 3(ac), 4(al), 5(al), 6(al)**
    Rationale: Central nervous system depression is seen with respiratory acidosis. This is observed as restlessness, apathy, weakness, disorientation, stupor, and coma. With respiratory acidosis, there is retention of carbon dioxide (PCO_2) and a pH less than 7.35. The lungs are not blowing off enough CO_2. In an attempt to compensate, the kidneys exchange H^+ for Na^+. While the hydrogen ion is excreted, HCO_3 is reabsorbed and there is an excess of carbonic acid (H_2CO_3). Flushing of the skin is the result of sympathetic nervous system depression. As potassium shifts out of the cells, dysrhythmias can occur resulting in a decreased cardiac output. Eventually, the respiratory center is stimulated to increase respiratory rate and depth to blow off water and carbon dioxide (CO_2). Exacerbation of chronic obstructive pulmonary disease (COPD) may be the initial cause of the acidosis with retention of carbon dioxide. Respiratory alkalosis occurs when the PCO_2 falls and the pH is greater than 7.35. Central nervous system excitability occurs with respiratory alkalosis. This is observed as irritability, confusion, tetany-like symptoms, and hyperactive reflexes. Chronic respiratory alkalosis is uncommon.
    Cognitive Level: Analysis
    Nursing Process: Assessment
    NCLEX-RN Test Plan: PHYS
    Reference: LeFever Kee, J., Paulanka, B., & Purnell, L. D. (2004). *Fluids and electrolytes with clinical applications: A programmed approach* (7th ed.). Newark, NJ: Thompson.

Unit 4 Answers and Rationales

Test 8 Answers and Rationales

1. **Answer: 3**

   Rationale: Digoxin (Lanoxin) will decrease the heart rate. Therefore, observe the monitor for bradycardia and/or arrhythmias, or count the apical pulse for at least one minute before administering the drug. Hold the medication if the heart rate is below 60 or if an arrhythmia occurs.

   Cognitive Level: Application

   Nursing Process: Assessment

   NCLEX-RN Test Plan: PHYS

   Reference: Karch, A. M. (2005). *2005 Lippincott's nursing drug guide.* Philadelphia: Lippincott Williams & Wilkins..

2. **Answer: 3**

   Rationale: Headache is a common side effect of nitroglycerine. Over-the-counter preparations may or may not help. It is important to continue the medication for symptoms of angina.

   Cognitive Level: Analysis

   Nursing Process: Implementation

   NCLEX-RN Test Plan: PHYS

   Reference: Karch, A. M. (2005). *2005 Lippincott's nursing drug guide.* Philadelphia: Lippincott Williams & Wilkins.

3. **Answer: 4**

   Rationale: The usual recommended dose is one tablet taken sublingually, which can be followed at five minute intervals with two more doses. Clients should be taught not to carry nitroglycerine (NTG) in their pockets because heat from the body can cause a loss of potency of the tablets. Nitroglycerine can be taken prophylactically before undertaking an activity that the client knows will precipitate an anginal attack. Because NTG tend to lose potency once a bottle has been opened, the patient should be advised to purchase a new supply every 6 months.

   Cognitive Level: Analysis

   Nursing Process: Implementation

   NCLEX-RN Test Plan: PHYS

   Reference: Lewis, S. M., Heitkemper, M. M., & Dirksen, S. R. (2004). *Medical-surgical nursing: Assessment and management of clinical problems* (6th ed.). St. Louis, MO: Elsevier Mosby.

4. **Answer: 3**

   Rationale: Protamine sulfate is a heparin antagonist. Vitamin K is a warfarin (Coumadin) antagonist. Iron is used to treat anemia, and platelets are given to increase platelet count.

   Cognitive Level: Application

   Nursing Process: Planning

   NCLEX-RN Test Plan: PHYS

   Reference: Karch, A. M. (2005). *2005 Lippincott's nursing drug guide.* Philadelphia: Lippincott Williams & Wilkins.

5. **Answer:**

   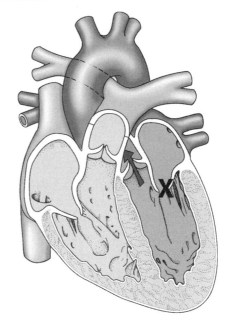

   Rationale: The heart contains two atrioventricular valves (the mitral and the tricuspid) and two semilunar valves (the aortic and the pulmonic), which are located in four strategic locations to control unidirectional blood flow. The mitral valve is located between the left atria and left ventricle.

   Cognitive Level: Application

Nursing Process: Assessment

NCLEX-RN Test Plan: PHYS

Reference: Lewis, S. M., Heitkemper, M. M., & Dirksen, S. R. (2004). *Medical-surgical nursing: Assessment and management of clinical problems* (6th ed.). St. Louis, MO: Elsevier Mosby.

6. **Answer: 1**

Rationale: The insertion site must have direct pressure and the client must remain supine for approximately six hours with the affected leg straight. Palpation of pedal pulses and observation of the access site are important nursing assessments that are made frequently after the procedure.

Cognitive Level: Analysis

Nursing Process: Assessment

NCLEX-RN Test Plan: PHYS

Reference: Wagner, D. W., Johnson, K., & Kidd, P. S. (2006). *High acuity nursing.* Upper Saddle River, NJ: Pearson Prentice Hall.

7. **Answer: 90**

Rationale: One method of calculating heart rate on an EKG strip is based on a six second strip. ECG paper is marked at the top margin in three second intervals. QRS complexes in a six second strip (30 large blocks) are multiplied by 10 to get the heart rate by minute (6 × 10 = 60 seconds). Therefore, 9 QRS complexes in a six second strip multiplied by 10 equals a rate of 90.

Cognitive Level: Analysis

Nursing Process: Assessment

NCLEX-RN Test Plan: PHYS

Reference: Wagner, D. W., Johnson, K., & Kidd, P. S. (2006). *High acuity nursing.* Upper Saddle River, NJ: Pearson Prentice Hall.

8. **Answers: 2, 3, 4, 5, 6, and 7**

Rationale: Modifiable risk factors include elevated serum lipids, hypertension, cigarette smoking, obesity, physical inactivity, diabetes mellitus, and a stressful lifestyle.

Unmodifiable risk factors include age, gender (men have a greater risk than women until age 60), ethnicity (African Americans have a greater risk than Whites), genetic predisposition, and a family history of heart disease.

Cognitive Level: Application

Nursing Process: Assessment

NCLEX-RN Test Plan: PHYS

Reference: Lewis, S. M., Heitkemper, M. M., & Dirksen, S. R. (2004). *Medical-surgical nursing: Assessment and management of clinical problems* (6th ed.). St. Louis, MO: Elsevier Mosby.

9. **Answer: 3**

Rationale: Fatigue is one of the earliest symptoms of CHF. Tachycardia may be one of the first clinical manifestations, as well. Dyspnea and edema are common side effects of CHF.

Cognitive Level: Application

Nursing Process: Assessment

NCLEX-RN Test Plan: PHYS

Reference: Lewis, S. M., Heitkemper, M. M., & Dirksen, S. R. (2004). *Medical-surgical nursing: Assessment and management of clinical problems* (6th ed.). St. Louis, MO: Elsevier Mosby.

10. **Answer: 15 ml/hr**

Rationale: Weight: 80 kg

Order: 300 mcg/kg/hr

Solution: 250 ml D_5W w/400 mg dopamine

$$80 \text{ kg} \times 300 \text{ mcg/kg} \times \text{hr} \times 250 \text{ ml/400 mg} \times 1 \text{ mg/1000 mcg} = 15 \text{ ml/hr}$$

Cognitive Level: Application

Nursing Process: Implementation

NCLEX-RN Test Plan: PHYS

Reference: Curren, A. (2006). *Dimensional analysis for meds* (3rd ed.). Clifton Park, NY: Thompson Delmar.

11. **Answer: 2**

Rationale: An increase in venous hydrostatic pressure, which develops when fluid accumulates in the veins, causes fluid to leak out into the tissues and causes edema. The other three choices refer to the manifestations of *arterial* insufficiency.

Cognitive Level: Analysis

Nursing Process: Evaluation

NCLEX-RN Test Plan: PHYS

Reference: Crutchlow, E. M., Dudac, P. J., MacAvoy, S., & Madara, B. R. (2002). *Quick look nursing: Pathophysiology.* Thorofare, NJ: Slack, Inc.

12. **Answer: 1**

Rationale: Dehydration increases the blood viscosity, and immobility leads to stasis of blood. Certain

oral contraceptives increase the coagulability of blood. Diabetes, hypertension, and high intake of calcium do not increase the risk of clotting.
Cognitive Level: Analysis
Nursing Process: Evaluation
NCLEX-RN Test Plan: PHYS
Reference: Crutchlow, E. M., Dudac, P. J., MacAvoy, S., & Madara, B. R. (2002). *Quick look Nursing: Pathophysiology.* Thorofare, NJ: Slack, Inc.

13. **Answer: 8 ml/hour**
    Rationale: 10,000 units/100 ml = 100 units/ml
    100 units/1 ml = 800 units/X ml
    X = 8 ml/hour
    Cognitive Level: Application
    Nursing Process: Planning
    NCLEX-RN Test Plan: PHYS
    Reference: Curren, A. (2006). *Dimensional analysis for meds* (3rd ed.). Clifton Park, NY: Thompson Delmar.

14. **Answer: Sinus bradycardia**
    Rationale: The rhythm is regular. The atrial and ventricular rates are less than 60 beats/minute. There is a P wave before each QRS complex. The QRS is of normal duration, and the PR interval is normal.
    Cognitive Level: Analysis
    Nursing Process: Assessment
    NCLEX-RN Test Plan: PHYS
    Reference: Baird, M. S., Keen, J. H., & Swearingen, P. L. (2005). *Manual of critical care nursing: Nursing interventions and collaborative management* (5th ed.). St. Louis, MO: Elsevier Mosby.

15. **Answer: 1**
    Rationale: Cardiac murmurs are turbulent sounds characterized by loudness, pitch, shape, quality, duration, and timing, which occur between normal heart sounds. S3 is an extra heart sound, is low pitched, ends in *early* diastole, and is similar to the sound of a gallop. S4 is an extra heart sound, is low pitched, ends in *late* diastole, and is similar to the sound of a gallop.
    Cognitive Level: Analysis
    Nursing Process: Assessment
    NCLEX-RN Test Plan: PHYS
    Reference: Lewis, S. M., Heitkemper, M. M., & Dirksen, S. R. (2004). *Medical-surgical nursing: Assessment and management of clinical problems* (6th ed.). St. Louis, MO: Elsevier Mosby.

16. **Answer: 3**
    Rationale: The P wave indicates Atrial depolarization, stimulated by the firing of the SA node traveling to the AV node.
    Cognitive Level: Analysis
    Nursing Process: Evaluation
    NCLEX-RN Test Plan: PHYS
    Reference: Wagner, D., Johnson, K., & Kidd, P. S. (2006). *High acuity nursing.* Upper Saddle River, NJ: Pearson Prentice Hall.

17. **Answer: 1**
    Rationale: Age is the only unmodifiable risk factor listed. All others are modifiable risk factors.
    Cognitive Level: Application
    Nursing Process: Assessment
    NCLEX-RN Test Plan: PHYS
    Reference: Lewis, S. M., Heitkemper, M. M., & Dirksen, S. R. (2004). *Medical-surgical nursing: Assessment and management of clinical problems* (6th ed.). St. Louis, MO: Elsevier Mosby.

18. **Answer: 3**
    Rationale: Responses 1, 2, and 4 are associated with a client having a myocardial infarction when cellular damage has occurred. Anginal pain usually lasts for only a few minutes (between three and five minutes) and commonly subsides when the precipitation factor (usually exertion) is relieved. Pain at rest is unusual.
    Cognitive Level: Application
    Nursing Process: Evaluation
    NCLEX-RN Test Plan: PHYS
    Reference: Lewis, S. M., Heitkemper, M. M., & Dirksen, S. R. (2004). *Medical-surgical nursing: Assessment and management of clinical problems* (6th ed.). St. Louis, MO: Elsevier Mosby.

19. **Answer: 1**
    Rationale: Recent studies indicate that up to a 50% reduction in unstable angina progression to MI occurs with the use of aspirin.
    Cognitive Level: Application
    Nursing Process: Implementation
    NCLEX-RN Test Plan: PHYS
    Reference: Lewis, S. M., Heitkemper, M. M., & Dirksen, S. R. (2004). *Medical-surgical nursing, Assessment and management of clinical problems* (6th ed.). St. Louis, MO: Elsevier Mosby.

20. **Answer: 2**

    Rationale: The client will need another NTG since there is still chest pain. However, the *first* thing is to assess another BP. If the systolic BP remains above 100, another NTG should be administered. If the systolic BP decreases below 100, the physician should be notified.

    Cognitive Level: Analysis

    Nursing Process: Implementation

    NCLEX-RN Test Plan: PHYS

    Reference: Karch, A. M. (2005). *2005 Lippincott's nursing drug guide.* Philadelphia: Lippincott Williams & Wilkins.

21. **Answer: 2**

    Rationale: Symptoms of patients with heart failure are a result of impaired ventricular function, which decreases the pumping ability of the heart and increases fluid volume. The other answers are all conditions that can trigger heart failure.

    Cognitive Level: Analysis

    Nursing Process: Assessment

    NCLEX-RN Test Plan: PHYS

    Reference: Wagner, D. W., Johnson, K., & Kidd, P. S. (2006). *High acuity nursing.* Upper Saddle River, NJ: Pearson Prentice Hall.

22. **Answer: 4**

    Rationale: Spironilactone (Aldactone) is a potassium sparing diuretic. It blocks the effects of aldosterone in the renal tubule, causing a loss of sodium and water and retention of potassium.

    Cognitive Level: Application

    Nursing Process: Analysis

    NCLEX-RN Test Plan: PHYS

    Reference: Karch, A. M. (2005). *2005 Lippincott's nursing drug guide.* Philadelphia: Lippincott Williams & Wilkins.

23. **Answer: 2**

    Rationale: Enoxaparin (Lovonox) is a low molecular heparin that inhibits thrombus and clot formation, requires less laboratory monitoring, and is often used to prevent DVT following surgery.

    Cognitive Level: Analysis

    Nursing Process: Analysis

    NCLEX-RN Test Plan: PHYS

    Reference: Karch, A. M. (2005). *2005 Lippincott's nursing drug guide.* Philadelphia: Lippincott Williams & Wilkins.

24. **Answer: 4**

    Rationale: Protamine sulfate is the treatment of heparin overdose. Vitamin K is the treatment for a warfarin (Coumadin) overdose. Protamine zinc is insulin given for hyperglycemia. Vitamin E is an antioxidant.

    Cognitive Level: Application

    Nursing Process: Implementation

    NCLEX-RN Test Plan: PHYS

    Reference: Karch, A. M. (2005). *2005 Lippincott's nursing drug guide.* Philadelphia: Lippincott Williams & Wilkins.

25. **Answer: 4**

    Rationale: Loss of appetite, nausea, vomiting, and blurred or yellow vision may be signs of digoxin toxicity. The client should be instructed to eat foods high in potassium to prevent hypokalemia, which increases the chances of developing digoxin toxicity. An apical pulse should be taken for a full minute prior to administering digoxin. The medication should be held and the physician should be contacted if the apical pulse is less than 60 beats per minute.

    Cognitive Level: Analysis

    Nursing Process: Implementation

    NCLEX-RN Test Plan: PHYS

    Reference: Karch, A. M. (2005). *2005 Lippincott's nursing drug guide.* Philadelphia: Lippincott Williams & Wilkins.

26. **Answer: 4**

    Rationale: The diagnosis of ventricular tachycardia is made when a run of three or more PVCs occurs. The ventricular rate is 100 to 250 beats per minute.

    Cognitive Level: Analysis

    Nursing Process: Analysis

    NCLEX-RN Test Plan: PHYS

    Reference: Lewis, S. M., Heitkemper, M. M., & Dirksen, S. R. (2004). *Medical-surgical nursing: Assessment and management of clinical problems* (6th ed.). St. Louis, MO: Elsevier Mosby.

27. **Answer: 3**

    Rationale: Ventricular fibrillation is a severe derangement of the heart rhythm characterized on an ECG by irregular undulations of varying contour and amplitude. Mechanically, the ventricle is simply "quivering," and no effective contraction or CO occurs.

    Cognitive Level: Analysis

    Nursing Process: Analysis

NCLEX-RN Test Plan: PHYS

Reference: Lewis, S. M., Heitkemper, M. M., &
    Dirksen, S. R. (2004). *Medical-surgical nursing:
    Assessment and management of clinical problems*
    (6th ed.). St. Louis, MO: Elsevier Mosby.

28. **Answer: 2**
    Rationale: Anginal pain usually lasts for only a few
    minutes (three to five minutes) and commonly sub-
    sides when the precipitation factor (usually exertion)
    is relieved. Pain at rest is unusual.
    Cognitive Level: Application
    Nursing Process: Evaluation
    NCLEX-RN Test Plan: PHYS
    Reference: Lewis, S. M., Heitkemper, M. M., &
        Dirksen, S. R. (2004). *Medical-surgical nursing:
        Assessment and management of clinical problems*
        (6th ed.). St. Louis, MO: Elsevier Mosby.

29. **Answer: 2**
    Rationale: Jugular vein distension is a symptom of
    right-sided heart failure. The other choices are
    symptoms of left-sided heart failure.
    Cognitive Level: Analysis
    Nursing Process: Assessment
    NCLEX-RN Test Plan: PHYS
    Reference: Lewis, S. M., Heitkemper, M. M., &
        Dirksen, S. R. (2004). *Medical-surgical nursing:
        Assessment and management of clinical problems*
        (6th ed.). St. Louis, MO: Elsevier Mosby.

30. **Answer: 1**
    Rationale: A measure used for assessing arterial flow
    to the extremities is the capillary filling time. The
    client's nail beds are squeezed to produce blanching
    and observed for the return of color. With normal
    arterial capillary perfusion, the color will return
    within three seconds.
    Cognitive Level: Analysis
    Nursing Process: Evaluation
    NCLEX-RN Test Plan: PHYS
    Reference: Lewis, S. M., Heitkemper, M. M., &
        Dirksen, S. R. (2004). *Medical-surgical nursing:
        Assessment and management of clinical problems*
        (6th ed.). St. Louis, MO: Elsevier Mosby.

31. **Answer: 4**
    Rationale: Patients with atrial fibrillation are at an
    increased risk for thrombus formation and subse-
    quent embolization to the brain. Anticoagulants are

used to prevent thrombosis formation. They do not
dissolve clots.
Cognitive Level: Analysis
Nursing Process: Evaluation
NCLEX-RN Test Plan: PHYS
Reference: Lewis, S. M., Heitkemper, M. M., &
    Dirksen, S. R. (2004). *Medical-surgical nursing:
    Assessment and management of clinical problems*
    (6th ed.). St. Louis, MO: Elsevier Mosby.

32. **Answer: 4**
    Rationale: This is an oral anticoagulant that pro-
    longs clotting times. Avoid situations in which you
    could be easily injured and that would cause bleed-
    ing, for example, shaving with a straight razor.
    Increased bleeding tendencies occur with aspirin.
    Monitor PT ratio or INR regularly to adjust dose.
    Cognitive Level: Analysis
    Nursing Process: Evaluation
    NCLEX-RN Test Plan: PHYS
    Reference: Karch, A. M. (2005). *2005 Lippincott's
        nursing drug guide.* Philadelphia: Lippincott
        Williams & Wilkins.

33. **Answer: 1, 2, 3, 4, 5, 6, 7, 8**
    Rationale: The steps for one-rescuer CPR are
    as follows:

    1. Assess the patient/victim for unresponsiveness
    2. Activate emergency medical system (EMS)
    3. Open victims airway
    4. Assess for breathing
    5. Give 2 breaths
    6. Assess for circulation
    7. Begin compressions
    8. Continue ventilation and compressions at a
       ratio of 2 ventilations : 30 compressions for
       2 minutes.
    9. Reassess victim
    10. Continue CPR until EMS or automatic
        external defibrillator (AED) arrives

    Cognitive Level: Application
    Nursing Process: Planning
    NCLEX-RN Test Plan: SECE
    Reference: American Heart Association. (2005). *BLS
        for healthcare providers.* Dallas, TX: Author.

34. **Answer: 2**
    Rationale: Family members should understand CPR
    due to the patient's probable history of cardiac

arrhythmias. Routine ICD checks are needed every two to three months. When traveling, airport security should be informed of the presence of the ICD because it may set off the metal detectors. If a hand-held screening wand is used, it should not be placed over the ICD. The ICD is placed in a subcutaneous pocket over the pectoralis muscle.
Cognitive Level: Analysis
Nursing Process: Implementation
NCLEX-RN Test Plan: PHYS
Reference: Lewis, S. M., Heitkemper, M. M., & Dirksen, S. R. (2004). *Medical-surgical nursing: Assessment and management of clinical problems* (6th ed.). St. Louis, MO: Elsevier Mosby.

35. **Answer: 2**
Rational: The client should understand the significance of the prescribed prophylactic antibiotic therapy before any invasive procedure. This includes all dental procedures likely to produce gingival or mucosal bleeding, including professional cleaning. It would not include a simple adjustment of orthodontic appliances or shedding of deciduous teeth. All dental procedures, chest X-rays, and exercise programs do not put the client at increased risk for effective endocarditis.
Cognitive Level: Application
Nursing Process: Evaluation
NCLEX-RN Test Plan: PHYS
Reference: Lewis, S. M., Heitkemper, M. M., & Dirksen, S. R. (2004). *Medical-surgical nursing: Assessment and management of clinical problems* (6th ed.). St. Louis, MO: Elsevier Mosby.

36. **Answer: 4**
Rationale: The patient with DVT may have no symptoms or may have unilateral leg edema, extremity pain, warm skin, erythema, and a systemic temperature greater than 100.4° F. If the calf is involved, tenderness may be present on palpation. A positive Homan's sign is a classic sign but very unreliable and appears in only 10% of clients.
Cognitive Level: Analysis
Nursing Process: Assessment
NCLEX-RN Test Plan: PHYS

Reference: Lewis, S. M., Heitkemper, M. M., & Dirksen, S. R. (2004). *Medical-surgical nursing: Assessment and management of clinical problems* (6th ed.). St. Louis, MO: Elsevier Mosby.

37. **Answer: 3**
Rationale: Enoxaparin (Lovenox) is a low molecular weight heparin (LMWH). Routine coagulation tests typically are not required. Do not expel the air bubble before administering it subcutaneously. Protamine sulfate partially reverses the effects of LMWH.
Cognitive Level: Application
Nursing Process: Planning
NCLEX-RN Test Plan: PHYS
Reference: Lewis, S. M., Heitkemper, M. M., & Dirksen, S. R. (2004). *Medical-surgical nursing: Assessment and management of clinical problems* (6th ed.). St. Louis, MO: Elsevier Mosby.

38. **Answer: 4**
Rationale: In preparation for the exercise stress test, the patient is instructed not to eat, smoke, or drink beverages containing caffeine for several hours prior to the test. Certain drugs, such as beta blockers, may be held for 24 hours prior to the procedure.
Cognitive Level: Analysis
Nursing Process: Assessment
NCLEX-RN Test Plan: PHYS
Reference: Wagner, D. W., Johnson, K., & Kidd, P. S. (2006). *High acuity nursing.* Upper Saddle River, NJ: Pearson Prentice Hall.

39. **Answer: 4**
Rationale: The landmark for proper hand placement for chest compressions is two fingers above the xyphoid-sternal notch.
Cognitive Level: Application
Nursing Process: Implementation
NCLEX-RN Test Plan: SECE
Reference: Lewis, S. M., Heitkemper, M. M., & Dirksen, S. R. (2004). *Medical-surgical nursing: Assessment and management of clinical problems* (6th ed.). St. Louis, MO: Elsevier Mosby.

Unit 4 Answers and Rationales

Test 9 Answers and Rationales

1. **Answer: 3**
   Rationale: When the gallbladder is inflamed as with cholecystitis, there is an intolerance to fatty foods. The inflamed gallbladder does not produce enough bile to the small intestine to aid in fat digestion. Fiber, sodium, and acid-ash diets are not influenced by the inflamed gallbladder in chronic cholecystitis.
   Cognitive Level: Application
   Nursing Process: Implementation
   NCLEX-RN Test Plan: HPM
   Reference: Lewis, S. M., Heitkemper, M. M., & Dirksen, S. R. (2004). *Medical-surgical nursing: Assessment and management of clinical problems* (6th ed.). St. Louis, MO: Elsevier Mosby.

2. **Answer: 1**
   Rationale: In the United States, alcohol abuse is the major cause of acute pancreatitis. Although it is not completely clear how alcohol causes pancreatitis, thoughts are that it stimulates secretion of hydrochloric acid, which leads to the release of hormones thereby stimulating further pancreatic enzyme secretion. Diabetes, CHF, and COPD are not factors that are consistent with acute pancreatitis.
   Cognitive Level: Analysis
   Nursing Process: Assessment
   NCLEX-RN Test Plan: PHYS
   Reference: Lewis, S. M., Heitkemper, M. M., & Dirksen, S. R. (2004). *Medical-surgical nursing: Assessment and management of clinical problems* (6th ed.). St. Louis, MO: Elsevier Mosby.

3. **Answer: 4**
   Rationale: Hemorrhage is the most serious complication of those listed. Bleeding occurs due to the loss of the protective mucosal barrier, which leads to tissue damage as the gastric acids further damage the epithelial wall. Anorexia may occur with ulcers but it is not as serious as hemorrhage. Esophagitis and pulmonary embolism are not usual complications of ulcer disease.
   Cognitive Level: Analysis
   Nursing Process: Analysis

NCLEX-RN Test Plan: PHYS
Reference: Black, J., & Hawks, J. H. (2005). *Medical-surgical nursing: Clinical management for positive outcomes* (7th ed.). St. Louis, MO: Elsevier Saunders.

4. **Answer: 1**
   Rationale: Both bowel conditions are inflammatory. While both involve inflammation, each has different populations affected, degrees of mucosal penetration, and different distribution patterns in the bowel.
   Cognitive Level: Analysis
   Nursing Process: Assessment
   NCLEX-RN Test Plan: PHYS
   Reference: Black, J., & Hawks, J. H. (2005). *Medical-surgical nursing: Clinical management for positive outcomes* (7th ed.). St. Louis, MO: Elsevier Saunders.

5. **Answer: 4**
   Rationale: Medications ordered as sublingual are given this way to be readily absorbed in the vascular area under the tongue. A nasogastric tube in place does not alter the desired effect of sublingual medications. The nurse should not change the form of sublingual medications nor are these medications to be crushed or dissolved.
   Cognitive Level: Application
   Nursing Process: Implementation
   NCLEX-RN Test Plan: PHYS
   Reference: Potter, P. A., & Perry, A. G. (2005). *Fundamentals of nursing* (6th ed.). St. Louis, MO: Elsevier Mosby.

6. **Answers: 1, 3, 4, 6, and 8**
   Rationale: Wound dehiscence refers to the opening of a skin wound if the collagen fibers are not mature enough to hold the incision closed. By reviewing the possible risk factors for dehiscence and being aware, the nurse can better plan the approach to implementing the activity order. Distention of the abdominal region with pressure, obesity, or infection can lead to weakening of the healing tissues. The effects of dehydration on the newly formed collagen

can weaken incision lines. The remaining options are not risk factors for wound dehiscence.
Cognitive Level: Application
Nursing Process: Assessment
NCLEX-RN Test Plan: PHYS
Reference: Lutz, C. A., & Przytulski, K. R. (2006). *Nutrition and diet therapy: Evidence-based application* (4th ed.). Philadelphia: F.A. Davis.

7. **Answer: 1**
Rationale: Normally the abdomen's shape is symmetrical. Asymmetry may indicate an underlying pathological condition that may require further investigation. The remaining options could be part of normal abdominal assessment.
Cognitive Level: Analysis
Nursing Process: Assessment
NCLEX-RN Test Plan: PHYS
Reference: Potter, P. A., & Perry, A. G. (2005). *Fundamentals of nursing* (6th ed.). St. Louis, MO: Elsevier Mosby.

8. **Answer: 4**
Rationale: To prevent aspiration of tube feeding, the client should be sitting up or lying with the head of bed elevated 30–45°. The client position of comfort does not guarantee it will prevent aspiration, nor is a 10° elevation enough to prevent aspiration.
Cognitive Level: Application
Nursing Process: Evaluation
NCLEX-RN Test Plan: HPM
Reference: Lewis, S. M., Heitkemper, M. M., & Dirksen S. R. (2004). *Medical-surgical nursing: Assessment and management of clinical problems* (6th ed.). St. Louis, MO: Elsevier Mosby.

9. **Answer: 3**
Rationale: With malabsorption there is impaired absorption of vitamins and minerals (e.g. iron), therefore the hemoglobin and hematocrit will be decreased, as the correct option denotes. The remaining options are not consistent with malabsorption. Infiltrates are seen with respiratory aliments, while reduced levels of calcium and potassium often may be seen with malabsorption syndrome.
Cognitive Level: Analysis
Nursing Process: Assessment
NCLEX-RN Test Plan: PHYS

References: Pagana, K. D., & Pagana, T. J. (2002). *Mosby's manual of diagnostic and laboratory tests.* St. Louis, MO: Mosby.

Lewis, S. M., Heitkemper, M. M., & Dirksen, S. R. (2004). Medical-surgical nursing: Assessment and management of clinical problems (6th ed.). St. Louis, MO: Elsevier Mosby.

10. **Answer: Potassium**
Rationale: A normal serum potassium level is 3.5–5 mEq/L. The 2.2 mEq/L potassium result is severe hypokalemia. Hypokalemia may result in cardiac abnormalities or even cardiac arrest, therefore this would be the most important lab value to report. While the sodium level is slightly low, is not severe. The glucose level is above normal, but it is not severe enough at this point to report.
Cognitive Level: Analysis
Nursing Process: Assessment
NCLEX-RN Test Plan: PHYS
Reference: Munden, J. (Ed.). (2006). *Fluids and electrolytes.* Philadelphia: Lippincott Williams and Wilkins.

11. **Answer: 2**
Rationale: Stool left in the bowel does not allow for adequate visualization and could be confused as polyps. A laxative will help to evacuate the bowel contents. The remaining responses are not appropriate nor do they reveal an understanding of the procedure.
Cognitive Level: Application
Nursing Process: Planning
NCLEX-RN Test Plan: PHYS
Reference: Pagana, K. D., & Pagana, T. J. (2002). *Mosby's manual of diagnostic and laboratory tests.* St. Louis, MO: Mosby.

12. **Answer: 2**
Rationale: An ileostomy is created from an opening in the ileum of the intestine. The contents contain digestive enzymes that are very irritating to the skin. Ileostomy bags do not need to be sterile since they are placed on the skin, but do require a skin barrier for protection from leakage of the continual fecal contents as with an ileostomy.
Cognitive Level: Application
Nursing Process: Planning
NCLEX-RN Test Plan: HPM

Reference: Lewis, S. M., Heitkemper, M. M., & Dirksen, S. R. (2004). *Medical-surgical nursing: Assessment and management of clinical problems* (6th ed.). St. Louis, MO: Elsevier Mosby.

13. **Answer: 3**

    Rationale: An adynamic obstruction results from the lack of peristaltic activity, thereby causing an accumulation of fluids and air proximal to the problem site. A nasogastic tube will suction the fluid and air until the bowel begins to function. Also, the tube will prevent further distention and break up the obstruction. The remaining options are not appropriate for treating an ileus.

    Cognitive Level: Analysis
    Nursing Process: Implementation
    NCLEX-RN Test Plan: PHYS
    Reference: Black, J., & Hawks, J. H. (2005). *Medical-surgical nursing: Clinical management for positive outcomes* (7th ed.). St. Louis, MO: Elsevier Saunders.

14. **Answer: 2525 ml infused during surgery**
    Rationale:

IV fluid at 150 ml times 9 hours =	1350 ml
Cefazolin sodium (Ancef) piggyback =	100 ml
1 unit of blood =	275 ml
1 unit of blood =	250 ml
Bolus of 250 ml normal saline × 2 =	500 ml
Ranitidine (Zantac) IV =	50 ml
Total	2525 ml

15. **Answer: 2**

    Rationale: The sequence of examination for the abdomen differs somewhat from other assessments. Auscultation is done before palpation and percussion because palpation and percussion may alter the frequency and character of bowel sounds.

    Cognitive Level: Application
    Nursing Process: Assessment
    NCLEX-RN Test Plan: HPM
    Reference: Potter, P. A., & Perry, A. G. (2005). *Fundamentals of nursing* (6th ed.). St. Louis, MO: Elsevier Mosby.

16. **Answer: 4**

    Rationale: The client is placed on one side to prevent aspiration while the sedation and local anesthe-

sia wear off. The other positions are not considered the safest postprocedure.

Cognitive Level: Application
Nursing Process: Implementation
NCLEX-RN Test Plan: PHYS
Reference: Black, J., & Hawks, J. H. (2005). *Medical-surgical nursing: Clinical management for positive outcomes* (7th ed.). St. Louis, MO: Elsevier Saunders.

17. **Answers: 1 and 5**

    Rationale: A client with cirrhosis is often given a diuretic (Lasix) to aid in fluid reduction. Common lab studies include liver function tests. Coumadin is not administered to a client with liver problems due to the backup of blood from the portal vein, which causes an increased removal of blood cells from the circulation. Daily chest X-rays are not necessary for the cirrhosis client. A diet high in calories, high in carbohydrates, and low in fat and protein are ordered for the liver diseased client. With cirrhosis, the metabolic demands of the liver are high, therefore, limited activity is necessary for the liver cells to recover.

    Cognitive Level: Analysis
    Nursing Process: Planning
    NCLEX-RN Test Plan: PHYS
    Reference: Lewis, S. M., Heitkemper, M. M., & Dirksen, S. R. (2004). *Medical-surgical nursing: Assessment and management of clinical problems* (6th ed.). St. Louis, MO: Elsevier Mosby.

18. **Answer: 4**

    Rationale: Giving the client the correct information about discomfort aids in the development of rapport. It is correct that the client may experience shoulder or subcostal discomfort from the pneumoperitoneum. The other responses do not display the nurse's knowledge.

    Cognitive Level: Analysis
    Nursing Process: Implementation
    NCLEX-RN Test Plan: PHYS
    Reference: Pagana, K. D., & Pagana, T. J. (2002). *Mosby's manual of diagnostic and laboratory tests.* St. Louis, MO: Mosby.

19. **Answer: Appendicitis**

    Rationale: The complaints listed are representative of classic clinical manifestations of appendicitis.

Appendicitis is an inflammation of the appendix and most commonly caused by obstruction, tumor, or intramural thickening.
Cognitive Level: Analysis
Nursing Process: Assessment
NCLEX-RN Test Plan: PHYS
Reference: Lewis, S. M., Heitkemper, M. M., & Dirksen, S. R. (2004). *Medical-surgical nursing: Assessment and management of clinical problems* (6th ed.). St. Louis, MO: Elsevier Mosby.

20. **Answer: 3**
Rationale: Headache is a side effect of ranitidine therapy. Usual GERD symptoms do not include headache. It cannot be assumed that a client has a brain tumor just by complaints of a headache.
Cognitive Level: Analysis
Nursing Process: Assessment
NCLEX-RN Test Plan: PHYS
Reference: Hodgson, B. B., & Kizior, R. J. (2006). *Saunders nursing drug handbook 2006.* St. Louis, MO: Elsevier Saunders.

21. **Answer: 1**
Rationale: Infection with *Clostridium difficile* is commonly seen in clients over 65 and those who have been in the hospital treated with antibiotics. Also, *C. difficile* occurs often in clients with COPD. The symptoms identified are consistent with bacterial infections of the gastrointestinal tract, not urinary tract. While a client with the flu may have nausea, the listed factors are all present with *C. difficile.*
Cognitive Level: Analysis
Nursing Process: Assessment
NCLEX-RN Test Plan: PHYS
Reference: Black, J., & Hawks, J. H. (2005). *Medical-surgical nursing: Clinical management for positive outcomes* (7th ed.). St. Louis, MO: Elsevier Saunders.

22. **Answer: 1**
Rationale: Diverticula most frequently occur in the sigmoid colon because of the high pressure required to move stool into the rectum. Therefore, the pain associated with this disease is found in the lower left quadrant. Generally, it is not found in the other quadrants.
Cognitive Level: Application
Nursing Process: Assessment

NCLEX-RN Test Plan: PHYS
Reference: Black, J., & Hawks, J. H. (2005). *Medical-surgical nursing: Clinical management for positive outcomes* (7th ed.). St. Louis, MO: Elsevier Saunders.

23. **Answer: 3**
Rationale: A diet high in fiber helps to pull water into the stool, thus creating bulkier, softer stools that are easier to pass. Other aids to preventing constipation include physical activity and fluid intake of at least 1500 L/day.
Cognitive Level: Application
Nursing Process: Planning
NCLEX-RN Test Plan: HPM
Reference: Potter, P. A., & Perry, A. G. (2005). *Fundamentals of nursing* (6th ed.). St. Louis, MO: Elsevier Mosby.

24. **Answer: 4**
Rationale: One of the treatments for cholecystitis is to educate clients on a low fat diet. By lowering the fat intake, biliary colic is prevented, therefore, the education provided was effective. Intake and output values and serum albumin are not factors in cholecystitis. With proper treatment of cholecystitis there may actually be improvement on an ultrasound.
Cognitive Level: Application
Nursing Process: Evaluation
NCLEX-RN Test Plan: PHYS
Reference: Black, J., & Hawks, J. H. (2005). *Medical-surgical nursing: Clinical management for positive outcomes* (7th ed.). St. Louis, MO: Elsevier Saunders.

25. **Answer: 300 ml**
Rationale: The time span in question is two and one half hours. 120+120+60=300 ml infused.
Cognitive Level: Application
Nursing Process: Implementation
NCLEX-RN Test Plan: PHYS
Reference: Brown, M., & Mulholland, J. (2004). *Drug Calculations.* St. Louis, MO: Elsevier Mosby.

26. **Answer: 4**
Rationale: Gastroesophageal reflux disease is caused by inappropriate relaxation of the lower esophageal

sphincter (LES). When sleeping, the LES will weaken and nocturnal reflux can occur. Elevating the head of the bed for sleep is recommended to prevent reflux. The remaining statements do not reflect an understanding about GERD education.
Cognitive Level: Application
Nursing Process: Evaluation
NCLEX-RN Test Plan: HPM
Reference: Black, J., & Hawks, J. H. (2005).
   Medical-surgical nursing: Clinical management for positive outcomes (7th ed.). St. Louis, MO: Elsevier Saunders.

27. **Answer: 1**
    Rationale: The function of the sigmoid colon is to remove water from the stool, thus making it formed. Therefore, a colostomy placed in the sigmoid colon will produce formed stool. The other responses are for ostomies in different areas of the bowel.
    Cognitive Level: Application
    Nursing Process: Implementation
    NCLEX-RN Test Plan: HPM
    Reference: Black, J., & Hawks, J. H. (2005).
       Medical-surgical nursing: Clinical management for positive outcomes (7th ed.). St. Louis, MO: Elsevier Saunders.

28. **Answers: 1, 3, 4**
    Rationale: An open cholecystectomy creates an upper abdominal incision, therefore it may be more difficult for the client to take deep breaths and cough. An incentive spirometer assists the client in expanding their lungs to prevent respiratory complications. Postoperatively, a client will be NPO with a nasogastric tube. Ensuring proper functioning is essential to the healing process of the incision. Administering pain medications allows for improved rest for healing as well as maintaining vital signs within normal limits. The remaining responses are not measures to prevent complications in a postoperative open cholecystectomy client.
    Cognitive Level: Analysis
    Nursing Process: Implementation
    NCLEX-RN Test Plan: PSYC
    Reference: Black, J., & Hawks, J. H. (2005).
       Medical-surgical nursing: Clinical management for positive outcomes (7th ed.). St. Louis, MO: Elsevier Saunders.

29. **Answer: 3**
    Rationale: The option of gelatin, water, and toast is the most bland selection. A bland diet is necessary while the mucosal barrier is healing itself, such as after an acute attack of gastritis. The remaining options are not all bland selections.
    Cognitive Level: Application
    Nursing Process: Implementation
    NCLEX-RN Test Plan: HPM
    Reference: Black, J., & Hawks, J. H. (2005).
       Medical-surgical nursing: Clinical management for positive outcomes (7th ed.). St. Louis, MO: Elsevier Saunders.

30. **Answer: 3**
    Rationale: Hepatitis A is caused by infected water or food sources as occur in many third world countries. The remaining options are not factors associated with Hepatitis A.
    Cognitive Level: Application
    Nursing Process: Assessment
    NCLEX-RN Test Plan: PHYS
    Reference: Black, J., & Hawks, J. H. (2005).
       Medical-surgical nursing: Clinical management for positive outcomes (7th ed.). St. Louis, MO: Elsevier Saunders.

31. **Answer: 2**
    Rationale: Portal hypertension causes the dilation of esophagogastric veins. Any irritation, increase in intrathoracic pressure, or reflux of gastric juices can lead to a rupture of these enlarged vessels. Rupture of the veins of the esophagus constitutes a medical emergency.
    Cognitive Level: Analysis
    Nursing Process: Assessment
    NCLEX-RN Test Plan: PSYC
    Reference: Black, J., & Hawks, J. H. (2005).
       Medical-surgical nursing: Clinical management for positive outcomes (7th ed.). St. Louis, MO: Elsevier Saunders.

32. **Answer: 4**
    Rationale: The client with hepatitis has severe fatigue from tremendous metabolic demands. Such a taxing activity order would not be in a plan of care for a client with hepatitis. The other options are appropriate orders for a client for hepatitis.

Cognitive Level: Analysis
Nursing Process: Implementation
NCLEX-RN Test Plan: PHYS
Reference: Black, J., & Hawks, J. H. (2005).
Medical-surgical nursing: Clinical management for positive outcomes (7th ed.). St. Louis, MO: Elsevier Saunders.

33. **Answer: 4**
    Rationale: The use of garlic may potentiate the action of anticoagulant medications. The nurse should report this information to the physician. The remaining options do not have an effect with anticoagulants.
    Cognitive Level: Analysis
    Nursing Process: Assessment
    NCLEX-RN Test Plan: HPM
    Reference: Hodgson, B. B., & Kizior, R. J. (2006). *Saunders nursing drug handbook 2006*. St. Louis, MO: Elsevier Saunders.

34. **Answer: 3**
    Rationale: Prevacid is best absorbed before meals. Food diminishes absorption. The other options are not correct to deliver the best therapeutic response.
    Cognitive Level: Application
    Nursing Process: Planning
    NCLEX-RN Test Plan: PHYS
    Reference: Hodgson, B. B., & Kizior, R. J. (2006). *Saunders nursing drug handbook 2006*. St. Louis, MO: Elsevier Saunders.

35. **Answer: 1**
    Rationale: Colace is a stool softener and can decrease constipation, thus regulating bowel movements. The other options are not seen with colace.
    Cognitive Level: Application
    Nursing Process: Evaluation
    NCLEX-RN Test Plan: PHYS
    Reference: Hodgson, B. B., & Kizior, R. J. (2006). *Saunders nursing drug handbook 2006*. St. Louis, MO: Elsevier Saunders.

36. **Answer: 1**
    Rationale: The first priority would be the assessment of vital signs. This will indicate the amount of

blood lost and also document a baseline from which to monitor the effectiveness of any treatments implemented. The nurse cannot be sure what diagnostic tests will be ordered, and therefore should not deliver any instructions. The remaining options may be appropriate, but are not a first priority.
Cognitive Level: Application
Nursing Process: Assessment
NCLEX-RN Test Plan: PHYS
Reference: Lewis, S. M., Heitkemper, M. M., & Dirksen, S. R. (2004). *Medical-surgical nursing: Assessment and management of clinical problems* (6th ed.). St. Louis, MO: Mosby.

37. **Answer: 4**
    Rationale: A "high" enema refers to the height from which enema fluid is delivered. Generally it is 12–18 inches above the anus. The higher the fluid, the stronger the pressure of fluid flow to cleanse the entire colon. The other options are not appropriate levels for a "high" enema delivery.
    Cognitive Level: Application
    Nursing Process: Implementation
    NCLEX-RN Test Plan: PHYS
    Reference: Potter, P. A., & Perry, A. G. (2005). *Fundamentals of nursing* (6th ed.). St. Louis, MO: Elsevier Mosby.

38. **Answer: 3**
    Rationale: By giving the client a knowledgeable answer, the nurse answers the real question the client is asking. The remaining responses are not the best answers for delivering prudent nursing care using therapeutic communication.
    Cognitive Level: Application
    Nursing Process: Implementation
    NCLEX-RN Test Plan: PSYC
    Reference: Black, J., & Hawks, J. H. (2005). *Medical-surgical nursing: Clinical management for positive outcomes* (7th ed.). St. Louis, MO: Elsevier Saunders.

Unit 4 Answers and Rationales

Test 10 Answers and Rationales

1. **Answer: 1**
   Rationale: The client with renal failure would be in metabolic acidosis (low HCO_3, low pH) and respiratory alkalosis (low PCO_2) as a compensatory mechanism. Normal lab values include pH 7.35–7.45, HCO_3 23–27, and PCO_2 35–45.
   Cognitive Level: Analysis
   Nursing Process: Assessment
   NCLEX-RN Test Plan: PSYC
   Reference: Ignatavicius, D. D, & Workman, M. L. (2006). *Medical-surgical nursing* (5th ed.). St. Louis, MO: Elsevier Saunders.

2. **Answer: 2**
   Rationale: During the denial stage of Kübler-Ross's stages of dying (grief theory), a client acts as though nothing has happened and may refuse to believe or understand that a loss has occurred. The other stages of this theory include anger, bargaining, depression, and acceptance; they do not apply to the client's situation presented in this question.
   Cognitive Level: Analysis
   Nursing Process: Assessment
   NCLEX-RN Test Plan: PSYC
   Reference: Potter, P. A, & Perry, A. G. (2005). *Fundamentals of nursing* (6th ed.). St. Louis, MO: Mosby.

3. **Answer: 3**
   Rationale: Kayexalate (sodium polystyrene sulfonate) and dialysis are the only two types of treatments that actually remove potassium from the body. All other answers are incorrect.
   Cognitive Level: Analysis
   Nursing Process: Implementation
   NCLEX-RN Test Plan: PHYS
   Reference: Lewis, S. M., Heitkemper, M. M, & Dirksen, S. R. (2004). *Medical-surgical nursing: Assessment and management of clinical problems* (6th ed.). St. Louis, MO: Mosby.

4. **Answer: 4**
   Rationale: When both the BUN and serum creatinine levels rise and the ratio between the two remain constant, renal failure is present. Normal serum level include a BUN level of 8–25 mg/dl and creatinine levels of 0.6–1.5 mg/dl. All other answers are incorrect.
   Cognitive Level: Analysis
   Nursing Process: Assessment
   NCLEX-RN Test Plan: PHYS
   Reference: Corbett, J. V. (2004). *Laboratory tests and diagnostic procedures* (6th ed.). Upper Saddle River, NJ: Pearson Prentice Hall.

5. **Answer: 3**
   Rationale: During the oliguric phase of acute renal failure (ARF), the urinary output is less than 400 ml per 24 hours and the BUN and serum creatinine levels increase. Renal tubular function is reestablished in the diuretic phase of ARF. All other answers occur in other phases of acute renal failure.
   Cognitive Level: Analysis
   Nursing Process: Assessment
   NCLEX-RN Test Plan: PHYS
   Reference: Ignatavicius, D. D, & Workman, M. L. (2006). *Medical-surgical nursing* (5th ed.). St. Louis, MO: Elsevier Saunders.

6. **Answers: 1, 2, 3, and 5**
   Rationale: Monitoring potassium intake is crucial because hyperkalemia can cause cardiac dysrthymias. Potassium intake should be limited to 60–70 mEq/day. Orange juice, tomatoes, bananas and raisins are foods considered to be high in potassium. They should be avoided as much as possible to keep the serum potassium in control for a client in CRF.
   Cognitive Level: Application
   Nursing Process: Planning
   NCLEX-RN Test Plan: PHYS
   Reference: Ignatavicius, D. D, & Workman, M. L. (2006). *Medical-surgical nursing* (5th ed.). St. Louis, MO: Elsevier Saunders.

7. **Answer: 3**

   Rationale: Ischemia occurs in a few clients with vascular access when the fistula decreases arterial blood flow to areas distal to the fistula. Ischemia symptoms (known as Steal syndrome) vary from cold fingers to gangrene. If the collateral circulation is inadequate, the fistula may need to be tied off and a new one created in another area to preserve extremity circulation. Rash and bleeding are not signs or symptoms of Steal syndrome. Foul smelling drainage from the vascular access site would indicate a possible infection.

   Cognitive Level: Application

   Nursing Process: Assessment

   NCLEX-RN Test Plan: HPM

   Reference: Ignatavicius, D. D, & Workman, M. L. (2006). *Medical-surgical nursing* (5th ed.). St. Louis, MO: Elsevier Saunders.

8. **Answer: 1**

   Rationale: Dialysis disequilibrium syndrome may develop during or after hemodialysis (HD) has been completed. The cause is thought to be the rapid decrease in fluid volume and BUN levels during HD. The change in urea levels can cause cerebral edema and increased intracranial pressure. Neurological symptoms include nausea, vomiting, restlessness, decreased levels of consciousness, seizures, coma, or death. Steal syndrome occurs when the hemodialysis vascular access (fistula) decreases arterial blood flow to areas distal to the access, causing ischemia to occur. Peritonitis is a major complication of peritoneal dialysis (PD) in which the peritoneum becomes infected due to contamination at the PD connection site. Septicemia is known as system sepsis (systemic infection).

   Cognitive Level: Application

   Nursing Process: Assessment

   NCLEX-RN Test Plan: HPM

   Reference: Ignatavicius, D. D, & Workman, M. L. (2006). *Medical-surgical nursing* (5th ed.). St. Louis, MO: Elsevier Saunders.

9. **Answer: 4**

   Rationale: Advantages of hemodialysis include rapid fluid removal, rapid removal of urea and creatinine, effective potassium removal, less protein loss and lowering of serum triglycerides. Hct, Hgb, calcium, and ammonia levels are not affected throughout the process of hemodialysis.

   Cognitive Level: Application

   Nursing Process: Evaluation

   NCLEX-RN Test Plan: PHYS

   Reference: Lewis, S. M., Heitkemper, M. M, & Dirksen, S. R. (2004). *Medical-surgical nursing: Assessment and management of clinical problems* (6th ed.). St. Louis, MO: Mosby.

10. **Answers: 1 and 2**

    Rationale: Phosphorus intake is monitored closely in CRF clients to avoid osteodystrophy. Dietary phosphorus restrictions and drugs are used to assist with phosphate control. Milk and nuts are considered to be foods that contain high levels of phosphorus and should be avoided as much as possible to keep the serum phosphorus level in control for a client in CRF.

    Cognitive Level: Application

    Nursing Process: Planning

    NCLEX-RN Test Plan: PHYS

    Reference: Ignatavicius, D. D, & Workman, M. L. (2006). *Medical-surgical nursing* (5th ed.). St. Louis, MO: Elsevier Saunders.

11. **Answer: 3**

    Rationale: PD's advantages include fewer fluid and dietary restrictions as compared to hemodialysis (HD). HD is a treatment that uses a dialyzer to filter the blood. PD is contraindicated for clients who have had abdominal surgery or trauma to the abdomen. Continuous renal replacement therapy (CRRT) is the treatment of choice for acute conditions.

    Cognitive Level: Application

    Nursing Process: Planning

    NCLEX-RN Test Plan: HPM

    Reference: LeFever Kee, J., Paulanka, B. J., & Purnell, L. D. (2004). *Fluids and electrolytes with clinical application* (7th ed.). Clifton Park, NY: Thomson Delmar Learning.

12. **Answer: 3**

    Rationale: Clients at risk for calculi (stone) formation who ingest large amounts of calcium-containing foods or have a poor fluid intake may form new stones. A client with history of kidney stones is

encouraged to eat a low protein, low phosphorus diet and increase their fluid intake.
Cognitive Level: Analysis
Nursing Process: Planning
NCLEX-RN Test Plan: PSYC
Reference: Ignatavicius, D. D, & Workman, M. L. (2006). *Medical-surgical nursing* (5th ed.). St. Louis, MO: Elsevier Saunders.

13. **Answer: 3**
Rationale: When blood volume is deficient (dehydration), the BUN level rises more rapidly than the serum creatinine. In dehydration, there is an increased specific gravity. Ketones do not apply in this question.
Cognitive Level: Analysis
Nursing Process: Analysis
NCLEX-RN Test Plan: PHYS
Reference: Ignatavicius, D. D, & Workman, M. L. (2006). *Medical-surgical nursing* (5th ed.). St. Louis, MO: Elsevier Saunders.

14. **Answer: 4**
Rationale: Serum creatinine is an end product of muscle and protein metabolism. No common pathologic condition other than renal disease increases the serum creatinine level. Bilirubin is the primary pigment in bile, which is excreted by the liver and biliary system. Specific gravity of urine is the density of urine to water and is part of a urinalysis test. BUN is the measure of renal excretion of urea nitrogen, which is a by-product of protein metabolism in the liver.
Cognitive Level: Analysis
Nursing Process: Analysis
NCLEX-RN Test Plan: PHYS
Reference: Ignatavicius, D. D, & Workman, M. L. (2006). *Medical-surgical nursing* (5th ed.). St. Louis, MO: Elsevier Saunders.

15. **Answer: 1, 2, 4**
Rationale: CRF is a multisystem disease. Multiple metabolic disturbances contribute to clinical manifestations with every system of the body. Possible metabolic disturbances of CRF include sleep disturbances, restless leg syndrome, pericardial effusion, pruritus, and dry skin.
Cognitive Level: Analysis

Nursing Process: Assessment
NCLEX-RN Test Plan: HPM
Reference: Baumberger, H. M. (2005). *Quick look nursing: Fluid and electrolytes.* Sudbury, MA: Jones and Bartlett.

16. **Answer: 4**
Rationale: After a percutaneous biopsy, the major risk is bleeding from the biopsy site. Infection, flank pain, and urinary retention are also common complications from a renal biopsy.
Cognitive Level: Analysis
Nursing Process: Analysis
NCLEX-RN Test Plan: PHYS
Reference: Ignatavicius, D. D, & Workman, M. L. (2006). *Medical-surgical nursing* (5th ed.). St. Louis, MO: Elsevier Saunders.

17. **Answer: 4**
Rationale: After the procedure, force fluids (if permitted) to flush out the contrast material. All other interventions are not appropriate for care of a client post IVP.
Cognitive Level: Application
Nursing Process: Implementation
NCLEX-RN Test Plan: PHYS
Reference: Lewis, S. M., Heitkemper, M. M, & Dirksen, S. R. (2004). *Medical-surgical nursing: Assessment and management of clinical problems* (6th ed.). St. Louis, MO: Mosby.

18. **Answer: 4**
Rationale: Contraindications to transplantation include disseminated malignancies, refractory or untreated cardiac disease, chronic respiratory failure, extensive vascular disease, chronic infection, and unresolved psychosocial disorders (for example, noncompliance with medical regimes, alcoholism, or drug addiction). The presence of hepatitis B or C is not a contraindication to transplantation.
Cognitive Level: Application
Nursing Process: Assessment
NCLEX-RN Test Plan: HPM
Reference: Lewis, S. M., Heitkemper, M. M., & Dirksen, S. R. (2004). *Medical-surgical nursing: Assessment and management of clinical problems* (6th ed.). St. Louis, MO: Mosby.

19. **Answers: 1, 2, 4, 5, and 7**

    Rationale: Before the procedure, ascertain the client's coagulation status through client history, medication history, CBC, hematocrit, prothrombin time, and bleeding and clotting time. Type and crossmatch the client for blood. Ensure that the consent form is signed. The client will not receive any iodine or type of dye during this procedure. There are no restriction on metal objects for this type of procedure since there is no magnetic imaging being done during a renal biopsy. A full bladder is not required for a renal biopsy.

    Cognitive Level: Application

    Nursing Process: Implementation

    NCLEX-RN Test Plan: SECE

    Reference: Lewis, S. M., Heitkemper, M. M., & Dirksen, S. R. (2004). *Medical-surgical nursing: Assessment and management of clinical problems* (6th ed.). St. Louis, MO: Mosby.

20. **Answer: 2**

    Rationale: Finasteride (Proscar, Propecia) is a 5-alpha-reductase inhibitor, used to treat BPH. Danazol (Danocrine) is an anabolic steroid that is used to treat endometriosis. Fluoxymesterone (Halotestin) and methyltestosterone (Android) are synthetic testosterone hormones.

    Cognitive Level: Analysis

    Nursing Process: Analysis

    NCLEX-RN Test Plan: PHYS

    Reference: Herbert-Ashton, M. J., & Clarkson, N. (2005). *Quick look nursing: Pharmacology.* Sudbury, MA: Jones and Bartlett.

21. **Answer: 2**

    Rationale: Phenazopyridine (Pyridium) is an OTC drug that provides a soothing effect on the urinary tract mucosa. It also stains the urine a reddish orange that may be mistaken for blood in the urine, and it may permanently stain underclothing. Pyridium is used to treat urinary pain during urination. Hematuria and hypertension are not side effects of this drug.

    Cognitive Level: Application

    Nursing Process: Evaluation

    NCLEX-RN Test Plan: PHYS

    Reference: Lewis, S. M., Heitkemper, M. M., & Dirksen, S. R. (2004). *Medical-surgical nursing: Assessment and management of clinical problems* (6th ed.). St. Louis, MO: Mosby.

22. **Answer: 3**

    Rationale: Anticipatory grieving related to loss of kidney function is manifested by expression of feelings of sadness, anger, inadequacy, and hopelessness. All other answers do not apply to that nursing diagnosis.

    Cognitive Level: Application

    Nursing Process: Assessment

    NCLEX-RN Test Plan: PSYC

    Reference: Lewis, S. M., Heitkemper M. M., & Dirksen, S. R. (2004). *Medical-surgical nursing: Assessment and management of clinical problems* (6th ed.). St. Louis, MO: Mosby.

23. **Answers: 1, 2, and 8**

    Rationale: The patient should be assessed for flank pain, hypotension, decreasing hematocrit, and temperature elevation. Serial urine specimens should be inspected frequently for bleeding. Extravasation is an infiltrate of dye or medication around an IV site. The client is to be on bedrest after the procedure. All other answers are incorrect.

    Cognitive Level: Application

    Nursing Process: Implementation

    NCLEX-RN Test Plan: SECE

    Reference: Lewis, S. M., Heitkemper, M. M., & Dirksen, S. R. (2004). *Medical-surgical nursing: Assessment and management of clinical problems* (6th ed.). St. Louis, MO: Mosby.

24. **Answer: 4**

    Rationale: When taking furosemide, the client should use sunscreen or protective clothing to prevent photosensitivity. On this medication, a diet high in potassium and an increased fluid intake is advised. A side effect of Lasix is hypotension.

    Cognitive Level: Application

    Nursing Process: Evaluation

    NCLEX-RN Test Plan: PHYS

    Reference: Mosby's (2004) *Nursing Drug Reference.* St. Louis, MO: Mosby, pgs. 476, 477, 478.

25. **Answer: 3**

    Rationale: The symptoms of BPH experienced by the client result from urinary obstruction. Symptoms are usually gradual in onset and may not be noticed until prostatic enlargement has been present for some time. Early symptoms are usually minimal because the bladder can compensate for a small amount of resistance to urine flow. The symptoms

gradually worsen as the degree of urethral obstruction increases. Symptoms fall into one of two groups: voiding symptoms and irritative symptoms. The majority of complications that develop in BPH are related to urinary obstruction. Acute urinary retention is a common complication and is an indication for surgical intervention.
Cognitive Level: Application
Nursing Process: Assessment
NCLEX-RN Test Plan: HPM
Reference: Lewis, S. M., Heitkemper, M. M., & Dirksen, S. R. (2004). *Medical-surgical nursing: Assessment and management of clinical problems* (6th ed.). St. Louis, MO: Mosby.

26. **Answer: 1**
Rationale: A common early symptom of adult PKD is abdominal or flank pain, which is steady and dull or abrupt in onset. Other clinical manifestations include hematuria, UTI, and hypertension.
Cognitive Level: Application
Nursing Process: Assessment
NCLEX-RN Test Plan: PHYS
Reference: Lewis, S. M., Heitkemper, M. M., & Dirksen, S. R. (2004). *Medical-surgical nursing: Assessment and management of clinical problems* (6th ed.). St. Louis, MO: Mosby.

27. **Answer: 2**
Rationale: A UTI may occur during the course of IC management. A UTI is likely to produce an acute exacerbation of lower urinary tract symptoms and urinary frequency, as well as dysuria (not typically associated with IC) and oderous urine, possibly with hematuria. The client needs to be instructed on maintaining good nutrition and abiding by dietary restrictions. Bladder irritants such as caffeine, alcohol, citrus products, aged cheeses, nuts, vinegar, or hot peppers should be eliminated from the diet. The client may also be advised to avoid taking a high-potency vitamin because these formulas may irritate the bladder.
Cognitive Level: Application
Nursing Process: Implementation
NCLEX-RN Test Plan: HPM
Reference: Lewis, S. M., Heitkemper, M. M., & Dirksen, S. R. (2004). *Medical-surgical nursing: Assessment and management of clinical problems* (6th ed.). St. Louis, MO: Mosby.

28. **Answer: Costovertebral angle (CVA)**
Rationale: A landmark useful in locating the kidneys is the costovertebral angle (CVA), which is formed by the rib cage and vertebral column.
Cognitive Level: Application
Nursing Process: Assessment
NCLEX-RN Test Plan: HPM
Reference: Lewis, S. M., Heitkemper, M. M., & Dirksen, S. R. (2004). *Medical-surgical nursing: Assessment and management of clinical problems* (6th ed.). St. Louis, MO: Mosby.

29. **Answer: 3**
Rationale: The management of APSGN focuses on symptomatic relief. Edema is treated by restricting sodium and fluid intake and by administering diuretics. Hypertension is treated with antihypertensives. Dietary protein intake may be restricted if there is evidence of an increase in nitrogenous wastes. Corticosteroids and cytotoxic drugs have not been shown to be of value.
Cognitive Level: Application
Nursing Process: Implementation
NCLEX-RN Test Plan: SECE
Reference: Lewis, S. M., Heitkemper, M. M., & Dirksen, S. R. (2004). *Medical-surgical nursing: Assessment and management of clinical problems* (6th ed.). St. Louis, MO: Mosby.

30. **Answer: 4**
Rationale: Clinical manifestations of a UTI include flank pain, chills, and the presence of a fever. It is important to remember that these symptoms are often absent in older adults. Older adults tend to experience nonlocalized abdominal discomfort rather than dysuria and suprapubic pain. In addition, they may have cognitive impairment. Older adults are also less likely to experience a fever with infection of the upper urinary tract. People with significant bacteriuria may have no symptoms or may have nonspecific symptoms such as fatigue or anorexia.
Cognitive Level: Analysis
Nursing Process: Assessment
NCLEX-RN Test Plan: HPM
Reference: Lewis, S. M., Heitkemper, M. M., & Dirksen, S. R. (2004). *Medical-surgical nursing: Assessment and management of clinical problems* (6th ed.). St. Louis, MO: Mosby.

31. **Answer: 2, 3, 1, 4**

    Rationale: The phases of oliguric acute renal failure are the onset phase, the oliguric phase, the diuretic phase (high output phase), and the recovery phase (convalescent phase).

    Cognitive Level: Application

    Nursing Process: Implementation

    NCLEX-RN Test Plan: PHYS

    Reference: Ignatavicius, D. D, & Workman, M. L. (2006). *Medical-surgical nursing* (5th ed.). St. Louis, MO: Elsevier Saunders.

32. **Answer: 2**

    Rationale: Recurrent UTIs are treated with a course of three to five days of antibiotics such as trimethoprim-sulfamethoxazole (Bactrim, Septra) or nitrofurantoin (Macrodantin, Furadantin). A simple, uncomplicated UTI is treated with a one to three day regimen of antibiotic therapy. In comparison, a complicated UTI will require longer treatment, lasting from 7 to 14 days, or even longer. Pyridium is an OTC drug that may be used in combination with antibiotic agents to provide a soothing effect on the urinary tract mucosa and relieve the transient acute discomfort associated with a UTI.

    Cognitive Level: Application

    Nursing Process: Implementation

    NCLEX-RN Test Plan: PHYS

    Reference: Lewis, S. M., Heitkemper, M. M., & Dirksen, S. R. (2004). *Medical-surgical nursing: Assessment and management of clinical problems* (6th ed.). St. Louis, MO: Mosby.

33. **Answer: 1**

    Rationale: Health promotion activities, including teaching preventive measures, are needed to help decrease the incidence of UTIs. Some of these principles include emptying the bladder regularly and completely, evacuating the bowel regularly, wiping the perineal area from front to back after urination or defecation, and drinking an adequate amount of liquids each day.

    Cognitive Level: Analysis

    Nursing Process: Evaluation

    NCLEX-RN Test Plan: HPM

    Reference: Lewis, S. M., Heitkemper, M. M., & Dirksen, S. R. (2004). *Medical-surgical nursing: Assessment and management of clinical problems* (6th ed.). St. Louis, MO: Mosby.

34. **Answers: 1, 2, 3, and 4**

    Rationale: All of the listed nursing diagnoses would be appropriate while planning care for a client with an ileal conduit. Anxiety would be related to effects of the ileal conduit on lifestyle and relationships, lack of knowledge, and its use. Disturbed body image relates to effects of the change in body function, lifestyle, and relationships. Risk for impaired skin integrity is related to an ill-fitting appliance, poor hygiene, and lack of knowledge. Risk for infection is related to the surgical procedure, possible obstruction, or inadequate stoma care.

    Cognitive Level: Application

    Nursing Process: Planning

    NCLEX-RN Test Plan: PHYS

    Reference: Lewis, S. M., Heitkemper, M. M., & Dirksen, S. R. (2004). *Medical-surgical nursing: Assessment and management of clinical problems* (6th ed.). St. Louis, MO: Mosby.

35. **Answer: 2**

    Rationale: Diabetes mellitus is a predisposing factor to urinary tract infections (UTIs). Persons with underlying diseases (such as diabetes) that compromise host immune responses are at high risk for UTIs.

    Cognitive Level: Application

    Nursing Process: Assessment

    NCLEX-RN Test Plan: HPM

    Reference: Lewis, S. M., Heitkemper, M. M., & Dirksen, S. R. (2004). *Medical-surgical nursing: Assessment and management of clinical problems* (6th ed.). St. Louis, MO: Mosby.

36. **Answers: 1, 2, and 4**

    Rationale: Answers 1, 2 and 4 are all correct nursing interventions for this type of client. Option 3 is incorrect because it is normal for the stoma to shrink within the first two weeks after surgery. The patient with an ileal conduit is fitted for a permanent appliance 7–10 days after surgery and may need to be refitted at a later time, depending on the degree of stoma shrinkage.

    Cognitive Level: Application

    Nursing Process: Implementation

    NCLEX-RN Test Plan: PHYS

    Reference: Lewis, S. M., Heitkemper, M. M., & Dirksen, S. R. (2004). *Medical-surgical nursing: Assessment and management of clinical problems* (6th ed.). St. Louis, MO: Mosby.

37. **Answer: 4**

    Rationale: Clinical manifestations of nephrotic syndrome include peripheral edema, massive proteinuria, hyperlipidemia, and hypoalbuminemia. Blood chemistries include decreased serum albumin, decreased total serum protein, and elevated serum cholesterol. The increased glomerular membrane permeability found with this disease is responsible for the massive excretion of protein in the urine. This results in decreased serum protein and edema formation. Treatment of this disease is aimed at relieving edema (ACE inhibitors, NSAIDs) and a low-sodium (2 to 3 g per day), low-to-moderate protein diet (0.5 to 0.6 kg per day). Treatment of hyperlipidemia includes use of lipid-lowering agents such as colestipol (Colestid) and lovastatin (Mevacor).

    Cognitive Level: Analysis

    Nursing Process: Evaluation

    NCLEX-RN Test Plan: HPM

    Reference: Lewis, S. M., Heitkemper, M. M., & Dirksen, S. R. (2004). *Medical-surgical nursing: Assessment and management of clinical problems* (6th ed.). St. Louis, MO: Mosby.

38. **Answers: 1 and 3**

    Rationale: Options 1 and 3 are correct indications for use of urinary catheterization. Catheterization should never be used for obtaining a routine urine sample or for nursing/family member convenience since it does carry serious risks, such as UTIs.

    Cognitive Level: Application

    Nursing Process: Implementation

    NCLEX-RN Test Plan: SECE

    Reference: Lewis, S. M., Heitkemper, M. M., & Dirksen, S. R. (2004). *Medical-surgical nursing: Assessment and management of clinical problems* (6th ed.). St. Louis, MO: Mosby.

39. **Answer: 3**

    Rationale: Overflow incontinence is a condition that occurs when the pressure of urine in an overfull bladder overcomes sphincter control. Symptoms may include leakage of small amounts of urine frequently throughout the day and night, urinating frequently in small amounts, and a distended and usually palpable bladder. Stress incontinence is caused by a sudden increase in abdominal pressure. Urge incontinence occurs randomly when involuntary urination is preceded by a warning of a few seconds to a few minutes. Reflex incontinence occurs when no warning or stress precedes periodic involuntary urination.

    Cognitive Level: Application

    Nursing Process: Assessment

    NCLEX-RN Test Plan: PHYS

    Reference: Lewis, S. M., Heitkemper, M. M., & Dirksen, S. R. (2004). *Medical-surgical nursing: Assessment and management of clinical problems* (6th ed.). St. Louis, MO: Mosby.

40. **Answers: 1, 2, and 3**

    Rationale: Treatment methods used for urge incontinence include treatment of the underlying cause, instructions to have the client urinate more frequently, anticholinergic drugs that reduce overactive bladder contractions at bedtime, calcium channel blockers that reduce smooth muscle contraction strength, or vaginal estrogen creams that, when locally applied, reduce urethral irritation and increase client defenses against UTIs.

    Cognitive Level: Application

    Nursing Process: Implementation

    NCLEX-RN Test Plan: PHYS

    Reference: Lewis, S. M., Heitkemper, M. M., & Dirksen, S. R. (2004). *Medical-surgical nursing: Assessment and management of clinical problems* (6th ed.). St. Louis, MO: Mosby.

Unit 4 Answers and Rationales

Test 11 Answers and Rationales

1. **Answer: 1**

   Rationale: An oral glucose tolerance test (OGTT) is a fasting test and the client will be NPO after midnight prior to the test. All the other responses identify appropriate client responses regarding to the test.

   Cognitive Level: Application

   Nursing Process: Evaluation

   NCLEX-RN Test Plan: PHYS

   Reference: Pagana, K. D., & Pagana, T. J. (2006). *Mosby's manual of diagnostic and laboratory tests* (3rd ed.). St. Louis, MO: Elsevier Mosby.

2. **Answer: 2**

   Rationale: In hypopituitarism, there is decreased cardiac output, decreased blood pressure, and decreased energy level (fatigue). These symptoms occur due to an absence of hormones resulting from the decreased pituitary activity and truncal obesity is commonly associated with this disorder.

   Cognitive Level: Analysis

   Nursing Process: Assessment

   NCLEX-RN Test Plan: PHYS

   Reference: Lewis, S. M., Heitkemper, M. M., & Dirksen, S. R. (2004). *Medical-surgical nursing: Assessment and management of clinical problems* (6th ed.). St Louis, MO: Mosby.

3. **Answers: 1, 2, 3, 4, 5, 7, and 8**

   Rationale: Acromegaly is due to excessive excretion of growth hormone. There is thickening and enlargement of bony and soft tissue resulting in increasing size of hands and feet, thickening and protruding of the jaw, dysphagia, arthritic changes, and increase in organ size. Hypotension occurs as a result of cardiovascular system changes.

   Cognitive Level: Analysis

   Nursing Process: Assessment

   NCLEX-RN Test Plan: PHYS

   Reference: Lewis, S. M., Heitkemper, M. M., & Dirksen, S. R. (2004). *Medical-surgical nursing: Assessment and management of clinical problems* (6th ed.). St Louis, MO: Mosby.

4. **Answer: 3**

   Rationale: A cerebral spinal leak is suspected and testing the fluid for the presence of glucose would confirm this. Most leaks heal spontaneously, but occasionally surgical repair is needed. Packing the nose will not heal the leak at this site. The head of the bed should be elevated to decrease pressure on the graph site and blowing the nose is contraindicated.

   Cognitive Level: Application

   Nursing Process: Implementation

   NCLEX-RN Test Plan: SECE

   Reference: Lemone, P., & Burke, K. (2004). *Medical surgical nursing: Critical thinking in client care* (3rd ed.). Upper Saddle River, NJ: Prentice Hall.

5. **Answers: 1, 2, 3, 5, and 6**

   Rationale: Addison's crisis is a life-threatening disorder caused by acute adrenal insufficiency. There is a severe deficit of all three classes of adrenal corticosteroids (glucorticoids, mineral corticoids, and androgens). Addison's crisis is commonly precipitated by major stressors, especially if the disease is poorly controlled.

   Cognitive Level: Analysis

   Nursing Process: Assessment

   NCLEX-RN Test Plan: PHYS

   Reference: Lemone, P., & Burke, K. (2004). *Medical surgical nursing: Critical thinking in client care* (3rd ed.). Upper Saddle River, NJ: Prentice Hall.

6. **Answer: 4**

   Rationale: After a hypophysectomy (surgical removal of the pituitary gland) there is a return to normal pituitary secretion. Hypopituitarism can cause a deficit of growth hormone, gonadotropins, thyroid stimulating hormones, and ACTH. The client needs to watch for changes in mental status, energy level, muscle strength, and cognitive function. Cushing's disease is a disorder of hypersecretion. Grave's disease is a hypersecretion of the thyroid gland. Diabetes mellitus is related to the function of the pancreas and is not related to the function of the pituitary.

   Cognitive Level: Application

Nursing Process: Implementation
NCLEX-RN Test Plan: HPM
Reference: Lemone, P., & Burke, K. (2004). *Medical surgical nursing: Critical thinking in client care* (3rd ed.). Upper Saddle River, NJ: Prentice Hall.

7. **Answer: 3**
   Rationale: Vasopressin (Pitressin) is an antidiuretic hormone and is given to a client with diabetes insipidus to increase urine concentration by increasing the tubular reabsorption of water. Vasopressin does not increase blood pressure or affect either insulin production or intestinal absorption of glucose.
   Cognitive Level: Analysis
   Nursing Process: Planning
   NCLEX-RN Test Plan: PHYS
   Reference: Springhouse nurse's drug guide. (2007). Philadelphia: Lippincott Williams & Wilkins.

8. **Answer: 1, 2, 3, 4, 6**
   Rationale: Manifestations of Cushing's syndrome result from ACTH or cortisol excess and cortisol actions. This results in obesity and redistribution of body fat, causing central obesity, buffalo hump, and moon face. Changes in protein metabolism cause the muscle weakness and wasting, thinning and bruising of the skin. Hypertension, not hypotension, is seen in patient's with Cushing's syndrome.
   Cognitive Level: Analysis
   Nursing Process: Assessment
   NCLEX-RN Test Plan: PHYS
   Reference: Lemone, P., & Burke, K. (2004). *Medical surgical nursing: Critical thinking in client care* (3rd ed.). Upper Saddle River, NJ: Prentice Hall.

9. **Answer: 1**
   Rationale: Excess corticoids in the individual with Addison's disease contribute to weight gain and calcium and protein loss. So the recommended diet for these individuals is one of high protein and calcium intake while maintaining lower caloric intake to prevent weight gain.
   Cognitive Level: Analysis
   Nursing Process: Implementation
   NCLEX-RN Test Plan: PHYS
   Reference: Lewis, S. M., Heitkemper, M. M., & Dirksen, S. R. (2004). *Medical-surgical nursing: Assessment and management of clinical problems* (6th ed.). St Louis, MO: Mosby.

10. **Answer: 1**
    Rationale: Glucocorticoid medication therapy is established with a basal dose. The typical regimen begins with two-thirds of the daily dose taken in the morning (8 AM) and the remaining one-third later (4 PM) in the day. This regimen closely resembles the diurnal pattern of secretion. Glucocorticoid medications do not have a cumulative effect and must be taken daily. Glucocorticoid needs fluctuate according to daily life events and/or stressors.
    Cognitive Level: Application
    Nursing Process: Evaluation
    NCLEX-RN Test Plan: PHYS
    Reference: Lemone, P., & Burke, K. (2004). *Medical surgical nursing: Critical thinking in client care* (3rd ed.). Upper Saddle River, NJ: Prentice Hall.

11. **Answer: 3**
    Rationale: Decreased hepatic glucosneogenesis and increased glucose uptake in the tissue cause hypoglycemia, not hyperglycemia. Elevated glucose is associated with cortisol excess, as in Cushing's disease. Hyperkalemia and hyponatremia are characteristic of Addison's disease. There is decreased renal perfusion and excretion of waste products, which cause an elevated BUN.
    Cognitive Level: Analysis
    Nursing Process: Analysis
    NCLEX-RN Test Plan: PHYS
    Reference: Lemone, P., & Burke, K. (2004). *Medical surgical nursing: Critical thinking in client care* (3rd ed.). Upper Saddle River, NJ: Prentice Hall.

12. **Answer: 3**
    Rationale: With adrenocortical insufficiency, muscle weakness, fatigue, nausea and vomiting, irritability, and mood changes are all signs and symptoms that occur. The other options listed are not symptoms of Addison's disease.
    Cognitive Level: Application
    Nursing Process: Assessment
    NCLEX-RN Test Plan: PHYS
    Reference: Lemone, P., & Burke, K. (2004). *Medical surgical nursing: Critical thinking in client care* (3rd ed.). Upper Saddle River, NJ: Prentice Hall.

13. **Answer: 1, 2, 3, 4**
    Rationale: Monitoring intake and output and electrolytes is very important postoperatively as adrenal

insufficiency occurs following an adrenalectomy. Addison's crisis and hypovolemic shock may occur. It is important to assess temperature and WBC levels as impaired postoperative wound healing increases the risk of infection in clients with adrenal disorders.
Cognitive Level: Application
Nursing Process: Implementation
NCLEX-RN Test Plan: SECE
Reference: Lemone, P., & Burke, K. (2004). *Medical surgical nursing: Critical thinking in client care* (3rd ed.). Upper Saddle River, NJ: Prentice Hall.

14. **Answer: 1**
Rationale: In Cushing's disease, skin bruising occurs caused by hypersecretion of glucocorticoids. Fluid retention causes hypertension. Hair on the head thins, while body hair increases. Weight gain also occurs.
Cognitive Level: Analysis
Nursing Process: Assessment
NCLEX-RN Test Plan: HPM
Reference: Lewis, S. M., Heitkemper, M. M., & Dirksen, S. R. (2004). *Medical-surgical nursing: Assessment and management of clinical problems* (6th ed.). St. Louis, MO: Mosby.

15. **Answer: 4**
Rationale: Urine tests that are positive for glucose and ketones as well as BG levels less than 450 mg/dl are diagnostic for diabetes mellitus rather than diabetes insipidus. A urinary output of 1–2 liters is a normal daily output. Polyuria is a manifestation of diabetes insipidus. In diabetes insipidus, there is a lack of antidiuretic hormone (ADH), which causes insufficient water reabsorption in the kidneys. This causes polyuria and results in decreased urine specific gravity (1.001–1.010). The client may consume and excrete 5–40 L of fluid a day.
Cognitive Level: Application
Nursing Process: Assessment
NCLEX-RN Test Plan: PHYS
Reference: McCance, K. L., & Huether, S. E. (2006). *Pathophysiology: The biologic basis for disease in adults and children* (5th ed.). St. Louis, MO: Elsevier Mosby.

16. **Answers: 1, 5, 7, 8, and 9**
Rationale: Clinical manifestations of hyperthyroidism are related to the effects of excessive thyroid hormones. There is a direct effect of hormones on

increasing metabolism. There is also increased tissue sensitivity to stimulation by the sympathetic nervous system causing increased sensitivity to the action of catecholamines (epinephrine and norepinephrine).The other options indicate signs and symptoms associated with decreased metabolism.
Cognitive Level: Analysis
Nursing Process: Assessment
NCLEX-RN Test Plan: PHYS
Reference: Lewis, S. M., Heitkemper, M. M., & Dirksen, S. R. (2004). *Medical-surgical nursing: Assessment and management of clinical problems* (6th ed.). St. Louis, MO: Mosby.

17. **Answer: 4**
Rationale: Clients with Cushing's disease have hypernatremia, not hyponatremia, and this sodium retention is typically accompanied by potassium depletion. Bone reabsorption of calcium increases the urine calcium level. The secretion of aldosterone results in hypertension, hypokalema, and edema. In addition, hyperglycemia rather than hypoglycemia is seen due to alteration in glucose metabolism.
Cognitive Level: Application
Nursing Process: Analysis
NCLEX-RN Test Plan: HPM
Reference: Lemone, P., & Burke, K. (2004). *Medical surgical nursing: Critical thinking in client care* (3rd ed.). Upper Saddle River, NJ: Prentice Hall.

18. **Answer: 4**
Rationale: Decreased thyroid (T_3, T_4) hormone levels and increased thyroid stimulating hormone (TSH) levels are indicative of hypothyroidism. Increased TSH levels indicate an elevation of production of this hormone directly related to decreased levels of circulation of thyroid (T_3, T_4) hormones.
Cognitive Level: Application
Nursing Process: Analysis
NCLEX-RN Test Plan: HPM
Reference: McCance, K. L., & Huether, S. E. (2006). *Pathophysiology: The biologic basis for disease in adults and children* (5th ed.). St. Louis, MO: Elsevier Mosby.

19. **Answers: 2, 6, 8, 9, and 10**
Rationale: Hypothyroidism has systemic effects characterized by an insidious and nonspecific slowing of body processes. It is associated with decreased

cardiac output and decreased cardiac contractility. Weight gain is due to the client's decreased metabolism. The other options would be seen in an individual with hyperthyroidism.
Cognitive Level: Analysis
Nursing Process: Assessment
NCLEX-RN Test Plan: PHYS
Reference: Lewis, S. M., Heitkemper, M. M., & Dirksen, S. R. (2004). *Medical-surgical nursing: Assessment and management of clinical problems* (6th ed.). St. Louis, MO: Mosby.

20. **Answer: 4**
Rationale: Hyperthyroidism, or Grave's disease, is characterized by increased metabolism. This increased metabolism increases the body's heat production and increases the heart rate (tachycardia). There is an increased appetite, and weight loss occurs even with the increased appetite as a result of the increased metabolism. Cool skin is associated with the slowing of metabolism and is seen with hypothyroidism. With the increased metabolism, the body's heat production increases and the patient may complain of feeling warm rather than cold..
Cognitive Level: Application
Nursing Process: Analysis
NCLEX-RN Test Plan: HPM
Reference: Lemone, P., & Burke, K. (2004). *Medical surgical nursing: Critical thinking in client care* (3rd ed.). Upper Saddle River, NJ: Prentice Hall.

21. **Answer: 4**
Rationale: Radioactive iodine destroys thyroid tissue so hormones are no longer produced. Radioactive iodine is used in place of a thyroidectomy (removal of the thyroid gland). RAI has no effect on thyroxine uptake.
Cognitive Level: Analysis
Nursing Process: Implementation
NCLEX-RN Test Plan: HPM
Reference: Lemone, P., & Burke, K. (2004). *Medical surgical nursing: Critical thinking in client care* (3rd ed.). Upper Saddle River, NJ: Prentice Hall.

22. **Answer: 3**
Rationale: Levothyroxene sodium (Synthroid) is a synthetic hormone that increases cellular metabolism. Synthroid should be taken once in the morning to

prevent sleeplessness at night. The medication should not be used prn and needs to be given at the same time each day to maintain adequate drug levels.
Cognitive Level: Application
Nursing Process: Evaluation
NCLEX-RN Test Plan: PHYS
Reference: Lemone, P., & Burke, K. (2004). *Medical surgical nursing: Critical thinking in client care* (3rd ed.). Upper Saddle River, NJ: Prentice Hall.

23. **Answer: 3**
Rationale: Methimazole (Tapazol) is a medication that should be taken at a consistent time each day to ensure adequate therapeutic blood levels of the medication. It should not be taken prn.
Cognitive Level: Application
Nursing Process: Evaluation
NCLEX-RN Test Plan: PHYS
Reference: Springhouse nurse's drug guide (8th ed.). (2007). Philadelphia: Lippincott Williams & Wilkins.

24. **Answer: 1, 5, 8, 2, 4, 6, 7, 3**
Rationale: This order of steps identifies the correct sequence for drawing up and administering a single dose of insulin.
Cognitive Level: Application
Nursing Process: Implementation
NCLEX-RN Test Plan: PHYS
Reference: Lewis, S. M., Heitkemper, M. M., & Dirksen, S. R. (2004). *Medical-surgical nursing: Assessment and management of clinical problems* (6th ed.). St. Louis, MO: Mosby.

25. **Answer: 4**
Rationale: Action of the medication is hormone replacement for deficient thyroid hormone. The other options are not the correct action of the medication.
Cognitive Level: Application
Nursing Process: Implementation
NCLEX-RN Test Plan: PHYS
Reference: Lemone, P., & Burke, K. (2004). *Medical surgical nursing: Critical thinking in client care* (3rd ed.). Upper Saddle River, NJ: Prentice Hall.

26. **Answer: 4**
Rationale: Obesity is the most controllable risk factor. Obesity increases insulin resistance, which is a

major contributing factor in Type 2 diabetes. Hypertension and cigarette smoking are not predisposing factors, but are risk factors for developing complications. A family history of Type 2 diabetes is a risk factor for developing diabetes, but it is not a controllable risk factor.

Cognitive Level: Application

Nursing Process: Planning

NCLEX-RN Test Plan: HPM

Reference: McCance, K. L., & Huether, S. E. (2006). *Pathophysiology: The biologic basis for disease in adults and children* (5th ed.). St. Louis, MO: Elsevier Mosby.

27. **Answer: 2**

Rationale: In hyperosmolar hyperglycemic nonketotic syndrome (HHNKS), glycosuria and polyuria occur as a result of extreme serum glucose elevation. This causes severe dehydration in the client. Ketosis and acidosis do not occur with HHNKS as insulin levels are sufficient to prevent excessive lipolysis but not for glucose utilization.

Cognitive Level: Analysis

Nursing Process: Assessment

NCLEX-RN Test Plan: PHYS

Reference: McCance, K. L., & Huether, S. E. (2002). *Pathophysiology: The biologic basis for disease in adults and children* (5th ed.). St. Louis, MO: Elsevier Mosby.

28. **Answer: 3, 1, 5, 4, 2, 6, 7, 9, 10, 8**

Rationale: When done in this order, these steps identify the correct sequence of drawing up and administering a mixed dose (Humulin R and Humulin N) of insulin. When drawing up both regular (R) and intermediate (N) insulin, the regular (R) insulin needs to be drawn up into the syringe first. If intermediate (N) acting insulin is ever injected into a vial of rapid-acting (Regular R) insulin, the entire vial needs to be discarded.

Cognitive Level: Application

Nursing Process: Implementation

NCLEX-RN Test Plan: PHYS

Reference: Lewis, S. M., Heitkemper, M. M., & Dirksen, S. R. (2004). *Medical-surgical nursing: Assessment and management of clinical problems* (6th ed.). St. Louis, MO: Mosby.

29. **Answer: 3**

Rationale: Illness, stress, and infection increase the body's insulin requirement. At this time, the patient should increase the frequency of blood and urine testing. Adequate fluid intake is required to counteract the dehydration that occurs with hyperglycemia. The client should maintain his/her normal dose of insulin and notify the physician if ketonemia occurs for more than 24 hours, if the client has an inability to take food and/or fluids for four hours, or if the illness persists for more than two days.

Cognitive Level: Application

Nursing Process: Implementation

NCLEX-RN Test Plan: SECE

Reference: Lewis, S. M., Heitkemper, M. M., & Dirksen, S. E. (2004). *Medical-surgical nursing: Assessment and management of clinical problems* (6th ed.). St. Louis, MO: Mosby.

30. **Answer: 3**

Rationale: NPH is an intermediate acting insulin. NPH insulin's onset of action is in 1–2 hours, the peak is in 6–8 hours, and the duration of action is 12–16 hours. Hypoglycemic reactions are most likely to occur during peak action hours.

Cognitive Level: Application

Nursing Process: Implementation

NCLEX-RN Test Plan: SECE

Reference: Lewis, S. M., Heitkemper, M. M., & Dirksen, S. R. (2004). *Medical-surgical nursing: Assessment and management of clinical problems* (6th ed.). St. Louis, MO: Mosby.

31. **Answer: 2**

Rationale: Regular insulin is a short acting insulin with an onset of action in ½–1 hour, a peak that occurs in 2–3 hours, and a duration of action of 4–8 hours. Hypoglycemia is most likely to occur during peak insulin times.

Cognitive Level: Application

Nursing Process: Implementation

NCLEX-RN Test Plan: SECE

Reference: Lewis, S. M., Heitkemper, M. M., & Dirksen, S. R. (2004). *Medical-surgical nursing: Assessment and management of clinical problems* (6th ed.). St. Louis, MO: Mosby.

32. **Answer: 1**

    Rationale: Second-generation oral hypoglycemic agents act to lower blood glucose level by stimulating the functioning beta cells of the pancreas to release insulin. They also work to increase the body cells' receptiveness to insulin. The medication does not alter the renal threshold of glucose.

    Cognitive Level: Application

    Nursing Process: Implementation

    NCLEX-RN Test Plan: PHYS

    Reference: Lewis, S. M., Heitkemper, M. M., & Dirksen, S. R. (2004). *Medical-surgical nursing: Assessment and management of clinical problems* (6th ed.). St. Louis, MO: Mosby.

33. **Answer: 1, 2, 3, 4, 5, 6, 7, 8**

    Rationale: Symptoms of hypoglycemia result from activation of the sympathetic nervous system (adrenergic symptoms), from an abrupt cessation of glucose delivery to the brain (neuroglycopenic symptoms), or both.

    Cognitive Level: Analysis

    Nursing Process: Assessment

    NCLEX-RN Test Plan: PHYS

    Reference: McCance, K. L., & Huether, S. E. (2002). *Pathophysiology: The biologic basis for disease in adults and children* (5th ed.). St. Louis, MO: Elsevier Mosby.

34. **Answer: 4**

    Rationale: The external insulin pump is a continuous subcutaneous insulin delivery system. It consists of a syringe in the pump attached to a long, thin, narrow-lumen plastic tubing with either a needle or Teflon catheter at the end. The needle/catheter is inserted into the subcutaneous tissue (usually in the abdomen). The syringe, tubing, and site are changed every three days. The pump uses regular buffered insulin. (Lispo may be prescribed). The pump delivers a continual (basal) infusion of insulin and additional low (bolus) doses of insulin are administered by the patient at meal times. The pump provides flexibility for the patient. The pump is worn continuously and is not disconnected for more than one hour at a time. Most pumps are now waterproof and can be worn during showers, swimming, etc.

    Cognitive Level: Application

    Nursing Process: Evaluation

    NCLEX-RN Test Plan: SECE

    Reference: Lewis, S. M., Heitkemper, M. M., & Dirksen, S. R. (2004). *Medical-surgical nursing: Assessment and management of clinical problems* (6th ed.). St. Louis, MO: Mosby.

35. **Answer: 4**

    Rationale: When the same site is used for insulin injections over an extended period of time, lipodystrophy (hypertrophy or atrophy of the tissue) can occur. The other options describe appropriate insulin injection administration techniques.

    Cognitive Level: Analysis

    Nursing Process: Assessment

    NCLEX-RN Test Plan: HPM

    Reference: Lewis, S. M., Heitkemper, M. M., & Dirksen, S. R. (2004). *Medical-surgical nursing: Assessment and management of clinical problems* (6th ed.). St. Louis, MO: Mosby.

36. **Answers: 1, 2, 3, and 5**

    Rationale: The clinical manifestations of hyperglycemia include polyuria and polydypsia, which result from osmotic changes occurring in response to hyperglycemia. Polyphagia results from depletion of cellular stores of carbohydrates, fats, and proteins. Metabolic changes result in poor dietary metabolism, which causes lethargy and fatigue.

    Cognitive Level: Analysis

    Nursing Process: Assessment

    NCLEX-RN Test Plan: PHYS

    Reference: McCance, K. L., & Huether, S. E. (2002). *Pathophysiology: The biologic basis for disease in adults and children.* (5th ed.). St. Louis, MO: Elsevier Mosby.

37. **Answer: 4**

    Rationale: HHNKS occurs in patients with Type 2 diabetes mellitus. The symptoms include polyuria, polydypsia, polyphagia, dehydration, weakness, and changes in mental status. DKA occurs in Type 1 diabetes mellitus. Porphyria is a group of inherited disorders in which there is an abnormal production of porphyrins. It can be of either the erythropoietic or hepatic type. Pheochronocytoma is a vascular tumor of the adrenal medulla characterized by hypersecretion of epinephrine and norepinephrine that cause persistent or intermittent hypertension.

Cognitive Level: Application
Nursing Process: Assessment
NCLEX-RN Test Plan: HPM
Reference: Lewis, S. M., Heitkemper, M. M., & Dirksen, S. R. (2004). *Medical-surgical nursing: Assessment and management of clinical problems* (6th ed.). St. Louis, MO: Mosby.

38. Answer: 2

Rationale: Diabetes mellitus is a disorder of abnormal insulin production and/or impaired utilization resulting in elevated blood glucose levels. Normal fasting blood glucose levels are 70–110 mg/dl. All other results are within normal limits.
Cognitive Level: Application
Nursing Process: Analysis
NCLEX-RN Test Plan: HPM
Reference: Lewis, S. M., Heitkemper, M. M., & Dirksen, S. R. (2004). *Medical-surgical nursing: Assessment and management of clinical problems* (6th ed.). St. Louis, MO: Mosby.

39. Answer: 3

Rationale: The glycosylated hemoglobin (HBA$_1$C) is a measure of blood/plasma glucose concentration over time. Over the 120-day life span of the red blood cell, glucose molecules attach to the hemoglobin forming glycosylated hemoglobin. A build-up of glycosylated hemoglobin within the red cell reflects the "average" level of glucose to which the cell has been exposed during its life cycle. Measuring HBA$_1$C monitors the long-term glucose regulation. Nondiabetic values should range from 2.2%–4.8%, good diabetic control will range from 2.5%–5.9%, fair control of diabetes will be 6%–8%, and poor control will be greater than or equal to 8%.
Cognitive Level: Application
Nursing Process: Analysis
NCLEX-RN Test Plan: HPM
Reference: McCance, K. L., & Huether, S. E. (2002). *Pathophysiology: The biologic basis for disease in adults and children* (5th ed.). St. Louis, MO: Elsevier Mosby..

40. Answer:

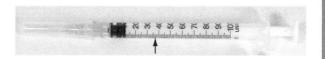

Rationale: The mark at 37 units indicates the correct positioning for drawing up a dose of insulin using a 1 cc (100 unit) syringe.
Cognitive Level: Application
Nursing Process: Implementation
NCLEX-RN Test Plan: SECE
Reference: Smith, S., Duell, D., & Martin, B. (2000). *Clinical nursing skills: Basic to advanced skills* (5th ed.). Upper Saddle River, NJ: Prentice Hall.

Unit 4 Answers and Rationales

Test 12 Answers and Rationales

1. **Answer: 3**
   Rationale: DIC causes a complex series of events leading to abnormal activation of the clotting cascade, resulting in excessive life-threatening simultaneous clotting and bleeding. DIC can be acute or chronic, but is not always controllable. Elevated platelet counts are not a characteristic of DIC and platelet counts are generally decreased due to platelet consumption. DIC does not involve a genetic vitamin K deficiency.
   Cognitive Level: Analysis
   Nursing Process: Analysis
   NCLEX-RN Test Plan: PHYS
   References: Smeltzer, S. C., & Bare, B. G. (2004). *Textbook of medical-surgical nursing* (10th ed.). Philadelphia: Lippincott Williams & Wilkins.

   Lewis, S. M., Heitkemper, M. M., & Dirksen, S. R. (2004). *Medical-surgical nursing: Assessment and management of clinical problems* (6th ed.). St. Louis, MO: Mosby.

   Black, J. M., & Hawks, J. H. (2005). *Medical-surgical nursing: Clinical management for positive outcomes* (7th ed.). St. Louis, MO: Elsevier Saunders.

2. **Answer: 1**
   Rationale: DIC causes a complex series of events leading to abnormal activation of the clotting cascade, resulting in excessive life-threatening simultaneous clotting and bleeding. Platelet counts are generally decreased due to platelet consumption, but platelet production is not affected. Sodium and fluid retention are not immediate manifestations of DIC. Thromboplastin and fibrinogen levels will be decreased in DIC.
   Cognitive Level: Analysis
   Nursing Process: Analysis
   NCLEX-RN Test Plan: PHYS
   References: Smeltzer, S. C., & Bare, B. G. (2004). *Textbook of medical-surgical nursing* (10th ed.). Philadelphia: Lippincott Williams & Wilkins.

   Lewis, S. M., Heitkemper, M. M., & Dirksen, S. R. (2004). *Medical-surgical nursing: Assessment and management of clinical problems* (6th ed.). St. Louis, MO: Mosby

   Black, J. M., & Hawks, J. H. (2005). *Medical-surgical nursing: Clinical management for positive outcomes* (7th ed.). St. Louis, MO: Elsevier Saunders.

3. **Answer: 2**
   Rationale: PTT, PT, and TT are elevated or prolonged in acute DIC due to the consumption of the key clotting factors and resulting clotting dysfunction. Chronic types of DIC may have varying levels of these values.
   Cognitive Level: Analysis
   Nursing Process: Assessment
   NCLEX-RN Test Plan: PHYS
   References: Smeltzer, S. C., & Bare, B. G. (2004). *Textbook of medical-surgical nursing* (10th ed.). Philadelphia: Lippincott Williams & Wilkins.

   Lewis, S. M., Heitkemper, M. M., & Dirksen, S. R. (2004). *Medical-surgical nursing: Assessment and management of clinical problems* (6th ed.). St. Louis, MO: Mosby.

   Black, J. M., & Hawks, J. H. (2005). *Medical-surgical nursing: Clinical management for positive outcomes* (7th ed.). St. Louis, MO: Elsevier Saunders.

   Pagana, K. D., & Pagana, T. J. (2002). *Manual of diagnostic and laboratory tests* (2nd ed.). St. Louis, MO: Mosby.

4. **Answers: 1, 2, 3, 4, 5, and 7**
   Rationale: A thrombocytopenic client is at risk for spontaneous and abnormal bleeding. Therefore, the client should avoid situations that could potentially cause injury or bleeding such as IM injections; rectal temps, meds, and exams; flossing teeth, straight razor usage, and contact sports. Using a soft toothbrush or swab, blowing the nose gently, and using an electric shaver are appropriate options for such a client. Fresh fruits and vegetables are not an issue with thrombocytopenia.

Cognitive Level: Application
Nursing Process: Implementation
NCLEX-RN Test Plan: PHYS

References: Lewis, S. M., Heitkemper, M. M., &
Dirksen, S. R. (2004). *Medical-surgical nursing:
Assessment and management of clinical problems*
(6th ed.). St. Louis, MO: Mosby.

Smeltzer, S. C., & Bare, B. G. (2004). *Textbook
of medical-surgical nursing* (10th ed.).
Philadelphia: Lippincott Williams & Wilkins.

5. **Answer: 4**

Rationale: ITP is an autoimmune disease that causes
destruction of circulating platelets resulting in
decreased platelet counts. White blood cells, red
blood cells, and granulocytes are not directly
affected by ITP.
Cognitive Level: Analysis
Nursing Process: Analysis
NCLEX-RN Test Plan: PHYS

References: Lewis, S. M., Heitkemper, M. M., &
Dirksen, S. R. (2004). *Medical-surgical nursing:
Assessment and management of clinical problems*
(6th ed.). St. Louis, MO: Mosby.

Smeltzer, S. C., & Bare, B. G. (2004). *Textbook
of medical-surgical nursing* (10th ed.).
Philadelphia: Lippincott Williams & Wilkins.

6. **Answer: 3**

Rationale: Notifying the dentist or any other healthcare provider of a platelet disorder is essential to prevent bleeding complications from an invasive
procedure. Using a rectal suppository, injections,
and medications that can affect platelets and increase
the risk for bleeding are contraindicated for thrombocytopenic clients.
Cognitive Level: Application
Nursing Process: Implementation
NCLEX-RN Test Plan: PHYS

References: Lewis, S. M., Heitkemper, M. M., &
Dirksen, S. R. (2004). *Medical-surgical nursing:
Assessment and management of clinical problems*
(6th ed.). St. Louis, MO: Mosby.

Smeltzer, S. C., & Bare, B. G. (2004). *Textbook
of medical-surgical nursing* (10th ed.).
Philadelphia: Lippincott Williams & Wilkins.

7. **Answer: 2 hours or 120 minutes**

Rationale:

42 gtt : 1 min :: 10 gtt : X min
$42X = 1 \times 10 = 10$
$X = 0.238 = 0.24$ min/ml
0.24 min/ml $\times 500$ ml $= 120$ min or 2 hours

Cognitive Level: Analysis
Nursing Process: Planning
NCLEX-RN Test Plan: SECE

References: Brown, M., & Mulholland, J. M. (2004).
*Drug calculations: Process and problems for
clinical practice* (7th ed.). St. Louis, MO: Mosby.

Kozier, B., Erb, G., Berman, A., & Snyder, S. J.
(2004). *Fundamentals of nursing: Concepts,
process, and practice* (7th ed.). Upper Saddle
River, NJ: Pearson Prentice Hall.

8. **Answer: 1**

Rationale: A platelet count of $9,000/mm^3$ is critically low, resulting in a high risk for spontaneous
bleeding. Head trauma can cause bleeding, but is
not a risk of a low platelet count. Anemia and
increased susceptibility to infection are not risks of a
low platelet count.
Cognitive Level: Application
Nursing Process: Assessment
NCLEX-RN Test Plan: PHYS

References: Lewis, S. M., Heitkemper, M. M., &
Dirksen, S. R. (2004). *Medical-surgical nursing:
Assessment and management of clinical problems*
(6th ed.). St. Louis, MO: Mosby.

Smeltzer, S. C., & Bare, B. G. (2004). *Textbook
of medical-surgical nursing* (10th ed.).
Philadelphia: Lippincott Williams & Wilkins.

Pagana, K. D., & Pagana, T. J. (2002). *Manual
of diagnostic and laboratory tests* (2nd ed.). St.
Louis, MO: Mosby.

9. **Answer: 4**

Rationale: Hemophilia A is an X-linked genetic
clotting disorder that results in Factor VIII deficiency with potential hemorrhagic episodes that
require Factor VIII replenishment. Hemophilia B,
not A, is associated with Factor IX deficiency that is
not asymptomatic. Neither type of hemophilia is a
Y-linked disorder. Some hemophilia patients have

developed HIV as a result of receiving frequent transfusions and blood products prior to HIV testing for blood products, but hemophilia is not always associated with a simultaneous diagnosis of HIV.
Cognitive Level: Analysis
Nursing Process: Analysis
NCLEX-RN Test Plan: PHYS
References: Black, J. M., & Hawks, J. H. (2005). *Medical-surgical nursing: Clinical management for positive outcomes* (7th ed.). St. Louis, MO: Elsevier Saunders.

Smeltzer, S. C., & Bare, B. G. (2004). *Textbook of medical-surgical nursing* (10th ed.). Philadelphia: Lippincott Williams & Wilkins.

10. **Answer: 2**
Rationale: Vitamin K is needed for prothrombin formation within the liver. Without vitamin K, essential clotting factors will be affected and bleeding can occur. Vitamin K does not regulate the utilization of Factors VIII and IX, does not stimulate platelets, and does not assist with iron absorption.
Cognitive Level: Analysis
Nursing Process: Analysis
NCLEX-RN Test Plan: PHYS
References: Black, J. M., & Hawks, J. H. (2005). *Medical-surgical nursing: Clinical management for positive outcomes* (7th ed.). St. Louis, MO: Elsevier Saunders.

Smeltzer, S. C., & Bare, B. G. (2004). *Textbook of medical-surgical nursing* (10th ed.). Philadelphia: Lippincott Williams & Wilkins.

11. **Answer: 3**
Rationale: All types of blood cells are manufactured in the bone marrow, developing from the pluripotent stem cell. The thymus and spleen have a role in immunity and blood cell destruction but do not produce blood cells. The central nervous system is not part of blood cell production or utilization.
Cognitive Level: Application
Nursing Process: Implementation
NCLEX-RN Test Plan: HPM
References: Black, J. M., & Hawks, J. H. (2005). *Medical-surgical nursing: Clinical management for positive outcomes* (7th ed.). St. Louis, MO: Elsevier Saunders.

Lewis, S. M., Heitkemper, M. M., & Dirksen, S. R. (2004). *Medical-surgical nursing: Assessment and management of clinical problems* (6th ed.). St. Louis, MO: Mosby.

Smeltzer, S. C., & Bare, B. G. (2004). *Textbook of medical-surgical nursing* (10th ed.). Philadelphia: Lippincott Williams & Wilkins.

12. **Answer: 1**
Rationale: Humoral immunity is the result of the activation of B-lymphocytes that produce antibodies in response to an invading antigen. Cellular immunity is mediated by T-lymphocytes. NK cells play an essentially unknown role in immunity. Humoral immunity can defend against viral, bacterial, and fungal infections.
Cognitive Level: Application
Nursing Process: Analysis
NCLEX-RN Test Plan: PHYS
References: Black, J. M., & Hawks, J. H. (2005). *Medical-surgical nursing: Clinical management for positive outcomes* (7th ed.). St. Louis, MO: Elsevier Saunders.

Lewis, S. M., Heitkemper, M. M., & Dirksen, S. R. (2004). *Medical-surgical nursing: Assessment and management of clinical problems* (6th ed.). St. Louis, MO: Mosby.

Smeltzer, S. C., & Bare, B. G. (2004). *Textbook of medical-surgical nursing* (10th ed.). Philadelphia: Lippincott Williams & Wilkins.

13. **Answer: 2, 4, 1, 3, 5**
Rationale: Upon suspecting a blood product transfusion reaction, the nurse should perform the actions in the following order: stop the infusion but maintain venous patency with saline solution; assess vital signs and airway patency; notify the physician and blood bank; treat the symptoms per physician order; then return the unused product, bag, and tubing to the blood bank.
Cognitive Level: Application
Nursing Process: Implementation
NCLEX-RN Test Plan: SECE
References: Black, J. M., & Hawks, J. H. (2005). *Medical-surgical nursing: Clinical management for positive outcomes* (7th ed.). St. Louis, MO: Elsevier Saunders.

Lewis, S. M., Heitkemper, M. M., & Dirksen, S. R. (2004). *Medical-surgical nursing: Assessment and management of clinical problems* (6th ed.). St. Louis, MO: Mosby.

Smeltzer, S. C., & Bare, B. G. (2004). *Textbook of medical-surgical nursing* (10th ed.). Philadelphia: Lippincott Williams & Wilkins.

Kozier, B., Erb, G., Berman, A., & Snyder, S. J. (2004). *Fundamentals of nursing: Concepts, process, and practice* (7th ed.). Upper Saddle River, NJ: Pearson Prentice Hall.

14. **Answer: 4**

Rationale: A transplant rejection is the result of cellular immunity and T-cell activation. Humoral immunity is not affected by a transplant procedure. An inflammatory response is a symptom, not a cause, of an immune response. An immune response aimed at a virus does not affect a transplant procedure.

Cognitive Level: Analysis
Nursing Process: Evaluation
NCLEX-RN Test Plan: PHYS

References: Black, J. M., & Hawks, J. H. (2005). *Medical-surgical nursing: Clinical management for positive outcomes* (7th ed.). St. Louis, MO: Elsevier Saunders.

Lewis, S. M., Heitkemper, M. M., & Dirksen, S. R. (2004). *Medical-surgical nursing: Assessment and management of clinical problems* (6th ed.). St. Louis, MO: Mosby.

Smeltzer, S. C., & Bare, B. G. (2004). *Textbook of medical-surgical nursing* (10th ed.). Philadelphia: Lippincott Williams & Wilkins.

15. **Answer: 2**

Rationale: Exposure to a virus in the environment is natural and active immunity. Passive immunity refers to immunity between a mother and infant. Artificial immunity refers to immunity received from an artificial source, such as a vaccination.

Cognitive Level: Analysis
Nursing Process: Analysis
NCLEX-RN Test Plan: HPM

Reference: Lewis, S. M., Heitkemper, M. M., & Dirksen, S. R. (2004). *Medical-surgical nursing: Assessment and management of clinical problems* (6th ed.). St. Louis, MO: Mosby.

16. **Answer: 3**

Rationale: HIV is transmitted through infected body fluids such as blood, semen, and vaginal secretions. Dirty needles can harbor HIV. HIV has not been shown to be transmitted through casual contact, such as kissing or touching, or through tears or saliva.

Cognitive Level: Analysis
Nursing Process: Analysis
NCLEX-RN Test Plan: HPM

References: Lewis, S. M., Heitkemper, M. M., & Dirksen, S. R. (2004). *Medical-surgical nursing: Assessment and management of clinical problems* (6th ed.). St. Louis, MO: Mosby.

Smeltzer, S. C., & Bare, B. G. (2004). *Textbook of medical-surgical nursing* (10th ed.). Philadelphia: Lippincott Williams & Wilkins.

Kozier, B., Erb, G., Berman, A., & Snyder, S. J. (2004). *Fundamentals of nursing: Concepts, process, and practice* (7th ed.). Upper Saddle River, NJ: Pearson Prentice Hall.

17. **Answer: Client B**

Rationale: Client B is the reservoir, the needle is the vehicle or mode of transmission, and Client A is the susceptible host.

Cognitive Level: Analysis
Nursing Process: Analysis
NCLEX-RN Test Plan: HPM

Reference: Kozier, B., Erb, G., Berman, A., & Snyder, S. J. (2004). *Fundamentals of nursing: Concepts, process, and practice* (7th ed.). Upper Saddle River, NJ: Pearson Prentice Hall.

18. **Answer: 2**

Rationale: Early HIV infection can be asymptomatic or symptoms can be vague and flu-like, such as fever, night sweats, aching, fatigue, malaise, and nausea. PCP, wasting syndrome, and KS are signs and symptoms of advancing HIV infection.

Cognitive Level: Analysis
Nursing Process: Implementation
NCLEX-RN Test Plan: PHYS

References: Black, J. M., & Hawks, J. H. (2005). *Medical-surgical nursing: Clinical management for positive outcomes* (7th ed.). St. Louis, MO: Elsevier Saunders.

Lewis, S. M., Heitkemper, M. M., & Dirksen, S. R. (2004). *Medical-surgical nursing: Assessment and management of clinical problems* (6th ed.). St. Louis, MO: Mosby.

Smeltzer, S. C., & Bare, B. G. (2004). *Textbook of medical-surgical nursing* (10th ed.). Philadelphia: Lippincott Williams & Wilkins.

19. Answer: 4

Rationale: A client experiencing fevers and night sweats will have resulting interrupted sleep. Every effort should be made to wake the client only when necessary to avoid further sleep interruption. Oral fluids help to maintain adequate hydration. Changing linens and using a plastic pillow cover assist with providing comfort.
Cognitive Level: Application
Nursing Process: Implementation
NCLEX-RN Test Plan: PHYS
References: Black, J. M., & Hawks, J. H. (2005). *Medical-surgical nursing: Clinical management for positive outcomes* (7th ed.). St. Louis, MO: Elsevier Saunders.

Lewis, S. M., Heitkemper, M. M., & Dirksen, S. R. (2004). *Medical-surgical nursing: Assessment and management of clinical problems* (6th ed.). St. Louis, MO: Mosby.

Smeltzer, S. C., & Bare, B. G. (2004). *Textbook of medical-surgical nursing* (10th ed.). Philadelphia: Lippincott Williams & Wilkins.

20. Answers: 1, 2, 4, 6, 7, and 8

Rationale: Among other nursing diagnoses, a new diagnosis of HIV can be expected to potentially produce fear, spiritual distress, ineffective coping, knowledge deficits, ineffective protection, and anxiety. The risk for poisoning and disturbed thought processes are not immediate or appropriate diagnoses to be used upon initial diagnosis of HIV infection.
Cognitive Level: Application
Nursing Process: Planning
NCLEX-RN Test Plan: PSYC
References: Ackley, B. J., & Ladwig, G. B. (2004). *Nursing diagnosis handbook: A guide to planning care* (6th ed.). St. Louis, MO: Mosby.

Lewis, S. M., Heitkemper, M. M., & Dirksen, S. R. (2004). *Medical-surgical nursing: Assessment and management of clinical problems* (6th ed.). St. Louis, MO: Mosby.

21. Answer: 3

Rationale: Hemoglobin contains iron and is affected by iron depletion or deficiency, resulting in anemia. Emphysema, PVD, and gestational diabetes are not direct causes of decreased hemoglobin levels.
Cognitive Level: Analysis
Nursing Process: Analysis
NCLEX-RN Test Plan: PHYS
References: Black, J. M., & Hawks, J. H. (2005). *Medical-surgical nursing: Clinical management for positive outcomes* (7th ed.). St. Louis, MO: Elsevier Saunders.

Pagana, K. D., & Pagana, T. J. (2002). *Manual of diagnostic and laboratory tests* (2nd ed.). St. Louis, MO: Mosby.

22. Answer: 1

Rationale: The American Association of Blood Banks recommends that two qualified persons check the identifying blood product labels and patient information for the purpose of verifying information and identifying potential incompatibilities. Another registered nurse is qualified to assist with blood product verification. A radiology technician, medical student, and phlebotomist are not qualified to assist with blood product verification.
Cognitive Level: Application
Nursing Process: Planning
NCLEX-RN Test Plan: SECE
References: Black, J. M., & Hawks, J. H. (2005). *Medical-surgical nursing: Clinical management for positive outcomes* (7th ed.). St. Louis, MO: Elsevier Saunders.

Lewis, S. M., Heitkemper, M. M., & Dirksen, S. R. (2004). *Medical-surgical nursing: Assessment and management of clinical problems* (6th ed.). St. Louis, MO: Mosby.

Smeltzer, S. C., & Bare, B. G. (2004). *Textbook of medical-surgical nursing* (10th ed.). Philadelphia: Lippincott Williams & Wilkins.

23. Answer: 3

Rationale: A change in vital signs can be one of the first symptoms of a blood transfusion reaction. Obtaining baseline vital signs and assessing vital signs throughout and at completion of the transfusion are critical nursing actions. Height, weight, intake output, and hemoglobin/hematocrit levels are also helpful components of a nursing assessment prior to a blood transfusion, but are not necessarily obtained immediately prior to the start of a transfusion.

Cognitive Level: Application
Nursing Process: Assessment
NCLEX-RN Test Plan: SECE
References: Black, J. M., & Hawks, J. H. (2005). *Medical-surgical nursing: Clinical management for positive outcomes* (7th ed.). St. Louis, MO: Elsevier Saunders.

Lewis, S. M., Heitkemper, M. M., & Dirksen, S. R. (2004). *Medical-surgical nursing: Assessment and management of clinical problems* (6th ed.). St. Louis, MO: Mosby.

Smeltzer, S. C., & Bare, B. G. (2004). *Textbook of medical-surgical nursing* (10th ed.). Philadelphia: Lippincott Williams & Wilkins.

24. **Answer: 2**

    Rationale: A PRBC transfusion should be initiated within 30 minutes after receiving them from the blood bank; any longer predisposes the blood cells to break down and requires the blood to be returned to the blood bank.

    Cognitive Level: Application
    Nursing Process: Planning
    NCLEX-RN Test Plan: SECE
    References: Black, J. M., & Hawks, J. H. (2005). *Medical-surgical nursing: Clinical management for positive outcomes* (7th ed.). St. Louis, MO: Elsevier Saunders.

    Lewis, S. M., Heitkemper, M. M., & Dirksen, S. R. (2004). *Medical-surgical nursing: Assessment and management of clinical problems* (6th ed.). St. Louis, MO: Mosby.

    Smeltzer, S. C., & Bare, B. G. (2004). *Textbook of medical-surgical nursing* (10th ed.). Philadelphia: Lippincott Williams & Wilkins.

25. **Answers: 1, 2, 3, 5, and 7**

    Rationale: Immunosuppression requires the nurse and staff to take necessary precautions to prevent infection of the client. Proper handwashing before and after care, utilizing personal protective equipment, restricting visitors, avoiding crowds, and cooking food thoroughly are all actions that can help limit the transmission of infection. The client

should be encouraged to bathe at least daily to prevent self-contamination. Fresh fruits and vegetables may need to be avoided, not encouraged, to limit the possibility of exposure to organisms. Disposing of linens in the trash is not necessary for an immunosuppressed client.

Cognitive Level: Application
Nursing Process: Implementation
NCLEX-RN Test Plan: PHYS
References: Smeltzer, S. C., & Bare, B. G. (2004). *Textbook of medical-surgical nursing* (10th ed.). Philadelphia: Lippincott Williams & Wilkins.

Pagana, K. D., & Pagana, T. J. (2002). *Manual of diagnostic and laboratory tests* (2nd ed.). St. Louis, MO: Mosby.

26. **Answer: 4**

    Rationale: A transfusion of PRBCs should not be longer than four hours due to inconsistent temperature of the blood and the possibility of infection.

    Cognitive Level: Analysis
    Nursing Process: Implementation
    NCLEX-RN Test Plan: SECE
    References: Black, J. M., & Hawks, J. H. (2005). *Medical-surgical nursing: Clinical management for positive outcomes* (7th ed.). St. Louis, MO: Elsevier Saunders.

    Lewis, S. M., Heitkemper, M. M., & Dirksen, S. R. (2004). *Medical-surgical nursing: Assessment and management of clinical problems* (6th ed.). St. Louis, MO: Mosby.

    Smeltzer, S. C., & Bare, B. G. (2004). *Textbook of medical-surgical nursing* (10th ed.). Philadelphia: Lippincott Williams & Wilkins.

27. **Answer: 3**

    Rationale: Most transfusion reactions will occur in the first 10–15 minutes of a transfusion. The nurse should remain with the patient during this time to assess for any complications.

    Cognitive Level: Application
    Nursing Process: Implementation
    NCLEX-RN Test Plan: SECE
    References: Black, J. M., & Hawks, J. H. (2005). *Medical-surgical nursing: Clinical management for positive outcomes* (7th ed.). St. Louis, MO: Elsevier Saunders.

Lewis, S. M., Heitkemper, M. M., & Dirksen, S. R. (2004). *Medical-surgical nursing: Assessment and management of clinical problems* (6th ed.). St. Louis, MO: Mosby.

Smeltzer, S. C., & Bare, B. G. (2004). *Textbook of medical-surgical nursing* (10th ed.). Philadelphia: Lippincott Williams & Wilkins.

28. **Answer: 1**

    Rationale: If the nurse suspects a client is having a transfusion reaction regardless of exact symptoms, the first action is to stop the transfusion. The blood transfusion should be completely stopped to allow for proper evaluation and to avoid possibly furthering the reaction by allowing the transfusion to continue. Physician notification is a critical element, but only after the transfusion has been stopped and the patient assessed. Covering the client with a blanket will maintain comfort but will not stop a transfusion reaction from occurring.
    Cognitive Level: Application
    Nursing Process: Implementation
    NCLEX-RN Test Plan: SECE
    References: Black, J. M., & Hawks, J. H. (2005). *Medical-surgical nursing: Clinical management for positive outcomes* (7th ed.). St. Louis, MO: Elsevier Saunders.

    Lewis, S. M., Heitkemper, M. M., & Dirksen, S. R. (2004). *Medical-surgical nursing: Assessment and management of clinical problems* (6th ed.). St. Louis, MO: Mosby.

    Smeltzer, S. C., & Bare, B. G. (2004). *Textbook of medical-surgical nursing* (10th ed.). Philadelphia: Lippincott Williams & Wilkins.

29. **Answers: 1, 3, 5, and 6**

    Rationale: Blood is connective tissue and is composed of 55% plasma and 45% formed elements. Blood transports oxygen, hormones, nutrients, and other elements throughout the body and helps to maintain fluid and electrolyte balance. Blood helps to protect against infection with white blood cells. All blood cells originate from the pluripotent stem cell within the bone marrow.
    Cognitive Level: Application
    Nursing Process: Analysis

NCLEX-RN Test Plan: HPM
References: Black, J. M., & Hawks, J. H. (2005). *Medical-surgical nursing: Clinical management for positive outcomes* (7th ed.). St. Louis, MO: Elsevier Saunders.

Lewis, S. M., Heitkemper, M. M., & Dirksen, S. R. (2004). *Medical-surgical nursing: Assessment and management of clinical problems* (6th ed.). St. Louis, MO: Mosby.

Smeltzer, S. C., & Bare, B. G. (2004). *Textbook of medical-surgical nursing* (10th ed.). Philadelphia: Lippincott Williams & Wilkins.

30. **Answer: 4**

    Rationale: A red, butterfly-shaped rash is a classic skin manifestation of SLE. Facial pallor, nail problems, and alopecia are cutaneous in nature, but not classic symptoms of SLE.
    Cognitive Level: Analysis
    Nursing Process: Assessment
    NCLEX-RN Test Plan: PHYS
    References: Black, J. M., & Hawks, J. H. (2005). *Medical-surgical nursing: Clinical management for positive outcomes* (7th ed.). St. Louis, MO: Elsevier Saunders.

    Lewis, S. M., Heitkemper, M. M., & Dirksen, S. R. (2004). *Medical-surgical nursing: Assessment and management of clinical problems* (6th ed.). St. Louis, MO: Mosby.

    Smeltzer, S. C., & Bare, B. G. (2004). *Textbook of medical-surgical nursing* (10th ed.). Philadelphia: Lippincott Williams & Wilkins.

31. **Answer: 3**

    Rationale: Leukocytosis is an elevated total WBC count. Elevations in the WBC count are associated with infection and inflammation. Anemia is reflected in the RBC count. Coagulation and renal or hepatic disorders are not detectable in the WBC count.
    Cognitive Level: Analysis
    Nursing Process: Analysis
    NCLEX-RN Test Plan: PHYS
    Reference: Pagana, K. D., & Pagana, T. J. (2002). *Manual of diagnostic and laboratory tests* (2nd ed.). St. Louis, MO: Mosby.

32. Answer: 2

Rationale: A total WBC count is normally between 4,000 and 10,000/mm^3. A WBC count of 1,700/mm^3 is a critically low value, necessitating physician notification. A hemoglobin level of 12.7 g/dl is normal or slightly low. A platelet count of 140,000/mm^3 is within normal limits or slightly low.

Cognitive Level: Analysis

Nursing Process: Analysis

NCLEX-RN Test Plan: PHYS

Reference: Pagana, K. D., & Pagana, T. J. (2002). *Manual of diagnostic and laboratory tests* (2nd ed.). St. Louis, MO: Mosby.

33. Answers: 1, 3, and 5

Rationale: Chemotherapy is myelosuppressive, causing a potential decrease in all blood cell counts. Acute leukemia is cancer of the blood and affects bone marrow production of blood cells. Therefore, this client is at risk for a decrease in platelet count, white blood cell counts, and red blood cell counts. BUN and creatinine can be affected by treatments, but are not blood counts.

Cognitive Level: Analysis

Nursing Process: Assessment

NCLEX-RN Test Plan: PHYS

References: Black, J. M., & Hawks, J. H. (2005). *Medical-surgical nursing: Clinical management for positive outcomes* (7th ed.). St. Louis, MO: Elsevier Saunders.

Lewis, S. M., Heitkemper, M. M., & Dirksen, S. R. (2004). *Medical-surgical nursing: Assessment and management of clinical problems* (6th ed.). St. Louis, MO: Mosby.

Smeltzer, S. C., & Bare, B. G. (2004). *Textbook of medical-surgical nursing* (10th ed.). Philadelphia: Lippincott Williams & Wilkins.

Lilley, L. L., Harrington, S., & Snyder, J. S. (2005). *Pharmacology and the nursing process* (4th ed.). St. Louis, MO: Mosby.

34. Answer: 4

Rationale: Maintaining comfort and managing pain are appropriate goals for end-of-life care. Verbalizing an understanding of disease transmission is appropriate at the time of initial diagnosis. Weight gain and attendance at social activities, although desirable, may not be possible at the end-of-life.

Cognitive Level: Application

Nursing Process: Planning

NCLEX-RN Test Plan: PSYC

References: Black, J. M., & Hawks, J. H. (2005). *Medical-surgical nursing: Clinical management for positive outcomes* (7th ed.). St. Louis, MO: Elsevier Saunders.

Lewis, S. M., Heitkemper, M. M., & Dirksen, S. R. (2004). *Medical-surgical nursing: Assessment and management of clinical problems* (6th ed.). St. Louis, MO: Mosby.

Smeltzer, S. C., & Bare, B. G. (2004). *Textbook of medical-surgical nursing* (10th ed.). Philadelphia: Lippincott Williams & Wilkins.

35. Answer: 1

Rationale: Organs involved in immune response include the thymus, spleen, and lymph nodes. These organs do not all play a role in digestion, electrolyte balance, and vitamin absorption.

Cognitive Level: Analysis

Nursing Process: Analysis

NCLEX-RN Test Plan: HPM

References: Black, J. M., & Hawks, J. H. (2005). *Medical-surgical nursing: Clinical management for positive outcomes* (7th ed.). St. Louis, MO: Elsevier Saunders.

Smeltzer, S. C., & Bare, B. G. (2004). *Textbook of medical-surgical nursing* (10th ed.). Philadelphia: Lippincott Williams & Wilkins.

36. Answer: 3

Rationale: Sepsis is an overwhelming systemic infectious process that can affect many vital organs, leading to symptoms that include oliguria, disorientation, and changes in cardiac output and function. Renal failure, pneumothorax, and compartment syndrome may have some, but not all, of these symptoms.

Cognitive Level: Analysis

Nursing Process: Assessment

NCLEX-RN Test Plan: PHYS

References: Black, J. M., & Hawks, J. H. (2005). *Medical-surgical nursing: Clinical management for positive outcomes* (7th ed.). St. Louis, MO: Elsevier Saunders.

Smeltzer, S. C., & Bare, B. G. (2004). *Textbook of medical-surgical nursing* (10th ed.). Philadelphia: Lippincott Williams & Wilkins.

37. **Answer: Hemoglobin**
   Rationale: Hemoglobin is the element of an RBC that contains iron and carries oxygen throughout the blood. It is essential to monitor hemoglobin in clients with iron-deficiency anemia.
   Cognitive Level: Analysis
   Nursing Process: Analysis
   NCLEX-RN Test Plan: PHYS
   References: Black, J. M., & Hawks, J. H. (2005). *Medical-surgical nursing: Clinical management for positive outcomes* (7th ed.). St. Louis, MO: Elsevier Saunders.

   Pagana, K. D., & Pagana, T. J. (2002). *Manual of diagnostic and laboratory tests* (2nd ed.). St. Louis, MO: Mosby.

38. **Answer: 1**
   Rationale: Pernicious anemia is caused by vitamin B_{12} deficiency; therefore, vitamin B_{12} supplementation by way of injection or oral administration are the usual treatments. Iron deficiency and vitamin B_6 deficiency are not related to pernicious anemia. Blood transfusions are not utilized unless the blood counts warrant blood replacement.
   Cognitive Level: Analysis
   Nursing Process: Implementation
   NCLEX-RN Test Plan: PHYS
   References: Lutz, C., & Przytulski, K. (2006). *Nutrition and diet therapy: Evidence-based applications* (4th ed.). Philadelphia: F.A. Davis Company.

   Lewis, S. M., Heitkemper, M. M., & Dirksen, S. R. (2004). *Medical-surgical nursing: Assessment and management of clinical problems* (6th ed.). St. Louis, MO: Mosby.

   Lilley, L. L., Harrington, S., & Snyder, J. S. (2005). *Pharmacology and the nursing process* (4th ed.). St. Louis, MO: Mosby.

39. **Answer: Anaphylaxis**
   Rationale: Anaphylaxis is a life-threatening and quickly progressing systemic immune response to an antigen. Anaphylaxis can cause all the symptoms this client is experiencing, along with many others. Life-saving measures may be necessary with this client.
   Cognitive Level: Analysis
   Nursing Process: Assessment
   NCLEX-RN Test Plan: PHYS
   References: Black, J. M., & Hawks, J. H. (2005). *Medical-surgical nursing: Clinical management for positive outcomes* (7th ed.). St. Louis, MO: Elsevier Saunders.

   Lewis, S. M., Heitkemper, M. M., & Dirksen, S. R. (2004). *Medical-surgical nursing: Assessment and management of clinical problems* (6th ed.). St. Louis, MO: Mosby.

   Smeltzer, S. C., & Bare, B. G. (2004). *Textbook of medical-surgical nursing* (10th ed.). Philadelphia: Lippincott Williams & Wilkins.

40. **Answer: 2**
   Rationale: Splenomegaly is an enlargement of the spleen that allows a larger capacity for filtering blood cells, which can lead to decreased levels of circulating blood cells, especially platelets. The spleen does not directly produce blood cells. Thrombocytopenia, not anemia, can be caused by disorders of the spleen.
   Cognitive Level: Analysis
   Nursing Process: Analysis
   NCLEX-RN Test Plan: PHYS
   References: Lewis, S. M., Heitkemper, M. M., & Dirksen, S. R. (2004). *Medical-surgical nursing: Assessment and management of clinical problems* (6th ed.). St. Louis, MO: Mosby.

   Smeltzer, S. C., & Bare, B. G. (2004). *Textbook of medical-surgical nursing* (10th ed.). Philadelphia: Lippincott Williams & Wilkins.

Unit 4 Answers and Rationales

Test 13 Answers and Rationales

1. **Answer: 4**
   Rationale: Sun exposure and tanning increases susceptibility to skin cancer and can have serious consequences, so the use of sunscreen products is encouraged year round. Allergies, diet, and pets can contribute to skin disorders, but with less serious consequences.
   Cognitive Level: Application
   Nursing Process: Planning
   NCLEX-RN Test Plan: HPM
   Reference: Lewis, S. M., Heitkemper, M. M., & Dirksen, S. R. (2004). *Medical-surgical nursing: Assessment and management of clinical problems* (6th ed.). St. Louis, MO: Mosby.

2. **Answer: 3**
   Rationale: Stress can play a role in creating or exacerbating a skin condition, but this open-ended question would not obtain specific stress information in relation to their skin disorder. It would be more important for the nurse to assess and question how much stress the client has and/or whether they feel that stress plays a role in their skin disorder. The other questions obtain specific health history information important in assessing a client with a skin disorder.
   Cognitive Level: Analysis
   Nursing Process: Assessment
   NCLEX-RN Test Plan: PHYS
   Reference: Lewis, S. M., Heitkemper, M. M., & Dirksen, S. R. (2004). *Medical-surgical nursing: Assessment and management of clinical problems* (6th ed.). St. Louis, MO: Mosby.

3. **Answers: 1, 2, 3, 5, and 6**
   Rationale: Psoriasis treatments include coal tar preparations, corticosteroids, intralesional injections, moisturizing creams, and phototherapy with ultraviolet light. Laser therapy is used for the removal of tumors, warts, and keloids.
   Cognitive Level: Analysis
   Nursing Process: Implementation
   NCLEX-RN Test Plan: PHYS

   Reference: Smeltzer, S. C., & Bare, B. G. (2004). *Brunner & Suddarth's textbook of medical-surgical nursing.* Philadelphia: Lippincott Williams & Wilkins.

4. **Answer: 2**
   Rationale: A biopsy is one of the most common diagnostic tests used in the evaluation of skin lesions. It is indicated in all conditions in which malignancy is suspected or a specific diagnosis is questionable. Even though a health history can not be obtained, inspection is the main diagnostic technique related to skin disorders. Topical medications are just one of the many treatments for skin lesions, and if they fail, other medications or therapies are initiated.
   Cognitive Level: Application
   Nursing Process: Implementation
   NCLEX-RN Test Plan: HPN
   Reference: Lewis, S. M., Heitkemper, M. M., & Dirksen, S. R. (2004). *Medical-surgical nursing: Assessment and management of clinical problems* (6th ed.). St. Louis, MO: Mosby.

5. **Answer: 3**
   Rationale: Turgor is properly assessed by pinching an area of skin. Skin generally becomes drier with increasing age but no flaking, scaling, or cracking should be present. It is important to inspect the client's general skin condition first, as this data can aid in assessing the skin lesions. Bright light from a penlight or flashlight can distort the characteristics of various skin lesions. A room with exposure to daylight is preferred.
   Cognitive Level: Application
   Nursing Process: Assessment
   NCLEX-RN Test Plan: PHYS
   Reference: Smeltzer, S. C., & Bare, B. G. (2004). *Brunner & Suddarth's textbook of medical-surgical nursing.* Philadelphia: Lippincott Williams & Wilkins.

6. **Answer: 1**
   Rationale: Hypothermia causes vasoconstriction, which can result in skin damage. Turning frequently

will help to reduce skin damage but will not reduce shivering or the amount of time that they may need therapy. Also, turning promotes client comfort, but it is not as important as preventing skin damage.

Cognitive Level: Analysis

Nursing Process: Implementation

NCLEX-RN Test Plan: PHYS

Reference: Lewis, S. M., Heitkemper, M. M., & Dirksen, S. R. (2004). *Medical-surgical nursing: Assessment and management of clinical problems* (6th ed.). St. Louis, MO: Mosby.

7. **Answers: 2, 3, 4, and 5**

Rationale: Skin cancer risk factors include light skin, light hair, and blue eyes; blistering sunburns; chronic skin irritation; and genetic predisposition. Dark skinned individuals have more melanin in their skin, which forms a natural sun shield just as the regular use of sunscreen does for others.

Cognitive Level: Analysis

Nursing Process: Assessment

NCLEX-RN Test Plan: HPM

Reference: Smeltzer, S. C., & Bare, B. G. (2004). *Brunner & Suddarth's textbook of medical-surgical nursing.* Philadelphia: Lippincott Williams & Wilkins.

8. **Answer: 2**

Rationale: If the client previously had a reaction to a bee sting, especially trouble breathing, immediate treatment may be needed. Reddened, swollen areas and fever and chills are mild reactions to the sting and should be monitored. Blood pressure can rise from the pain of the sting.

Cognitive Level: Analysis

Nursing Process: Assessment

NCLEX-RN Test Plan: PHYS

Reference: Lewis, S. M., Heitkemper, M. M., Dirksen, S. R. (2004). *Medical-surgical nursing: Assessment and management of clinical problems* (6th ed.). St. Louis, MO: Mosby.

9. **Answer: 4**

Rationale: A pustular inflammation is commonly caused by staphylococcus aureus. Using a new cosmetic pad each time with makeup will decrease the risk of reinfection. Moist compresses and dietary

changes may decrease some of the inflammation but not the infection. Squeezing pustules will spread the bacteria and cause more damage to already irritated skin.

Cognitive Level: Analysis

Nursing Process: Implementation

NCLEX-RN Test Plan: PHYS

Reference: Smeltzer, S. C., & Bare, B. G. (2004). *Brunner & Suddarth's textbook of medical-surgical nursing.* Philadelphia: Lippincott Williams & Wilkins.

10. **Answer: 1**

Rationale: Since a wart is a virus-induced epidermal tumor, it may reappear at the original site or in another body area despite the fact that the original wart was removed. They are mildly contagious by autoinoculation and all age groups may be infected, but it is most frequent between the ages of 12 and 16. As noted above, warts can spread even if treated.

Cognitive Level: Application

Nursing Process: Planning

NCLEX-RN Test Plan: HPM

Reference: Lewis, S. M., Heitkemper, M. M., & Dirksen, S. R. (2004). *Medical-surgical nursing: Assessment and management of clinical problems* (6th ed.). St. Louis, MO: Mosby.

11. **Answer: 1**

Rationale: Pediculosis capitis is head lice, and nits are cemented to the hair shaft. The nits are silvery to white in color, similar to dandruff. They are most commonly seen on hair on the back of the head near the nape of the neck. A papular rash may be present at the nape of the neck secondary to scratching. Seborrheic dermatitis is the term for dandruff, and scaling of the scalp can also be seen with psoriasis and tinea capitis (ringworm of the scalp). However, none of these disorders cause a rash on the back of the neck.

Cognitive Level: Application

Nursing Process: Assessment

NCLEX-RN Test Plan: PHYS

Reference: Smeltzer, S. C., & Bare, B. G. (2004). *Brunner & Suddarth's Textbook of medical-surgical nursing.* Philadelphia: Lippincott Williams & Wilkins.

12. **Answer: 2**

    Rationale: Contact dermatitis is an acute or chronic skin inflammation that results from direct skin contact with chemicals or allergens. Contact with plants (poison-ivy or poison-oak) would be a common exposure during a camping trip. It presents as a localized red, vesicular or papular rash, with pruritus often being a common complaint. Cellulitis is a localized area of inflammation with redness, warmth, swelling, and pain. Folliculitis is a grouping of pustules. Seborrheic dermatitis is an inflammation of the scalp with white to yellow scales.

    Cognitive Level: Application

    Nursing Process: Assessment

    NCLEX-RN Test Plan: PHYS

    Reference: Smeltzer, S. C., & Bare, B. G. (2004). *Brunner & Suddarth's textbook of medical-surgical nursing.* Philadelphia: Lippincott Williams & Wilkins.

13. **Answer: 1, 3, 2**

    Rationale: Basal cell carcinoma is the least severe because the nodules rarely metastasize and have well-defined borders, making excision easier. Squamous cell carcinoma is a more invasive cancer that can metastasize by the blood and lymphatic system. Malignant melanoma is an irregularly shaped, deeper lesion that is highly malignant and easily metastasizes to surrounding tissues and the lymphatic system. This makes it the most serious of the skin cancers.

    Cognitive Level: Analysis

    Nursing Process: Assessment

    NCLEX-RN Test Plan: PHY

    Reference: Smeltzer, S. C., & Bare, B. G. (2004). *Brunner & Suddarth's textbook of medical-surgical nursing.* Philadelphia: Lippincott Williams & Wilkins.

14. **Answer: 3**

    Rationale: Shoes, clothes, and equipment can all transfer the plant oils to the skin where it can begin another reaction. Items that have touched any part of the plant should be washed in hot water and detergent. The skin should be rinsed with cool water within fifteen minutes after exposure to neutralize the oil before it can bond to the skin. Do not scrub the skin because this will remove protective oils from normal skin and further spread the plant oil, increasing irritation. Although animals seem unaffected by these plants, their fur carries the oils and can become a source of contamination.

    Cognitive Level: Application

    Nursing Process: Analysis

    NCLEX-RN Test Plan: SECE

    Reference: Smeltzer, S. C., & Bare, B. G. (2004). *Brunner & Suddarth's textbook of medical-surgical nursing.* Philadelphia: Lippincott Williams & Wilkins.

15. **Answer: Basal cell carcinoma**

    Rationale: Basal cell carcinomas are found on the face. They are mostly nodules that are pink or pearly in color and are frequently without pain or pruritus.

    Cognitive Level: Application

    Nursing Process: Assessment

    NCLEX-RN Test Plan: PHYS

    Reference: Smeltzer, S. C., & Bare, B. G. (2004). *Brunner & Suddarth's textbook of medical-surgical nursing.* Philadelphia: Lippincott Williams & Wilkins.

16. **Answer: 4**

    Rationale: Warm compresses would cause vasodilatation releasing valuable water and oils from the skin, which would increase dryness and further increase pruritus. Cool compresses, cornstarch baths, and oatmeal preparations provide a soothing effect, decrease inflammation, and help remove crusts and scales.

    Cognitive Level: Analysis

    Nursing Process: Implementation

    NCLEX-RN Test Plan: PHYS

    Reference: Lewis, S. M., Heitkemper, M. M., Dirksen, S. R. (2004). *Medical-surgical nursing: Assessment and management of clinical problems* (6th ed.). St. Louis, MO: Mosby.

17. **Answer: 1**

    Rationale: Most frequently, contact dermatitis is an inflammation of the skin caused by direct contact with an irritating substance. Possible irritating substances need to be identified first. If there is no relief from removing possible causative agents, then allergy testing may be needed. Antihistamines and

hydrocortisone creams are treatment options but not first in the plan of care.
Cognitive Level: Application
Nursing Process: Implementation
NCLEX-RN Test Plan: PHYS
Reference: Smeltzer, S. C., & Bare, B. G. (2004). *Brunner & Suddarth's textbook of medical-surgical nursing.* Philadelphia: Lippincott Williams & Wilkins.

18. **Answer: 1**
Rationale: The virus can be spread by direct contact between an actively infected person and a susceptible host, especially when vesicles are open and draining, so isolation techniques are needed. Visitors must also take precautions.
Cognitive Level: Analysis
Nursing Process: Analysis
NCLEX-RN Test Plan: SECE
Reference: Smeltzer, S. C., & Bare, B. G. (2004). *Brunner & Suddarth's textbook of medical-surgical nursing.* Philadelphia: Lippincott Williams & Wilkins.

19. **Answer: 3**
Rationale: The virus can be spread by direct contact between an actively infected person and a susceptible host, especially when vesicles are open and draining. Preventing the spread of the virus to other clients is of most importance. Dressing changes, wound assessment, and repositioning are all needed for the skin care of this client, but are not the most important priority.
Cognitive Level: Application
Nursing Process: Planning
NCLEX-RN Test Plan: PHYS
Reference: Smeltzer, S. C., & Bare, B. G. (2004). *Brunner & Suddarth's textbook of medical-surgical nursing.* Philadelphia: Lippincott Williams & Wilkins.

20. **Answers: 1, 2, 4, and 6**
Rationale: Pruritus (itching) is one of the most common symptoms of a client with skin disorders. Acute pain and itching, disturbed body image, disturbed sleep patterns, and impaired skin integrity are applicable nursing diagnoses that would be appropriate in the care of a client with pruritus. Disturbed personal integrity applies more to gen-

der, ethnicity, occupation, and the various roles that one may have. Ineffective protection refers more to immuno-deficient conditions.
Cognitive Level: Analysis
Nursing Process: Planning
NCLEX-RN Test Plan: PHYS
Reference: Smeltzer, S. C., & Bare, B. G. (2004). *Brunner & Suddarth's textbook of medical-surgical nursing.* Philadelphia: Lippincott Williams & Wilkins.

21. **Answer: 3**
Rationale: The virus remains in the body in a dormant state in the nerve ganglia and the client is asymptomatic. Recurrence of herpes zoster is triggered by physical or psychological stressors such as trauma, fever, fatigue, etc. Herpes zoster is caused by reactivation of the varicella-zoster virus, which is contagious to people who have not been previously exposed to chicken pox (varicella). Lesions can shed the virus until they are crusted over and healing. Several days of discomfort are usually noted by the client before vesicles appear.
Cognitive Level: Application
Nursing Process: Implementation
NCLEX-RN Test Plan: HPM
Reference: Smeltzer, S. C., & Bare, B. G. (2004). *Brunner & Suddarth's textbook of medical-surgical nursing.* Philadelphia: Lippincott Williams & Wilkins.

22. **Answer: 4**
Rationale: The characteristic lesions of psoriasis are thick, erythematous plaques covered by silvery scales. Common sites are the scalp, elbows, knees, sacrum, and trunk. Some discomfort may be present with the lesions but it is not described as being intense.
Cognitive Level: Application
Nursing Process: Assessment
NCLEX-RN Test Plan: PHYS
Reference: Smeltzer, S. C., & Bare, B. G. (2004). *Brunner & Suddarth's textbook of medical-surgical nursing.* Philadelphia: Lippincott Williams & Wilkins.

23. **Answer: 3**
Rationale: Soft brushing while the lesions are moist will help debride some of the scales so the moisturizers and other topical medications can penetrate the

lesions easier. Constant occlusion may increase effects of some of the topical medications and increase infection. Warm baths and compresses promote moisture loss from the skin, which would further increase scales.

Cognitive Level: Application
Nursing Process: Implementation
NCLEX-RN Test Plan: HPM
Reference: Smeltzer, S. C., & Bare, B. G. (2004). *Brunner & Suddarth's textbook of medical-surgical nursing.* Philadelphia: Lippincott Williams & Wilkins.

24. **Answer: 2**
Rationale: Psoriasis has been shown to respond to phototherapy with ultraviolet light. Laser treatments are used for removal of tumors, warts, or keloids. Radiation therapy is used for cutaneous malignancies. Topical 5-FU (Fluorouracil) is a cytotoxic agent for premalignant conditions such as actinic keratosis.

Cognitive Level: Analysis
Nursing Process: Analysis
NCLEX-RN Test Plan: PHYS
Reference: Smeltzer, S. C., & Bare, B. G. (2004). *Brunner & Suddarth's textbook of medical-surgical nursing.* Philadelphia: Lippincott Williams & Wilkins.

25. **Answers: 2, 3, and 6**
Rationale: Cryosurgery (freezing), electrosurgery (removal of tissue by electrical energy), and surgical excision are the treatments used to remove basal cell carcinoma. Corticosteroids are used for treatment of several skin disorders but not removal of lesions. Immunotherapy has been used with some success for malignant melanoma but not basal cell carcinoma. Phototherapy is used for psoriasis.

Cognitive Level: Analysis
Nursing Process: Implementation
NCLEX-RN Test Plan: PHYS
Reference: Smeltzer, S. C., & Bare, B. G. (2004). *Brunner & Suddarth's Textbook of medical-surgical nursing.* Philadelphia: Lippincott Williams & Wilkins.

26. **Answer: 4**
Rationale: The client states that they are unable to work because of the horrible appearance of their

lesions, which demonstrates social isolation related to decreased activities and fear of rejection. The nursing diagnoses of anxiety, ineffective coping, and self-esteem could be applicable but the etiology data, lack of knowledge, and lack of social and financial support are not applicable to the information in the question.

Cognitive Level: Analysis
Nursing Process: Planning
NCLEX-RN Test Plan: HPM
Reference: Smeltzer, S. C. & Bare, B. G. (2004). *Brunner & Suddarth's textbook of medical-surgical nursing.* Philadelphia: Lippincott Williams & Wilkins.

27. **Answer: 4**
Rationale: Topical corticosteroid creams are lower doses and are absorbed slower so they can be used for a longer period of time without serious side effects. Topical creams should be applied in a thin layer to increase absorption of the medication. Do not rub the medication completely into the lesion as this could damage healing tissue. Psoriasis has exacerbations and remissions normally so discontinuing the medication will not cause an exacerbation.

Cognitive Level: Application
Nursing Process: Implementation
NCLEX-RN Test Plan: HPM
Reference: Lewis, S. M., Heitkemper, M. M., Dirksen, S. R. (2004). *Medical-surgical nursing: Assessment and management of clinical problems* (6th ed.). St. Louis, MO: Mosby.

28. **Answer: 3**
Rationale: Treatment for psoriasis involves a combination of therapies; ultraviolet light, tar preparations, and assisting with altered self-concept are frequently used. Liberal application of moisturizing creams is not used in psoriasis because it would interfere with the other topical medications. Pain management is rarely needed in psoriasis. Warm compresses and retinoid creams are not used.

Cognitive Level: Application
Nursing Process: Planning
NCLEX-RN Test Plan: PHYS
Reference: Smeltzer, S. C., & Bare, B. G. (2004). *Brunner & Suddarth's textbook of medical-surgical nursing.* Philadelphia: Lippincott Williams & Wilkins.

29. **Answer: Malignant melanoma**
    Rationale: Malignant melanoma frequently arises from preexisting moles. The lesions are very colorful with irregular borders.
    Cognitive Level: Application
    Nursing Process: Assessment
    NCLEX-RN Test Plan: PHYS
    Reference: Smeltzer, S. C., & Bare, B. G. (2004). *Brunner & Suddarth's textbook of medical-surgical nursing.* Philadelphia: Lippincott Williams & Wilkins.

30. **Answer: 1**
    Rationale: Signs that suggest malignant changes are referred to as the ABCDs of mole assessment: asymmetry, irregular borders, color changes, and diameter exceeding six centimeters. Clients are taught a self skin examination to be done monthly to check for these changes.
    Cognitive Level: Application
    Nursing Process: Assessment
    NCLEX-RN Test Plan: HPM
    Reference: Smeltzer, S. C., & Bare, B. G. (2004). *Brunner & Suddarth's textbook of medical-surgical nursing.* Philadelphia: Lippincott Williams & Wilkins.

31. **Answer: 2**
    Rationale: Almost all cases of skin cancer diagnosed each year are considered to be sun related. Ultraviolet rays are strongly suspected based on the increased incidence in countries near the equator and in people younger than thirty who have used a tanning bed more than ten times a year. Although fair-skinned individuals are more at risk for skin cancer, everyone needs to be aware of the risks of ultraviolet exposure. As with any cancer, a family history and genetic factors carry an increased risk.
    Cognitive Level: Application
    Nursing Process: Analysis
    NCLEX-RN Test Plan: HPM
    Reference: Lewis, S. M., Heitkemper, M. M., & Dirksen, S. R. (2004). *Medical-surgical nursing: Assessment and management of clinical problems* (6th ed.). St. Louis, MO: Mosby.

32. **Answer: 2, 4, 5, 6, 1, 3**
    Rationale: The usual presentation of herpes zoster begins with paresthesias, then redness and swelling

develops before the vesicles appear along the affected nerve. These vesicles usually open and begin to drain for a few days before they crust over and healing begins. Some clients develop postherpetic neuralgia (pain along the nerve) for months after the lesions disappear.
Cognitive Level: Analysis
Nursing Process: Assessment
NCLEX-RN Test Plan: PHYS
Reference: Smeltzer, S. C., & Bare, B. G. (2004). *Brunner & Suddarth's textbook of medical-surgical nursing.* Philadelphia: Lippincott Williams & Wilkins.

33. **Answer: 3**
    Rationale: Colors that may indicate malignancy are red, white, and blue. Shades of blue can vary from bluish-grey to bluish-black and purple. Pain, pruritus, and purulent drainage are important signs to note with skin lesions but are not typically seen at the onset of melanoma.
    Cognitive Level: Analysis
    Nursing Process: Assessment
    NCLEX-RN Test Plan: PHYS
    Reference: Smeltzer, S. C., & Bare, B. G. (2004). *Brunner & Suddarth's textbook of medical-surgical nursing.* Philadelphia: Lippincott Williams & Wilkins.

34. **Answer: 4**
    Rationale: Surgical excision is the treatment of choice for malignant melanoma. Cryosurgery (freezing) and radiation therapy is used more frequently for the less invasive skin cancers. Laser treatments are used for the removal of superficial tumors, warts, and keloids.
    Cognitive Level: Analysis
    Nursing Process: Analysis
    NCLEX-RN Test Plan: PHYS
    Reference: Smeltzer, S. C., & Bare, B. G. (2004). *Brunner & Suddarth's textbook of medical-surgical nursing.* Philadelphia: Lippincott Williams & Wilkins.

35. **Answer: Mouth or oral cavity**
    Rationale: Herpes simplex 1 is seen mostly on the mouth or oral cavity.
    Cognitive Level: Application
    Nursing Process: Assessment

NCLEX-RN Test Plan: PHYS

Reference: Smeltzer, S. C., & Bare, B. G. (2004). *Brunner & Suddarth's textbook of medical-surgical nursing.* Philadelphia: Lippincott Williams &Wilkins.

36. **Answer: 1**

Rationale: A high fiber diet is one of the ten preventative measures noted by the American Cancer Society to help reduce the risk of cancer, but it is more specific to cancers of the colon, prostate, and breast. Using sunscreen, monthly skin examination, and stopping smoking are more effective preventive measures for skin cancers.

Cognitive Level: Analysis

Nursing Process: Analysis

NCLEX-RN Test Plan: HPM

Reference: Smeltzer, S. C., & Bare, B. G. (2004). *Brunner & Suddarth's textbook of medical-surgical nursing.* Philadelphia: Lippincott Williams & Wilkins.

37. **Answer: 1**

Rationale: The most common presentation of basal cell carcinoma is a nodular lesion with well-defined borders that has a pearly or shiny appearance. Macules are small, flat lesions most commonly described as freckles. Rough, scaly tumors are usually squamous cell carcinoma. Weeping vesicles are usually some type of herpes lesion.

Cognitive Level: Application

Nursing Process: Assessment

NCLEX-RN Test Plan: PHYS

Reference: Lewis, S. M., Heitkemper, M. M., & Dirksen, S. R. (2004). *Medical-surgical nursing: Assessment and management of clinical problems* (6th ed.). St. Louis, MO: Mosby.

38. **Answer: 1**

Rationale: The white milky plaque is candidiasis (oral thrush) that often develops as a result of the overgrowth of bacteria after a client has been on antibiotics. Dermatitis is not found in the mouth. Herpes simplex lesions are painful with vesicles. Squamous cell carcinoma is a rough, scaly tumor.

Cognitive Level: Application

Nursing Process: Planning

NCLEX-RN Test Plan: PHYS

Reference: Lewis, S. M., Heitkemper, M. M., Dirksen, S. R. (2004). *Medical-surgical nursing: Assessment and management of clinical problems* (6th ed.). St. Louis, MO: Mosby.

39. **Answer: Fungal**

Rationale: Tinea is the most common fungal infection. It is also called ringworm and can affect the head, body, groin, feet, and nails.

Cognitive Level: Application

Nursing Process: Analysis

NCLEX-RN Test Plan: PHYS

Reference: Smeltzer, S. C., & Bare, B. G. (2004). *Brunner & Suddarth's textbook of medical-surgical nursing.* Philadelphia: Lippincott Williams & Wilkins.

Unit 4 Answers and Rationales

Test 14 Answers and Rationales

1. **Answers: 1, 2, 4, 5, 7, 8, and 9**
   Rationale: The nurse facilitates the education of the public in prevention and detection of cancer. Early detection and treatment increase survival rates. Since the seven warning signs detect fairly advanced cancer, the emphasis in public health education is prevention.
   Cognitive Level: Knowledge
   Nursing Process: Intervention
   NCLEX-RN Test Plan: HPM
   Reference: Lewis, S. M., Heitkemper, M. M., & Dirksen, S. R. (2004). *Medical-surgical nursing: Assessment and management of clinical problems* (6th ed.). St. Louis, MO: Mosby.

2. **Answer: 2**
   Rationale: Expected adverse outcomes of chemotherapy are those that result from destruction or altered synthesis of rapidly dividing cells. In addition to those targeted with the chemotherapy, these cells include all mucous membranes, hair follicles and blood cells originating in the bone marrow such as white blood cells, red blood cells, and platelets. When normal body defenses are lacking, the body's immune system is compromised. Candida albicans is an opportunistic organism that thrives when these defenses fail. Problems with mucousal integrity are not limited to visible areas of the mouth. Severity of lesions of the mouth, including thrush, provides a snapshot of the severity of infection throughout the gastrointestinal tract. Early identification and intervention of oral lesions permits treatment of the entire alimentary tract to prevent advanced candida infections. Additional instructions related to nausea and vomiting and avoiding persons with communicable diseases are also important for early symptom management. Labs in an outpatient setting are usually obtained one to three times a week depending on a client's stability.
   Cognitive Level: Synthesis
   Nursing Process: Intervention
   NCLEX-RN Test Plan: SECE
   Reference: Phillips, L. D. (2005). *Manual of i.v. therapeutics* (4th ed.). Philadelphia: F.A. Davis.

3. **Answer: 2**
   Rationale: Myelosuppression is the most common dose-limiting factor in chemotherapy administration. It is the inhibited production of blood cells and platelets in the bone marrow. A low platelet count can result in bleeding of the mucus membranes. The mucus membranes are at additional risk as these cells are rapidly dividing. The other symptoms listed, also side effects of chemotherapy, are not directly related to myelosuppression.
   Cognitive Level: Application
   Nursing Process: Evaluation
   NCLEX-RN Test Plan: PHYS
   Reference: Weinstein, S. (2001). *Plumer's principles and practice of intravenous therapy* (7th ed). Philadelphia: Lippincott Williams & Wilkins .

4. **Answer: 3**
   Rationale: In certain diseases when radiation is combined with surgery and chemotherapy, a cure is achieved. Cancer cells are permanently damaged with cumulative doses of radiation. Preoperatively, radiation causes tumor cells to lose their ability to proliferate (grow) and at the time of division, the cell dies. Radiation will reduce the tumor size to facilitate resection. Postoperatively, radiation will destroy the remaining tumor cells. It is essential and required that the nurse and physician provide complete information to a client regarding treatment options. Understanding the role of radiation in cancer treatment is included in the information necessary to make an informed decision to accept or refuse treatment or to seek a second opinion.
   Cognitive Level: Application
   Nursing Process: Intervention
   NCLEX-RN Test Plan: SECE
   Reference: Lewis, S. M., Heitkemper, M. M., & Dirksen, S. R. (2004). *Medical-surgical nursing: Assessment and management of clinical problems* (6th ed.). St. Louis, MO: Mosby.

5. **Answer: 2**
   Rationale: In a neutropenic client, there are not enough circulating neutrophils available to mount a

response against a potentially infectious agent. The client is immune-compromised and should avoid crowds. Ability to respond to an infectious process with redness, swelling, warmth, and purulence is lacking. These clients may experience only a one degree increase from their baseline temperature in attempts to mount an infectious response against an invading organism. Temperature should be done daily to track trends. Gardening will expose the client to invasive environmental organisms if they become injured. Even a small scratch that breaks their protective skin barrier will become a portal of entry. Fruits and vegetables are covered with environment organisms that are not normally harmful in individuals who are not immune-compromised. These foods should be served cooked.

Cognitive Level: Comprehension
Nursing Process: Intervention
NCLEX-RN Test Plan: PHYS
Reference: Phillips, L. D. (2005). *Manual of i.v. therapeutics* (4th ed.). Philadelphia: F.A. Davis.

6. **Answer: 1**
Rationale: Chemotherapeutic agents target cells that enter the replication (division) and proliferation (growth) cycles. These agents cannot distinguish between cancer and normal cells. Signs and symptoms of adverse reactions are the result of temporary damage to normal cells. Early detection and proper intervention can reverse and minimize the signs and symptoms associated with antineoplastic therapy and hospitalization can be avoided.

Cognitive Level: Application
Nursing Process: Intervention
NCLEX-RN Test Plan: PHYS
Reference: Weinstein, S. (2001). *Plumer's principles and practice of intravenous therapy* (7th ed.). Philadelphia: Lippincott Williams & Wilkins.

7. **Answer: 2**
Rationale: The sequence and fixed schedule of administered chemotherapy agents yields predictable toxicities. Neutropenia results when the bone marrow is depleted of neutrophils. A nadir is the lowest drop of the neutrophil blood count between cycles of chemotherapy. Depending on the protocol, this can occur from 7–28 days from the day of treatment. The nadir is evaluated prior to the next dose of chemotherapy. When the nadir is

below 1.5 ng/dL, or if the patient experiences an infection, the chemotherapy dose is reduced. Medications and maintaining hydration are important to treat side effects and to rid the body of metabolites of cellular destruction, but can be managed at home. Radiation therapy given concurrently will affect bone marrow in the treatment field. White blood cell production is affected in one week. Concurrent treatment emphasizes the need for laboratory monitoring of neutrophils.

Cognitive Level: Synthesis
Nursing Process: Intervention
NCLEX-RN Test Plan: PHYS
Reference: Weinstein, S. (2001). *Plumer's principles and practice of intravenous therapy* (7th ed.). Philadelphia: Lippincott Williams & Wilkins.

8. **Answer: 3**
Rationale: Most side effects of radiation therapy are related to exposure of the normal cells that fall within the targeted tumor treatment area. Fatigue is a common side effect that will occur in all instances of radiation therapy and is thought to be due to the accumulation of metabolites from cells destroyed during treatment. Alopecia occurs only in the targeted area. Cranial hair loss will occur when the head is irradiated. Diarrhea will occur when the epithelial lining of the intestines is denuded during abdominal exposure. Reproductive dysfunction will occur when the ova or testes are damaged from therapy.

Cognitive Level: Application
Nursing Process: Implementation
NCLEX-RN Test Plan: PHYS
Reference: Lewis, S. M., Heitkemper, M. M., & Dirksen, S. R. (2004). *Medical surgical nursing: Assessment and management of clinical problems* (6th ed.). St. Louis, MO: Mosby.

9. **Answer: 2**
Rationale: Multiple myeloma is also known as plasma cell myeloma. The malignant plasma cell infiltrates and destroys the bone. The client is at risk for pathological fractures. Hypercalcemia can result in gastric, renal, and neurological disorders. Adequate hydration is a primary nursing consideration. Neutrophils, platelets, white blood cells, as well as red blood cells, will decrease as the bone destruction affects the integrity of the bone marrow and pancytopenia develops.

Cognitive Level: Comprehension
Nursing Process: Evaluation
NCLEX-RN Test Plan: PHYS
Reference: Lewis, S. M., Heitkemper, M. M., & Dirksen, S. R. (2004). *Medical surgical nursing: Assessment and management of clinical problems* (6th ed.). St. Louis, MO: Mosby.

10. **Answer: 3**
   Rationale: A debulking is a surgical procedure that is done to remove as much tumor tissue as possible when the complete tumor cannot be removed. This is necessary when the tumor is attached to a vital organ and cannot be removed without significant damage or complete destruction of the organ. Debulking decreases the tumor burden and recruits resting cells to begin dividing. This procedure allows chemotherapy and radiation to be more effective by increasing cell sensitivity.
   Cognitive Level: Knowledge
   Nursing Process: Intervention
   NCLEX-RN Test Plan: PHYS
   Reference: Phillips, L. D. (2005). *Manual of i.v. therapeutics* (4th ed.). Philadelphia: F.A. Davis.

11. **Answer: 2**
   Rationale: The pain control dose will initially cause sedation. The sedative effects will subside with maintenance pain control. Additionally, clients in chronic, uncontrolled pain are usually sleep deprived and must catch up. Catching up is expected when pain is controlled. This adds to the perception of increased sedative effect of opioids. The client has woken, but has not complained of pain. Although it may be necessary at some point, there is no need to change the drug, alter the dose, or add additional opioids for pain control at this time.
   Cognitive Level: Comprehension
   Nursing Process: Evaluation
   NCLEX-RN Test Plan: PHYS
   Reference: Bourdeanu, L., Loseth, D. B., & Funk, M. (2005). Management of opioid-induced sedation in patients with cancer. *Clinical Journal of Oncology Nursing, 9*(6), 705.

12. **Answer: 2**
   Rationale: Vomiting results in the loss of hydrochloric acid as well as acids from extracellular fluids in the gastrointestinal tract. Signs include hyperreflexia, irritability, confusion, tetany-like symptoms, and shallow respirations. Metabolic acidosis is the result loss observed in losses from the lower gastrointestinal tract. Respiratory acidosis and alkalosis are related to respiratory alterations.
   Cognitive Level: Analysis
   Nursing Process: Evaluation
   NCLEX-RN Test Plan: PHYS
   Reference: LeFever Kee, J., Paulanka, B., & Purnell, L. D.(2004). *Fluids and electrolytes with clinical applications: A programmed approach* (7th ed.). Newark, NJ: Thompson.

13. **Answer: 1**
   Rationale: The side effects have occurred due to temporary or permanent damage to the cells in the treatment area. Dry skin should be lubricated with lotions that do not contain metal, alcohol, perfume, or irritating additives. Irradiated cells should be protected from extremes of temperature. Constricting garments, deodorants, soaps, and other harsh chemicals can further traumatize new epidermal cells.
   Cognitive Level: Application
   Nursing Process: Intervention
   NCLEX-RN Test Plan: PHYS
   Reference: Lewis, S. M., Heitkemper, M. M., & Dirksen, S. R. (2004). *Medical-surgical nursing: Assessment and management of clinical problems* (6th ed.) St. Louis, MO: Mosby.

14. **Answer: 3**
   Rationale: alpha-fetoprotein (AFP) is elevated in 70% of clients with hepatocellular carcinoma. It also helps to distinguish primary from metastatic cancer. CA 15-3 is a breast cancer associated antigen with higher levels found when metastasis is present. CEA or carcinoembryonic antigen is elevated in colon cancer and metastatic breast disease. A free PSA less than 25% of the total PSA supports the diagnosis of prostatic cancer, and it also differentiates it from benign prostatic hypertrophy (BPH).
   Cognitive Level: Knowledge
   Nursing Process: Assessment
   NCLEX-RN Test Plan: PHYS
   Reference: Corbett, J. (2004). *Laboratory tests and diagnostic procedures with nursing diagnosis* (6th ed.). Upper Saddle River, NJ: Pearson Prentice Hall.

15. **Answer: 3**

Rationale: Ovarian is the fifth leading cause of cancer deaths. Ovarian cancer can metastasize by shedding cells that may implant onto the uterus, bladder, bowel, and omentum. Several localized lymphatic systems are readily available to manage the abnormal cells, complimenting the metastatic process. Early stages of the disease are asymptomatic. In most cases, the disease is advanced at the time of diagnosis.

Cognitive Level: Comprehension

Nursing Process: Planning

NCLEX-RN Test Plan: PSYC

Reference: Lewis, S. M., Heitkemper, M. M., & Dirksen, S. R. (2004). *Medical-surgical nursing: Assessment and management of clinical problems* (6th ed.). St. Louis, MO: Mosby.

16. **Answer: 3**

Rationale: BRCA-1 is a gene on chromosome 17 and BRCA-2 is a gene found on chromomsome 11. Both of these are tumor suppressor genes that, when mutated, increase a woman's risk for breast cancer. Mutation of the BRCA-1 gene creates a 50–85% lifetime chance for a woman to develop breast cancer. This risk is similar for BRCA-2 gene mutations. High risk for ovarian cancer also exists with BRCA-1 and BRCA-2 gene mutations; 25–40% and 10–20%, respectively. An elective bilateral oopherectomy can decrease risk of both ovarian and breast cancers. An elective bilateral mastectomy can reduce a woman's risk of breast cancer by 90%. Additional genetic testing is available specific to Alzheimer's and Down's syndrome.

Cognitive Level: Analysis

Nursing Process: Planning

NCLEX-RN Test Plan: PHYS

Reference: Lewis, S. M., Heitkemper, M. M., & Dirksen, S.R. (2004). *Medical-surgical nursing: Assessment and management of clinical problems* (6th ed.). St. Louis, MO: Mosby.

17. **Answer: 4**

Rationale: In an autologous stem cell transplant, the patient's blood is collected by pharesis. Attached to a cell separator machine, the blood is collected from the client, the stem cells are removed, and the remaining blood is returned to the client. The stem cells are treated to kill cancer cells. They are then frozen and stored. The client receives intensive, high dose chemotherapy to treat the breast cancer. This process will ultimately destroy the rapidly dividing cells of the bone marrow. The stem cells will be infused as any other blood transfusion and seed into the bone marrow. Hematologic recovery is shorter with peripheral stem cell transplant than with a bone marrow transplant. If the client is compromised in a manner that requires blood transfusions and antibiotic therapy, transplant will be delayed in order to achieve positive client outcomes. Genetic counseling would involve the client's female offspring if indicated.

Cognitive Level: Synthesis

Nursing Process: Planning

NCLEX-RN Test Plan: PHYS

Reference: Lewis, S. M., Heitkemper, M. M., & Dirksen, S. R. (2004). *Medical-surgical nursing: Assessment and management of clinical problems* (6th ed.). St. Louis, MO: Mosby.

18. **Answer: 3**

Rationale: Age is a risk factor in both men and women that increases at age 40 and rises rapidly each decade thereafter. Family history should also be considered since there is a genetic predisposition in at least 6% of clients with colorectal cancer. Family history or client history of polyps, colorectal cancer, or adenomas is a risk factor. Chronic inflammatory bowel disease increases risk. Diets high in fat and/or those low in fiber remain controversial. If colorectal cancer is suspected after yearly tests for fecal occult blood, a sigmoidoscopy and double-contrast barium enema are performed. However, a sigmoidoscopy and barium enema are recommended every five years after age 50.

Cognitive Level: Comprehension

Nursing Process: Planning

NCLEX-RN Test Plan: SECE

Reference: Lewis, S. M., Heitkemper, M. M., & Dirksen, S. R. (2004). *Medical-surgical nursing: Assessment and management of clinical problems* (6th ed.). St. Louis, MO: Mosby.

19. **Answer: 4**

Rationale: Cell destruction that occurs with neoplasms will cause an increase in uric acid. Additionally, after chemotherapy and radiation, additional

cell death occurs and the significant hyperuricemia that occurs is treated with hydration and Zyloprim (allopurinol) to prevent renal damage. Increased ammonia levels result from liver dysfunction. Hemoblobin A1C measures glucose saturated hemoglobin. Lactic acid is a normal by-product of strenuous exercise.
Cognitive Level: Comprehension
Nursing Process: Assessment
NCLEX-RN Test Plan: PHYS
Reference: Lewis, S. M., Heitkemper, M. M., & Dirksen, S. R. (2004). *Medical-surgical nursing: Assessment and management of clinical problems* (6th ed.). St. Louis, MO: Mosby.

20. **Answer: 2**
Rationale: Elevated PSA (prostatic-specific antigen) is specific for both benign and malignant prostatic epithelium. Free PSA will be 25% lower than the total PSA in men with a prostatic malignancy. PKU (phenylketonuria) is a condition that occurs when an infant is lacking the enzyme necessary to metabolize phenylalanine (an amino acid). High serum levels of phenylalanine can cause brain damage. PTH (parathyroid hormone) is produced by the parathyroid gland and controls calcium and phosphorus levels.
Cognitive Level: Comprehension
Nursing Process: Assessment
NCLEX-RN Test Plan: PHYS
Reference: Corbett, J. (2004). *Laboratory tests and diagnostic procedures with nursing diagnosis* (6th ed.). Upper Saddle River, NJ: Pearson Prentice Hall.

21. **Answer: 4**
Rationale: Prostate cancer begins in the prostate gland in single or multiple areas. The cancer proliferates causing the gland to enlarge inward toward the urethra and outward toward the capsule. Initially, the cancer spreads by direct extension and involves the seminal vesicles, urethral mucosa, bladder wall, and external sphincter. As the cancer enters the lymphatics, the regional lymph nodes are involved. Metastasis, by way of the prostatic veins, is considered the mode of spread to the pelvis, femur, lumbar spine, liver, and lungs.
Cognitive Level: Comprehension

Nursing Process: Evaluation
NCLEX-RN Test Plan: PHYS
Reference: Hogan, M. A., & Hill, K. (2004). *Pathophysiology reviews and rationales.* Upper Saddle River, NJ: Prentice Hall.

22. **Answer: 2**
Rationale: A thoracotomy is required for a lobectomy. It is a major surgery with a large posterolateral or anterolateral incision into bone, muscle, and cartilage. Medial sternotomy is performed with heart surgery. Strong mechanical retractors are used to gain access to the lung, and pain is severe after surgery because muscles are severed. Chest tubes are placed to drain air and fluid for lung expansion. Pulmonary function studies are performed preoperatively.
Cognitive Level: Synthesis
Nursing Process: Planning
NCLEX-RN Test Plan: PHYS
Reference: Lewis, S. M., Heitkemper, M. M., & Dirksen, S. R. (2004). *Medical-surgical nursing: Assessment and management of clinical problems* (6th ed.). St. Louis, MO: Mosby.

23. **Answer: 4**
Rationale: Non-small cell lung cancer (NSCLC) includes squamous cell, adenocarcinoma, and large cell undifferentiated carcinoma. Small cell lung cancer (SCLC) includes oat cell. Squamous, large cell, and small cell are associated with smoking, but adenocarcinoma is not. Surgery is often attempted with squamous and adenocarcinoma but not usually attempted in large and small cell carcinomas. Small cell cancer has the poorest prognosis with an average median survival of 12–18 months.
Cognitive Level: Synthesis
Nursing Process: Planning
NCLEX-RN Test Plan: PSYC
Reference: Lewis, S. M., Heitkemper, M. M., & Dirksen, S. R. (2004). *Medical-surgical nursing: Assessment and management of clinical problems* (6th ed.). St. Louis, MO: Mosby.

24. **Answer: 2**
Rationale: All of the listed options are risk factors for pancreatic cancer. Cigarette smoking is the most firmly established risk factor with a two fold incidence with those smoking two packs per day as

compared to nonsmokers. It is thought that tobacco carcinogens reach the pancreas by way of the bloodstream and the pancreatic ducts and bile reflux.
Cognitive Level: Knowledge
Nursing Process: Assessment
NCLEX-RN Test Plan: SECE
Reference: Lewis, S. M., Heitkemper, M. M., & Dirksen, S. R. (2004). *Medical-surgical nursing: Assessment and management of clinical problems* (6th ed.). St. Louis, MO: Mosby.

25. **Answer: 3**
Rationale: The client is experiencing symptoms of pulmonary embolism which is a frequently occurring complication of liver cancer. Presenting symptoms of liver cancer are similar to those seen with early changes of cirrhosis, including weight loss, peripheral edema, portal hypertension, enlarged liver, and ascites. With the increase in malignant cells, the liver becomes enlarged and malformed. Congestion, varicies, and ascites occur throughout the portal circulation as blood is obstructed from passing through the liver. Spontaneous pneumothorax is not directly related to hepatic carcinoma. Fever and hemoptysis are not usually seen in chronic congestive heart failure in the absence of an acute exacerbation.
Cognitive Level: Analysis
Nursing Process: Evaluation
NCLEX-RN Test Plan: PHYS
Reference: Lewis, S. M., Heitkemper, M. M., & Dirksen, S. R. (2004). *Medical-surgical nursing: Assessment and management of clinical problems* (6th ed.). St. Louis, MO: Mosby.

26. **Answers: 1, 2, and 4**
Rationale: Cancer of the kidney is twice as common in males age 50–70 than in females. Although cigarette smoking is the greatest risk factor, obesity, exposure to asbestos, cadmium, and gasoline, and use of analgesics containing phenacetin also contribute to an increase in risk. Early symptoms are not evident. As the disease progresses, clients complain of generalized symptoms of weight loss, weakness, and anemia. Late manifestations include gross hematuria, flank pain, and a palpable mass in the flank.
Cognitive Level: Knowledge
Nursing Process: Assessment

NCLEX-RN Test Plan: PSYC
Reference: Lewis, S. M., Heitkemper, M. M., & Dirksen, S. R. (2004). *Medical-surgical nursing: Assessment and management of clinical problems* (6th ed.). St. Louis, MO: Mosby.

27. **Answer: 3**
Rationale: Metastatic carcinoma is the most frequent type of hepatic cancer. All blood travels through the liver where cells from primary cancer sites become trapped in the hepatocytes. Primary hepatic carcinomas include hepatocellular carcinoma, cholaniomas, or bile duct carcinomas and are associated with cirrhosis and chronic liver diseases including hepatitis B and C.
Cognitive Level: Analysis
Nursing Process: Assessment
NCLEX-RN Test Plan: PHYS
Reference: Lewis, S. M., Heitkemper, M. M., & Dirksen, S. R. (2004). *Medical-surgical nursing: Assessment and management of clinical problems* (6th ed.). St. Louis, MO: Mosby.

28. **Answer: 2**
Rationale: The most common type of colon cancer is adenocarcinoma, which most often arises from adenomatous polyps. All tumors spread through the intestinal walls and enter the lymphatic system. Because colonic venous blood travels through the portal vein to the liver, it is the common site of metastasis. As the tumor penetrates, the bowel wall can spread retroperitoneally and into the pelvis. After surgical intervention and therapy involving radiation and chemotherapy, involvement of other organs will require evaluation and follow-up to determine loss of function.
Cognitive Level: Application
Nursing Process: Assessment
NCLEX-RN Test Plan: PHYS
Reference: Lewis, S. M., Heitkemper, M. M., & Dirksen, S. R. (2004). *Medical-surgical nursing: Assessment and management of clinical problems* (6th ed.). St. Louis, MO: Mosby.

29. **Answer: 3**
Rationale: By the second postoperative day, the nurse has an understanding of the surgical procedure, the planned hospital course of treatment, and

the expected recovery as determined by the physician. A double-barrel colostomy is when the proximal and distal ends of the resected colon are brought up through the abdominal wall as two separate stomas. The proximal is functional for elimination of stool; the distal stoma is referred to as a mucus fistula. This type of colostomy is usually temporary. There would be no indication to perform a colostomy (large intestine) and an ileostomy (small intestine) simultaneously. The construction of a temporary, double-barrel colostomy, which is reversible, instead of a single-barreled, permanent colostomy tends to indicate that the tumor was not larger than expected.

Cognitive Level: Analysis

Nursing Process: Evaluation

NCLEX-RN Test Plan: PSYC

Reference: Lewis, S. M., Heitkemper, M. M., & Dirksen, S. R. (2004). *Medical-surgical nursing: Assessment and management of clinical problems* (6th ed.). St. Louis, MO: Mosby.

30. **Answer: 3**

Rationale: The Billroth II operation results in removal of the antrum (bottom) and pylorus of the stomach along with the phyloric sphincter. The body of the stomach is attached to the jejunum. The reservoir capacity of the stomach is greatly reduced. Loss of the pyloric sphincter eliminates the stomach's ability to control the amount of gastric chyme entering the intestine. After the large amount of hypertonic food/fluid enters the intestine, fluid is drawn to the hypertonic intestinal fluid with a resultant decreased plasma volume. Clients complain of weakness, sweating, palpitations, and dizziness. The large amount of fluid that enters the intestines stimulates hyperactive intestinal peristalsis. Esophageal varicies and ascities result from obstruction of portal blood flow through the liver.

Cognitive Level: Analysis

Nursing Process: Assessment

NCLEX-RN Test Plan: PHYS

Reference: Lewis, S. M., Heitkemper, M. M., & Dirksen, S. R. (2004). *Medical-surgical nursing: Assessment and management of clinical problems* (6th ed.). St. Louis, MO: Mosby.

31. **Answer: 4**

Rationale: The client will complain of epigastric fullness and satiety after meals. Depending on the location within the stomach, clinical manifestations include burning or pressure and pain 1–4 hours after a meal. Antacids, antisecretory agents, and changes in diet help to relieve pain and discomfort. Along with the gastric distress or indigestion, the client will have symptoms of anemia caused by chronic blood loss, erosion of the tumor through the mucosa, or due to pernicious anemia (with loss of intrinsic factor). The primary symptom of esophageal cancer is dysphagia. Liver cancer symptoms are similar to cirrhosis. Myocardial infarction symptoms, including pain, nausea, vomiting, fatigue, and in some occasions, indigestion, leads to a diagnosis sooner than the sustained symptoms seen with gastric cancer. Often gastric cancers will invade adjacent organs before distressing symptoms develop.

Cognitive Level: Analysis

Nursing Process: Assessment

NCLEX-RN Test Plan: PHYS

Reference: Lewis, S. M., Heitkemper, M. M., & Dirksen, S. R. (2004). *Medical-surgical nursing: Assessment and management of clinical problems* (6th ed.). St. Louis, MO: Mosby.

32. **Answer: 4**

Rationale: Pancreatic cancer has a poor prognosis, with death occurring between 5–12 months from the initial diagnosis. Psychological support for anxiety and depression as well as helping client and family through the grieving process is essential. Surgery is the most effective treatment. Radiation is effective for pain, but does not alter survival. Chemotherapy offers very little effect on survival. The most firmly established risk factor for pancreatic cancer is cigarette smoking. Pancreatic cancer develops twice as often in heavy smokers than in nonsmokers. The anxiety related to smoking cessation may outweigh the benefit produced with such a short term survival rate.

Cognitive Level: Application

Nursing Process: Planning

NCLEX-RN Test Plan: PYSC

Reference: Lewis, S. M., Heitkemper, M. M., & Dirksen, S. R. (2004). *Medical-surgical nursing: Assessment and management of clinical problems* (6th ed.). St. Louis, MO: Mosby.

33. **Answers: 1, 2, 3, 4, 5, 6, 7, and 8**

Rationale: Cardiac tamponode results when fluid accumulates in the pericardial sac causing constrictive pressure of the pericardium. This can be caused by a tumor or pericarditis. Treatment includes establishing a pericardial window or an indwelling pericardial catheter. Carotid blow out or rupture is a complication seen with cancers of the head and neck secondary to arterial invasion of the tumor or erosion related to chemotherapy or radiation. Hypercalcemia occurs with bony metastasis or when a parathyroid-like substance is secreted by cancer cells. Aredia (biphosphonate pamidronate) is the treatment of choice. Syndrome of inappropriate antidiuretic hormone (SIADH) is the result of sustained production of antidiuretic hormone related to cancers whose cells are able to manufacture, store, and release ADH. Treatment includes fluid restrictions and administration of intravenous 3% sodium chloride. Spinal cord compression occurs from compression by a tumor on the epidural space of the spinal cord. Symptoms include veterbral tenderness, motor weakness and dysfunction, and sensory paresthesia. Loss of autonomic dysfunction is evident in a change in bladder and bowel dysfunction. Superior vena cava (SVC) syndrome presents with facial edema, periorbital edema, neck and chest vein distention, headache, and seizures caused by a mediastinal mass that obstructs the SVC. Third space syndrome results from a shift of vascular fluids into the interstitial spaces with signs of hypovolemia. Treatment includes fluid, electrolyte, and plasma replacement therapy. Tumor lysis syndrome (TLS) is usually triggered by chemotherapy after massive amounts of cancer cell kill when the intracellular components affect the extracellular acid base balance. Treatment includes measures to decrease serum phosphate, potassium, and uric acid and to increase serum calcium.

Cognitive Level: Evaluation

Nursing Process: Evaluation

NCLEX-RN Test Plan: PHYS

Reference: Lewis, S. M., Heitkemper, M. M., & Dirksen, S. R. (2004). *Medical-surgical nursing: Assessment and management of clinical problems* (6th ed.). St. Louis, MO: Mosby.

34. **Answer: 1**

Rationale: The client should be instructed to determine a consistent day of the month to exam his testicles. The nurse should identify the structure and discuss the normal shape and consistency of the testes within the scrotal sac. The epididymis should be differentiated from the testes, as well as the spermatic cord. The warmth of a shower permits the testes to hang lower in the scrotum for a thorough exam and is the easiest time to exam the testicles. Both hands should be used to exam each testes separately. The testes are rolled between the thumb and first three fingers. The client should assess for pain, lumps, irregularities, and a dragging sensation.

Cognitive Level: Synthesis

Nursing Process: Planning

NCLEX-RN Test Plan: PHYS

Reference: Lewis, S. M., Heitkemper, M. M., & Dirksen, S. R. (2004). *Medical-surgical nursing: Assessment and management of clinical problems* (6th ed.). St. Louis, MO: Mosby.

35. **Answer: 3**

Rationale: With the initiation of chemotherapy and tumor cell destruction, there is a rapid release of intracellular components including phosphorus, potassium, and uric acid. Calcium has an inverse relationship with phosphorus and is decreased. These are the hallmark signs of tumor lysis syndrome (TLS). Tumor lysis syndrome will begin within 1–5 days after initiation of chemotherapy for fast growing tumor cells. The treatment for TLS is aimed at prevention of renal failure and acute electrolyte imbalances with alkaline hydration, if indicated, to alkalinize acidic urine, Zyloprim (allopurinol) to decrease uric acid concentrations, calcium supplements, and preparation for hemodialysis, if necessary, to decrease uric acid, phosphorus, and potassium. Hematuria and cramps may accompany a urinary tract infection, but the changes in electrolyes do not support this as a primary diagnosis.

Cognitive Level: Analysis

Nursing Process: Evaluation

NCLEX-RN Test Plan: PHYS

Reference: Lewis, S. M., Heitkemper, M. M., & Dirksen, S. R. (2004). *Medical-surgical nursing: Assessment and management of clinical problems* (6th ed.). St. Louis, MO: Mosby.

36. **Answer: 3**

Rationale: Nitrogen mustard (M), Oncovin (O), Procarbazine (P), and Prednisone (P) comprise a combination protocol referred to as MOPP. These agents differ in action, toxic affects, and nadir. Their action is synergistic and the combination is effective in destroying the cancer cells present in early stages of Hodgkin's disease. Often clients and families receive distressing news and are unable to process all the information provided by the physician. It is important for the nurse to participate in the multi-disciplinary team so they may provide related support and teaching. Allowing them to verbalize distorted understanding and concerns related to treatment would support negative thought processes. The physician would expect the nurse to provide necessary teaching to support treatment. Hospice is provided for end of life care and is not necessary in this situation.

Cognitive Level: Synthesis
Nursing Process: Evaluation
NCLEX-RN Test Plan: PSYC
Reference: Lewis, S. M., Heitkemper, M. M., & Dirksen, S. R. (2004). *Medical-surgical nursing: Assessment and management of clinical problems* (6th ed.). St. Louis, MO: Mosby.

37. **Answers: 1, 2, 3, 5, 7, and 8**

Rationale: Leukemia is a general term to describe malignant disorders that affect the bone marrow, lymph, and spleen. These structures include the blood forming tissues. Dysfunctional cells disrupt regulation of cell division. Blood cells include red blood cells, white blood cells, and platelets. Clients are at risk for anemia, infection, bleeding disorders, and related symptoms.

Cognitive Level: Evaluation
Nursing Process: Evaluation
NCLEX-RN Test Plan: PHYS
Reference: Lewis, S. M., Heitkemper, M. M., & Dirksen, S. R. (2004). *Medical-surgical nursing: Assessment and management of clinical problems* (6th ed.). St. Louis, MO: Mosby.

38. **Answers: 1, 2, 3, and 4**

Rationale: Treatment of metastatic tumors with chemotherapy and radiation becomes difficult due to spontaneous genetic mutations that occur within tumor cells. Although both the primary and metastatic tumors may originate from a single cell the mutations cause them to become heterogeneous (different). Treatment protocols are developed specifically to the response of the primary cells. The heterogeneous characteristics of metastatic tumor create a challenge and unpredictable response to treatment. Positive outcomes with surgical resection are greatest when the tumor is small and invasion of surrounding tissues and organs is minimized.

Cognitive Level: Analysis
Nursing Process: Planning
NCLEX-RN Test Plan: PSYC
Reference: Lewis, S. M., Heitkemper, M. M., & Dirksen, S. R. (2004). *Medical-surgical nursing: Assessment and management of clinical problems* (6th ed.). St. Louis, MO: Mosby.

39. **Answers: 1**

Rationale: The smaller a tumor is, the easier it is to treat and the more responsive it is to chemotherapy. Radiation and many chemotherapy agents have the greatest effect when the cell is growing (proliferation) or dividing (mitosis). As a tumor grows, many cells convert to a resting (G_O) stage. These cells can escape death. Therefore both radiation and chemotherapy administration intervals are scheduled according to cell life and metabolic activity.

Cognitive Level: Comprehension
Nursing Process: Intervention
NCLEX-RN Test Plan: PHYS
Reference: Lewis, S. M., Heitkemper, M. M., & Dirksen, S. R. (2004). *Medical-surgical nursing: Assessment and management of clinical problems* (6th ed.). St. Louis, MO: Mosby.

Unit 4 Answers and Rationales

Test 15 Answers and Rationales

1. **Answer: 4**
   Rationale: Excessive exertion, overheating, and infections are all known stressors that can precipitate an exacerbation of multiple sclerosis. Clients should be encouraged to live as independently and normally as possible but a plan should be developed to reduce fatigue and conserve energy.
   Cognitive Level: Application
   Nursing Process: Implementation
   NCLEX-RN Test Plan: HPM
   Reference: Lewis, S. M., Heitkemper, M. M., & Dirkson, S. R. (2004). *Medical-surgical nursing: Assessment and management of clinical problems* (6th ed.). St. Louis, MO: Mosby.

2. **Answer: 2**
   Rationale: Most clients with Guillain-Barre Syndrome will give a history of a mild febrile illness 1–3 weeks prior to the onset of the neurological signs and symptoms. The predisposing febrile illness is usually a viral upper respiratory or gastrointestinal infection. Recent travel and immunizations may be additional information to gather.
   Cognitive Level: Analysis
   Nursing Process: Assessment
   NCLEX-RN Test Plan: PHYS
   Reference: Lewis, S. M., Heitkemper, M. M., & Dirkson, S. R. (2004). *Medical-surgical nursing: Assessment and management of clinical problems* (6th ed.). St. Louis, MO: Mosby.

3. **Answer: 1**
   Rationale: Fever, severe headache, and stiff neck are key signs of meningitis. Fever, chills and malaise are symptoms of infection. Deterioration of consciousness is indicative of increased intracranial pressure. Seizures indicate irritability of the cerebral cortex.
   Cognitive Level: Analysis
   Nursing Process: Assessment
   NCLEX-RN Test Plan: PHYS

   Reference: Lewis, S. M., Heitkemper, M. M., & Dirkson, S. R. (2004). *Medical-surgical nursing: Assessment and management of clinical problems* (6th ed.). St. Louis, MO: Mosby.

4. **Answer: 1**
   Rationale: It is important to stress to clients with Parkinson's disease that side effects are dose related and can be controlled by dose adjustment. Medication should be taken at the scheduled time and skipping doses may affect mobility. Adverse side effects need to be reported to the doctor immediately.
   Cognitive Level: Application
   Nursing Process: Implementation
   NCLEX-RN Test Plan: HPM
   Reference: Aschenbrenner, D., Cleveland, L. W., & Venable, S. (2002). *Drug therapy in nursing.* Philadelphia: Lippincott.

5. **Answer: 4**
   Rationale: Using a wide-based stance helps the client with bradykinesia, tremors, and rigidity to maintain balance and improve walking. Crepe-soled shoes stick to carpeting and can cause the client to fall. Clients with bradykinesia are unable to hurry; trying to hurry can precipitate falls. Clients should be taught to lift their feet and avoid shuffling to prevent falls.
   Cognitive Level: Application
   Nursing Process: Implementation
   NCLEX-RN Test Plan: SECE
   Reference: Phipps, W. J., Monahan, F. D, Sands, J. K., Marek, J. F., & Neighbors, M. (2003). *Medical-surgical nursing: Health and illness perspectives.* St. Louis, MO: Mosby.

6. **Answer: 1**
   Rationale: Clients' needs are met by staff and they need to provide for a safe, respectful environment. Clients should be encouraged to participate in activities for as long as possible and visitors are limited only when the visit is beyond what the client is able

to tolerate. Speech and hearing are separate senses; clients may lose speech but retain their ability to hear. Activities should be explained in short, easily understood sentences, breaking the task into small understandable units.

Cognitive Level: Application

Nursing Process: Implementation

NCLEX-RN Test Plan: PSYC

Reference: Lewis, S. M., Heitkemper, M. M., & Dirkson, S. R. (2004). *Medical-surgical nursing: Assessment and management of clinical problems* (6th ed.). St. Louis, MO: Mosby.

7. **Answers: 1, 2, 3, 5, and 7**

Rationale: Any cervical cord injury may impair breathing. Vital signs are needed for baseline information and cervical injuries may show signs of spinal shock (hypotension, bradycardia, and hypothermia). An estimation of cord involvement should be ascertained but a complete neurological assessment is not possible at this time. It is important to check for an associated head injury. The nurse should maintain alignment and stabilization of the cervical spine. An incomplete cord injury could cause a complete transaction of the cord if the client is allowed to move. Trauma frequently causes multiple organ damage and hemorrhage and visceral hemorrhage must be found and treatment initiated.

Cognitive Level: Application

Nursing Process: Implementation

NCLEX-RN Test Plan: IMP

Reference: Lewis, S. M., Heitkemper, M. M., & Dirkson, S. R. (2004). *Medical-surgical nursing: Assessment and management of clinical problems* (6th ed.). St. Louis, MO: Mosby.

8. **Answers: 2, 3, 4, and 5**

Rationale: Immobilization and paralysis contribute to the development of thrombophlebitis with or without pulmonary emboli. Manifestations of thrombophlebitis include redness, warmth, and swelling. Indications of arterial thrombi include coolness, paleness, and decreased pulses in the extremity. Range of motion, elastic compression stockings (TED), and intermittent compression devices (ICD) are used to improve blood return to the heart. An increase in circumference in one leg should be reported to the health care provider. Low

molecular weight or low dose heparin is given prophylactically but does not require daily coagulation studies. The legs need to be protected from injury and injections should be avoided.

Cognitive Level: Analysis

Nursing Process: Implementation

NCLEX-RN Test Plan: PHYS

Reference: Lewis, S. M., Heitkemper, M. M., & Dirkson, S. R. (2004). *Medical-surgical nursing: Assessment and management of clinical problems* (6th ed.). St. Louis, MO: Mosby.

9. **Answers: 1 and 3**

Rationale: Autonomic dysreflexia is a life-threatening emergency occurring in the rehabilitative phase of spinal cord injury usually above T_7. Nursing care is directed at preventing the noxious triggering mechanisms. A urinary catheter should be checked for patency and free flow of urine. The nurse needs to monitor and document bowel movements and promote soft stool evacuation. Rectal examination or insertion of a suppository or enema should not be done without anesthetizing the rectal sphincter. Autonomic dysreflexia is characterized by paroxysmal hypertension and is triggered by noxious stimuli. Clients should be encouraged to wear a medic alert bracelet to alert others to possible problems but it is not a prevention measure.

Cognitive Level: Application

Nursing Process: Implementation

NCLEX-RN Test Plan: PL

Reference: Lewis, S. M., Heitkemper, M. M., & Dirkson, S. R. (2004). *Medical-surgical nursing: Assessment and management of clinical problems* (6th ed.). St. Louis, MO: Mosby.

10. **Answers: 1, 2, 3, and 6**

Rationale: It is important to inspect the client's skin for sign of irritation and erythema being alert to sensitive pressure areas. Foam or gel pads can be used to protect bony prominences from direct pressure. Non-erythematous areas should be routinely massaged to promote circulation and prevent skin breakdown. Powder tends to cake in areas of moisture and can cause the skin to break down. Minimize skin exposure to moisture, cleanse incontinent clients, and keep the skin clean.

Cognitive Level: Application

Nursing Process: Planning
NCLEX-RN Test Plan: PHYS
Reference: Lewis, S. M., Heitkemper, M. M., & Dirkson, S. R. (2004). *Medical-surgical nursing: Assessment and management of clinical problems* (6th ed.). St. Louis: Mosby.

11. **Answer: UMN: Use reflex emptying 30 minutes after a meal. LMN: Use manual stool removal and small volume enemas.**
    Rationale: An injury in the cervical and thoracic cord segments interrupts upper motor neuron (UMN) voluntary muscle control of bladder and bowel. The $S_{2,3,4}$ reflex arcs remain intact allowing for reflex emptying of the bowel and bladder. With spinal cord injuries in the cervical area of the cord, clients should have a routine evacuation schedule time 30 minutes after a meal (breakfast) or after a warm drink. Stroking the abdomen and increased abdominal pressure may trigger reflex emptying of the bladder. The lower motor neurons (LMN) in the sacral spinal segments transmit motor impulses to the bowel and bladder. Injury to this area interrupts both voluntary control and reflex activity resulting in a flaccid bowel and bladder and loss of anal tone. This type of injury is usually managed with use of increased abdominal pressure techniques, manual removal of impaction and small volume enemas. UMNs are located in the cerebral cortex and transmit impulses from the brain down the spinal cord to the bowel and bladder. Injuries in the cord interrupt the transmission causing dysfunction in these areas. In most adults the spinal cord ends around T_{12} or L_1. LMN's are located in the anterior horn cells in each of the spinal segments. Increased fluid intake, a diet high in fiber and /or stool softeners should be used in both types of injuries to promote evacuation.
    Cognitive Level: Application
    Nursing Process: Planning
    NCLEX-RN Test Plan: PHYS
    Reference: Lewis, S. M., Heitkemper, M. M., & Dirkson, S. R. (2004). *Medical-surgical nursing: Assessment and management of clinical problems* (6th ed.). St. Louis, MO: Mosby.

12. **Answers: 1, 2, 3, 5, and 6**
    Rationale: The client and family along with the health team members collaborate in the development of the rehabilitative plan. Nurses spend more time with the client and family than any other health team member and a rapport must be established between the nurse, client, and family that is the basis for communication and teaching. The nurse needs to establish an atmosphere that allows free expression, recognizing that anger, denial, withdrawal, and demanding behavior may be adaptive coping responses, and that clients and families need to express feelings, concerns, and questions. It is important to talk often with client and family to evaluate comprehension of information, and refer to the appropriate source to answer questions if information is unknown. Discharge planning is a coordinated effort by all team members, and the client and families may benefit by discussing their concerns, fears, and adjustments. Involving the client in the decision-making process about their care helps to foster feelings of self-control.
    Cognitive Level: Application
    Nursing Process: Planning
    NCLEX-RN Test Plan: SECE
    Reference: Lewis, S. M., Heitkemper, M. M., & Dirkson, S. R. (2004*). Medical-surgical nursing: Assessment and management of clinical problems* (6th ed.). St. Louis, MO: Mosby.

13. **Answer: The level of consciousness**
    Rationale: Level of consciousness is the most reliable indicator of overall brain function.
    Cognitive Level: Analysis
    Nursing Process: Assessment
    NCLEX-RN Test Plan: PHYS
    Reference: Lewis, S. M., Heitkemper, M. M., & Dirkson, S. R. (2004*). Medical-surgical nursing: Assessment and management of clinical problems* (6th ed.). St. Louis, MO: Mosby.

14. **Answer: 1**
    Rationale: A score of 8 or less can be considered to be a generally accepted level of coma. A fully alert, well-oriented person would have a high score of 15. A client in deep coma would have the lowest possible score of 3.
    Cognitive Level: Application
    Nursing Process: Analysis
    NCLEX-RN Test Plan: PHYS
    Reference: Lewis, S. M., Heitkemper, M. M., & Dirkson, S. R. (2004*). Medical-surgical nursing: Assessment and management of clinical problems* (6th ed.). St. Louis, MO: Mosby.

15. **Answer: 1**

    Rationale: Dural tears are common in basal skull fractures and the suction catheter is a source of infection and can lead to the development of meningitis. Clients should be kept flat to decrease pressure and the amount of CSF draining from the dural tear. The lower extremities should never be used for intravascular access in any client problem because of the risk for thrombophlebitis and pulmonary emboli. Suctioning longer than 15 seconds should be avoided in all clients.

    Cognitive Level: Application

    Nursing Process: Implementation

    NCLEX-RN Test Plan: SECE

    Reference: Lewis, S. M., Heitkemper, M. M., & Dirkson, S. R. (2004*). Medical-surgical nursing: Assessment and management of clinical problems* (6th ed.). St. Louis, MO: Mosby.

16. **Answer: 1**

    Rationale: An epidural hematoma is most often due to a torn meningeal artery and symptoms of increased intracranial pressure develop quickly along with rapid deterioration of neurological status. Venous bleeding results in subdural hematomas and may be acute (within 48 hours), subacute (2 days to 2 weeks after injury), or chronic (several months after injury).

    Cognitive Level: Analysis

    Nursing Process: Analysis

    NCLEX-RN Test Plan: PHYS

    Reference: Lewis, S. M., Heitkemper, M. M., & Dirkson, S. R. (2004*). Medical-surgical nursing: Assessment and management of clinical problems* (6th ed.). St. Louis, MO: Mosby.

17. **Answer: 3**

    Rationale: Head trauma, as well as other body system problems, can cause abnormal respiratory patterns. Whatever the reason for the respiratory change, it requires immediate further assessment and intervention. Hypertension is common and often reflects an increase in intracranial pressure, but may also be due to pain, fear, or a pre-existing condition. Bradycardia is associated with rising intracranial pressure and widening pulse pressure. Multiple injuries and internal bleeding usually cause tachycar-

dia in a head injury. Variations in temperature can be associated with injury to the hypothalamus.

Cognitive Level: Analysis

Nursing Process: Assessment

NCLEX-RN Test Plan: PHYS

Reference: Hickey, J. V. (2003). *The clinical practice of neurological and neurosurgical nursing.* Philadelphia: Lippincott.

18. **Answer: 3**

    Rationale: Signs and symptoms of oculomotor (Cranial Nerve III) are noted on the ipsilateral (right) side of the brain. The optic nerve (Cranial Nerve II) is for vision.

    Cognitive Level: Analysis

    Nursing Process: Assessment

    NCLEX-RN Test Plan: HPM

    Reference: Lewis, S. M., Heitkemper, M. M., & Dirkson, S. R. (2004). *Medical-surgical nursing: Assessment and management of clinical problems* (6th ed.). St. Louis, MO: Mosby.

19. **Answer: 2**

    Rationale: Neck pain and stiffness occur as a result of blood that has come in contact with the meninges, causing symptoms of meningitis. At the time of rupture, many clients experience a violent "explosive" headache and other signs of increased intracranial pressure such as hemiparesis, hemiplegia, and vomiting.

    Cognitive Level: Analysis

    Nursing Process: Assessment

    NCLEX-RN Test Plan: PHYS

    Reference: Lewis, S. M., Heitkemper, M. M., & Dirkson, S. R. (2004). *Medical-surgical nursing: Assessment and management of clinical problems* (6th ed.). St. Louis, MO: Mosby.

20. **Answer: 2**

    Rationale: A positive Kernig's and Brudzinski confirm the presence of meningeal irritation. The Brudzinski is positive if flexion of the neck causes flexion of both legs. Briskly rotating the head assesses the intactness of the brain stem. Applying painful stimuli assesses purposeful motor response in the unconsciousness.

    Cognitive Level: Application

Nursing Process: Assessment
NCLEX-RN Test Plan: HPM
Reference: Lewis, S. M., Heitkemper, M. M., & Dirkson, S. R. (2004). *Medical-surgical nursing: Assessment and management of clinical problems* (6th ed.). St. Louis, MO: Mosby.

21. **Answer: 2**
    Rationale: Rebleed occurs most frequently from the 3rd to the 11th day, with the peak incidence around the 7th day after the original bleed.
    Cognitive Level: Application
    Nursing Process: Assessment
    NCLEX-RN Test Plan: PHYS
    Reference: Hickey, J. V. (2003). *The clinical practice of neurological and neurosurgical nursing.* Philadelphia: Lippincott.

22. **Answer: 1**
    Rationale: A quiet environment will help to keep the client calm and the blood pressure low. All care is given by personnel to prevent any exertion that would increase the blood pressure. The room lighting should be kept low because of photophobia. Visitors are limited to immediate family and only two at a time to keep the client as quiet as possible.
    Cognitive Level: Application
    Nursing Process: Implementation
    NCLEX-RN Test Plan: SECE
    Reference: Swearingen, P. L. (2003). *Manual of medical-surgical nursing care: Nursing interventions and collaborative management.* St.Louis, MO: Mosby.

23. **Answer: Corticosteroids help to decrease cerebral edema and intracranial pressure. Anticonvulsants are given to control or prevent seizures. Antihypertensives are given to keep the blood pressure normotensive. A low sodium, low cholesterol diet is used to control hypertension and atherosclerosis.**
    Rationale: Hemorrhagic CVA causes bleeding and cerebral edema leading to a large increase in intracranial pressure (ICP). Corticosteroids may be used to prevent or reduce cerebral edema. Anticonvulsant drugs are given to control and prevent seizures if present. Antihypertensive agents are used to control high blood pressure which may cause cerebral edema

and increased ICP. When the client is conscious and able to swallow, a diet may be prescribed to minimize risk factors of hypertension and atherosclerosis.
    Cognitive Level: Application
    Nursing Process: Implementation
    NCLEX-RN Test Plan: PHYS
    Reference: Swearingen, P.L. (2003). *Manual of medical-surgical nursing care: Nursing interventions and collaborative management.* St. Louis, MO: Mosby.

24. **Answer: 3**
    Rationale: Hydrocephalus is more common in an aneurysm client because blood from the aneurysm may obstruct the reabsorption of CSF in the arachnoid villi. Diabetes insipidus and SIADH are also a possibility since the pituitary gland is close to the operative site. Diabetes mellitus may have been a pre-existing condition but is not related to the specific surgery.
    Cognitive Level: Application
    Nursing Process: Analysis
    NCLEX-RN Test Plan: PHYS
    Reference: Phipps, W. J., Monahan, F. D, Sands, J. K., Marek, J. F., & Neighbors, M. (2003). *Medical-surgical nursing: Health and illness perspectives.* St. Louis, MO: Mosby.

25. **Answer: Impaired physical mobility related to limited ability to use of left arm and leg; unilateral neglect related to disturbed perceptual ability secondary to right brain damage; disturbed sensory perception related to loss of vision in the left visual field.**
    Rationale: Classically symptoms appear on the side of the body opposite the damaged site. Clients with right hemisphere injury may have decreased movement, sensation, and visual field deficit on the left side of the body. Neglect of and attention to stimuli on the affected side occurs more often with right hemisphere injury.
    Cognitive Level: Analysis
    Nursing Process: Analysis
    NCLEX-RN Test Plan: PHYS
    Reference: Phipps, W. J., Monahan, F. D, Sands, J. K., Marek, J. F., & Neighbors, M. (2003). *Medical-surgical nursing: Health and illness perspectives.* St. Louis, MO: Mosby.

26. **Answer: 3**

    Rationale: Persistent disregard of objects in part of the visual field should alert the nurse to the possibility of left homonymous hemianopsia. Initially the nurse might help the client by arranging the food tray so that all foods are on the right side. Later, the client learns to compensate for the visual deficit by scanning the left side. Weak extremities should be assessed for adequacy for self-care.

    Cognitive Level: Application

    Nursing Process: Implementation

    NCLEX-RN Test Plan: PHYS

    Reference: Lewis, S. M., Heitkemper, M. M., & Dirkson, S. R. (2004). *Medical-surgical nursing: Assessment and management of clinical problems* (6th ed.). St. Louis, MO: Mosby.

27. **Answer: 3**

    Rationale: Clients with right brain injury are more likely to have unilateral neglect and this client is exhibiting signs of self-neglect by attending to the unaffected side of the face. Confusion most likely would interfere with his ability to perform any self-care, not just shaving. Clients with depression generally lack desire to participate in hygiene activities.

    Cognitive Level: Application

    Nursing Process: Diagnosis

    NCLEX-RN Test Plan: PHYS

    Reference: Lewis, S. M., Heitkemper, M. M., & Dirkson, S. R. (2004). *Medical-surgical nursing: Assessment and management of clinical problems* (6th ed.). St. Louis, MO: Mosby.

28. **Answer: 4**

    Rationale: Aspiration can cause pneumonia and every precaution should be taken to prevent aspiration. The alternative choices are important to know and can help with feeding any client.

    Cognitive Level: Analysis

    Nursing Process: Implementation

    NCLEX-RN Test Plan: PHYS

    Reference: Phipps, W. J., Monahan, F. D, Sands, J. K., Marek, J. F., & Neighbors, M. (2003). *Medical-surgical nursing: Health and illness perspectives.* St. Louis, MO: Mosby.

29. **Answer: 1**

    Rationale: Global aphasia (Expressive and Receptive) is the complete inability to use or comprehend language and symbols. It does not result in impaired hearing or intelligence. Receptive aphasia is characterized by the inability to recognize or comprehend the spoken word and is often described as if a foreign language were being spoken. Expressive aphasia, the ability to understand and comprehend language, is retained but the client has difficulty expressing words.

    Cognitive Level: Analysis

    Nursing Process: Implementation

    NCLEX-RN Test Plan: SECE

    Reference: Phipps, W. J., Monahan, F. D, Sands, J. K., Marek, J. F., & Neighbors, M. (2003). *Medical-surgical nursing: Health and illness perspectives.* St. Louis, MO: Mosby.

30. **Answer: 4**

    Rationale: The corneal reflex can be elicited by stroking the cornea lightly with a wisp of cotton, and the normal response is bilateral blink. The pupils are examined using a penlight for the reaction to light. Instilling dye is sometimes done to determine if there are foreign bodies in the eye. The red reflex is found when visualizing the retina.

    Cognitive Level: Application

    Nursing Process: Assessment

    NCLEX-RN Test Plan: PHYS

    Reference: Hickey, J. V. (2003). *The clinical practice of neurological and neurosurgical nursing.* Philadelphia: Lippincott.

31. **Answer: 1**

    Rationale: An unconscious client purposeful response is to push the painful stimulus away. Other responses should be noted but are not appropriate.

    Cognitive Level: Analysis

    Nursing Process: Assessment

    NCLEX-RN Test Plan: PHYS

    Reference: Hickey, J. V. (2003). *The clinical practice of neurological and neurosurgical nursing.* Philadelphia: Lippincott.

32. **Answer: 2**

    Rationale: A common problem associated with loss of corneal reflex is corneal abrasion. The eye must be protected by taping or shielding and lubricating it with saline or tears. Corneal abrasion will not be prevented by keeping the room dark, applying compresses, or alternating eye patches.

Cognitive Level: Application
Nursing Process: Implementation
NCLEX-RN Test Plan: PHYS
Reference: Phipps, W. J., Monahan, F. D, Sands, J. K., Marek, J. F., & Neighbors, M. (2003). *Medical-surgical nursing: Health and illness perspectives.* St. Louis, MO: Mosby.

33. **Answer: 1**

Rationale: Tolerance to tube feedings is evaluated by the measurement of gastric residuals and the presence of abdominal distention, vomiting, and diarrhea. Residual should be less than 200 ml. Lab studies are helpful in monitoring clients receiving enteral feedings, the urine specific gravity, serum sodium and potassium are within normal requiring no intervention.
Cognitive Level: Application
Nursing Process: Evaluation
NCLEX-RN Test Plan: PHYS
Reference: Hickey, J. V. (2003). *The clinical practice of neurological and neurosurgical nursing.* Philadelphia: Lippincott.

34. **Answer: 1**

Rationale: Clients receiving continuous feedings require larger doses of phenytoin (Dilantin) to maintain therapeutic levels because the feedings bind to the protein, which results in decreased absorption. The dosage will need to be evaluated and probably decreased when the tube feeding is discontinued.
Cognitive Level: Application
Nursing Process: Planning
NCLEX-RN Test Plan: PHYS
Reference: Hickey, J. V. (2003). *The clinical practice of neurological and neurosurgical nursing.* Philadelphia: Lippincott.

35. **Answer: 2**

Rationale: Rapid administration can cause cardiac arrest. If the drug is given in a dextrose solution, it will precipitate into crystals. Clients receiving intravenous phenytoin should be observed for the development of phlebitis. Frequent administration causes discomfort.
Cognitive Level: Application
Nursing Process: Implementation
NCLEX-RN Test Plan: PHYS

Reference: Hickey, J. V. (2003). *The clinical practice of neurological and neurosurgical nursing.* Philadelphia: Lippincott.

36. **Answers: 1, 2, 3, 4, and 5**

Rationale: An airway may be needed during or immediately after seizure activity. Suction may be necessary to prevent airway obstruction and possible aspiration. Oxygen is provided as necessary. The client should be protected from injury by keeping the side rails up and the bed in the lowest position. Restraint during seizure activity may result in client injury. It is important to remain with the client and observe the seizure activity and the physician can be notified after the seizure.
Cognitive Level: Application
Nursing Process: Implementation
NCLEX-RN Test Plan: PHYS
Reference: Lewis, S. M., Heitkemper, M. M., & Dirkson, S. R. (2004). *Medical-surgical nursing: Assessment and management of clinical problems* (6th ed.). St. Louis, MO: Mosby.

37. **Answer: Cholinergic crisis is the result of excess acetylcholine causing parasympathetic nervous system stimulation. The client will have increased gastrointestinal activity with abdominal cramping and diarrhea. There is severe muscle weakness and the client may have respiratory distress. Myasthenic crisis is the result of decreased acetylcholine resulting in extreme muscle weakness and risk of respiratory failure. The client may have difficulty in swallowing, impaired speech, and ptosis. Both types of crises are life-threatening situations and require ventilator assistance.**
Cognitive Level: Analysis
Nursing Process: Evaluation
NCLEX-RN Test Plan: PHYS
Reference: Lewis, S. M., Heitkemper, M. M., & Dirkson, S. R. (2004). *Medical-surgical nursing: Assessment and management of clinical problems* (6th ed.). St. Louis: Mosby.

38. **Answer: 1**

Rationale: There is no standard dosage of Mestinon because of the great variations among clients and in the same client from time to time. An individualized dosage schedule needs to be established that allows for the maximum benefit with the least amount of side effects. All other answers are possible, but understanding dosage variation is the most important in nursing management.

Cognitive Level: Application
Nursing Process: Implementation
NCLEX-RN Test Plan: PHYS

Reference: Phipps, W. J., Monahan, F. D., Sands, J. K., Marek, J. F., & Neighbors, M. (2003). *Medical-surgical nursing: Health and illness perspectives.* St. Louis, MO: Mosby.

Rationale: The nurse can use a variety of methods to solve this problem. Dimensional analysis was used in this situation.

Cognitive Level: Application
Nursing Process: Implementation
NCLEX-RN Test Plan: PHYS

Reference: Curren, A. M. (2002). *Dimensional analysis for meds.* Clifton Park, NY: Delmar Thompson Learning.

39. **Answer: 2 mcg/min (the lower rate)**

$$\text{mL} = \frac{1000 \text{ mL}}{6 \text{ mg}} \times \frac{1 \text{mg}}{1000 \text{ mcg}} \times \frac{2 \text{ mcg}}{1 \text{ min}} \times \frac{60 \text{ min}}{1 \text{ hr}} = 20 \text{ mL/hr}$$

Upper rate of 4 mcg/ min:

$$\text{mL} = \frac{1000 \text{ mL}}{6 \text{ mg}} \times \frac{1 \text{ mg}}{1000 \text{ mcg}} \times \frac{4 \text{ mcg}}{1 \text{ min}} \times \frac{60 \text{ min}}{1 \text{ hr}} = 40 \text{ mL/hr}$$

Unit 4 Answers and Rationales

Test 16 Answers and Rationales

1. **Answer: 4**
   Rationale: With carpal tunnel syndrome, when a client holds the wrist in flexion for 60 seconds, it will produce tingling and numbness over the median nerve, the palmer surface of the thumb, the index finger, the middle finger, and part of the ring finger. This is called a positive Phalen's test. The other answers do not occur with carpal tunnel syndrome.
   Cognitive Level: Application
   Nursing Process: Assessment
   NCLEX-RN Test Plan: PHYS
   Reference: Lewis, S. M., Heitkemper, M. M., & Dirksen, S. R. (2004). *Medical-surgical nursing: Assessment and management of clinical problems* (6th ed.). St. Louis, MO: Mosby.

2. **Answer: 2**
   Rationale: A client that has a rotator cuff injury will complain of shoulder pain and inability to initiate or maintain abduction of the arm or shoulder. With a rotator cuff injury, the patient would also have a positive Neer's test not a negative test. Tinel's sign is present in carpal tunnel syndrome, and a rotator cuff injury would occur in someone who plays baseball, not golf.
   Cognitive Level: Application
   Nursing Process: Assessment
   NCLEX-RN Test Plan: PHYS
   Reference: Lewis, S. M., Heitkemper, M. M., & Dirksen, S. R. (2004). *Medical-surgical nursing: Assessment and management of clinical problems* (6th ed.). St. Louis, MO: Mosby.

3. **Answer: 3**
   Rationale: With bursitis, the immobilization of the affected part in a compression dressing or plaster splint can attempt to correct the cause. Also, with bursitis, rest and ice to the affected extremity should be used, not exercise and heat. NSAIDS are used first for the inflammation and then corticosteroids may also be used.
   Cognitive Level: Application
   Nursing Process: Implementation

NCLEX-RN Test Plan: PHYS
Reference: Lewis, S. M., Heitkemper, M. M., & Dirksen, S. R. (2004). *Medical-surgical nursing: Assessment and management of clinical problems* (6th ed.). St. Louis, MO: Mosby.

4. **Answer: 4**
   Rationale: This is the only bone tissue that contains pain receptors. Any process that disrupts or results in pressure on the periosteum will cause pain.
   Cognitive Level: Application
   Nursing Process: Analysis
   NCLEX-RN Test Plan: PHYS
   Reference: Crutchlow, E. M., Dudar, P. J., MacAvoy, S., & Madara, B. R. (2002). *Quick look nursing: Pathophysiology.* Thorofare, NJ: Slack, Inc.

5. **Answers: 2, 3, and 4**
   Rationale: Answers 2, 3, and 4 are all signs and symptoms of a herniated intervertebral disc. Coughing, sneezing, or bending would intensify the pain, not lessen it.
   Cognitive Level: Application
   Nursing Process: Assessment
   NCLEX-RN Test Plan: PHYS
   Reference: Tamparo, C. D., & Lewis, M. A. (2005). *Diseases of the human body.* Philadelphia: F.A. Davis.

6. **Answers: 1, 2, and 3**
   Rationale: Answers 1, 2, and 3 are all manifestations of Paget's disease. Bladder and bowel dysfunction may occur from immobility with progression of the disease. Fractures are common in patients with Paget's disease because of increased vascularity of the involved bones, and the long bones are the most susceptible to fractures. Hypercalcemia is common in immobilized patients because calcium deposits develop in the joint spaces which lead to excessive amounts of calcium in the blood stream. Answer 4 is a manifestation of osteoporosis.
   Cognitive Level: Application
   Nursing Process: Implementation
   NCLEX-RN Test Plan: PHYS

Reference: Lemone, P., & Burke, K. (2004). *Medical-surgical nursing: Critical thinking in client care.* Upper Saddle River, NJ: Prentice Hall.

7. **Answer: 2**

   Rationale: Degenerative disc disease results from fibrosis and thinning of the nucleus palposus, which is associated with aging. The other answers do not pertain to degenerative disc disease.

   Cognitive Level: Analysis

   Nursing Process: Analysis

   NCLEX-RN Test Plan: PHYS

   Reference: Crutchlow, E. M., Dudar, P. J., MacAvoy, S., & Madora, B. R. (2002). *Quick look nursing: Pathophysiology.* Thorofare, NJ: Slack Inc.

8. **Answer: 4**

   Rationale: Due to cytoxan being an antineoplastic drug, it causes immunosuppression. If a client has signs of infection, the physician needs to know for accurate treatment of the infection. Cytoxin causes neutropenia, not bleeding. It also causes fatigue, but not muscle weakness, and will cause dizziness, but is not associated with behavioral changes.

   Cognitive Level: Application

   Nursing Process: Implementation

   NCLEX-RN Test Plan: PHYS

   Reference: Lemone, P., & Burke, K. (2004). *Medical-surgical nursing: Critical thinking in client care.* Upper Saddle River, NJ: Prentice Hall.

9. **Answers: 2 and 3**

   Rationale: Skin care and avoiding exposure to infection are important factors that should be included for patients with SLE. Management of stiffness and pain and clothing options pertain to rheumatoid arthritis.

   Cognitive Level: Application

   Nursing Process: Implementation

   NCLEX-RN Test Plan: HPM

   Reference: Lemone, P., & Burke, K. (2004). *Medical-surgical nursing: Critical thinking in client care.* Upper Saddle River, NJ: Prentice Hall.

10. **Answer: 3**

    Rationale: Careful hand washing removes transient organisms from the skin, reducing the risk of transmission to the client. The client with SLE is at increased risk for infection and multi-organ system

problems because of this disease. Administration of preoperative medication, monitoring lab values, and providing appropriate skin care are all important interventions for a patient with SLE, but they are not the most important because proper hand washing reduces bacteria and prevents the spread of infection. These patients are already at risk of infection because this disease produces a large variety of autoantibodies against the body.

Cognitive Level: Application

Nursing Process: Implementation

NCLEX-RN Test Plan: HPM

Reference: Lemone, P., & Burke, K. (2004). *Medical-surgical nursing: Critical thinking in client care.* Upper Saddle River, NJ: Prentice Hall.

11. **Answers: 1, 2, 3, and 4**

    Rationale: All of the answers are multisystem effects of SLE.

    Cognitive Level: Application

    Nursing Process: Assessment

    NCLEX-RN Test Plan: PHYS

    Reference: Lemone, P., & Burke, K. (2004). *Medical-surgical nursing: Critical thinking in client care.* Upper Saddle River, NJ: Prentice Hall.

12. **Answers: 2 and 4**

    Rationale: Wrapping the amputated part in a clean cloth will keep it from getting infected and the saline will keep the part hydrated. Putting the body part on ice will vasoconstrict the blood vessels and prevent further bleeding. If measures are not done to preserve the amputated part, the area will die and not be viable. Placing the amputated part in warm water will cause vasodilation and cause further blood loss.

    Cognitive Level: Application

    Nursing Process: Implementation

    NCLEX-RN Test Plan: SECE

    Reference: Lemone, P., & Burke, K., (2004). *Medical-surgical nursing: Critical thinking in client care.* Upper Saddle River, NJ: Prentice Hall.

13. **Answer: 3**

    Rationale: Elevating the limb promotes venous return and decreases edema, which will decrease pain. Elevating the limb for longer periods increases the risk for contracture. Abducting the limb on a scheduled basis is important to prevent muscle atrophy but increases pain. Applying traction to the

limb would also increase pain. Keeping the limb flat is not necessary because it could lead to disuse syndrome from lack of use.
Cognitive Level: Analysis
Nursing Process: Implementation
NCLEX-RN Test Plan: PHYS
Reference: Lemone, P., & Burke, K. (2004). *Medical-surgical nursing: Critical thinking in client care.* Upper Saddle River, NJ: Prentice Hall.

14. **Answer: 4**
Rationale: Arthroplasty is the reconstruction or replacement of a joint. This surgical procedure is performed to relieve pain, improve or maintain range of motion, and correct the deformity.
Cognitive Level: Application
Nursing Process: Implementation
NCLEX-RN Test Plan: PHYS
Reference: Lewis, S. M., Heitkemper, M. M., & Dirksen, S. R. (2004). *Medical-surgical nursing: Assessment and management of clinical problems* (6th ed.). St. Louis, MO: Mosby.

15. **Answers: 1, 3, and 4**
Rationale: Excessive weight, decreased estrogen, and inactivity are all factors that contribute to osteoarthritis. Epstein Barr virus may play a role in initiating the autoimmune processes present in rheumatoid arthritis.
Cognitive Level: Application
Nursing Process: Implementation
NCLEX-RN Test Plan: PHYS
Reference: Lemone, P., & Burke, K. (2004). *Medical-surgical nursing: Critical thinking in client care.* Upper Saddle River, NJ: Prentice Hall.

16. **Answer: 4**
Rationale: Uricosurics are anti-inflammatory medications used with all of these conditions. The other choices are incorrect because narcotics are not used for long-term treatment of arthritis; under certain circumstances, steroids are sometimes used for RA; and NSAIDS are used only with gout.
Cognitive Level: Application
Nursing Process: Assessment
NCLEX-RN Test Plan: PHYS
Reference: Crutchlow, E. M., Dudar, P. J., MacAvoy, S., & Madora, B. R. (2002). *Quick look nursing: Pathophysiology.* Thorofare NJ: Slack Inc.

17. **Answer: 3**
Rationale: This is the only option that describes the pathophysiology of gout. With gout, you have hyperuricemia, not a reduction of uric acid. Tophi forms on the skin when kidney uric acid deposits in articular cartilage and leads to inflammation.
Cognitive Level: Application
Nursing Process: Assessment
NCLEX-RN Test Plan: PHYS
Reference: Crutchlow, E. M., Dudar, P. J., MacAvoy, S., & Madora, B. R. (2002). *Quick look nursing: Pathophysiology.* Thorofare, NJ: Slack Inc.

18. **Answers: 2 and 3**
Rationale: Antirheumatoids have immunomodulating effects and are indicated for short-term use. They are given at lower doses, not higher doses, during maintenance therapy, and have some severe, not minor, adverse effects including bone marrow suppression.
Cognitive Level: Application
Nursing Process: Assessment
NCLEX-RN Test Plan: PHYS
Reference: Herbert-Ashton, M. J., & Clarkson, N. E. (2005). *Quick look nursing: Pharmacology.* Sudbury, MA: Jones & Bartlett.

19. **Answer: 3**
Rationale: Clients should increase their fluid intake to at least 2000 ml to help with excretion to prevent formation of uric acid stones. Alcohol, turkey, organ meats, and high purine foods exacerbate gout. Diarrhea is a sign of toxicity and the medication should be stopped.
Cognitive Level: Application
Nursing Process: Implementation
NCLEX-RN Test Plan: PHYS
Reference: Herbert-Ashton, M. J., & Clarkson, N. E. (2005). *Quick look nursing: Pharmacology.* Sudbury, MA: Jones & Bartlett.

20. **Answers: 3 and 4**
Rationale: Answers 3 and 4 are important points the nurse should include when teaching patients and caregivers about bisphosphonates. Answers 1 and 2 are important points the nurse should include when teaching patients and caregivers about antigout medications.
Cognitive Level: Application
Nursing Process: Implementation

NCLEX-RN Test Plan: PHYS

Reference: Adams, M. P., Josephson, D. L., & Holland, L. N. (2005). *Pharmacology for nurses: A pathophysiologic approach.* Upper Saddle River, NJ: Pearson Prentice Hall.

21. **Answer: 3**

    Rationale: Long-term use of glucocorticoid hormones can commonly cause osteoporosis; the others do not.
    Cognitive Level: Application
    Nursing Process: Assessment
    NCLEX-RN Test Plan: PHYS
    Reference: Crutchlow, E. M., Dudar, P. J., MacAvoy, S., & Madora, B. R. (2002). *Quick look nursing: Pathophysiology.* Thorofare NJ: Slack Inc.

22. **Answer: 1**

    Rationale: The factors in answer 1 are risk factors for osteoporosis. A diet deficient in protein, obesity, a history of falls, and depression do not contribute to development of osteoporosis.
    Cognitive Level: Analysis
    Nursing Process: Assessment
    NCLEX-RN Test Plan: HPM
    Reference: Tamporo, C. D., & Lewis, M. A. (2005). *Diseases of the human body.* Philadelphia: F.A. Davis.

23. **Answer: 2**

    Rationale: Clinical manifestations of fibromyalgia overlap with those of CFS. The remaining answers are incorrect because more women are diagnosed with FMS, a definitive diagnosis is difficult to establish, and burning pain worsens and improves throughout the day.
    Cognitive Level: Application
    Nursing Process: Implementation
    NCLEX-RN Test Plan: HPM
    Reference: Lewis, S. M., Heitkemper, M. M., & Dirksen, S. R. (2004). *Medical-surgical nursing: Assessment and management of clinical problems* (6th ed.). St. Louis, MO: Mosby.

24. **Answer: 2**

    Rationale: The foot should be elevated with the heel off the floor to help reduce discomfort and prevent edema. The client should walk with proper weight distribution; walking on the heels would be improper weight distribution. If the feet were numb

for several days this would indicate a problem with neurovascular status. The patient may experience pain or a throbbing sensation when starting to ambulate. Soaking the feet in warn water is not a treatment for a bunion, because warm water would dilate the blood vessels and increase pain. Icing the site would constrict circulation and blood vessels and decrease pain.
    Cognitive Level: Application
    Nursing Process: Implementation
    NCLEX-RN Test Plan: HPM
    Reference: Lewis, S. M., Heitkemper, M. M., & Dirksen, S. R. (2004). *Medical-surgical nursing: Assessment and management of clinical problems* (6th ed.). St. Louis, MO: Mosby.

25. **Answers: 1 and 3**

    Rationale: Excess body weight places extra stress on the lower back and weakens the abdominal muscles that support the lower back. Sleeping in a side-lying position with knees flexed prevents unnecessary pressure on the support muscles and lumbosacral joints. Sleeping in a prone position produces excessive lumbar lordosis, causing excessive stresses on lower back. You should sleep with a firm mattress for added support.
    Cognitive Level: Application
    Nursing Process: Implementation
    NCLEX-RN Test Plan: SECE
    Reference: Lewis, S. M., Heitkemper, M. M., & Dirksen, S. R. (2004). *Medical-surgical nursing: Assessment and management of clinical problems* (6th ed.). St. Louis, MO: Mosby.

26. **Answer: 3**

    Rationale: A sprain is an injury to ligamentous structures surrounding a joint, usually caused by a wrenching or twisting motion. The other answers do not apply to the question.
    Cognitive Level: Application
    Nursing Process: Assessment
    NCLEX-RN Test Plan: PHYS
    Reference: Lewis, S. M., Heitkemper, M. M., & Dirksen, S. R. (2004). *Medical-surgical nursing: Assessment and management of clinical problems* (6th ed.). St. Louis, MO: Mosby.

27. **Answer: 4**

    Rationale: EMG consists of small gauge needles that are inserted into certain muscles. Needle probes are attached to leads that feed into the EMG machine. The other answers are incorrect with regard to an EMG.

Cognitive Level: Application

Nursing Process: Implementation

NCLEX-RN Test Plan: PHYS

Reference: Lewis, S. M., Heitkemper, M. M., & Dirksen, S. R. (2004). *Medical-surgical nursing: Assessment and management of clinical problems* (6th ed.). St. Louis, MO: Mosby.

28. **Answer: 1**

Rationale: Normal physical assessment of the musculoskeletal system would include a full range of motion for all joints without pain or laxity. A normal assessment would also include a muscle strength of 5, normal spinal curvature, and no muscle atrophy or asymmetry.

Cognitive Level: Application

Nursing Process: Assessment

NCLEX-RN Test Plan: PHYS

Reference: Lewis, S. M., Heitkemper, M. M., & Dirksen, S. R. (2004). *Medical-surgical nursing: Assessment and management of clinical problems* (6th ed.). St. Louis, MO: Mosby.

29. **Answer: 4**

Rationale: The donor site usually causes greater postoperative pain than the fused area. The other answers are incorrect. Body alignment is maintained by using a rigid orthosis. The spine is stabilized by creating an anlylosis (fusion) of contigious vertebrae with a bone graft. Earlier ambulation is not permitted because immobilization over an extended time is necessary to help heal the spine. Instruction in proper body mechanics and prevention of further back injuries is essential to the healing process.

Cognitive Level: Application

Nursing Process: Implementation

NCLEX-RN Test Plan: PHYS

Reference: Lewis, S. M., Heitkemper, M. M., & Dirksen, S. R. (2004). *Medical-surgical nursing: Assessment and management of clinical problems.* St. Louis, MO: Mosby.

30. **Answer: 2**

Rationale: A diminished or absent pulse distal to the injury can indicate vascular insufficiency. The nurse would assess the actual fracture site, the area proximal to the fracture, and the extremity not affected after the initial neurovascular assessment is made.

Cognitive Level: Application

Nursing Process: Assessment

NCLEX-RN Test Plan: PHYS

Reference: Lewis, S. M., Heitkemper, M. M., & Dirksen, S. R. (2004). *Medical-surgical nursing: Assessment and management of clinical problems* (6th ed.). St. Louis, MO: Mosby.

31. **Answers: 2, 3, and 4**

Rationale: Paresthesia, or numbness and tingling; pallor or coolness; and diminished/absent peripheral pulses are characteristics of impending compartment syndrome. Pain occurs distal to the injury, not proximal.

Cognitive Level: Application

Nursing Process: Assessment

NCLEX-RN Test Plan: PHYS

Reference: Lewis, S. M., Heitkemper, M. M., & Dirksen, S. R. (2004). *Medical-surgical nursing: Assessment and management of clinical problems* (6th ed.). St. Louis, MO: Mosby.

32. **Answer: 2**

Rationale: A clinical manifestation of hip fractures is external rotation. Additional signs would be a shortening of the affected extremity, muscle spasms, and severe pain and tenderness at the fracture site.

Cognitive Level: Application

Nursing Process: Assessment

NCLEX-RN Test Plan: PHYS

Reference: Lewis, S. M., Heitkemper, M. M., & Dirksen, S. R. (2004). *Medical-surgical nursing: Assessment and management of clinical problems* (6th ed.). St. Louis, MO: Mosby.

33. **Answer: 2**

Rationale: Putting on shoes and socks should be avoided because it predisposes the client to dislocation by reproducing greater than 90° of flexion, adduction, or internal rotation. Using a walker, a lifted toilet seat, and a pillow between the legs keeps the hips in abduction, thus preventing adduction.

Cognitive Level: Application

Nursing Process: Implementation

NCLEX-RN Test Plan: PHYS

Reference: Lewis, S. M., Heitkemper, M. M., & Dirksen, S. R. (2004). *Medical-surgical nursing: Assessment and management of clinical problems* (6th ed.). St. Louis, MO: Mosby.

34. **Answers: 2, 3, and 4**

    Rationale: Using an elevated toilet seat prevents dislocation by making it easier for the client to get off of the toilet; using a pillow between the legs also helps avoid dislocation. Informing the dentist of the presence of a prosthesis before dental work is also correct because the dentist can give prophylactic antibiotics. Crossing your legs is incorrect because it predisposes the client to dislocation.

    Cognitive Level: Application

    Nursing Process: Implementation

    NCLEX-RN Test Plan: PHYS

    Reference: Lewis, S. M., Heitkemper, M. M., & Dirksen, S. R. (2004). *Medical-surgical nursing: Assessment and management of clinical problems* (6th ed.). St. Louis, MO: Mosby.

35. **Answer: 2**

    Rationale: Drugs that cause gastric irritation are best taken after or with a meal, when stomach contents help minimize the local irritation.

    Cognitive Level: Application

    Nursing Process: Implementation

    NCLEX-RN Test Plan: HPM

    Reference: Hodgson, B., & Kizior, R. (2006). *Saunders nursing drug handbook 2006.* St Louis, MO: Elsevier.

36. **Answer: 3**

    Rationale: Flexeril is a centrally acting skeletal muscle relaxant. It relieves local skeletal muscle spasm. It has no effect on microorganisms, does not reduce itching, and does not reduce pain.

    Cognitive Level: Application

    Nursing Process: Implementation

    NCLEX-RN Test Plan: PHYS

    Reference: Hodgson, B., & Kizior, R. (2006). *Saunders nursing drug handbook 2006.* St. Louis, MO: Elsevier.

37. **Answer: 1**

    Rationale: Musculoskeletal injuries can cause changes in the neurovascular system. Application of a cast or the physiological response to an injury can cause nerve or vascular damage, usually distal to the injury. Assessing capillary refill and circulation is a priority assessment. Discussing proper cast care, pain management, and performing range of motion with the client are important to teach a client with a fractured tibia. Assessing capillary refill is the most important nursing action because it is necessary to identify/monitor changes in neurovascular status.

    Cognitive Level: Application

    Nursing Process: Implementation

    NCLEX-RN Test Plan: PHYS

    Reference: Lewis, S. M., Heitkemper, M. M., & Dirksen, S. R. (2004). *Medical-surgical nursing: Assessment and management of clinical problems* (6th ed.). St. Louis, MO: Mosby.

38. **Answer: 4**

    Rationale: Placing a foreign object inside the cast predisposes the client to skin breakdown and infection. Elevating the extremity above the heart promotes venous return and application of ice helps control or prevent edema. Drying a cast promotes the use of the cast, which is to ensure stability of the fracture.

    Cognitive Level: Application

    Nursing Process: Implementation

    NCLEX-RN Test Plan: SECE

    Reference: Lewis, S. M., Heitkemper, M. M., & Dirksen, S. R. (2004). *Medical-surgical nursing: Assessment and management of clinical problems* (6th ed.). St. Louis, MO: Mosby.

39. **Answer: 1**

    Rationale: Combining NSAIDs with alcohol or aspirin increases the risk of bleeding. Aspirin should be avoided in children under 17 to prevent Reye's syndrome. Enteric coated aspirin should not be taken with an antacid as this will decrease the effectiveness and defeat the purpose of the enteric coated aspirin. NSAIDs should be taken with food to decrease GI side effects.

    Cognitive Level: Application

    Nursing Process: Implementation

    NCLEX-RN Test Plan: PHYS

    Reference: Herbert-Ashton, M. J., & Clarkson, N. E. (2005). *Quick look nursing: Pharmacology.* Sudbury, MA: Jones & Bartlett.

Unit 5 • The Client Having Surgery

Perioperative Nursing Care

1. A 42-year-old female is in the postanesthesia care unit (PACU) following an abdominal hysterectomy. On admission, a priority would be assessment of which of the following?
   1. Airway.
   2. Dressing.
   3. Output.
   4. Pain.

2. An elderly client has been admitted to the postanesthesia care unit (PACU) after undergoing dissociate anesthesia with Ketalar. During his PACU stay, the nurse should do which of the following?
   1. Assume that the hallucinations and delirium are a normal part of emergence.
   2. Decrease verbal, tactile, and visual stimulation.
   3. Increase verbal, tactile, and visual stimulation.
   4. Place the client in a brightly lit area to shorten the recovery period.

3. During the preoperative interview, the client states that he takes ASA (acetylsalicylic acid) 81 mg. daily. In preparation for his upcoming surgery, the nurse instructs the client to do which of the following?
   1. Be only concerned about prescription medications.
   2. Continue the same dose of aspirin prior to surgery.
   3. Double the dose to prevent blood clots.
   4. Discontinue the aspirin two weeks prior to surgery.

4. In the preoperative area, the nurse notices that the surgical permit has not been signed; however, the client has been medicated with Ativan (lorazepam) and Demerol (meperidine). What should the nurse do?
   1. Have the client sign the permit.
   2. Have the client's friend sign the permit.
   3. Notify the doctor.
   4. Sign the permit for the client.

5. A postoperative client questions the need to ambulate on the first postoperative day. The nurse explains the importance to the client based on the rationale that early ambulation will do which of the following? Select all that apply.
   1. Decrease vital capacity and maintain respiratory function.
   2. Decrease muscle tone.
   3. Increase vital capacity.
   4. Increase circulation and prevent venous stasis.
   5. Increase gastrointestinal and urinary function.

6. The anesthesiologist has ordered IM Atropine (atropine sulfate) to be administered one hour preoperative. What is the purpose of this medication?
   1. To decrease the heart rate.
   2. To decrease tracheobronchial secretions.
   3. To increase peripheral vascular resistance.
   4. To increase vagal response.

7. The geriatric client undergoing surgery is at risk of which of the following? Select all that apply.

1. Having an increased ability to communicate.
2. Having a normal response to pain medication.
3. Having decreased skin elasticity.
4. Having complications from pre-existing osteoporosis and arthritis.
5. Having increased skin elasticity.
6. Having varying responses to medications.

8. The client was administered the neuromuscular blocking agent Norcuron (vercuronium bromide). It is important for the nurse to monitor which of the following for at least one hour after the effects of the drug have worn off?

1. Level of consciousness.
2. Respiration.
3. Temperature.
4. Urinary output.

9. After the administration of preoperative medications Versed (midazolam hydrochloride) and Demerol (meperidine hydrochloride), the client states the need to void. Which of the following is the most appropriate action by the nurse?

1. Assist the client to the bathroom.
2. Insert a Foley catheter.
3. Offer the client the bedpan.
4. Palpate the client's bladder.

10. With the administration of spinal anesthesia, the client will experience a loss of which of the following?

1. Consciousness.
2. Motor function.
3. Motor and sensory function.
4. Sensory function.

11. The client is unconscious on admission to the postanesthesia care unit (PACU). How should the nurse position the client?

1. In a lateral position.
2. In a prone position.
3. In a supine position.
4. With the head elevated.

12. To monitor and promote the respiratory status of a postoperative client, the nurse would do which of the following?

1. Draw arterial blood gases to check oxygen saturation.
2. Encourage the client to lay flat in bed.
3. Instruct the client to take short, shallow breaths.
4. Instruct the client and monitor the use of the incentive spirometer.

13. During the postoperative period, antiembolic stockings are used in which of the following ways?

1. Only when the client is in bed.
2. To prevent varicose veins.
3. To prevent venous stasis.
4. To replace the need for postoperative leg exercises.

14. What conditions are necessary for informed consent to be valid? Select all that apply.

1. Ability to pay for the consented procedure.
2. Ability to read the consent form.
3. Adequate disclosure of the diagnosis and treatment.
4. Demonstration of clear understanding and comprehension.
5. Voluntary consent.

15. **During the preoperative interview, the client states that her mother developed MH (malignant hyperthermia) after the administration of Anectine (succinylcholine chloride) during anesthesia. In planning care for the client, the nurse needs to be aware of which of the following?**
    1. A rise in body temperature is an early sign of MH.
    2. Malignant hyperthermia can be promptly treated with Dantrium (dantrolene).
    3. Tachycardia, tachypnea, and hypercarbia are definite indicators of MH.
    4. The patient will definitely develop MH.

16. **When positioning a client for a surgical procedure, which of the following should be a priority of care?**
    1. Access to the airway.
    2. Correct skeletal alignment.
    3. Modesty in exposure.
    4. Pooling of blood.

17. **A diabetic surgical client is at risk for the development of which of the following? Select all that apply.**
    1. Decreased healing time.
    2. Hyperthermia.
    3. Hypoglycemia.
    4. Increased healing time.
    5. Infection.

18. **The nurse identifies hypoventilation in the postoperative client who is exhibiting which of the following?**
    1. Increased PaO_2.
    2. Increased $PaCO_2$.
    3. A pH between 7.35 and 7.45.
    4. A respiratory rate of 18–24/min.

19. **Which of the following is a priority treatment of hypotension in the postanesthesia care unit (PACU)?**
    1. Analgesics.
    2. Antiarrhythmics.
    3. IV fluid bolus.
    4. Oxygen therapy.

20. **The physician has ordered Heparin (heparin sodium) 5000 units for a client with a DVT (deep vein thrombosis). Heparin is available in a 10 mL vial in a concentration of 20,000 units per milliliter. Which of the following is the correct dose?**
    1. 0.025 mL.
    2. 0.25 mL.
    3. 2.5 mL.
    4. 25 mL.

21. **A client has been diagnosed with a DVT (deep vein thrombosis). The nurse recognizes that which of the following was a predisposing factor for this client?**
    1. Decreased blood coagulability.
    2. Dietary deficiency of green leafy vegetables.
    3. Previous history of venous problems.
    4. Use of antiembolic stockings.

22. **Which of the following is a major advantage of regional anesthesia?**
    1. The client is able to undergo a lengthy surgical procedure.
    2. The client remains conscious.
    3. The client is rendered unconscious.
    4. The client retains all reflexes.

23. **Which of the following is true of surgical asepsis?**
    1. It is required only in invasive surgeries.
    2. It is a standard precaution in home health nursing.
    3. It is the absence of microorganisms.
    4. It is utilized when performing ADLs for the client.

24. **Identify the client who is a high risk for developing respiratory problems in the postoperative course.**
    1. The client is ambulatory.
    2. The client has no history of respiratory problems.
    3. The client has undergone genitourinary surgery.
    4. The client is obese.

25. **The nurse suspects the client may have developed a DVT after surgery. Which of the following was a predisposing factor?**
    1. Decreased blood coagulability due to dehydration.
    2. Lovenox ordered every 12 hours postoperatively.
    3. Passive range of motion exercises.
    4. Venous stasis due to decreased movement.

26. **Which of the following are predisposing factors that can cause acute urinary retention in the postoperative period?**
    1. Diminished pain.
    2. Increased IV fluids.
    3. Narcotics and anesthesia.
    4. Providing privacy.

27. **Which of the following will contribute to urinary retention in the postoperative client? Select all that apply.**
    1. Depression of the micturition reflex.
    2. Lack of skeletal muscle tone.
    3. Lower abdominal surgery.
    4. Pain.
    5. Supine position.
    6. Upper thoracic surgery.

28. **Versed (midazolam hydrochloride) 3 mg IM (intramuscularly) was ordered preoperatively. Versed is available as 5 mg/mL. The nurse would administer which of the following?**
    1. 0.06 mL.
    2. 0.6 mL.
    3. 6.0 mL.
    4. 60 mL.

29. **Twenty-four hours postoperatively, the nurse anticipates which of the following changes in the client based on the surgical stress response?**
    1. Decreased temperature.
    2. Decreased urinary output.
    3. Increased respiratory rate.
    4. Increased urinary output.

30. **Four days after undergoing an abdominal resection, a client presents with a temperature of 102.8°F and an incision that is red, warm, tender, and has purulent drainage. How would the nurse interpret this data?**
    1. It is abnormal because the client is not on antibiotics.
    2. It is abnormal because of the drainage, temperature, and tenderness.
    3. It is normal because the client is in the hospital.
    4. It is normal because of the surgical stress response.

31. **The circulating nurse is preparing the surgical suite for a procedure. The nurse notices that a sterile package has become wet with sterile normal saline. Select the most appropriate action.**
    1. Discard the package.
    2. Include it in the sterile field.
    3. Let the package dry and use it in the procedure.
    4. Save it for the next procedure.

32. A postoperative client has a decreased urinary output. The physician orders one liter of normal saline over six hours. How many mL/h would the nurse administer?

1. 0.167.
2. 1.67.
3. 16.7.
4. 167.
5. 1670.

33. Twenty-four hours after general surgery, the nurse notes a urinary output of 240 cc for an 8 hour shift for the client. How is this interpreted by the nurse?

1. A normal compensatory response as the client eliminates excess urine output.
2. A normal compensatory response resulting from decreased levels of Aldosterone and ADH (antidiuretic hormone).
3. A normal compensatory response resulting from an increased secretion of Aldosterone and ADH (antidiuretic hormone).
4. A normal compensatory response resulting from increased respiratory effort.

34. A client is ordered NPO (nothing by mouth) prior to surgery and questions why. The nurse responds with which of the following?

1. Eating before surgery will increase your appetite after surgery.
2. Preoperative medications may cause nausea.
3. The GI (gastrointestinal system) will decrease activity and decrease pain.
4. Refraining from food and fluids will decrease your risk of aspiration.

35. Which of the following describes the client during stage three of surgical anesthesia?

1. She will be euphoric, drowsy, and dizzy.
2. She will breathe irregularly and be susceptible to external stimuli.
3. She will have an absent or minimal heartbeat and be dilated.
4. She will have a regular breathing pattern and absent corneal reflexes.

36. During surgery, which of the following indicates the scrub nurse has broken sterile technique?

1. When arms are kept above waist level.
2. When hands are placed on the top level of the surgical drape.
3. When instruments are passed to the surgeon.
4. When the surgical hair cap is touched.

37. Fentanyl 0.1 mg was ordered to be given one hour preoperatively IM (intramuscular). Fentanyl is available as 50 mcg/mL. The nurse would administer which of the following?

1. 0.2 mL.
2. 0.02 mL.
3. 2 mL.
4. 22 mL.
5. 222 mL.

38. The goal of PCA (patient controlled analgesia) is which of the following?

1. To be cost effective.
2. To decrease respiratory depression.
3. To increase client independence.
4. To provide immediate analgesia.

Intravenous and TPN Therapies

1. Coagulase-negative staphylococcus is the most common organism responsible for catheter-related septicemia. In collaborating with the physician prior to and during central line placement on an extremely anxious client with limited venous access, the nurse would do which of the following?
   1. Allow the family to provide emotional support during the procedure.
   2. Encourage a quad-lumen catheter to avoid multiple sticks.
   3. Encourage placement in the internal jugular for easy access.
   4. Prepare for and monitor aseptic insertion and dressing protocol.

2. A client has an IV running at 150 ml/hr. in the left lower forearm and complains of swollen fingers. The nurse obtains a blood tinged flashback on squeezing the tubing, observes low infusion pressure on the screen of the infusion device, examines cool and pale fingers, determines both hands are slightly swollen, and elevates the hands on pillows. In two hours the swelling has progressed to the entire left hand and wrist. What information did the nurse gather that independently supported the nursing diagnosis of Risk for Injury?
   1. Blood tinged flashback.
   2. Both hands are slightly swollen.
   3. Cool and pale fingers.
   4. Low infusion pressure.

3. The nurse determines that an IV site is red 1.5" along the vein but only slightly swollen. The client denies pain and refuses an IV start because of "terrible veins". What is the most appropriate initial action the nurse should take?
   1. Explain that since the IV is important, it will not be removed unless a new one is placed in two attempts or less.
   2. Explain that the IV catheter may cause further vein damage; it must be removed and the client may refuse to have a new IV placed.
   3. Maintain the IV until the physician visits the client.
   4. Phone the physician and obtain an order to maintain the IV.

4. Place the steps for inserting an IV in the proper order.
   1. Catheter stabilization and application of dressing.
   2. Check physician's order.
   3. Insertion into vein.
   4. Assemble equipment.
   5. Don gloves.
   6. Documentation of procedure.
   7. Site preparation.
   8. Site selection and vein dilation.

5. Prior to administering an IV push medication, the nurse gathers information to prevent which of the following serious systemic complications of intravenous administration of medication into a vein?

1. Infiltration.
2. Phlebitis.
3. Speed shock.
4. Thrombophlebitis.

6. According to the hospital policy, IV site rotations and administration set changes are done every 72 hours. The client's IV is three days old, the current tubing and secondary tubing are 48 hours old, and 250 ml remains in the IV running at 42 ml/hr. Which of the following is the most appropriate action for the nurse?

1. Change the IV site and change both sets of tubing.
2. Change the IV site and maintain the primary and secondary tubing sets.
3. Change the IV site, change both tubing sets, and change the solution bag.
4. Obtain an order to maintain the site for one more day if it is without complications.

7. Which of the following are selection criteria and guidelines for autologous blood transfusions? Select all that apply.

1. Underweight clients can participate.
2. Blood typing and compatibility are required.
3. Freezing is not routinely recommended.
4. Donated hemoglobin should be 11 g/dL and hematocrit 33%.

8. Before starting an IV, the nurse should always do which of the following?

1. Apply a tourniquet.
2. Palpate the vein.
3. Select the largest cannula that the vein will accommodate.
4. Select the largest vein available.

9. After receiving TPN at 84 ml/hr continuously for five days, a client, in a state of confusion, pulled out their central line. Prior to notifying the physician, the nurse should start a peripheral IV and do which of the following?

1. Adapt the peripheral IV line to await further instructions from the physician.
2. Change the tubing and filter on the TPN and restart the infusion at 84 ml/hr.
3. Hang an infusion of 5–10% dextrose at 84 ml/hr.
4. Notify the pharmacy.

10. A client refuses to have an IV started. The nurse explains the rationale for the infusion and explains that without the IV, the client's condition will deteriorate rapidly. The client continues to resist. The nurse contacts the physician who is on another floor within the hospital and plans to visit shortly. The client begins to exhibit signs of decreased cardiac output including confusion, hypotension, tachycardia, diaphoresis, cool skin, and shortness of breath. What should the nurse do immediately?

1. Administer the ordered sedation and proceed with the IV start.
2. Ask for assistance, start the IV, and begin the infusion.
3. Notify the family.
4. Notify the physician.

11. While preparing to administer a new container of TPN as a total nutrient admixture (TNA) or a 3:1 solution at 84 ml/hr., the nurse checks the order with another nurse. The client has a patent designated central line and an electronic infusion device (EID) at the bedside. The nurse gathers tubing for the new container. What is the appropriate size final filter for this infusion?

1. 0.22 micron.
2. 0.45 micron.
3. 1.2 micron.
4. 170–260 micron.

12. **After two days of nausea, vomiting, and severe abdominal pain, a client is admitted with a diagnosis of acute pancreatitis. What size catheter and which vein should the nurse consider to accommodate therapy for this client?**
    1. An 18-gauge catheter in the antecubital vein.
    2. A 20-gauge catheter in the cephalic vein.
    3. A 22-gauge catheter in the digital vein.
    4. A 24-gauge catheter in the basilica vein.

13. **On entering the room of a client receiving 3:1 total parenteral nutrition (TPN), the nurse observes white streaking in the solution and gently agitates it. The streaking disappears. In two hours, the nurse discovers a dense white color at the top of the solution and is concerned that these are signs of instability. Which of the following phenomenon does *not* require that the TPN be discontinued immediately and returned to pharmacy for testing?**
    1. Aggregation.
    2. Cracking.
    3. Creaming.
    4. Oiling out.

14. **Which of the following symptoms are seen with metabolic alkalosis? Select all that apply.**
    1. Apathy.
    2. Bicarbonate excess.
    3. Cardiac dysrhythmias.
    4. Flushing.
    5. Irritability or hyperactive reflexes.
    6. Lethargy.
    7. Rapid deep respirations.
    8. Shallow breathing.

15. **For three weeks a client has received preservative-free morphine (Duramorph) through a tunneled epidural catheter as patient-controlled analgesia (PCA) with** good control of pain. Prior to catheter placement, this client was receiving a fentanyl (Duragesic) patch every 72 hours and oral oxycontin. The client admits to restlessness at night and sleeping poorly since the catheter was inserted. The current settings include a basal rate of 2 mg/hour and a patient-controlled bolus of 1 mg every 15 minutes/4 per hour. The nurse examines the program and determines that in the last 24 hours the client has received 88 boluses and a total of 136 mg of Duramorph. Which of the following would describe this client?
    1. She is anxious about the new therapy.
    2. She is having an adverse reaction to Duramorph.
    3. She requires a dosing adjustment.
    4. She requires a PRN sleeping pill.

16. **With significant third spacing, including 4+ pitting edema and bilateral pleural effusions, a client is ordered 25 grams of Albumin 25% IV to be followed by Lasix (furosemide) 40 mg IVP. Prior to administration, the nurse considers which of the following about this client?**
    1. The client is blood type AB negative.
    2. The client does not eat pork products.
    3. The client may become short of breath.
    4. The client must sign a consent form.

17. **Complications of intravenous therapy occur for various reasons. The nurse recognizes that with proper technique and therapy management, some that are preventable include hematoma from**

    _____,

    phlebitis from

    _____,

    thrombophlebitis from

    _____,

    and thrombus from

    _____.

1. Obstruction of flow, a large bore catheter in a small vein, a tourniquet that is too tight, the use of veins in the legs.

2. Obstruction of flow, a tourniquet that is too tight, the use of veins in the legs, a large bore catheter in a small vein.

3. A tourniquet that is too tight, a large bore catheter in a small vein, the use of veins in the legs, obstruction of flow.

4. A tourniquet that is too tight, obstruction of flow, the use of veins in the legs, a large bore catheter in a small vein.

18. **After a craniotomy for a subdural hematoma, a client becomes restless with a change in consciousness. The nurse recognizes Cushing's Triad for increased intracranial pressure. The client exhibits a widening pulse pressure (increased systolic and decreased diastolic blood pressure), a decrease in pulse rate, and altered respiratory pattern. Which of the following solutions should the nurse anticipate the doctor will order to decrease intracranial pressure?**

1. Albumin 25%.
2. Dextran 70.
3. Hydroxyethyl glucose (Hetastarch or Hespan).
4. Mannitol 25%.

19. **A client with a GI bleed has received several units of blood. The client is showing signs of hypovolemia including low blood pressure, rapid pulse, and shortness of breath. As two nurses check the next unit of blood and verify patient identifying information, the client, who is AB negative, notices the unit of blood is B negative and voices concern. In addition to psychosocial support to the client, what is the most appropriate action the primary nurse must take?**

1. Administer the blood as ordered.
2. Contact the physician for IV orders.
3. Notify the blood bank.
4. Notify the blood bank supervisor.

20. **Calculate the drops per minute of an IV of 500 ml of LR over 3 hours using 20 drop/ml tubing.**

21. **On entering the room the nurse sees the client lying on their left side on their left arm. The IV, in the left forearm, is infusing at 125 ml/hr. The IV site is blanched and four inches of edema surround the site, which is cool to the touch but not painful. The nurse recognizes this is which of the following?**

1. Dependent edema.
2. Extravasation.
3. Grade 1 infiltration.
4. Grade 2 infiltration.

22. **A nondiabetic client has had a recent seven pound weight loss. Vital signs include an oral temperature of 100°F, a blood pressure of 92/48, a heart rate of 112, and respirations 28 and shallow. Labs are as follows: BS 230, Na^+ 154, K^- 4.9, Cl^- 98, BUN 48, Creatinine 1.2. This client is demonstrating signs of which of the following?**

1. Hypertonic dehydration.
2. Hypotonic overhydration.
3. Isotonic dehydration.
4. Isotonic overhydration.

23. **The nurse entered a client's room to find a Grade IV infiltration of peripheral parenteral nutrition (PPN) administered through 1.25 inch peripheral infusion catheter in the right cephalic mid-forearm. The immediate appropriate action for the nurse is to discontinue the infusion and then do which of the following?**

1. Discontinue the catheter and apply cold.
2. Discontinue the catheter and apply heat.
3. Flush, then discontinue the catheter.
4. Maintain the catheter and notify the pharmacy.

24. The nurse enters the client's room and realizes that due to a shortage of EIDs on the unit, a client is receiving an IV that is infusing at 28 drops/min with 20 drop factor (drop/ml) tubing. How many ml of solution will this client receive at the end of a 12 hour shift?
    1. 84 ml.
    2. 672 ml.
    3. 1008 ml.
    4. 1680 ml.

25. After three days of nausea, vomiting, and other flu-like symptoms, a client presents with a blood pressure of 90/50, a heart rate of 118, and a respiratory rate of 10. Reflexes are hyperactive and the family reports a new onset of confusion. The nurse realizes that although mild cases are not treated, this patient will require IV therapy because they are in a state of which of the following?
    1. Metabolic acidosis.
    2. Metabolic alkalosis.
    3. Respiratory acidosis.
    4. Respiratory alkalosis.

26. An electronic infusion device (EID) was unavailable for an initial infusion of Vancocin (vancomycin hydrochloride). The nurse began the 90 minute infusion by regulating the flow with the tubing roller clamp. Within 15 minutes, the nurse found the client with hypotension; cool, clammy skin; fever; chills; numbness of fingers and toes; and erythema of the neck and back. What should the nurse recognize could occur with this client that is seen with rapid vancomycin hydrochloride infusions?
    1. Allergic reaction.
    2. Fluid overload.
    3. Hypersensitivity.
    4. Red neck syndrome.

27. A client admitted for severe abdominal pain with a hemoglobin of 7.2 g/dL and a hematocrit of 21.6% is to receive two units of packed red blood cells (RBCs). The nurse knows that usually after receiving one unit of blood, the hemoglobin will increase by

    _____

    and the hematocrit will increase by

    _____.
    1. 0.5 g/dL, 1%.
    2. 1 g/dL, 2%.
    3. 1 g/dL, 3%.
    4. 2 g/dL, 2%.

28. Discharge instructions for parents of an infant newly diagnosed with sickle cell anemia should include which of the following?
    1. Avoid high altitudes and provide plenty of fluids.
    2. Keep the infant very active to increase circulation.
    3. Pain medications are necessary only during a crisis.
    4. Proactively schedule monthly blood transfusions.

29. A new triple lumen catheter has been inserted into the left subclavian vein of a client who is septic. The nurse obtains vital signs and records T 103°F, BP 88/48, P 118 bpm, R 36 bpm, and O_2 Sat 88%. Blood, urine, and sputum cultures have been obtained. An order is written to begin IV fluids and initiate antibiotic therapy. Which of the following should the nurse do immediately?
    1. Initiate the IV therapy and begin the antibiotics.
    2. Notify the physician of the vital signs.
    3. Order a stat chest X-ray.
    4. Stat page respiratory.

30. **Which of the following apply when starting an IV? Select all that apply.**
    1. Avoid the antecubital vein.
    2. Do not use an extremity that has been impaired.
    3. It is not always necessary to palpate a vein.
    4. IVs may be placed in the leg of a child up to age 12.
    5. A tourniquet is necessary to cause vein distention.

31. **A client is admitted with an HCO_3 of 18 mEq (22–26), CO_2 of 28 mmHg (35–45). What pH value and acid base imbalance would most likely accompany these values?**
    1. Decreased pH and metabolic acidosis.
    2. Decreased pH and respiratory acidosis.
    3. Elevated pH and metabolic alkalosis.
    4. Elevated pH and respiratory alkalosis.

32. **Which of the following would be a dangerous outcome of intracellular fluid (ICF) overload?**
    1. Cellular dehydration.
    2. Cerebral cellular rupture.
    3. Congestive heart failure.
    4. Hypervolemia.

33. **An order is received to obtain a Garamycin (gentamycin) peak (4–8 mcg/ml) and trough (less than 2 mcg/ml) blood level. In seeking additional client and chart information for a peak result of 10 mcg/ml and a trough result of 3.3 mcg/ml, select all that apply.**
    1. Blood urea nitrogen.
    2. Complaints of ringing in the ears.
    3. Complaints of dizziness.
    4. Creatinine.
    5. White blood cells.

34. **An elderly client has been receiving and tolerating IV therapy at a rate of 150 ml/hr. On the night shift, the nurse and ancillary staff are involved with a complex, unstable client and family and did not hear the infusion pump alarming an empty container. After two hours, the nurse discovers the dry bag and a clotted IV. The client is restless with an increase in heart rate from 88 to 100 and a decrease in blood pressure from 110/76 to 100/60. The nurse restarted the IV without difficulty; what is the next best action for the nurse?**
    1. Notify the physician immediately and monitor the client.
    2. Restart the IV at 150 ml/hr and monitor the client.
    3. Restart the IV at 200 ml/hr for four hrs and monitor the client.
    4. Restart the IV at 300 ml/hr for two hours and monitor the client.

35. **A client with hemophilia presents with hemarthrosis and severe knee pain. In addition to starting an IV line immediately to administer factor, which of the following is appropriate?**
    1. Administer low dose aspirin (acetylsalicylic acid) to prevent DVT.
    2. Apply heat to the knee.
    3. Gently mobilize the joint to prevent contracture.
    4. Obtain a stool specimen.

36. **The nurse is pulled to the pediatric floor. A toddler client is lying quietly in bed and requires an IV to be started. The parents offer assistance to hold the child's arm during the procedure. The nurse decides to defer the IV start to a pediatric nurse. Which of the following clinical practice skills does the pediatric specialty nurse possess that supported this nurse's decision?**

1. Knowledge that parental presence is counterproductive.
2. Knowledge of appropriate catheter size for small veins.
3. Knowledge of stages of growth and development.
4. Knowledge of vein location in toddler clients.

37. **During the discussion with the oncologist, the nurse learns that the client will be receiving treatment for central nervous system (CNS) leukemia. In preparing a client for treatment, which of the following routes of chemotherapy administration should the nurse anticipate?**
    1. Intra-arterial.
    2. Intraperitoneal.
    3. Intrathecal.
    4. Intravenous.

38. **During IV therapy the nurse must monitor a compromised client. Select all of the following that are signs of left-sided heart failure.**
    1. Dyspnea.
    2. Gastrointestinal bloating.
    3. Jugular vein distention.
    4. Orthopnea.
    5. Paroxysmal noctural dyspnea.
    6. Peripheral edema.
    7. Pulmonary congestion.
    8. Pulmonary edema.
    9. Right upper quadrant pain.

39. **During an admission, a new client reports the following information. He had the flu one month ago and received treatment at home. Then two weeks ago he got the flu again and had to come into the hospital emergency room for intravenous fluids and a dose of antibiotics. Now he is back and said the symptoms are worse and he thinks the hospital "just didn't get rid of the bug the last time." Which of the following would most likely describe the client?**
    1. He's a carrier of a communicable disease.
    2. He's faking for healthcare worker attention.
    3. He's having an allergic reaction to foods.
    4. He's immunosuppressed.

Nutrition

1. A middle-aged woman relates in her history that she experiences bloating, flatulence, and diarrhea when she drinks milk. Which of the following does the nurse suspect as her problem?
   1. She is consuming too much milk.
   2. She is lactose intolerant.
   3. She is consuming too little milk.
   4. She is sucrose intolerant.

2. A client asks the nurse if there is a "real" danger in a high protein diet. The best response for the nurse to make is which of the following?
   1. Protein can be toxic to the liver.
   2. Excess protein is excreted, so there is no harm.
   3. Excess protein is retained to build muscle.
   4. Excess protein taxes the kidney since the overload of nitrogen needs to be excreted.

3. Which source of milk would the nurse suggest to the parents of a 3-year-old child who follows a vegetarian diet?
   1. Cow's milk.
   2. Evaporated milk.
   3. Soy milk.
   4. Goat's milk.

4. A client with severe hepatic failure is ordered a high calorie, low protein diet. Which selection is most appropriate for the client?
   1. Scrambled eggs, bacon, pancakes, orange slices.
   2. Grilled cheese sandwich, potato chips, chocolate pudding.
   3. Steak, french fries, corn, salad.
   4. Chicken breast, mashed potatoes, spinach.

5. The client complains of occasional mild heartburn. The nurse identifies foods that affect lower esophageal sphincter (LES) pressure that contribute to irritating the esophagus. Which statement from the client would indicate that additional teaching is needed?
   1. "I try to avoid eating after supper."
   2. "I drink four cups of coffee a day."
   3. "I drink milk when I get heartburn."
   4. "I avoid foods and candies made with chocolate."

6. A nurse is teaching a client with cholecystitis about the dietary modifications of a low-fat diet. Which meal selection indicates an understanding of these instructions?
   1. Creamed chicken on a biscuit with peas and carrots.
   2. Roast beef with gravy, mashed potatoes, and pudding.
   3. Macaroni and cheese, salad, and vanilla ice cream.
   4. Roast turkey, rice pilaf, green beans, and fruit cup.

7. The RN instructs the client with a colostomy about foods that are gas forming. Which food is *not* considered to be gas forming?
   1. Fish.
   2. Beer.
   3. Onions.
   4. Carbonated beverages.

8. To decrease dyspnea and conserve energy, the nurse recommends several options to the client with chronic obstructive pulmonary disease (COPD). Which of the following is *not* an appropriate instruction from the nurse?
   1. Rest for at least 30 minutes before eating.
   2. Use the bronchodilators after meals.
   3. Eat five to six small, frequent meals.
   4. Select foods that can be prepared in advance.

9. Which statement made by the client indicates an understanding of what types of foods protect against cardiovascular disease?
   1. "I eat plenty of fruits and vegetables each day."
   2. "I don't believe red meat is going to hurt anyone."
   3. "I love my scrambled eggs each morning."
   4. "I dislike skim milk. Only whole milk for me!"

10. A client complains of frequent constipation. The nurse identifies which of the following foods as being high in fiber? Select all that apply.
    1. Brown rice.
    2. Blackberries.
    3. Whole wheat bread.
    4. Beans.
    5. Turkey.

11. A client with a CVA is admitted to the rehab unit. At supper time, the nurse notices that the client experiences severe dysphagia and reports this to the physician. What form of nutritional support is most essential for this client?
    1. NPO until dysphagia subsides.
    2. Nasogastric tube feeding.
    3. Total parenteral nutrition (TPN).
    4. Soft residue diet.

12. A school nurse discusses optimal pregame meals with the high school track team. The best suggestions would include which of the following?
    1. Cheeseburgers, fries, and diet cola.
    2. Spaghetti and meatballs, bread, and fruit juice.
    3. Eggs, bacon, toast, and orange juice.
    4. Fish and chips, coleslaw, and coffee.

13. Hydration is important to the athlete. The nurse explains to the parents of the junior high school football team that which of the following liquids is the best choice to adequately provide hydration?
    1. Water.
    2. Vegetable juice.
    3. Energy drinks.
    4. Milk.

14. A young man visits the clinic for his annual physical exam. He states that he has been weight training for the past three months. He asks the nurse practitioner about starting creatine supplements. Her best response would be which of the following?
    1. Additional supplements are unnecessary because the body manufactures sufficient creatine.
    2. Supplements are very expensive; that is the only drawback.
    3. Supplements build a lot of muscle mass and are very good.
    4. Supplements are approved by the FDA.

15. Identify an appropriate nursing diagnosis for a patient with malnutrition.

_____

_____

16. The nurse recommends a diet low in residue, roughage, and fat, but high in calories and protein to a teenage client with Crohn's disease. Select the most appropriate food choice for this client's menu.
1. Vanilla milkshake.
2. Peanuts and popcorn.
3. Tossed green salad.
4. Toast with butter and jelly.

17. The nurse talks to her client with cancer about foods that can prevent fat and muscle loss. Which foods would help the client prevent protein or calorie malnutrition? Select all that apply.
1. Cottage cheese.
2. Milkshakes.
3. Tuna fish.
4. Strawberries and bananas.
5. Egg and ham omelet.

18. Dietary restrictions for a client who has gout include limiting the use of alcohol and foods high in purine. The nurse recommends avoiding which of the following foods high in purine? Select all that apply.
1. Sardines, herring, and mussels.
2. Cheese, milk, and ice cream.
3. Organ meats such as liver or kidneys.
4. Cabbage, beans, and lentils.
5. Bacon and pork.

19. The nurse explains to the parents of a 3-month-old that the American Association of Pediatrics recommends formula to be continued in a child's dietary intake until what age?

1. 6 months.
2. 12 months.
3. 18 months.
4. 24 months.

20. The pediatric nurse practitioner discusses with the mother of a 6-month-old infant about what should she begin to feed her daughter. Which of the following is the correct response?
1. Egg whites are the least allergenic food to be introduced into the baby's diet.
2. Rice cereal is the first solid introduced that is the least allergenic of the cereals.
3. Formula is the only source of nutrition given for the first year.
4. Fruits and vegetables are good sources of iron.

21. An 8-year-old child is at the 98th percentile for weight and at the 40th percentile for height. How would the school nurse interpret this information?
1. The child is underweight or small in stature.
2. The child is overweight or large in stature.
3. The child is experiencing a prepubescent growth spurt.
4. The child is normal for his size.

22. Two mothers ask the nurse how their 8-year-old children can be so different in height and weight. What is the appropriate response?
1. This is an abnormality that should be referred to the physician.
2. One of the children is displaying a "growth spurt."
3. Rates of growth vary and individual differences occur for each child.
4. The sequence of growth and development is unpredictable for each child.

23. A mother of a 2-year-old asks the nurse in the pediatric clinic what types of foods she should prepare for the child. Select the most appropriate menu for a nutritious dinner.
    1. 2% milk, hot dog, rice, and orange slices.
    2. Whole milk, chicken, mashed potatoes, carrots, and apple slices.
    3. Skim milk, beef, fried potatoes, peas, and pudding.
    4. Fruit punch, half a peanut butter sandwich, celery sticks, and ice cream.

24. The student nurse discusses the risk of aspiration with the parents of an 18-month-old. Which foods should be avoided?
    1. Apples, crackers, and applesauce.
    2. Cherries, peanuts, and hard candy.
    3. Cheerios, fruit juice, and raisins.
    4. Orange juice, toast, bananas.

25. The nurse explains to a group of parents attending a community lecture that which of the following is the *greatest* influence on a child's growth and development?
    1. Nutrition.
    2. Social income.
    3. Exposure to secondary smoke.
    4. Ethnic background.

26. The nurse practitioner explains to the parents the risks of iron deficiency anemia for their infant. Identify the most appropriate recommendation the nurse should include.
    1. Limit milk to no more than 32 oz/day.
    2. Increase fat-soluble vitamins in the diet.
    3. Include grains and legumes in the daily intake.
    4. Limit foods that are high in protein in the daily caloric requirement.

27. The nurse discusses discharge planning instructions with a patient who recently had a partial gastric resection. The nurse explains that the patient will have monthly injections of vitamin B_{12} for the rest of his life. Why is this the case?
    1. The client needs to replace vitamin B_{12} to prevent pernicious anemia as a result of the lack of the intrinsic factor.
    2. Vitamin B_{12} promotes healing and prevents complications in the postoperative period.
    3. Vitamin B_{12} prevents the chance of gastric reflux from secretion of hydrochloric acid in the stomach.
    4. Vitamin B_{12} supplies a required daily allowance of all fat-soluble vitamins.

28. The client who has chronic renal failure for the past two years has a recent blood test that reveals his creatinine clearance rate is 45 ml/min. Based on his lab value, his healthcare provider would most likely do which of the following to his protein consumption per day?
    1. Unrestrict his protein intake.
    2. Limit his protein intake to 60 g/day.
    3. Limit his protein intake to 40 g/day.
    4. Limit his protein intake to 20 g/day.

29. Women diagnosed with diabetes mellitus, based on average height and weight, should have a total calorie count of how many kcal/day?

    _____

30. The nurse speaks to a community group about the positive effects of antioxidants, enzymatic, and immune biologic agents. Which vitamin should be recommended?
    1. Vitamin A.
    2. Vitamin B.
    3. Vitamin C.
    4. Vitamin D.

31. The nurse reviews the monthly dietary recall journal of a geriatric client who has recently been diagnosed with anemia. Which foods *best* identify essential nutrients that promote erythropoiesis?
    1. Roast beef, broccoli, and whole grain bread.
    2. Lasagna, garlic toast, and creamed corn.
    3. Tacos, spanish rice, and cherry cobbler.
    4. French toast, sausage, and figs.

32. The nurse discusses medications with a patient diagnosed with Type 1 diabetes. The nurse explains that the client prescribed chlorpropamide (Diabinese) should avoid which of the following?
    1. Chocolate.
    2. Milk.
    3. Alcohol.
    4. Shellfish.

33. A physician informs the client that her cholesterol level is 250. The client is prescribed atorvastatin (Lipitor). Which food would the client be instructed to *avoid* while taking this medication?
    1. Milk or milk products.
    2. Grapefruit or grapefruit juice.
    3. Poultry.
    4. Legumes.

34. You are the nurse in charge of a 12-patient module on the evening shift. Dinner trays arrive and there are two patients requiring assistance with their meal. Which of the following scenarios would be the most appropriate?
    1. UAP to feed patient with shortness of breath.
    2. UAP to feed patient with complaints of chest pain.
    3. UAP to feed patient with new tracheotomy.
    4. UAP to feed patient with Parkinson's disease.

35. The nurse midwife recommends to the pregnant client that during the second and third trimester of pregnancy she will need to increase her daily total number of calories by which of the following?
    1. 200.
    2. 300.
    3. 400.
    4. 500.

36. The client lives alone in a small one bedroom apartment. Which of the following is the easiest method to assess his nutritional status?
    1. Call his physician.
    2. Check the contents of his refrigerator.
    3. Assess his nail beds.
    4. Ask his neighbors.

37. The client who has fibrocystic breast disease asks the nurse if there are specific foods she should avoid. What is the nurse's best response?
    1. Do not eat spicy foods.
    2. Do not drink alcoholic beverages.
    3. Increase caffeine and decrease vitamin B_6.
    4. Decrease caffeine and increase vitamin B_6.

38. The nurse discusses the use of herbal therapies. He explains that the client who is taking a hypoglycemic agent for their Type 2 diabetes must not use which of the following commonly used herbs or supplements?
    1. Chamomile.
    2. Goldenseal.
    3. Garlic.
    4. St. John's wort.

39. **Identify the correct sequence in which the nurse would administer an enteral feeding via a nasogastric tube.**

1. Adjust the flow rate of the drip or pump.
2. Aspirate for stomach contents.
3. Flush the tube with water.
4. Assess for bowel sounds.
5. Elevate the head of the bed 30–45°.

Unit 5 Answers and Rationales

Test 17 Answers and Rationales

1. **Answer: 1**
   Rationale: When the client is admitted to the postanesthesia care unit, the assessment begins with the ABC status. A priority is respiratory assessment including airway patency, respiratory rate, quality and pattern, and breath sounds. After establishment of this system, the other options would be assessed.
   Cognitive Level: Application
   Nursing Process: Implementation
   NCLEX-RN Test Plan: PHYS
   Reference: Lewis, S. M., Heitkemper, M. M., & Dirksen, S. R. (2004). *Medical-surgical nursing: Assessment and management of clinical problems* (6th ed.). St. Louis, MO: Mosby.

2. **Answer: 2**
   Rationale: Ketalar (ketamine) is a phenylcyclidine derivative and can cause hallucinations and nightmares. To decrease and prevent these responses, the patient needs to be placed in a quiet, dimly lit recovery area. Limiting stimulation is also essential. All other options are incorrect.
   Cognitive Level: Analysis
   Nursing Process: Implementation
   NCLEX-RN Test Plan: PHYS
   Reference: Lewis, S. M., Heitkemper, M. M., & Dirksen, S. R. (2004). *Medical-surgical nursing: Assessment and management of clinical problems* (6th ed.). St. Louis, MO: Mosby.

3. **Answer: 4**
   Rationale: ASA (acetylsalicylic acid) can contribute to postoperative bleeding as a result of increased coagulation resulting from inhibition of platelet aggregation. It is recommended to decrease ASA for at least two weeks prior to surgery. Although it is not considered a prescription medication, it is considered a medication that will affect the patient's physiologic clotting status. Increasing the dose will increase the risk of bleeding. Both prescription and non-prescription medications can contribute to bleeding and drug interaction with anesthesia.
   Cognitive Level: Analysis
   Nursing Process: Assessment
   NCLEX-RN Test Plan: PHYS
   Reference: Lewis, S. M., Heitkemper, M. M., & Dirksen, S. R. (2004). *Medical-surgical nursing: Assessment and management of clinical problems* (6th ed.). St. Louis, MO: Mosby.

4. **Answer: 3**
   Rationale: Preoperative medications can alter a client's state of consciousness and comprehension. For the surgical permit to be valid, the client must have adequate disclosure, be able to demonstrate clear understanding and comprehension of the information, and give the consent voluntarily. The client of legal age is the only person able to consent to surgery. The exception would be if a life-threatening emergency is present. A minor is not legally able to sign the permit for the client.
   Cognitive Level: Analysis
   Nursing Process: Implementation
   NCLEX-RN Test Plan: SECE
   Reference: Lewis, S. M., Heitkemper, M. M., & Dirksen, S. R. (2004). *Medical-surgical nursing: Assessment and management of clinical problems* (6th ed.). St. Louis, MO: Mosby.

5. **Answers: 3, 4, and 5**
   Rationale: Early ambulation will increase, not decrease, muscle tone, prevent venous stasis, increase circulation, and enhance wound healing. The respiratory system will benefit by increasing the client's vital capacity and mobilizing secretions. Increased muscle tone will improve gastrointestinal and urinary function to re-establish normal patterns.
   Cognitive Level: Analysis
   Nursing Process: Implementation
   NCLEX-RN Test Plan: PHYS
   Reference: Lewis, S. M., Heitkemper, M. M., & Dirksen, S. R. (2004). *Medical-surgical nursing: Assessment and management of clinical problems* (6th ed.). St. Louis, MO: Mosby.

6. **Answer: 2**

   Rationale: Atropine (atropine sulfate) is an anticholinergic medication. It is used as a preoperative medication to reduce secretions. Atropine can cause an increase in heart rate. Atropine will increase the heart rate. It is used to treat a decrease in heart rate as a result of vagal response. Stimulation of the vagus nerve will decrease the heart rate.

   Cognitive Level: Analysis

   Nursing Process: Implementation

   NCLEX-RN Test Plan: PHYS

   Reference: Lewis, S. M., Heitkemper, M. M., & Dirksen, S. R. (2004). *Medical-surgical nursing: Assessment and management of clinical problems* (6th ed.). St. Louis, MO: Mosby.

7. **Answers: 3, 4, and 6**

   Rationale: As the client ages, there is a decrease in skin elasticity. With aging, a decline in auditory and visual acuity may present barriers to communication and comprehension. Pre-existing conditions such as arthritis and osteoporosis can be potential complications for mobility, comfort, and safety. A decline in cardiac, renal, or liver function may interfere or delay the metabolism or excretion of medications.

   Cognitive Level: Analysis

   Nursing Process: Assessment

   NCLEX-RN Test Plan: PHYS

   Reference: Lewis, S. M., Heitkemper, M. M., & Dirksen, S. R. (2004). *Medical-surgical nursing: Assessment and management of clinical problems* (6th ed.). St. Louis, MO: Mosby.

8. **Answer: 2**

   Rationale: Neuromuscular blocking agents are used to facilitate intubation and to promote paralysis and skeletal muscle relaxation during surgery. Prolonged paralysis of respiratory muscles can occur. Respiratory monitoring of the client's rate and pattern is essential until the client is able to cough and return to his preoperative status and muscle strength. It is essential to make sure the client has a patent airway. The agents will not alter level of consciousness and do not interfere with perfusion of internal organs that would be reflected by urinary output.

   Cognitive Level: Analysis

   Nursing Process: Implementation

   NCLEX-RN Test Plan: PHYS

   Reference: Lewis, S. M., Heitkemper, M. M., & Dirksen, S. R. (2004). *Medical-surgical nursing: Assessment and management of clinical problems* (6th ed.). St. Louis, MO: Mosby.

9. **Answer: 3**

   Rationale: Preoperative medications can alter a client's level of consciousness (LOC) and impair mobility. All clients should be instructed to void before the administration of preoperative medications. Voiding before surgery can also prevent involuntary elimination under anesthesia and reduces the chance of urinary retention immediately postoperatively. Impaired LOC can alter a patient's ability to ambulate and result in a fall or impaired mobility. Foley catheters are not routinely inserted as they can be a source of infection. Palpating the bladder does not assist the patient with urination.

   Cognitive Level: Analysis

   Nursing Process: Implementation

   NCLEX-RN Test Plan: PHYS

   Reference: Lewis, S. M., Heitkemper, M. M., & Dirksen, S. R. (2004). *Medical-surgical nursing: Assessment and management of clinical problems* (6th ed.). St. Louis, MO: Mosby.

10. **Answer: 3**

    Rationale: Spinal anesthesia is the injection of a local anesthetic agent into the subarachnoid space. The interaction of anesthetic and cerebrospinal fluid results in a motor, sensory, and autonomic blockade. The client will not have a loss of consciousness. Epidural anesthesia, in low concentration, generally blocks only sensory impulse.

    Cognitive Level: Analysis

    Nursing Process: Evaluation

    NCLEX-RN Test Plan: PHYS

    Reference: Lewis, S. M., Heitkemper, M. M., & Dirksen, S. R. (2004). *Medical-surgical nursing: Assessment and management of clinical problems* (6th ed.). St. Louis, MO: Mosby.

11. **Answer: 1**

    Rationale: Airway maintenance is essential for the postanesthetic client. To facilitate airway maintenance, correct positioning of the client is essential. Unconscious clients, unless contraindicated, are positioned in the lateral/recovery position. This position reduces the risk of aspiration if the client vomits. When the client resumes consciousness, the head of the bed can be elevated if it is not contraindicated.

Cognitive Level: Analysis

Nursing Process: Implementation

NCLEX-RN Test Plan: PHYS

Reference: Lewis, S. M., Heitkemper, M. M., & Dirksen, S. R. (2004). *Medical-surgical nursing: Assessment and management of clinical problems* (6th ed.). St. Louis, MO: Mosby.

12. **Answer: 4**

Rationale: Respiratory intervention is an essential component of the care plan for the postoperative client. The use of the incentive spirometer will help to prevent alveolar collapse, atelectasis, and stasis of secretions. To evaluate the effectiveness of the incentive spirometer, the nurse needs to adequately instruct the client, observe a return demonstration, document the frequency of use, and assess the client's respiratory staus. Lack of ambulation will cause stasis of fluid with a potential for infection. Lack of adequate thoracic expansion will result in hypoventilation and atelectasis. Blood gas analysis is not a routine component of respiratory assessment.

Cognitive Level: Analysis

Nursing Process: Assessment

NCLEX-RN Test Plan: PHYS

Reference: Lewis, S. M., Heitkemper, M. M., & Dirksen, S. R. (2004). *Medical-surgical nursing: Assessment and management of clinical problems* (6th ed.). St. Louis, MO: Mosby.

13. **Answer: 3**

Rationale: In the postoperative period, the cardiovascular system is at risk for developing complications. With increased blood coagulability, decreased activity and body positioning is important to institute measures to prevent stasis of blood in the lower extremities. Venous stasis can result in a deep vein thrombosis, which can be life threatening. Antiembolic stockings are ordered to enhance and stimulate the milking and massaging action of veins. The stockings should be worn when the client ambulates and do not replace the need for postoperative leg exercises.

Cognitive Level: Analysis

Nursing Process: Implementation

NCLEX-RN Test Plan: PHYS

Reference: Lewis, S. M., Heitkemper, M. M., & Dirksen, S. R. (2004). *Medical-surgical nursing: Assessment and management of clinical problems* (6th ed.). St. Louis, MO: Mosby.

14. **Answers: 3, 4, and 5**

Rationale: Informed consent protects the client, doctor, and institution/employees. For informed consent to be valid, three criteria are necessary. The client must have adequate disclosure of the diagnosis including risks and benefits. The client must also be able to demonstrate clear understanding and comprehension. The client must also give consent voluntarily without influence. If a client is unable to read the consent form, it can be read to him or her and a demonstration of understanding must be obtained. Financial status does not contribute to the validity of informed consent.

Cognitive Level: Analysis

Nursing Process: Assessment

NCLEX-RN Test Plan: SECE

Reference: Lewis, S. M., Heitkemper, M. M., & Dirksen, S. R. (2004). *Medical-surgical nursing: Assessment and management of clinical problems* (6th ed.). St. Louis, MO: Mosby.

15. **Answer: 2**

Rationale: Dantrium (dantrolene) is the definitive treatment of malignant hyperthermia. The treatment protocol is available at www.mhaus.com. If a patient is known or suspected to be at risk for malignant hyperthermia, they can be anesthetized with minimal risks if proper precautions are implemented. A rise in body temperature is not an early indicator of the condition. Tachycardia, hypercarbia, tachypnea and ventricular abnormalities can be seen with the malignant hyperthermic patient but are nonconclusive. Malignant hyperthermia is autosomal dominant in inheritance, but is variable in its genetic penetrance. Predictions based on family history are important but inconsistent.

Cognitive Level: Analysis

Nursing Process: Asesment

NCLEX-RN Test Plan: PHYS

Reference: Lewis, S. M., Heitkemper, M. M., & Dirksen, S. R. (2004). *Medical-surgical nursing: Assessment and management of clinical problems* (6th ed.). St. Louis, MO: Mosby.

16. **Answer: 1**

    Rationale: Although all options are important to the client's well-being and safety when undergoing surgery, the ABCs are a priority. It is essential to provide and maintain the client's airway.

    Cognitive Level: Analysis

    Nursing Process: Implementation

    NCLEX-RN Test Plan: PHYS

    Reference: Lewis, S. M., Heitkemper, M. M., & Dirksen, S. R. (2004). *Medical-surgical nursing: Assessment and management of clinical problems* (6th ed.). St. Louis, MO: Mosby.

17. **Answers: 3, 4, and 5**

    Rationale: The diabetic client is at high risk for developing a wound infection and/or increased healing time. Alteration in postoperative nutritional status, IV fluid replacement, and the influence of the surgical stress response can alter blood sugar levels. Delayed healing time in diabetes mellitus results from decreased collagen synthesis, impaired phagocytosis, decreased oxygenation, and nutrient supply. Hypothermia may be present in the immediate post-op period up to 12 hours. Fever may occur at any time during the post-op period.

    Cognitive Level: Analysis

    Nursing Process: Assessment

    NCLEX-RN Test Plan: PHYS

    Reference: Lewis, S. M., Heitkemper, M. M., & Dirksen, S. R. (2004). *Medical-surgical nursing: Assessment and management of clinical problems* (6th ed.). St. Louis, MO: Mosby.

18. **Answer: 2**

    Rationale: A common complication in the PACU (postanesthesia care unit) is hypoventilation. Hallmarks of hypoventilation are a decreased respiratory rate or effort, an increasing $PaCO_2$ (hypercapnia), and a decreased PaO_2 (hypoxemia). Abnormal O_2 (oxygen) and CO_2 (carbon dioxide) levels will alter the blood pH. A normal blood pH is 7.35 to 7.45. Respiratory alteration will alter the normal pH. A normal respiratory rate is 18 to 20 breaths per minute. Alteration of this respiratory rate may affect the blood pH.

    Cognitive Level: Analysis

    Nursing Process: Assessment

    NCLEX-RN Test Plan: PHYS

Reference: Lewis, S. M., Heitkemper, M. M., & Dirksen, S. R. (2004). *Medical-surgical nursing: Assessment and management of clinical problems* (6th ed.). St. Louis, MO: Mosby.

19. **Answer: 4**

    Rationale: Oxygen therapy is the first line treatment for hypotension in the PACU (postanesthetic care unit). The purpose of oxygen therapy is to promote oxygenation of the hypoperfused organs. Once the cause of hypotension is identified, additional therapy will be instituted. Fluid loss during surgery is a common cause of hypertension in the PACU. Cardiac dysfunction may result from fluid and electrolyte imbalance. Analgesics are generally used to treat hypertension from sympathetic stimulation.

    Cognitive Level: Analysis

    Nursing Process: Implementation

    NCLEX-RN Test Plan: PHYS

    Reference: Lewis, S. M., Heitkemper, M. M., & Dirksen, S. R. (2004). *Medical-surgical nursing: Assessment and management of clinical problems* (6th ed.). St. Louis, MO: Mosby.

20. **Answer: 2**

    Rationale: $mL = 1\ mL/20000 \times 5000 = 0.25\ mL$

    Cognitive Level: Analysis

    Nursing Process: Implementation

    NCLEX-RN Test Plan: SECE

    Reference: Gray Morris, D.(2006). *Calculating with confidence* (4th ed.). St. Louis, MO: Mosby.

21. **Answer: 3**

    Rationale: A client who has had previous endothelial damage from a DVT (deep vein thrombosis) has a higher risk for developing another DVT. Another contributing factor would be increased blood coagulability to promote clotting. Antiembolic stockings are used to prevent stasis and clot formation. Dietary modifications are necessary if the patient is on anticoagulant therapy.

    Cognitive Level: Analysis

    Nursing Process: Evaluation

    NCLEX-RN Test Plan: PHYS

    Reference: Lewis, S. M., Heitkemper, M. M., & Dirksen, S. R. (2004). *Medical-surgical nursing: Assessment and management of clinical problems* (6th ed.). St. Louis, MO: Mosby.

22. **Answer: 2**

Rationale: Regional anesthesia involves the injection of anesthetic agents in or around a group of nerves. As a result, autonomic nervous system blockade and skeletal muscle paralysis of the affected nerve will occur. The operative procedure is performed without loss of consciousness or sedation. A disadvantage of regional anesthesia is the inability to match the duration of the agent administered to the duration of the surgical procedure.

Cognitive Level: Analysis

Nursing Process: Assessment

NCLEX-RN Test Plan: PHYS

Reference: Lewis, S. M., Heitkemper, M. M., & Dirksen, S. R. (2004). *Medical-surgical nursing: Assessment and management of clinical problems* (6th ed.). St. Louis, MO: Mosby.

23. **Answer: 3**

Rationale: Surgical asepsis is achieved by sterilization. Aseptic technique is utilized in the operating room and it is based on the basic aseptic principles. Medical asepsis is a clean technique utilizing standard precautions when helping clients perform ADLs. All surgical procedures are invasive in nature.

Cognitive Level: Analysis

Nursing Process: Implementation

NCLEX-RN Test Plan: SECE

Reference: Lewis, S. M., Heitkemper, M. M., & Dirksen, S. R. (2004). *Medical-surgical nursing: Assessment and management of clinical problems* (6th ed.). St. Louis, MO: Mosby.

24. **Answer: 4**

Rationale: The obese client is at a higher risk for developing obstruction, hypoxemia, and/or hypoventilation in the immediate postanesthetic period. Obesity can prevent lung expansion, resulting in mechanical restriction and hypoventilation. The client who is ambulatory will facilitate lung expansion and gas exchange to aid in respiration. Surgery on areas above the waist can affect the rate and depth of respiration and contribute to atelectasis.

Cognitive Level: Analysis

Nursing Process: Assessment

NCLEX-RN Test Plan: PHYS

Reference: Lewis, S. M., Heitkemper, M. M., & Dirksen, S. R. (2004). *Medical-surgical nursing: Assessment and management of clinical problems* (6th ed.). St. Louis, MO: Mosby.

25. **Answer: 4**

Rationale: Venous stasis, damage to the endothelium or inner lining of the vein, and hypercoagulability of blood are factors that contribute to the development of a DVT (deep vein thrombosis). These three factors are known as Virchow's triangle. Patients at risk for developing DVTs generally have these predisposing conditions. Dehydration will increase blood viscosity and contribute to dehydration. Range of motion exercise (active or passive) will improve circulation and blood flow that will prevent venous stasis. Lovenox LMWH is effective for prevention and treatment of DVT.

Cognitive Level: Analysis

Nursing Process: Assessment

NCLEX-RN Test Plan: PHYS

Reference: Lewis, S. M., Heitkemper, M. M., & Dirksen, S. R. (2004). *Medical-surgical nursing: Assessment and management of clinical problems* (6th ed.). St. Louis, MO: Mosby.

26. **Answer: 3**

Rationale: Anesthesia and narcotics can lead to acute urinary retention in the postoperative period. Voluntary micturition can be impeded by anesthesia because anesthesia depresses the micturition reflex. Narcotics and anticholinergics may also interfere with the ability to initiate voiding. Pain may alter the client's perception of pain and interfere with the patient's awareness of the pain sensation. IV fluids are used to treat a decrease in urinary output.

Cognitive Level: Analysis

Nursing Process: Assessment

NCLEX-RN Test Plan: PHYS

Reference: Lewis, S. M., Heitkemper, M. M., & Dirksen, S. R. (2004). *Medical-surgical nursing: Assessment and management of clinical problems* (6th ed.). St. Louis, MO: Mosby.

27. **Answers: 1, 2, 3, 4, and 5**

Rationale: Retention is more likely to occur after lower abdominal and pelvic surgery because of spasm or guarding of the abdominal and pelvic muscle.

This may interfere with micturition. Pain may alter the client's perception and interfere with the patient's sensation of a full bladder. The supine position decreases the ability to relax the perineal muscles and external sphincter to initiate voiding. All other options are incorrect.

Cognitive Level: Analysis

Nursing Process: Assessment

NCLEX-RN Test Plan: PHYS

Reference: Lewis, S. M., Heitkemper, M. M., & Dirksen, S. R. (2004). *Medical-surgical nursing: Assessment and management of clinical problems* (6th ed.). St. Louis, MO: Mosby.

28. **Answer: 2**

    Rationale: mL = 1 mL/5 mg × 3 mg = 3/5 = 0.6 mL

    Cognitive Level: Analysis

    Nursing Process: Implementation

    NCLEX-RN Test Plan: SECE

    Reference: Gray Morris, D. (2006). *Calculating with confidence* (4th ed.). St. Louis, MO: Mosby.

29. **Answer: 2**

    Rationale: Aldosterone and ADH (anti-diuretic hormone) are released as a response by the body to the stress of surgery. The surgical stress response is an adaptive response to maintain circulating fluid volume. Preoperative fluid restriction, fluid loss during surgery, drainage, and diaphoresis may also contribute to this. Regardless of fluid intake, a low urine output of 800–1500 mL in the first 24 hours is expected. An increased temperature (up to 100.4°F) within 24 hours post-op may result from the inflammatory response to surgical stress. Temperatures above 100.4°F may result from respiratory congestion and atelectasis. Increased respiratory rate is an abnormal response that may occur because of pain or anxiety.

    Cognitive Level: Analysis

    Nursing Process: Assessment

    NCLEX-RN Test Plan: PHYS

    Reference: Lewis, S. M., Heitkemper, M. M., & Dirksen, S. R. (2004). *Medical-surgical nursing: Assessment and management of clinical problems* (6th ed.). St. Louis, MO: Mosby.

30. **Answer: 2**

    Rationale: The assessment data is abnormal. After 48 hours, a temperature elevation greater than 99.9°F may signify a wound infection. Drainage is expected

to change from sanguineous to serosanguineous to serous over a period of days. The incision may be red, however the area surrounding the incision should not be tender and warm. All other options are incorrect.

Cognitive Level: Analysis

Nursing Process: Assessment

NCLEX-RN Test Plan: PHYS

Reference: Lewis, S. M., Heitkemper, M. M., & Dirksen, S. R. (2004). *Medical-surgical nursing: Assessment and management of clinical problems* (6th ed.). St. Louis, MO: Mosby.

31. **Answer: 1**

    Rationale: Aseptic technique is practiced in the operating room to prevent infections. The principles of aseptic technique state that a contaminated item must be removed from the sterile field. Once the package was permeated with fluid, even though it was sterile saline, the sterility was challenged allowing a potential for bacteria and contamination. All other options are incorrect.

    Cognitive Level: Analysis

    Nursing Process: Implementation

    NCLEX-RN Test Plan: SECE

    Reference: Lewis, S. M., Heitkemper, M. M., & Dirksen, S. R. (2004). *Medical-surgical nursing: Assessment and management of clinical problems* (6th ed.). St. Louis, MO: Mosby.

32. **Answer: 4**

    Rationale: mL = 1000 mL/1 L × 1 L/6 hr = 1000/6 = 167 mL/hr

    Cognitive Level: Analysis

    Nursing Process: Implementation

    NCLEX-RN Test Plan: SECE

    Reference: Gray Morris, D. (2006). *Calculating with confidence* (4th ed.). St. Louis, MO: Mosby.

33. **Answer: 3**

    Rationale: A decreased urinary output for the first 24 hours after surgery is a normal response. Activation of the surgical stress response to meet the postanesthetic needs of the client result in an increased secretion of aldosterone and ADH (anti-diuretic hormone). As a result, low urinary output (800–1500 mL) in the first 24 hours is expected. All other options are incorrect.

    Cognitive Level: Analysis

    Nursing Process: Assessment

NCLEX-RN Test Plan: PHYS

Reference: Lewis, S. M., Heitkemper, M. M., & Dirksen, S. R. (2004). *Medical-surgical nursing: Assessment and management of clinical problems* (6th ed.). St. Louis, MO: Mosby.

34. **Answer: 4**

    Rationale: The preoperative restriction of food and fluid is designed to decrease the risk of postoperative nausea and vomiting. The restriction will also decrease the chance of aspiration. All other options are incorrect.

    Cognitive Level: Analysis

    Nursing Process: Assessment

    NCLEX-RN Test Plan: PHYS

    Reference: Lewis, S. M., Heitkemper, M. M., & Dirksen, S. R. (2004). *Medical-surgical nursing: Assessment and management of clinical problems* (6th ed.). St. Louis, MO: Mosby.

35. **Answer: 4**

    Rationale: Stage three is the stage of surgical anesthesia in which the client will have a regular breathing pattern, absent corneal reflexes, and can safely stay in this stage as surgery is performed. In stage one, the client will be euphoric and drowsy. In stage two, the client will breathe irregularly and be susceptible to external stimuli. In stage four, the client may have an absent or minimal heartbeat.

    Cognitive Level: Analysis

    Nursing Process: Assessment

    NCLEX-RN Test Plan: PHYS

    Reference: Spry, C. (2005). *Essentials of perioperative nursing* (3rd ed.). Sudbury, MA: Jones and Bartlett.

36. **Answer: 4**

    Rationale: The scrub nurse must adhere to the basic principles of aseptic technique. When she touches her cap with her sterile glove, she has now contaminated her glove. All other options adhere to the principles of aseptic technique.

    Cognitive Level: Analysis

    Nursing Process: Implementation

    NCLEX-RN Test Plan: SECE

    Reference: Lewis, S. M., Heitkemper, M. M., & Dirksen, S. R. (2004). *Medical-surgical nursing: Assessment and management of clinical problems* (6th ed.). St. Louis, MO: Mosby.

37. **Answer: 3**

    Rationale: mL = 1 mL/50 mcg × 1000 mcg/1 mg × 0.1 mg = 100/50 = 2 mL

    Cognitive Level: Analysis

    Nursing Process: Implementation

    NCLEX-RN Test Plan: SECE

    Reference: Gray Morris, D. (2006). *Calculating with confidence* (4th ed.). St. Louis, MO: Mosby.

38. **Answer: 4**

    Rationale: PCA (patient controlled analgesia) is utilized as an alternative intervention for pain control. The goal of PCA is to provide immediate analgesia. The client is able to self administer a predetermined dose for effective pain management when necessary. The dose is predetermined to prevent overdosage. All other options are incorrect.

    Cognitive Level: Analysis

    Nursing Process: Planning

    NCLEX-RN Test Plan: PHYS

    Reference: Lewis, S. M., Heitkemper, M. M., & Dirksen, S. R. (2004). *Medical-surgical nursing: Assessment and management of clinical problems* (6th ed.). St. Louis, MO: Mosby.

Unit 5 Answers and Rationales

Test 18 Answers and Rationales

1. **Answer: 4**
   Rationale: Primary risk factors for catheter related infections are associated with a break in aseptic insertion techniques and aseptic dressing change procedures as well as site election and number of catheter lumens. Catheter securement and occlusive dressings are difficult to maintain with internal jugular catheters due to the bending and twisting motion of the neck, the gravitational pull of the catheter, and proximity to the hairline. These factors permit catheter manipulation and increased exposure to skin and hair flora as well as environmental pathogens. Exposure to extrinsic (healthcare workers) and endogenous (flora) sources of contaminants increases with multiple catheter hubs and injection ports. Presence of nonessential personnel during aseptic procedures increases the air flow of environmental pathogens.
   Cognitive Level: Analysis
   Nursing Process: Planning
   NCLEX-RN Test Plan: SECE
   Reference: Phillips, L. D. (2005). *Manual of IV therapeutics* (4th ed.). Philadelphia: F.A. Davis.

2. **Answer: 2**
   Rationale: Depending on the amount of fluid that infiltrates, blanching and a sensation of coolness are additional symptoms that support infiltration. The infusate is room temperature, much cooler than the human body, and cools the surrounding tissue when infiltrated. The infiltrate causes localized edema, putting pressure on microvessels, leaving the affected area pale. An infiltrate in one hand would not cause swelling in the opposite. In this case the client may have edema unrelated to the infusion. A blood tinged flashback helps to support that an IV is in a vein when running at 150 ml/hr, but does not necessarily prove it. If an IV has slipped out of a vein and blood from the puncture of the vein leaks into the surrounding tissue, a blood tinged flashback could represent that leak. An electronic infusion device (EID) will monitor occlusive pressures. When an infusion is delivered to the tissues, the EID will not show high pressure or sound an alarm until the pressure exceeds that pressure set on the EID to detect obstruction of flow.
   Cognitive Level: Analysis
   Nursing Process: Evaluation
   NCLEX-RN Test Plan: PHYS
   Reference: Josephson, D. (2004). *Intravenous infusion therapy for nurses: Principles & practice* (2nd ed.). Clifton Park, NJ: Delmar.

3. **Answer: 2**
   Rationale: The nurse must provide sufficient information for the client to make an informed, rational decision to accept or refuse treatment. An option that maintains a venous catheter that is producing an adverse effect on the vein without explaining the consequences of such action is a breach of duty to inform by the nurse. Explaining that an IV is important will support the need to restart the IV. By bargaining that the problem catheter will not be removed until a new one is started within two attempts prolongs an adverse event and may jeopardize any IV restart. The nurse does not require the permission of a physician to discontinue an IV catheter that is problematic. It is within the scope of nursing judgment to determine that an IV catheter is creating more harm than good. It would be prudent of the nurse to refuse to continue infusing medication into an IV catheter with questionable integrity.
   Cognitive Level: Synthesis
   Nursing Process: Intervention
   NCLEX-RN Test Plan: SECE
   Reference: Phillips, L. D. (2005). *Manual of IV therapeutics* (4th ed.). Philadelphia: F.A. Davis.

4. **Answer: 2, 4, 5, 8, 7, 3, 1, 6**
   Rationale: Although there are many aseptic approaches to venipuncture techniques, mastery of psychomotor clinical skills and knowledge of infusion therapy are fundamental. Beginning practitioners must follow a step-by-step approach to venipuncture.
   Cognitive Level: Synthesis
   Nursing Process: Implementation

NCLEX-RN Test Plan: SECE
Reference: Phillips, L. D. (2005). *Manual of IV therapeutics* (4th ed.). Philadelphia: F.A. Davis.

5. **Answer: 3**
   Rationale: Speed shock is a systemic complication and occurs when organs with a rich blood supply, including the heart, brain and liver, are flooded with medications in toxic proportions. Speed shock requires immediate intervention. Progressive symptoms include syncope, hypotension, dysrhythmias and shock. Infiltration, phlebitis, and thrombophlebitis are local complications seen at or near the infusion site and may be easily corrected. However, serious complications can occur if left untreated.
   Cognitive Level: Analysis
   Nursing Process: Planning
   NCLEX-RN Test Plan: SECE
   Reference: Weinstein, S. (2001). *Plumer's principles and practice of intravenous therapy* (7th ed.). Philadelphia: Lippincott.

6. **Answer: 3**
   Rationale: Primary administration set change should coincide with a peripheral catheter change and initiation of a new container of IV solution. Secondary continuous extension sets, filters, stopcocks, and needleless devices should coincide with primary administration set changes. When a client has available venous access sites, rotation of the site will tend to preserve the integrity of the vein in use for future access by removing potentially irritating solutions and catheter materials.
   Cognitive Level: Synthesis
   Nursing Process: Planning
   NCLEX-RN Test Plan: SECE
   Reference: Infusion Nurses Society. (2006). Infusion nursing standards of practice. *Journal of Infusion Nursing, 29*(Suppl. 1S), S48.

7. **Answers: 1, 3, and 4**
   Rationale: Homologous blood donation is blood that is donated by one individual for someone other than themselves. Autologous blood donation is blood that is collected from the donor for the donor. Blood typing is not necessary since it is the client's own blood. Underweight clients are disqualified for homologous donations, due to specific volumes that are required per unit. The underweight client can donate for themselves but proportionately smaller units would be withdrawn with each donation. Red blood cells have a 42-day shelf life and can be frozen, but due to the expense and limitations of some blood banks, it is not recommended for autologous donations. Clients can donate weekly with the last donation occurring minimally 72 hours, but preferably a week, prior to surgery to avoid hypovolemia during surgery. With homologous donations, hemoglobin and hematocrit must be at least 12.5 g/dL and 38% for males and 12.0 g/dL and 36% for females, but autologous must be at least 11 g/dL and 33% except in special circumstances.
   Cognitive Level: Comprehension
   Nursing Process: Analysis
   NCLEX-RN Test Plan: PHYS
   Reference: Phillips, L. D. (2005). *Manual of IV therapeutics* (4th ed.). Philadelphia: F.A. Davis.

8. **Answer: 2**
   Rationale: A vein must be palpated to determine stability, pliability, and presence of sclerosed valves, contour, and refill potential. Tourniquets should be avoided if client exhibits fragile veins or is taking anticoagulants. Allowing fragile veins to overdistend may cause vein damage, vessel hemorrhage, or subcutaneous bleeding after puncturing. The smallest size and shortest length cannula should be selected that would accommodate the prescribed therapy. Areas of flexion are to be avoided for IV therapy. The large veins in the antecubital fossa are not necessary for all types of therapy and should be reserved for PICC and midline placement and for blood draws.
   Cognitive Level: Application
   Nursing Process: Planning
   NCLEX-RN Test Plan: HPM
   Reference: Phillips, L. D. (2005). *Manual of IV therapeutics* (4th ed.). Philadelphia: F.A. Davis.

9. **Answer: 3**
   Rationale: There is an increase in endogenous (from the pancreas) insulin secretion in response to high serum glucose levels with administration of TPN formulas. A sudden withdrawal of the hypertonic solution will cause a client to experience sudden hypoglycemia. Initiation of either a 5% or 10% dextrose solution, determined by institutional policy,

will prevent the drop in blood sugar. To discontinue a TPN solution, the rate of administration is gradually decreased to allow the body to adjust to the change in glucose levels and insulin demand. The TPN formula administered through a central line is not appropriate for peripheral infusion and will cause severe phlebitis and vein damage. A delay in hanging a 5–10% solution, while awaiting instruction from the physician, may create a dangerous hypoglycemic event for the client. The pharmacy will require notification, but it is not a priority event in this circumstance.

Cognitive Level: Synthesis
Nursing Process: Intervention
NCLEX-RN Test Plan: PHYS
Reference: Weinstein, S. (2001). *Plumer's principles and practice of intravenous therapy* (7th ed.). Philadelphia: Lippincott.

10. **Answer: 4**
Rationale: The client or their power of attorney should be notified of benefits and risks of therapy and that they have the right to either accept or refuse treatment. The nurse explained the rationale and consequences to the client. By administering sedation and proceeding with the IV placement and the infusion, the nurse would violate the client's right to refuse treatment. The designated family member should have been notified at the time the physician was notified. At the point of physiological deterioration, the physician becomes the client advocate who must determine the proper course of immediate action.

Cognitive Level: Evaluation
Nursing Process: Implementation
NCLEX-RN Test Plan: SECE
Reference: Infusion Nurses Society (2006). Infusion nursing standards of practice. *Journal of Infusion Nursing. 29*(Suppl. 1S), S18–S19.

11. **Answer: 3**
Rationale: A 1.2 air-eliminating final filter set is required for nutrient admixtures that contain lipids for removal of inadvertent debris and fungi. A .22 micron filter is used for nutrient mixtures that do not contain lipids. Lipids infused separately require a .45 micron final filter to remove inadvertent air, debris, and microbes. If either a .22 or .45 micron

filter was used for a TNA/3:1 solution, the filter would trap larger nutrient molecules and clog the filter, causing the EID alarm to signal an occlusion. A 170–260 micron filter is used as the standard clot filter for blood administration.

Cognitive Level: Comprehension
Nursing Process: Planning
NCLEX-RN Test Plan: SECE
Reference: Phillips, L. D. (2005). *Manual of IV therapeutics* (4th ed.). Philadelphia: F.A. Davis.

12. **Answer: 2**
Rationale: The larger the gauge, the smaller the catheter diameter in IV cannulas. A client with acute pancreatitis who has been vomiting for two days will have evidence of altered fluids and electrolytes due to gastrointestinal loss as well as the inability to replace fluids orally. Amylase and lipase are enzymes secreted by the pancreas to aid in the digestion of starch and lipids. In acute pancreatitis, these enzymes attack the pancreas and surrounding tissue causing inflammation. If left untreated, pancreatitis can result in scarring and permanent loss of tissue. In order to reverse this process, the client is kept NPO to minimize the excretion of amylase and lipase. IV replacement fluids are initiated at higher rates to support losses and correct electrolyte imbalances. Both 18- and 20-gauge catheters are appropriate for hypertonic or isotonic solutions with additives or for blood administration. The cephalic vein is the second largest vein in the forearm and can accommodate high infusion rates. Both 22- and 24-gauge catheters are appropriate for pediatric clients, and 22-gauge catheters are used for frail veins in elderly clients or if the nurse is unable to place a 20-gauge. Areas of flexion such as the antecubital and wrist areas should be avoided. Digital veins should be avoided with isotonic solutions that contain additives due to a high rate of infiltration. The basilic is the largest vein in the forearm and moves easily with rotation of the arm. A 24-gauge catheter in the basilic vein is too small to deliver a high volume of fluid per hour.

Cognitive Level: Application
Nursing Process: Planning
NCLEX-RN Test Plan: PHYS
Reference: Phillips, L. D. (2005). *Manual of IV therapeutics* (4th ed.). Philadelphia: F.A. Davis.

13. **Answer: 1**

    Rationale: Aggregation is observed as rare white streaks and is an early sign of creaming. Aggregation is reversible with gentle agitation and is not harmful to the patient. Although creaming is reversible as a dense white color at the top of the solution, it may indicate an unstable emulsion if it reappears within two hours. Oiling out or cracking is irreversible. It is the appearance of yellow streaking or oil globules on the surface. These globules will coalesce (fuse together) and form larger oil droplets throughout the solution. This solution should be discontinued immediately to prevent fat embolism.

    Cognitive Level: Evaluation

    Nursing Process: Evaluation

    NCLEX-RN Test Plan: SECE

    Reference: Weinstein, S. (2001). *Plumer's principles and practice of intravenous therapy* (7th ed.). Philadelphia: Lippincott.

14. **Answers: 2, 5, and 8**

    Rationale: Central nervous system excitability occurs with metabolic alkalosis. This is observed as irritability, confusion, tetany-like symptoms, and hyperactive reflexes. With metabolic alkalosis, there is an excess of bicarbonate (HCO_3). The respiratory system compensates with hypoventilation to conserving hydrogen ions. Nausea and vomiting may be the initial cause of the alkalosis with a loss of potassium and chloride ions. The kidneys exchange HCO_3 for H^+ and hydrogen is retained. Central nervous system depression is seen with metabolic acidosis. This is observed as restlessness, apathy, weakness, disorientation, stupor, and coma. With metabolic acidosis, there is an excess of carbonic acid (H_2CO_3) or a bicarbonate (HCO_3) deficit. The respiratory system compensates with Kussmaul respirations (deep and rapid). The kidneys exchange H^+ for Na^+ and the hydrogen ion is excreted. Flushing of the skin is the result of sympathetic nervous system depression. As potassium shifts out of cells, dysrhythmias can occur resulting in a decreased cardiac output.

    Cognitive Level: Evaluation

    Nursing Process: Diagnosis

    NCLEX-RN Test Plan: PHYS

    Reference: LeFever Kee, J., Paulanka, B., Purnell, L. D. (2004). *Fluids and electrolytes with clinical applications: A programmed approach* (7th ed.). Newark, NJ: Thompson.

15. **Answer: 3**

    Rationale: In the last 24 hours, this client received 48 mg of morphine at a basal rate of 2 mg per hour, and self administered an additional 88 mg (1 mg/ 15 minutes) to obtain pain control. During most hours, including the night, the client received up to 6 mg/hr. Bolus or PRN administration of opioids is not meant to be included in basal dosing for pain control. PRN dosing is intended to manage breakthrough pain. Individuals who have received opioids for an extended period of time develop an opioid tolerance, not to be confused with opioid addiction. Periodic dosage adjustments are necessary. It is the nurse's responsibility to obtain all dosing and assessment information when collaborating with the physician for pain management.

    Cognitive Level: Evaluation

    Nursing Process: Evaluation

    NCLEX-RN Test Plan: PHYS

    Reference: Gordon, D. B., Dahl, J., Phillips, P., Frandsen, J., Cowley, C., Foster, R. L., Fine, P. G., Miaskowski, C., Fishman, S., & Finley, R. S. (2004). The use of 'as-needed' range orders for opioid analgesics in the management of acute pain: A consensus statement of the American Society for Pain Management Nursing and the American Pain Society [Electronic version]. *Pain Management Nursing, 5*, 53–58. Retrieved March 17, 2006, from http://www.ampainsoc.org/pub/bulletin/jul04/consensus1.htm

16. **Answer: 3**

    Rationale: Although it is a human derived blood product, a special consent form is not required for administration of Albumin. Albumin is not blood type specific. It can be given to all blood types. Serum albumin (a colloid) helps to maintain the plasma colloidal osmotic pressure within the capillary bed. Interstitial albumin helps to maintain interstitial osmotic pressure within the tissues. Osmotic pressure is the force that draws water to the side of a semipermeable membrane that has a higher concentration of colloids (nondiffusible substances). Without serum albumin, fluids would readily leak into the interstitial spaces (surrounding tissues) and cause edema; without interstitial albumin, fluid would be drawn into the capillaries and cause circulatory overload. Additionally, hydrostatic pressures within the capillaries and the tissues work in tandem with osmotic pressures to maintain equilibrium at the capillary membrane. Hydrostatic pressures are the pressures exerted by stationary fluids. Hydrostatic pressures move fluid out of the capillaries at the arterial end and plasma oncotic pressure pulls fluid into the capillaries at the venous end. When administered intravenously, Albumin 25% expands the vascular volume by four times the amount infused and draws interstitial fluid into the vasculature to establish oncotic equilibrium. Albumin has immediate onset and peaks at the end of the infusion. Even if administered to diminish third spacing, clients are at risk for circulatory overload.

Cognitive Level: Analysis
Nursing Process: Evaluation
NCLEX-RN Test Plan: PHYS
Reference: LeFever Kee, J., Paulanka, B., & Purnell, L. D. (2004). *Fluids and electrolytes with clinical applications: A programmed approach* (7th ed.). Newark, NJ: Thompson.

17. **Answer: 3**
Rationale: Hematoma occurs when blood leaks from a puncture site into the surrounding tissue. It can occur with nicking of a vein, discontinuing an IV without applying pressure, applying a tourniquet too tightly, or anything that prevents return of blood to systemic circulation. Phlebitis is the inflammation of the vein and can be caused by mechanical, chemical, bacterial or post-infusion irritation. It can be caused by insertion technique, duration of cannulation, host factors, infrequent dressing changes, patient or vein conditions, poor filtration or incompatibility of solutions, and needle size or gauge. Thrombophlebitis is both thrombosis and inflammation due to chemical or mechanical irritants. It is related to the use of veins in the legs, infusion of hypertonic or highly acid solutions, insertion techniques, patient or vein conditions, poor filtration or incompatibility of solutions, and needle size or gauge. Thrombosis formation occurs when trauma to endothelial cells causes red blood cells to adhere to the vein wall with formation of a clot. This clot usually occludes the circulation of blood. The IV drip rate must be taken not to propel the clot into the bloodstream.

Cognitive Level: Analysis

Nursing Process: Evaluation
NCLEX-RN Test Plan: PHYS
Reference: Phillips, L. D. (2005). *Manual of IV therapeutics* (4th ed.). Philadelphia: F.A. Davis.

18. **Answer: 4**
Rationale: Mannitol is a sugar alcohol. It is used to reduce excess cerebral spinal fluid (CSF), promote diuresis, and will promote excretion of toxic blood substances. Albumin is a human donor plasma protein colloid and is used to treat hypovolemic shock, acute blood loss, erythroblastosis fetalis, and hypoproteinemic states. Dextran is a polysaccharide that behaves as a colloid and is used as a plasma substitute or expander. The intravascualar space is expanded in excess of volume infused. Hetastarch is a synthetic colloid made from starch and is used as adjunct therapy for shock due to hemorrhage, burns, surgery, or trauma.

Cognitive Level: Synthesis
Nursing Process: Planning
NCLEX-RN Test Plan: PHYS
Reference: Phillips, L. D. (2005). *Manual of IV therapeutics* (4th ed.). Philadelphia: F.A. Davis.

19. **Answer: 1**
Rationale: An antigen is any substance that is able to stimulate production of an antibody and then react with that antibody. Blood type A has A antigens on the RBC membrane and B antibodies in the plasma. Type B has B antigens on the RBC membrane and A antibodies in the plasma. Type O has no antigens on the red blood cells membrane and has both A and B antibodies in their plasma. Type AB blood has both A and B antigens on the red blood cells but neither A nor B antibodies in the plasma. Since antibodies are absent in the plasma, a person with AB blood can receive all blood types and is considered a universal recipient. Likewise, type O blood has no antigens on the red blood cells and can be administered to persons with all blood types. A Type O blood donor is considered a universal donor.

Cognitive Level: Analysis
Nursing Process: Planning
NCLEX-RN Test Plan: PHYS
Reference: Phillips, L. D. (2005). *Manual of IV therapeutics* (4th ed.). Philadelphia: F.A. Davis.

20. **Answer: 56 gtts/min**

    Rationale: The formula for calculating drops per minute is ml per hour, times the drops per ml, divided by 60 minutes per hour.

    $$\frac{\text{gtt}}{\text{min}} = \frac{20 \text{ gtts}}{1 \text{ ml}} \times \frac{500 \text{ ml}}{3 \text{ hrs}} \times \frac{1 \text{ hr}}{60 \text{ min}} = \frac{56 \text{ gtts}}{\text{min}}$$

    Cognitive Level: Application
    Nursing Process: Implementation
    NCLEX-RN Test Plan: PHYS
    Reference: Phillips, L. D. (2005). *Manual of IV therapeutics* (4th ed.). Philadelphia: F.A. Davis.

21. **Answer: 4**

    Rationale: Infiltration is related to distal vein wall puncture, puncture from mechanical friction of the catheter, dislodgement of the needle from the vein, poor securement of the catheter, overmanipulation of the IV device, high delivery rates, or high pressure from an electronic infusion device. If a client lies on the arm in which an IV is infusing, return venous circulation is impeded. If arterial flow is uninterrupted while the infusion continues, the pressure within the vein increases. The solution takes the path of least resistance and it will leak into the surrounding tissue through the puncture site in the vein. If the edema on this client was dependent, it would cover an area larger than 4 inches. All infiltrations should be rated on a 0 to 4 scale. Grade 1, the earliest identification of infiltration, is blanched, cool to touch, with or without pain, and edema is less than one inch. A Grade 2 infiltration includes the same symptoms as Grade 1 but the edema is 1–6 inches. Infiltrations of Grade 3–4 including extravasations are painful, with swelling greater than 6 inches, and translucence of skin with local neurological and circulatory impairment.
    Cognitive Level: Synthesis
    Nursing Process: Evaluation
    NCLEX-RN Test Plan: PHYS
    Reference: Phillips, L. D. (2005). *Manual of IV therapeutics* (4th ed.). Philadelphia: F.A. Davis.

22. **Answer: 1**

    Rationale: Hypertonic fluid dehydration results from inadequate fluid intake. In situations when clients cannot respond to a thirst (for example, if they are bedridden or an infant) a decrease in fluid intake will cause a decrease in vascular volume and a concentration of vascular solutes. Fluid will shift from the interstitial tissues and eventually from the cells to maintain circulatory volume. Solute concentration and serum osmolarity is reflected in labs with elevated blood sugar, sodium, and blood urea nitrogen. Isotonic dehydration results when blood or fluids are lost in equal proportion to electrolytes and proteins. Isotonic dehydration is seen with hemorrhage, gastrointestinal losses, diaphoresis, burns, third spacing, and with diuretics that cause fluid and electrolyte losses proportionately. Isotonic overhydration occurs when excess amounts of fluids and solutes of equal proportions are retained or administered. This is seen with renal failure, heart failure with stasis and venous congestion, isotonic IV administrations, high corticosteroid levels with sodium and water retention, and high aldosterone levels. Hypotonic overhydration or water intoxication occurs when more fluids are gained than solutes, plain water enemas, hypotonic fluid administration, poor infant formulas, syndrome of inappropriate antidiuretic hormone.
    Cognitive Level: Analysis
    Nursing Process: Diagnosis
    NCLEX-RN Test Plan: PHYS
    Reference: Phillips, L. D. (2005). *Manual of IV therapeutics* (4th ed.). Philadelphia: F.A. Davis.

23. **Answer: 4**

    Rationale: A vesicant is a drug or solution that, when permitted to leak into the tissue, will cause blistering, tissue necrosis, and sloughing. All infiltrations must be graded. A vesicant infiltration, or extravasation, is classified as a Grade IV Infiltration. Severity of damage is related to pH, osmolarity, type, concentration, and volume of fluid infiltrated into the tissues. Endothelial and cellular damage caused by irritation stimulates an inflammatory response. Release of proteins with an increase in capillary permeability allows fluids and protein to shift to the interstitial space. Edema, ischemia, vasoconstriction, pain, and erythema increases lead to tissue necrosis. Treatment includes stopping the infusion, maintaining the catheter, and withdrawing any residual medication and blood. Without delay, an antidote, particular to the vesicant, is instilled into the tissues. The catheter is then removed and the appropriate thermal pack to the particular vesicant is applied. If the needle is withdrawn prior to instillation of the antidote, the antidote is injected in a pinwheel pattern in the area of the infiltration. A photograph of the area is taken. Elevation is controversial and in some clients may be uncomfortable. Use of heat or cold is controversial and is specific to individual infiltrates. The physician is notified and a plastic surgery consult is requested. Pharmacy provides information resources specific to antidote administration.

Cognitive Level: Evaluation
Nursing Process: Evaluation
NCLEX-RN Test Plan: PHYS
Reference: Phillips, L. D. (2005). *Manual of IV therapeutics* (4th ed.). Philadelphia: F.A. Davis.

24. **Answer: 3**
Rationale: The formula for calculating ml using dimensional analysis allows the nurse to find the ml per hour and multiply by 12, the number of hours in the shift. To calculate ml per hour, multiply ml per drops times drops per minute and then multiply by 60 minutes per hour.

$$\frac{mL}{hr} = \frac{1 \; mL}{20 \; \cancel{gtts}} \times \frac{28 \; \cancel{gtts}}{1 \; \cancel{min}} \times \frac{60 \; \cancel{min}}{1 \; hr} = \frac{84 \; mL}{hr} \times 12 \; hrs = 1008 \; mL$$

Cognitive Level: Application
Nursing Process: Implementation
NCLEX-RN Test Plan: PHYS
Reference: Josephson, D. (2004). *Intravenous infusion therapy for nurses: Principles & practice* (2nd ed.). Clifton Park, NJ: Delmar.

25. **Answer: 2**
Rationale: Central nervous system irritability occurs with metabolic alkalosis. The renal and pulmonary systems attempt to compensate for the alkaline state. The kidneys excrete alkali ions (HCO_3) in exchange for hydrogen (H^+) and the respiratory rate and depth diminish as the lungs attempt to retain carbon dioxide (CO_2). In this patient, the heart rate is elevated with a low blood pressure due to hypovolemia related to high gastric output from vomiting for three days. In addition to metabolic alkalosis, this client is in fluid volume deficit and a state of isotonic dehydration.

Cognitive Level: Analysis
Nursing Process: Assessment
NCLEX-RN Test Plan: PHYS

Reference: LeFever Kee, J., Paulanka, B., Purnell, L. D. (2004). *Fluids and electrolytes with clinical applications: A programmed approach* (7th ed.). Newark, NJ: Thompson.

26. **Answer: 4**
Rationale: "Red neck syndrome" or "red man syndrome" is the most common toxicity seen with vancomycin. Symptoms of the "red man syndrome" occur due to a histamine-like reaction that occurs when vancomycin is given by direct or rapid injection of larger than normal dose. Symptoms include chills; fever; fainting; tachycardia; hives; itching; hypotension; nausea; vomiting; maculopapular rash of the face, base of neck, upper body, back, and arms; and, rarely, cardiac arrest. If symptoms have not progressed to decompensation, the syndrome is reversible with a slowing of the infusion.

Cognitive Level: Synthesis
Nursing Process: Evaluation
NCLEX-RN Test Plan: PHYS
Reference: Murray, B. E. (2005). Clinical implications of glycopeptide use: Pros and cons [Electronic version]. *Clinical Updates in Infectious Diseases, 8,* 1–4. Retrieved March 5, 2006 from http://www.nfid.org/pdf/id_archive/glycopeptides.pdf

27. **Answer: 3**
Rationale: In the absence of bleeding, administration of one unit of packed RBCs or one unit of whole blood will both raise the hemoglobin by 1 g/dL. The hematocrit will increase by 3% with RBCs and 3–4% with whole blood. Packed cells have 80% less plasma than whole blood. Both units contain the same amount of RBCs.

Cognitive Level: Comprehension
Nursing Process: Evaluation
NCLEX-RN Test Plan: PHYS
Reference: Josephson, D. (2004). *Intravenous infusion therapy for nurses: Principles & practice* (2nd ed.). Clifton Park, NJ: Delmar.

28. **Answer: 1**
Rationale: In a client with sickle cell anemia, hemoglobin within an erythrocyte is in an abnormal form. In periods of hypoxia, the sickle cell hemoglobin S (HbS) aggregates (gather) into long chains, causing the

red blood cell to stiffen and elongate into a crescent (sickle) shape. Precipitating factors include viral or bacterial infection (most common), high altitudes, emotional or physical stress, surgery, blood loss, dehydration, acidosis, and hypothermia. Crisis can also occur for other reasons that are not obvious. Symptoms are related to vaso-occlusive crisis. Sickled cells block capillaries causing vasospasm, and blood flow is impeded. Capillary hypoxia alters membrane permeability. Plasma leaks into the interstitial spaces. Hemoconcentration and thrombus formation increase stagnation. Tissue ischemia, infarction, and necrosis with irreversible alterations in function can occur in all tissues and organs throughout the body. Pain results from the tissue ischemia and is described as deep, gnawing, and throbbing. The degree of ischemia determines the level of pain suffered and oral narcotic analgesics are required after crisis resolution. Blood transfusions are not routinely used between crisis events and should be used wisely to treat crisis. Clients with sickle cell disease (SCD) have exercise intolerance due to the increased metabolic demand for oxygen. Rest is a treatment intervention. In addition to oxygen, pain medication, and rest, intravenous fluids and electrolytes are administered to decrease blood viscosity. If necessary, antibiotic treatment is initiated. Hydroxyurea (Droxia), an antisickling agent, increases fetal hemoglobin, reduces hemolysis, increases hemoglobin concentration, and decreases sickled cells.

Cognitive Level: Synthesis
Nursing Process: Implementation
NCLEX-RN Test Plan: SECE
Reference: Lewis, S. M., Heitkemper, M. M., & Dirksen, S. R. (2004). *Medical-surgical nursing: Assessment and management of clinical problems* (6th ed.). St. Louis, MO: Mosby.

29. **Answer: 3**
Rationale: After insertion of any central venous catheter, final verification of tip placement and absence of insertion related complications is required. Radiographic confirmation of placement in the superior vena cava (SVC) is to occur prior to administration of any vesicant, fluid, or if the tip placement is in question. Hemothorax, pneumothorax, chylothorax, and extravascular malposition should be ruled out. Hemothorax occurs when blood enters the pleural cavity after trauma or tran-

section of a vein. Pneumothorax is the collection of air in the pleural space after puncture of the parietal pleura. Chylothorax is the collection of lymph fluid in the pleural cavity after the transection of the thoracic duct where it enters the left subclavian vein. Extravascular malposition occurs when the catheter exits the vein with the tip lying outside of the vasculature. Additionally, a catheter that is threaded into position can inadvertently be threaded into the internal jugular, external jugular, innominate, or mammary veins. The vital signs obtained are typical in a client with sepsis. Anticipating the need for the required X-ray would expedite verification of the tip placement, initiation of fluids, and antibiotics.

Cognitive Level: Application
Nursing Process: Planning
NCLEX-RN Test Plan: SECE
Reference: Phillips, L. D. (2005). *Manual of IV therapeutics* (4th ed.). Philadelphia: F.A. Davis.

30. **Answers: 1 and 2**
Rationale: Tourniquets should be avoided on fragile veins because the pressure can cause rupture of the vein wall with needle puncture, resulting in a hematoma. Veins in the antecubital fossa, and all areas of flexion, should be avoided due to difficulty in immobilization. Damage to the antecubital vein limits access to distal veins. Use of the legs should be avoided in adults and children that are walking. Veins should be avoided in an extremity that is on the side of a mastectomy, lymph node dissection or stripping, that is impaired from a cerebral vascular accident (CVA), that has been partially amputated, that has had reconstructive or orthopedic surgery, or one that has sustained third degree burns.

Cognitive Level: Comprehension
Nursing Process: Planning
NCLEX-RN Test Plan: SECE
Reference: Josephson, D. (2004). *Intravenous infusion therapy for nurses: Principles & practice* (2nd ed.). Clifton Park, NJ: Delmar.

31. **Answer: 1**
Rationale: pH (7.35–7.45) determines acid or base status. Decreased pH (less than 7.35) indicates acidosis. A decreased HCO_3 and a decreased (partially compensated) or normal (acute) CO_2 occur with metabolic acidosis (pH less than 7.35). An elevated

HCO_3 and an increased (partially compensated) or normal (acute) CO_2 would occur with metabolic alkalosis (pH more than 7.35). In respiratory acidosis (pH less than 7.35), an increased CO_2 and an increased (partially compensated) or normal (acute) HCO_3 occurs. A decreased CO_2 and a decreased (partially compensated) or normal (acute) HCO_3 would accompany respiratory alkalosis (pH more than 7.35).

Cognitive Level: Synthesis

Nursing Process: Evaluation

NCLEX-RN Test Plan: PHYS

Reference: Corbett, J. (2004). *Laboratory tests and diagnostic procedures with nursing diagnosis* (6th ed.). Upper Saddle River, NJ: Pearson Prentice Hall.

32. **Answer: 2**

Rationale: When intracellular osmolality is greater than the extracellular osmolality, fluid moves by osmosis into the cell. Cells can rupture from too much fluid. The cells in the brain are the most vulnerable to this. Hypervolemia is too much fluid in the vascular compartment. Cellular dehydration is the opposite of fluid overload. Congestive heart failure results from a weakened left ventricle, possibly from too much fluid in the vascular compartment, not in the cells.

Cognitive Level: Analysis

Nursing Process: Diagnosis

NCLEX-RN Test Plan: PHYS

Reference: Baumberger-Henry, M. (2005). *Fluid and electrolytes.* Sudbury, MA: Jones and Bartlett.

33. **Answers: 1, 2, 3, 4, and 5**

Rationale: Aminoglycosides can cause eighth cranial nerve damage (neurotoxicity). Ototoxicity manifests as vestibular dysfunction and will affect equilibrium as well as irreversible hearing loss. Nephrotoxicity can also occur especially with underlying impaired renal function. Hematologically, red blood cells, white blood cells and platelet counts can be affected by aminoglycosides.

Cognitive Level: Analysis

Nursing Process: Evaluation

NCLEX-RN Test Plan: PHYS

Reference: Corbett, J. (2004). *Laboratory tests and diagnostic procedures with nursing diagnosis* (6th ed.). Upper Saddle River, NJ: Pearson Prentice Hall.

34. **Answer: 2**

Rationale: It is not recommended to "catch up" on IV fluids that are behind schedule. After consideration of cardiovascular history and medical condition, a recalculation of the infusion rate may be feasible in some clients. However, elderly clients neither have the fluid reserves of younger clients nor do they have the ability to adapt to rapid changes. In the elderly, renal changes associated with aging cause a decrease in glomerular filtration rate. Rapid infusion of solutions with dextrose can lead to cerebral edema. The elderly must be assessed frequently for signs of fluid overload. Since the IV was off for only two hours, the IV was started without difficulty. As long as the client's vital signs remained within normal limits, the nurse could safely restart the IV at the same rate, monitor the patient for further compromise, and discuss rate changes with the physician in the morning.

Cognitive Level: Synthesis

Nursing Process: Planning

NCLEX-RN Test Plan: PHYS

Reference: Phillips, L. D. (2005). *Manual of IV therapeutics* (4th ed.). Philadelphia: F.A. Davis.

35. **Answer: 4**

Rationale: Gastrointestinal bleeding is evidenced in hematemesis, gastric and abdominal pain, and occult blood in stools. Aspirin is never given to a hemophilia client. Heat and movement would increase the bleeding in the joint. Ice and rest are appropriate treatment options.

Cognitive Level: Synthesis

Nursing Process: Planning

NCLEX-RN Test Plan: PHYS

Reference: Hogan, M. A., Hill, K. (2004). *Pathophysiology reviews and rationales.* Upper Saddle River, NJ: Prentice Hall.

36. **Answer: 3**

Rationale: Nursing management of the pediatric client includes age-appropriate instructions during procedures. A nurse must develop these communication and interaction skills to ensure consistent positive outcomes with a toddler client. Parents provide comfort and are encouraged to participate in client care. An IV would not be placed in the scalp or lower extremity of a walking client. Knowledge of appropriate vein selection, vein size, infusion rate and type,

client level of activity, and catheter size is a standard
for nurses initiating IV therapy in any client.
Cognitive Level: Comprehension
Nursing Process: Planning
NCLEX-RN Test Plan: PSYC
Reference: Phillips, L. D. (2005). *Manual of IV
therapeutics* (4th ed.). Philadelphia: F.A. Davis.

37. **Answer: 3**
Rationale: Intrathecal administration allows delivery
of chemotherapy directly into the cerebral spinal
fluid (CSF) when delivery does not require passage
through the blood-brain barrier. Intravenous is the
most common route and provides quick therapeutic
blood levels and are not absorbed in the gastrointestinal tract. Intra-arterial delivery allows high concentrations of chemotherapy to be administered
directly to tumor sites. The intraperitoneal route
delivers chemotherapy into body cavities, including
the bladder, peritoneum, pleura, and pericardium.
Cognitive Level: Comprehension
Nursing Process: Planning
NCLEX-RN Test Plan: PHYS
Reference: Phillips, L. D. (2005). *Manual of IV
therapeutics* (4th ed.). Philadelphia: F.A. Davis.

38. **Answer: 1, 4, 5, 7, 8**
Rationale: Left-sided heart failure results when the
left ventricle of the heart can no longer pump blood
effectively to supply the tissues. Blood backs up into
the left atrium and the pulmonary vasculature.
Dyspnea occurs as a result of engorged pulmonary
vasculature and pulmonary interstitial edema
referred to as pulmonary edema. Orthopnea, parox-

ysmal nocturnal dyspnea, and dry hacking cough are
accompanying symptoms. In right-sided heart failure, blood backs up into the systemic venous circulation causing jugular venous distention, peripheral
edema, and gastrointestinal vascular congestion.
Cognitive Level: Evaluation
Nursing Process: Evaluation
NCLEX-RN Test Plan: PHYS
Reference: Baumberger-Henry, M. (2005). *Fluid and
electrolytes.* Sudbury, MA: Jones and Bartlett.

39. **Answer: 4**
Rationale: Persons with impaired host defenses are
referred to as compromised or immunosuppressed
hosts. The clinical picture of immune dysfunction
includes frequent infections, more severe infections,
infections with opportunistic or unusual organisms,
and an incomplete response to a normal course of
treatment in which the infecting organism is not
eliminated. A carrier can transmit the disease without becoming ill themselves. This client is at risk for
contracting a communicable disease. An allergic
reaction would include other symptoms related to
histamine release that are not reported by this client.
There is no evidence to support faking a medical
condition in this client and it is unethical to pre-
judge ulterior motives before differential diagnosing
is completed.
Cognitive Level: Synthesis
Nursing Process: Assessment
NCLEX-RN Test Plan: PHYS
Reference: Phillips, L. D. (2005). *Manual of IV
therapeutics* (4th ed.). Philadelphia: F.A. Davis.

Unit 5 Answers and Rationales

Test 19 Answers and Rationales

1. **Answer: 2**
   Rationale: Bloating, flatulence, and diarrhea are common symptoms experienced by individuals who are lactose intolerant. Lactose-free products should be recommended. Ingestion of sucrose does not contribute to the symptoms of lactose intolerance.
   Cognitive Level: Analysis
   Nursing Process: Assessment
   NCLEX-RN Test Plan: PHYS
   Reference: Farrell, M., & Nicoteri, J. A. (2001). *Quick look nursing: Nutrition.* Thorofare, NJ: Slack Inc.

2. **Answer: 4**
   Rationale: The kidney acts as a filter for the by-products of protein metabolism, and excess protein can cause renal damage. With ingestion of a high protein diet, renal blood flow increases 20% to 30% within 1 to 2 hours. The liver is essential for protein synthesis, conversion of amino acids into tissue in plasma, nucleic acids, ketone bodies, and glucose. Excess protein is not recommended in late stage hepatic failure.
   Cognitive Level: Application
   Nursing Process: Analysis
   NCLEX-RN Test Plan: PHYS
   Reference: Porth, C. M. (2005). *Pathophysiology: Concepts of altered health states* (7th ed.). Philadelphia: Lippincott.

3. **Answer: 3**
   Rationale: Milk made from soy beans is an excellent protein source for the vegetarian family. Dietary practices influenced by religious or cultural influences need to be respected. A well-planned diet can be developed to prevent vitamin and protein deficiencies.
   Cognitive Level: Application
   Nursing Process: Implementation
   NCLEX-RN Test Plan: HPM
   Reference: Lewis, S. M., Heitkemper, M. M., & Dirksen, S. R. (2004). *Medical-surgical nursing: Assessment and management of clinical problems* (6th ed.). St. Louis, MO: Mosby.

4. **Answer: 4**
   Rationale: Chicken is a low-fat protein food; mashed potatoes add calories, and spinach is recommended to prevent bleeding. The other options are high in calorie and protein contents.
   Cognitive Level: Application
   Nursing Process: Implementation
   NCLEX-RN Test Plan: HPM
   Reference: Lewis, S. M., Heitkemper, M. M., & Dirksen, S. R. (2004). *Medical-surgical nursing: Assessment and management of clinical problems* (6th ed.). St. Louis, MO: Mosby.

5. **Answer: 2**
   Rationale: Heartburn may occur following ingestion of caffeine, which decreases the LES pressure. Clients should be advised to limit intake of foods and fluids prior to sleep in order to decrease LES pressure. Heartburn is relieved by milk or milk products. Chocolate irritates the esophagus and ingestion should be limited or avoided.
   Cognitive Level: Analysis
   Nursing Process: Evaluation
   NCLEX-RN Test Plan: PHYS
   Reference: Lewis, S. M., Heitkemper, M. M., & Dirksen, S. R. (2004). *Medical-surgical nursing: Assessment and management of clinical problems* (6th ed.). St. Louis, MO: Mosby.

6. **Answer: 4**
   Rationale: Roast turkey is a low-fat protein that is an excellent choice for this diet. Low-fat food decreases stimulation of the gallbladder. Creams, gravies, ice cream, cheese, nuts, and fried food should be avoided.
   Cognitive Level: Analysis
   Nursing Process: Evaluation
   NCLEX-RN Test Plan: PHYS
   Reference: Lewis, S. M., Heitkemper, M. M., & Dirksen, S. R. (2004). *Medical-surgical nursing: Assessment and management of clinical problems* (6th ed.). St. Louis, MO: Mosby.

7. **Answer: 1**

   Rationale: Fish is not considered to be a gas forming food for the client with a colostomy. However, fish is an odor producing food. Beer, onions, and carbonated beverages are gas forming foods and should be consumed in moderation for a client with a stoma.

   Cognitive Level: Application

   Nursing Process: Evaluation

   NCLEX-RN Test Plan: PHYS

   Reference: Lewis, S. M., Heitkemper, M. M., & Dirksen, S. R. (2004). *Medical-surgical nursing: Assessment and management of clinical problems* (6th ed.). St. Louis, MO: Mosby.

8. **Answer: 2**

   Rationale: Bronchodilators should be used before meals to reduce the amount of breathlessness and enable the client to eat with ease. Other options are correct and should be recommended to the client with COPD. Clients with COPD should try to keep their body weight for height in the standard range.

   Cognitive Level: Analysis

   Nursing Process: Implementation

   NCLEX-RN Test Plan: PHYS

   Reference: Lewis, S. M., Heitkemper, M. M., & Dirksen, S. R. (2004). *Medical-surgical nursing: Assessment and management of clinical problems* (6th ed.). St. Louis, MO: Mosby.

9. **Answer: 1**

   Rationale: Evidence-based research finds that clients who eat fruits and vegetables reduce their risk of cardiovascular disease. A higher intake of fruit and vegetables may be protective against CVD. Data supports current dietary guidelines to increase fruit and vegetable intake. Red meats, eggs, and milk products are major sources of saturated fats and cholesterol, which contribute to CVD.

   Cognitive Level: Analysis

   Nursing Process: Evaluation

   NCLEX-RN Test Plan: PHYS

   Reference: Lewis, S. M., Heitkemper, M. M., & Dirksen, S. R. (2004). *Medical-surgical nursing: Assessment and management of clinical problems* (6th ed.). St. Louis, MO: Mosby.

10. **Answer: 1, 2, 3, 4**

    Rationale: Foods high in fiber are brown rice, blackberries, whole wheat bread, and beans. Teaching the client dietary measures such as increasing fluid intake, regular exercise, and the importance of a high fiber diet are essential to the nursing management of a client with constipation. Option 5 is incorrect; turkey is not a food high in fiber.

    Cognitive Level: Application

    Nursing Process: Planning

    NCLEX-RN Test Plan: HPM

    Reference: Lewis, S. M., Heitkemper, M. M., & Dirksen, S. R. (2004). *Medical-surgical nursing: Assessment and management of clinical problems* (6th ed.). St. Louis, MO: Mosby.

11. **Answer: 2**

    Rationale: Nasogastric tube feedings to provide enteral nutrition are used for clients who are at risk of aspiration caused by a diminished gag reflex or difficulty swallowing. Other options are inappropriate for the client with dysphagia. Making a client NPO provides no source of nutrition. TPN is used when the GI tract cannot be used for the ingestion, digestion, and absorption of essential nutrients. A soft residue diet would place the client at risk of aspiration due to their difficulty to swallow solids.

    Cognitive Level: Analysis

    Nursing Process: Assessment

    NCLEX-RN Test Plan: PHYS

    Reference: Lewis, S. M., Heitkemper, M. M., & Dirksen, S. R. (2004). *Medical-surgical nursing: Assessment and management of clinical problems* (6th ed.). St. Louis, MO: Mosby.

12. **Answer: 2**

    Rationale: Adolescence is a period of accelerated physical growth. There is a need to double the intake of iron, calcium, zinc, and protein. However, the teen's active lifestyle may alter food selections. Spaghetti and meatballs are an excellent source of providing complex carbohydrates prior to a track meet. Increasing the intake of carbohydrates prior to an activity that is physically challenging will provide energy for the adolescent. Cheeseburgers and french-fries provide excess fats and diet cola provides empty calories with little energy. Eggs, bacon, and toast provide adequate nutrition but miss necessary complex carbohydrates. Fish and chips are high in fat content. Coffee is a caffeinated beverage.

    Cognitive Level: Application

    Nursing Process: Planning

NCLEX-RN Test Plan: HPM
Reference: Farrell, M., & Nicoteri, J. A. (2001). *Quick look nursing: Nutrition.* Thorofare, NJ: Slack Inc.

13. **Answer: 1**
    Rationale: Water is the best fluid choice to supply adequate hydration and satisfy thirst. Other options will increase fluid intake, but they are not the best choice. Vegetable juice provides essential vitamins but excess sodium. Energy drinks are not recommended because they provide a high sugar content which leads to rapid heart rates and elevated blood sugar.
    Cognitive Level: Application
    Nursing Process: Planning
    NCLEX-RN Test Plan: HPM
    Reference: Farrell, M., & Nicoteri, J. A. (2001). *Quick look nursing: Nutrition.* Thorofare, NJ: Slack Inc.

14. **Answer: 1**
    Rationale: Clients should discuss with their health care provider before beginning any supplement. The body's pool of creatine can be replenished either from food (or supplements) or through synthesis from precursor amino acids. Dietary sources include beef, tuna, cod, salmon, herring, and pork. The normal dietary intake of creatine is 1–2 g/day, although vegetarians may consume less. Athletes with high creatine stores do not appear to benefit from supplementation, whereas individuals with the lowest levels, such as vegetarians, have the most pronounced increases following supplementation. Without supplementation, the body can replenish muscle creatine at the rate of about 2 g/day.
    Cognitive Level: Application
    Nursing Process: Implementation
    NCLEX-RN Test Plan: HPM
    Reference: Farrell, M., & Nicoteri, J. A. (2001). *Quick look nursing: Nutrition.* Thorofare, NJ: Slack Inc.
    Lulinski, B. (1999). *Creatine supplementation.* Retrieved July 23, 2006 from http://www.quackwatch.org/01QuackeryRelatedTopics/DSH/creatine.html

15. **Answer: Imbalanced nutrition**
    Rationale: Imbalanced nutrition means less than body requirements related to decreased access, inges-

tions, digestion or absorption of food, or to anorexia. This is an acceptable nursing diagnosis as defined in the NANDA classification system.
Cognitive Level: Application
Nursing Process: Assessment
NCLEX-RN Test Plan: PHYS
Reference: Lewis, S. M., Heitkemper, M. M., & Dirksen, S. R. (2004). *Medical-surgical nursing: Assessment and management of clinical problems* (6th ed.). St. Louis, MO: Mosby.

16. **Answer: 4**
    Rationale: Toast with butter and jelly would be easily digested and present no risk of inflammation to the damaged mucosa. Foods containing leafage, nuts, seeds, or grains may cause intestinal inflammation and discomfort. Milk and milk products should be avoided due to the inability of damaged mucosa to produce the primary disaccharide, lactose.
    Cognitive Level: Application
    Nursing Process: Implementation
    NCLEX-RN Test Plan: PHYS
    Reference: Lewis, S. M., Heitkemper, M. M., & Dirksen, S. R. (2004). *Medical-surgical nursing: Assessment and management of clinical problems* (6th ed.). St. Louis, MO: Mosby.

17. **Answers: 1, 2, 3, and 5**
    Rationale: Protein-rich foods with high biologic value such as whole milk, eggs, cheese, meat, poultry, or fish are recommended for patients with cancer who experience protein and calorie malnutrition. Increasing protein helps to facilitate regeneration of cells and provide energy. Fruits such as bananas and strawberries are excellent sources of potassium.
    Cognitive Level: Application
    Nursing Process: Implementation
    NCLEX-RN Test Plan: PHYS
    Reference: Lewis, S. M., Heitkemper, M. M., & Dirksen, S. R. (2004). *Medical-surgical nursing: Assessment and management of clinical problems* (6th ed.). St. Louis, MO: Mosby.

18. **Answers: 1, 3, and 5**
    Rationale: Clients are counseled to avoid sardines, herring, mussels, and organ meats, which are high in purine. Bacon and pork are moderately high in purine and should be consumed in moderation. Traditional

dietary restrictions in combination with drug therapy (Allopurinol) are useful in the treatment of gout to maintain or prevent elevation of uric acid.

Cognitive Level: Application
Nursing Process: Implementation
NCLEX-RN Test Plan: PHYS
Reference: Lewis, S. M., Heitkemper, M. M., & Dirksen, S. R. (2004). *Medical-surgical nursing: Assessment and management of clinical problems* (6th ed.). St. Louis, MO: Mosby.

19. **Answer: 2**
    Rationale: The American Academy of Pediatrics (AAP) recommends that all formulas be fortified with iron and continued for the first 12 months. Whole milk should not be introduced to infants until after 1 year of age. Pasteurized cow's milk is deficient in iron, zinc, and vitamin C, and has a high renal solute load. Solid foods are introduced between 4 and 6 months of age.
    Cognitive Level: Application
    Nursing Process: Implementation
    NCLEX-RN Test Plan: HPM
    Reference: Wong, D. (2005). *Wong's essentials of pediatric nursing* (7th ed.). St. Louis, MO: Mosby.

20. **Answer: 2**
    Rationale: The introduction of solid food is recommended for the infant between 4 to 6 months old, when the gastrointestinal system has matured sufficiently to handle complex nutrients. The suck reflex and tongue thrust reflex diminishes at 4 months of age. Rice cereal is the first solid food because it is a rich source of iron and rarely induces allergic reactions. Fruits and vegetables, good sources of vitamins, and fiber are introduced after cereal one at a time to determine allergic reactions. Egg whites are highly allergic.
    Cognitive Level: Application
    Nursing Process: Planning
    NCLEX-RN Test Plan: PHYS
    Reference: Wong, D. (2005). *Wong's essentials of pediatric nursing* (7th ed.). St. Louis, MO: Mosby.

21. **Answer: 2**
    Rationale: The NCHS growth charts use the 5th and 95th percentiles as criteria for determining those children who fall outside the normal limits for

growth. Children whose height and weight are above the 95th percentile are considered overweight or large for stature. Prepubescent growth spurts are between 10–12 years for girls and 12–14 years for boys. The percentiles in this question are not normal proportions for height and weight for this 8-year-old.
Cognitive Level: Analysis
Nursing Process: Assessment
NCLEX-RN Test Plan: HPM
Reference: Wong, D. (2005). *Wong's essentials of pediatric nursing* (7th ed.). St. Louis, MO: Mosby.

22. **Answer: 3**
    Rationale: Because growth is a continuous but uneven process, the most reliable evaluation is to compare growth measurements over time. Normal growth patterns vary among children at the same age. The sequence of growth and development is predictable. The child's height and weight are plotted on percentiles and compared with the general population. Middle childhood is a time of gradual growth and development.
    Cognitive Level: Application
    Nursing Process: Assessment
    NCLEX-RN Test Plan: HPM
    Reference: Wong, D. (2005). *Wong's essentials of pediatric nursing* (7th ed.). St. Louis, MO: Mosby.

23. **Answer: 2**
    Rationale: Whole milk is recommended to provide the chief source of calcium and phosphorus. A balanced diet, which includes choices from the basic food groups, is recommended. Skim milk or 2% milk should not be offered until after age 2. Excess carbohydrates, fats, and sugars should be avoided.
    Cognitive Level: Application
    Nursing Process: Planning
    NCLEX-RN Test Plan: HPM
    Reference: Wong, D. (2005). *Wong's essentials of pediatric nursing* (7th ed.). St. Louis, MO: Mosby.

24. **Answer: 2**
    Rationale: Toddlers chew well, but may have difficulty swallowing large pieces of food. Young children cannot discard pits (such as from cherries). Hard foods such as peanuts and hard candy are easily aspirated. Other options are softer in consistency which would be less likely to be aspirated.

Cognitive Level: Application
Nursing Process: Assessment
NCLEX-RN Test Plan: SECE
Reference: Wong, D. (2005). *Wong's essentials of pediatric nursing* (7th ed.). St. Louis, MO: Mosby.

25. **Answer: 1**
Rationale: Nutrition is the greatest influence on growth and development. Dietary factors regulate growth and development. Adequate nutrition provides essential nutrients to sustain physiological needs. Other factors such as income, exposure to secondary smoke, and ethnic background have significant influence on growth and development, but not as much as nutrition.
Cognitive Level: Analysis
Nursing Process: Assessment
NCLEX-RN Test Plan: HPM
Reference: Wong, D. (2005). *Wong's essentials of pediatric nursing* (7th ed.). St. Louis, MO: Mosby.

26. **Answer: 1**
Rationale: Excessive milk consumption should be discouraged, especially more than 1 liter/day (32 oz). Milk is a poor source of iron. Iron fortified rice cereal should be introduced into the diet at 4–6 months of age. Fat soluble vitamins do not provide iron. Foods high in protein, such as meats, spinach, nuts, and whole grains, would not be limited because they are major sources of iron in a balanced diet.
Cognitive Level: Application
Nursing Process: Implementation
NCLEX-RN Test Plan: HPM
Reference: Wong, D. (2005). *Wong's essentials of pediatric nursing* (7th ed.). St. Louis, MO: Mosby.

27. **Answer: 1**
Rationale: Intrinsic factor is secreted by gastric glands in the stomach and is specifically needed for the absorption of vitamin B_{12}. Many patients have a lack of intrinsic factor after partial removal of the stomach, resulting in a deficiency in vitamin B_{12}.
Cognitive Level: Application
Nursing Process: Implementation
NCLEX-RN Test Plan: PHYS
Reference: Farrell, M., & Nicoteri, J. A. (2001). *Quick look nursing: Nutrition.* Thorofare, NJ: Slack Inc.

28. **Answer: 1**
Rationale: Creatinine clearance rate of 40 mL/min and above is sufficient to metabolize unrestricted protein level (within reason) and does not increase the progression of renal disease.
Cognitive Level: Analysis
Nursing Process: Analysis
NCLEX-RN Test Plan: PHYS
Reference: Farrell, M., & Nicoteri, J. A. (2001). *Quick look nursing: Nutrition.* Thorofare, NJ: Slack Inc.

29. **Answer: 1,200**
Rationale: 1,200 kcal/day are recommended for the woman of normal height and weight according to the American Diabetes Association.
Cognitive Level: Application
Nursing Process: Implementation
NCLEX-RN Test Plan: PHYS
Reference: Farrell, M., & Nicoteri, J. A. (2001). *Quick look nursing: Nutrition.* Thorofare, NJ: Slack Inc.

30. **Answer: 3**
Rationale: Vitamin C is a water soluble vitamin, antioxidant, enzymatic, and an immune biologic agent. Sources of vitamin C include citrus fruits such as oranges, lemons, tangerines, and grapefruits. In fact, vitamin C comes almost exclusively from fruits and vegetables. Other good sources are tomatoes, strawberries, raspberries, peppers, broccoli, asparagus, brussel sprouts, cauliflower, cabbage, peas, rutabagas, cantaloupe, kiwi, papayas, potato, paprika, and watermelon. Vitamin A is essential for normal retinal function and cell growth differentiation. Vitamin D promotes ossification of bones and teeth. B-complex vitamins are essential in the metabolism of nutrients.
Cognitive Level: Application
Nursing Process: Implementation
NCLEX-RN Test Plan: HPM
Reference: The Liquid Vitamin C Supplements Store. (n.d.) Retrieved July 23, 2006 from http://www.vitamin-supplements-store.net/vitamins/vitamin-c.html

31. **Answer: 1**

    Rationale: Anemia is common in older adults. Red meats, especially liver, provide the necessary nutrient cobalamin (vitamin B_{12}) to promote RBC maturation. Green leafy vegetables provide iron needed for hemoglobin synthesis and folic acid for RBC maturation. Milk, milk products, cheese, and ice cream provide essential amino acids for synthesis of nucleoproteins. Other necessary nutrients include vitamin C, which is found in citrus fruits, green leafy vegetables, strawberries, and cantaloupe.

    Cognitive Level: Analysis

    Nursing Process: Evaluation

    NCLEX-RN Test Plan: PHYS

    Reference: Lewis, S. M., Heitkemper, M. M., & Dirksen, S. R. (2004). *Medical-surgical nursing: Assessment and management of clinical problems* (6th ed.). St. Louis, MO: Mosby.

32. **Answer: 3**

    Rationale: Alcohol can cause serious adverse effects when used in conjunction with certain oral medications used to treat diabetes. It may produce effects similar to that of antabuse (nausea, vomiting, flushing, respiratory distress, or chest pain when ingested with sulfonylurea medications). Alcohol is high in calories with no nutritive value and promotes hyperglyceridemia.

    Cognitive Level: Application

    Nursing Process: Implementation

    NCLEX-RN Test Plan: SECE

    Reference: Lewis, S. M., Heitkemper, M. M., & Dirksen, S. R. (2004). *Medical-surgical nursing: Assessment and management of clinical problems* (6th ed.). St. Louis, MO: Mosby.

33. **Answer: 2**

    Rationale: Atorvastatin (Lipitor) is an HMG-CoA reductase inhibitor, also known as a "statin," used in combination with a low-cholesterol and low-fat diet to decrease cholesterol and triglyceride levels and to raise good cholesterol (HDL) levels in the blood. It may also be used for children 10 to 17 who have genetically inherited hypercholesteremia. People taking Lipitor are advised not to eat grapefruit or grapefruit juice. Grapefruit has a chemical that blocks certain drugs from being absorbed properly. All other options are acceptable in the diet prescribed Lipitor.

    Cognitive Level: Application

    Nursing Process: Implementation

    NCLEX-RN Test Plan: PHYS

    References: Lewis, S. M., Heitkemper, M. M., & Dirksen, S. R. (2004). *Medical-surgical nursing: Assessment and management of clinical problems* (6th ed.). St. Louis, MO: Mosby.

    American Society of Health-System Pharmacists Inc. (2006). *Atorvastatin.* Retrieved July 23, 2006 from http://www.nlm.nih.gov/medlineplus/druginfo/medmaster/a600045.html

34. **Answer: 4**

    Rationale: The most appropriate choice is to delegate the UAP to assist the patient with Parkinson's disease, after the RN assesses the condition and complexity of the patient. The RN must follow the State Nurse Practice Act and hospital policy in regard to delegation of tasks assigned to the unlicensed assistive personnel (UAP) or the LPN. If the client is stable and the task is routine and standard in nature, the UAP may be delegated to perform the task. The RN is responsible to explain the task, ensure the UAP understands the expected goals, and to provide supervision and/or feedback to the UAP as necessary.

    Cognitive Level: Application

    Nursing Process: Implementation

    NCLEX-RN Test Plan: SECE

    Reference: State of Ohio Board of Nursing. (2006). *Chapter 4723-13: Delegation of nursing tasks.* Retrieved November 18, 2006, from http://nursing.ohio.gov/PDFS/NewLawRules/4723-13DelegationbyLicensedNurses.pdf

35. **Answer: 2**

    Rationale: The recommended additional 300 calories during the second and third semester is necessary for maternal and fetal development and nutrition during pregnancy. The expected weight gain for a woman during pregnancy is 25–30 lbs.

    Cognitive Level: Application

    Nursing Process: Implementation

    NCLEX-RN Test Plan: PHYS

    Reference: Farrell, M., & Nicoteri, J. A. (2001). *Quick look nursing: Nutrition.* Thorofare, NJ: Slack Inc.

36. **Answer: 2**
    Rationale: By checking his refrigerator, you can determine the amounts of fresh foods he has, frequency of his shopping, sanitation habits, and his ability to care for himself. Other options will be helpful to validate or identify any data collected.
    Cognitive Level: Analysis
    Nursing Process: Assessment
    NCLEX-RN Test Plan: SECE
    Reference: Farrell, M., & Nicoteri, J. A. (2001). *Quick look nursing: Nutrition.* Thorofare, NJ: Slack Inc.

37. **Answer: 4**
    Rationale: By decreasing caffeine and increasing vitamin B_6, these dietary changes may alleviate some of the discomfort associated with fibrocystic changes. Other options are incorrect. Caffeine, cola, chocolate, and tea are foods that contain xanthines. Women are advised to avoid these foods in their daily diet, especially in the pre-menstrual period. Vitamin E may be helpful in reducing breast pain (mastalgia).
    Cognitive Level: Application
    Nursing Process: Implementation
    NCLEX-RN Test Plan: PHYS
    Reference: Porth, C. M. (2005). *Pathophysiology: Concepts of altered health states* (7th ed.). Philadelphia: Lippincott.

38. **Answer: 3**
    Rationale: Garlic may cause a mild increase in serum insulin levels, so it should not be used with hypoglycemic agents. In addition, garlic inhibits platelet aggregation. All other options have no known contraindications with hypoglycemics.
    Cognitive Level: Application
    Nursing Process: Implementation
    NCLEX-RN Test Plan: SECE
    Reference: Lewis, S. M., Heitkemper, M. M., & Dirksen, S. R. (2004). *Medical-surgical nursing: Assessment and management of clinical problems* (6th ed.). St. Louis, MO: Mosby.

39. **Answer: 4, 2, 5, 3, 1**
    Rationale: The nurse would first assess for the client's bowel sounds, then aspirate for stomach contents to determine residual amounts and pH of contents. After elevating the head of the bed to prevent aspiration prior to starting the feeding the nurse would then flush the tube with water to assure patency, then adjust the flow rate and begin to administer the feeding. Flush water may be given to assure the patency of the tube once feeding is completed.
    Cognitive Level: Application
    Nursing Process: Implementation
    NCLEX Test Plan: SECE
    Reference: Lewis, S. M., Heitkemper, M. M., & Dirksen, S. R. (2004). *Medical-surgical nursing: Assessment and management of clinical problems* (6th ed.). St. Louis, MO: Mosby.

Unit 6 • Nursing Care of Specific Groups

Maternal-Newborn

1. Using Leopold's maneuvers, the nurse palpates a round, firm, moveable part in the fundal portion of the uterus and a long, smooth surface on the mother's right side. In which maternal quadrant should the nurse expect to auscultate fetal heart tones?
   1. The lower left.
   2. The lower right.
   3. The upper left.
   4. The upper right.

2. During her prenatal visit, a woman at 12 weeks gestation asks the nurse about the cause of her indigestion and heartburn. What is the best explanation?
   1. Increased pancreatic activity results in digestive tract fat intolerance.
   2. Increased estrogen production causes increased secretion of hydrochloric acid, leading to peptic ulcer formation.
   3. Pressure from the growing uterus displaces the stomach and intestines.
   4. Progesterone, produced by the placenta, causes decreased motility of smooth muscle.

3. A pregnant woman's history reveals one pregnancy, terminated by elective abortion at 9 weeks; the birth of twins at 36 weeks; and a spontaneous abortion at 15 weeks. According to the TPAL system, which of the following describes her present parity?
   1. 0-1-2-2.
   2. 0-2-2-2.
   3. 1-0-2-2.
   4. 2-0-2-2.

4. When teaching a class of pregnant women about fetal development, the nurse should include which of the following?
   1. "The baby's heart beat is audible by doppler at 12 weeks of pregnancy."
   2. "The sex of the baby is determined by week 8 of pregnancy."
   3. "Very fine hairs, called lanugo, cover your baby's entire body by week 36 of pregnancy."
   4. "You will first feel your baby move by week 24 of pregnancy."

5. Mark the place where the fundus should be located at 20 weeks gestation.

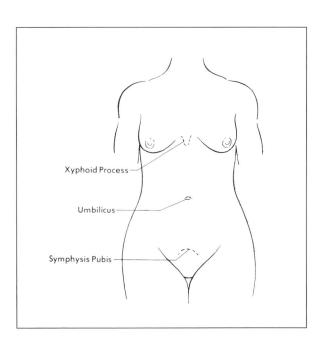

Xyphoid Process —

Umbilicus —

Symphysis Pubis —

6. **The date of a client's last menstrual period was May 4, 2007. Using Naegele's Rule, calculate the estimated date of birth.**
   1. February 11, 2008.
   2. February 27, 2008.
   3. April 27, 2008.
   4. August 11, 2008.

7. **A client visits the prenatal clinic stating that she thinks she may be pregnant. She states that she is able to feel the baby move. The nurse explains that this is a**

   _____

   sign of pregnancy.
   1. Presumptive.
   2. Probable.
   3. Possible.
   4. Positive.

8. **A woman in the first stage of labor is using pattern-paced breathing. She complains of feeling lightheaded and states that her fingers are tingling. Which of the following actions should the nurse take?**
   1. Administer oxygen via nasal cannula.
   2. Help the client breathe into a paper bag.
   3. Notify the client's physician.
   4. Tell the client to slow the rate of her breathing.

9. **When evaluating a fetal heart rate (FHR) pattern on an external electronic fetal monitor, the nurse notes that the FHR begins to decelerate after the contraction has started and the lowest point of the deceleration occurs after the peak of the contraction. What is the nurse's first priority?**
   1. Change the client's position.
   2. Document the findings as benign decelerations.
   3. Insert a scalp electrode.
   4. Prepare for an amnioinfusion.

10. **Which of the following nursing actions reflects application of the gate control theory during labor?**
    1. Administer the prescribed medication when the client is dilated to 4 cm.
    2. Encourage the client to rest between contractions.
    3. Massage the client's back.
    4. Turn the client onto her left side.

11. **A laboring client delivers two hours after receiving meperidine (Demerol) IV. Which of the following medications should be available to counteract the effects of meperidine (Demerol) in the newborn?**
    1. Beractant (Survanta).
    2. Betamethasone.
    3. Fentanyl (Sublimaze).
    4. Naloxone (Narcan).

12. **After vaginal examination, assessment of a laboring client is documented as 3 cm, 30%, and –1. The nurse's interpretation of this assessment is which of the following?**
    1. The cervix is dilated 3 cm, it is effaced 30%, and the presenting part is 1 cm above the ischial spines.
    2. The cervix is dilated 3 cm, it is effaced 30%, and the presenting part is 1 cm below the ischial spines.
    3. The cervix is effaced 3 cm, it is dilated 30%, and the presenting part is 1 cm above the ischial spines.
    4. The cervix is effaced 3 cm, it is dilated 30%, and the presenting part is 1 cm below the ischial spines.

13. **Which of the following factors could negatively affect labor?**
    1. The fetal attitude is in general flexion.
    2. The fetal lie is longitudinal.
    3. The maternal pelvis is gynecoid.
    4. The presenting part is sacrum.

14. **Place in order the seven cardinal movements of the mechanism of labor that occur in a vertex presentation.**
    1. Descent.
    2. Engagement.
    3. Flexion.
    4. Expulsion.
    5. Extension.
    6. External rotation.
    7. Internal rotation.

15. **Immediately after a laboring client's membranes rupture, which of the following is the priority nursing care?**
    1. Assess the client's blood pressure.
    2. Assess the fetal heart rate pattern.
    3. Take the client's temperature.
    4. Time the client's contractions.

16. **A client at 35 weeks gestation is admitted to labor and delivery with a diagnosis of preeclampsia. Which of the following orders should be questioned?**
    1. Assess reflexes every shift.
    2. Take a daily weight.
    3. Perform a nonstress test.
    4. Let the client up as desired.

17. **A client who is at 36 weeks gestation is admitted to labor and delivery with painless, bright red vaginal bleeding. Which of the following does the nurse suspect?**
    1. Abruptio placentae.
    2. Placenta previa.
    3. Preterm labor.
    4. Threatened abortion.

18. **Which of the following variables are assessed during a biophysical profile? Select all that apply.**
    1. Biparietal diameter of the fetal skull.
    2. Fetal breathing movements.
    3. Fetal tone.
    4. Gross body movements.
    5. Contraction stress test.
    6. Qualitative amniotic fluid volume.
    7. Reactive fetal heart rate on a nonstress test.

19. **Which of the following pregnant women should have amniotic fluid alpha-fetoprotein (AFP) screening?**
    1. A woman who has a cardiac anomaly.
    2. A woman who has been exposed to AIDS.
    3. A woman who has had a child with spina bifida.
    4. A woman who is in preterm labor.

20. **During a nonstress test, the nurse notes that the fetal heart rate decelerates about 15 beats during a period of fetal movement. The decelerations occur twice during the test and last 20 seconds each time. The nurse realizes that these results will be interpreted as which of the following?**
    1. A negative test.
    2. A nonreactive test.
    3. A positive test.
    4. A reactive test.

21. **A pregnant client who is at 36 weeks gestation is scheduled for an amniocentesis. Prior to the procedure, the client has an ultrasound done. The nurse explains that which of the following is the purpose of an ultrasound at this time?**
    1. To determine if there is more than one fetus.
    2. To estimate fetal age.
    3. To locate the placenta and fetus.
    4. To prescreen the fetus for gross congenital anomalies.

22. **Which of the following results would suggest that the fetal lungs are mature enough for birth?**
    1. The absence of phosphatidylglycerol (PG).
    2. A fetal biophysical profile score of 8.
    3. A lecithin/sphingomyelin (L/S) ratio of 2:1.
    4. A reactive nonstress test.

23. **After birth, the nurse immediately dries off the newborn with a sterile towel. This action prevents heat loss through which of the following?**
    1. Conduction.
    2. Convection.
    3. Evaporation.
    4. Radiation.

24. **A sudden loud noise produced the following response in a newborn: symmetric abduction and extension of the arms with the fingers fanning out and forming a "C" with the thumb and forefinger. A slight tremor was also noted. The nurse would document this finding as a positive**

    _____

    reflex.
    1. Babinski.
    2. Moro.
    3. Rooting.
    4. Tonic neck.

25. **A new mother asks about the swollen area that she noticed on her newborn's head. The edema crosses the suture line. The newborn was delivered vaginally, with a vacuum assist. Based on the nurse's assessment of the newborn, the mother is told that this is called which of the following?**
    1. A mongolian spot.
    2. Caput succedaneum.
    3. Cephalhematoma.
    4. Erythema toxicum.

26. **A newborn is placed under a radiant heat warmer after birth. The nurse evaluates the newborn's body temperature every hour. These actions are done to prevent which of the following?**
    1. Cold stress.
    2. Respiratory depression.
    3. Tachycardia.
    4. Thermogenesis.

27. **A client's blood is type A, Rh negative. Her newborn's blood is type O, Rh positive. Why would a direct Coombs test be done?**
    1. To determine if kernicterus has occurred in the newborn.
    2. To detect Rh negative antibodies in the newborn.
    3. To detect Rh positive antibodies in the mother's blood.
    4. To measure the presence of maternal antibodies in the fetal blood.

28. **Which of the following lab values need to be monitored when providing care for an infant of a diabetic mother (IDM)? Select all that apply.**
    1. Blood glucose.
    2. Direct Coombs test.
    3. Red blood cell count.
    4. Serum bilirubin.
    5. Serum calcium.
    6. White blood cell count.

29. **Of the following nursing diagnoses pertaining to the newborn, which would require immediate nursing intervention?**
    1. Altered urinary elimination related to postcircumcision status.
    2. An ineffective breathing pattern related to mucus obstruction.
    3. An ineffective infant feeding pattern related to the inability to coordinate sucking and swallowing.
    4. A risk for infection related to immature immunologic defenses and environmental exposure.

30. After delivery, the following assessments were noted: Heart rate of 110; slow, weak cry; some flexion of extremities; cries with gentle taps on the soles of the feet; and pink color. Based on these findings, the APGAR score is

    _____.

31. A postpartum client delivered a healthy baby girl two days ago. Document the expected type of lochia at this time.

    _____

32. A client delivered a 7-pound, 6-ounce healthy newborn 12 hours ago. Where should the nurse expect to palpate the fundus?
    1. Approximately 1 cm above the umbilicus.
    2. Approximately at the level of the umbilicus.
    3. Approximately 1 cm below the umbilicus.
    4. Approximately 2 cm below the umbilicus.

33. The nurse assesses a postpartum client and finds the fundus slightly boggy and displaced to the right. Based on these findings, which of the following would be an appropriate nursing diagnosis?
    1. Acute pain related to postpartum physiologic changes.
    2. Risk for deficient fluid volume related to uterine atony secondary to a distended bladder.
    3. Risk for impaired urinary elimination related to effects of anesthesia.
    4. Risk for infection related to invasive procedures during labor and delivery.

34. The nurse assesses a postpartum client's fundus and finds it to be firm, 3 cm above the umbilicus, and displaced to the right. Which of the following is an appropriate nursing intervention?

    1. Assist the client to the bathroom to void, then reassess the fundus.
    2. Document the findings as within normal limits.
    3. Gently massage the fundus every 15 minutes.
    4. Encourage the client to ambulate to aid in the involution process.

35. A 26-year-old gravida 3, para 2-0-0-2 gave birth 5 hours ago to a 9-pound, 6-ounce girl after augmentation of labor with oxytocin (Pitocin). This client is at risk for postpartum hemorrhage due to which of the following conditions?
    1. Puerperal infection.
    2. Retained placental fragments.
    3. Unrepaired vaginal lacerations.
    4. Uterine atony.

36. The nurse is assessing a client who delivered vaginally four hours ago. The client has saturated a perineal pad within 20 minutes. Which of the following should be the nurse's first action?
    1. Assess the client's blood pressure.
    2. Notify the primary health care provider.
    3. Palpate the client's fundus.
    4. Prepare to administer an oxytocic preparation.

37. Identify which nursing diagnoses are appropriate for a client experiencing an uncomplicated vaginal delivery. Select all that apply.
    1. Acute pain related to postpartum physiologic changes.
    2. Deficient diversional activity related to bed rest.
    3. Disturbed sleep pattern related to excitement, discomfort, and newborn needs.
    4. Ineffective tissue perfusion related to hypovolemia.
    5. Risk for deficient fluid volume related to uterine atony/hemorrhage.
    6. Risk for impaired urinary elimination related to perineal trauma.
    7. Interrupted family processes related to separation from newborn.

38. When instructing a breastfeeding mother regarding diet, the nurse should stress that which of the following nutritional requirements is higher during lactation than during pregnancy?
   1. Calcium.
   2. Energy (kcal).
   3. Folic acid.
   4. Iron.

39. While caring for a postpartum client who experienced abruptio placentae, the nurse notices petechiae and bleeding around the IV site. The nurse should monitor her for which of the following?
   1. Amniotic fluid embolism.
   2. Disseminated intravascular coagulation.
   3. Preeclampsia.
   4. Puerperal infection.

Women's Health

1. **Medications for a client with polycystic ovarian syndrome (PCOS) include which of the following?**
   1. Insulin, oral contraceptives, and Glucophage (metformin).
   2. Glucophage (metformin) and Clomid (clomiphene).
   3. Oral contraceptives, Glucophage (metformin), and Clomid (clomiphene).
   4. Oral contraceptives and Glucophage (metformin).

2. **A client is experiencing urinary incontinence. The nurse suggests that the client should do which of the following? Select all that apply.**
   1. Decrease dietary fiber.
   2. Discontinue doing daily Kegel exercises.
   3. Restrict her daily fluid intake to 1.5 liters per day.
   4. Reduce her intake of foods such as chocolate, caffeine, carbonated beverages, alcohol, orange juice, and tomatoes, which can irritate her bladder.

3. **A client expresses concern about her need to have gynecological surgery. She states, "I'm not sure I want to undergo surgery." The nurse recognizes that the woman's statement warrants further assessment to determine which of the following?**
   1. The woman has both general concerns about surgery and specific concerns about gynecological surgery.
   2. The woman is afraid of surgery.
   3. The woman has financial problems.
   4. The woman is concerned about her surgical risk.

4. **The client states, "I'm a little nervous because I have never had a pelvic examination before." The nurse recognizes the client is anxious and explains which of the following about the exam?**
   1. The examiner will use a plastic speculum to visualize and inspect the woman's vulva, vagina, and cervix.
   2. The woman's cervix will be inspected using a speculum.
   3. The examiner will perform both a bimanual examination and an inspection that will include palpation of the cervix, uterus, and ovaries.
   4. The exam will include an inspection of the vulva, vagina, and cervix using a speculum.

5. **A perimenopausal woman complains of transient shortness of breath and dizziness over the last several days, especially when performing her household activities. The nurse recognizes which of the following?**
   1. This client is depressed.
   2. This client may have symptoms of coronary artery disease (CAD).
   3. This woman is reacting to a stressful home environment.
   4. This woman is anxious.

6. When reviewing the lab work for an obese perimenopausal woman, the nurse notes that the LDL/HDL ratio is 6. Which of the following statements is a correct description of an LDL/HDL ratio?
   1. A ratio of 4 or less is considered acceptable.
   2. A ratio of 6 or higher is acceptable.
   3. A ratio of less than 4 is unacceptable and warrants an aggressive approach.
   4. A ratio of 6 or higher is serious and warrants an aggressive approach.

7. A client expresses concern about her risk for coronary artery disease. The nurse explains that there are both modifiable and nonmodifiable risk factors. Which of the following are modifiable risk factors?
   1. Cigarette smoking, obesity, and gender.
   2. Obesity, hypertension, and diabetes.
   3. Physical inactivity, hypertension, and hyperlipidemia.
   4. Family history, age, and gender.

8. When developing a plan of care for a client with a nursing diagnosis of pain related to relaxation of the pelvic support and elimination, the nurse would obtain a thorough pain history by doing which of the following? Select all that apply.
   1. Assessing the location, frequency, severity, and duration of the pain.
   2. Educate the client about prescribed medications.
   3. Provide the client with information about regular toileting.
   4. Ask the client to decrease fluids and fiber in her diet.

9. Discussion of nonsurgical interventions for pelvic organ prolapse includes which of the following? Select all that apply.
   1. A Kegel exercises regimen.
   2. The use of pessories.
   3. The use of estrogen replacement therapy.
   4. Encouraging high aerobic exercise activity.

10. Which of the following symptoms is common to all types of pelvic organ prolapse?
   1. Stress incontinence.
   2. Incontinence of flatus and liquid or solid stool.
   3. Dyspareunia.
   4. Feeling of dragging, a lump in the vagina, or something "coming down".

11. Which of the following medications are used to prevent osteoporosis in menopausal women?
   1. Levothyroxine (Synthroid).
   2. Vitamin E.
   3. Raloxiphine (Evista).
   4. Alendronate sodium (Fosamax).

12. A postmenopausal client asks the nurse practitioner what she can do to prevent osteoporosis. The nurse responds with which of the following? Select all that apply.
   1. Eat a well balanced diet that includes adequate amounts of citrus fruit.
   2. Take a 1200 mg calcium supplement daily.
   3. Take a 1500 mg calcium supplement and a vitamin D supplement daily and eat a well balanced diet that is rich in calcium.
   4. Decrease the use of dairy products, fish, and whole wheat bread in her diet.

13. A menopausal client is complaining of vaginal dryness and itching and is refusing hormone therapy. The nurse suggests that the client try alternative therapies to relieve the symptoms. Which of the following would be a good suggestion for the client?
   1. Use valerian (a natural tranquilizer).
   2. Use a natural diuretic (such as parsley).
   3. Add more walnuts, bran, and brown rice in her diet.
   4. Apply vitamin E to her skin.

14. **The client is experiencing menopausal symptoms and questions the nurse about the use of herbs to relieve or reduce her symptoms. Which of the following is an appropriate response from the nurse? Select all that apply.**

   1. Many herbal products have not undergone long term testing for safety and efficacy.
   2. Herbal therapies do not have any benefits and will not help your symptoms.
   3. You should begin immediately as they will help you.
   4. There are no ill effects involved with the use of herbal therapies.

15. **Which of these diagnostic tests is most commonly used to diagnose and screen for osteoporosis?**

   1. DEXA scan (dual-energy X-ray absorbtiometry).
   2. Pelvic spine X-ray.
   3. Abdominal cat scan.
   4. Bone biopsy.

16. **A nonpregnant woman has been diagnosed with bacterial vaginosis (BV). The nurse is aware that this increases the woman's risk for which of the following?**

   1. Endometriosis.
   2. Uterine cancer.
   3. Pelvic inflammatory disease and abnormal cervical cytology.
   4. Irregular menstrual cycles.

17. **Hysteroscopy is a common diagnostic procedure used to view the uterine cavity and diagnose fibroid tumors. The nurse's client discharge instructions following this procedure would include all *except* which of the following?**

   1. The client should expect possible shoulder pain, uterine cramping, and mild vaginal spotting for one to three days.
   2. The client should abstain from sexual intercourse, douching, and tampon use for two weeks.
   3. The client should notify health care providers if she experiences heavy bleeding, odor, or fever.
   4. The client should be on a liquid diet for one to two days following the procedure.

18. **A client presents with a mass in the left ovarian area but does not have an elevated Ca-125. Which of the following should the nurse know about Ca-125 levels?**

   1. Ca-125 is elevated in only 50% of the cases of early stage ovarian cancer.
   2. Endometriosis does not cause Ca-125 elevations.
   3. Ca-125 is always used to diagnose ovarian cancer.
   4. All ovarian tumors give elevations in Ca-125.

19. **The nurse is presenting an educational program on cancer risk to a group of mothers. A young mother asks if there are any factors that reduce ovarian cancer risk. The nurse responds that women who do which of the following have a reduction in ovarian cancer risk? Select all that apply.**

   1. Exercise regularly.
   2. Breast feed and use oral contraceptives.
   3. Have had one or more term pregnancies.
   4. Are menopausal.

20. A sixty-year-old postmenopausal client presents with complaints of bright red vaginal bleeding. Which of the following data will the nurse collect? Select all that apply.
1. Postmenopausal status and date of last menstrual period.
2. A description of the frequency and duration of the bleeding.
3. Hormone therapy use, type of hormones, and history.
4. Use of herbs and dietary supplements.

21. The client is ordered a SERM (Arimidex). The nurse explains to the client that she may experience which of the following side effects?
1. Nausea, hot flashes, and fatigue.
2. Hot flashes, bone pain, and diarrhea.
3. Nausea, vomiting, and diarrhea.
4. Hot flashes, weight gain, and vaginal bleeding.

22. A client has just been given the diagnosis of breast cancer. Which of the following nursing diagnoses would take precedence?
1. Disturbed body image.
2. Fear related to breast cancer.
3. Knowledge deficit.
4. Interrupted family processes.

23. A postmenopausal client is diagnosed with an estrogen positive and progesterone positive breast tumor. The nurse is aware that this patient will most likely be treated with a SERM (hormone therapy). SERMs are used for which of the following?
1. To block or counter the effect of estrogen.
2. To increase the effect of estrogen.
3. To increase the woman's quality of life.
4. To decrease the woman's risk for endometrial cancer.

24. When rounding, the nurse observes that a six-hour postoperative hysterectomy client's Foley catheter drainage is becoming increasingly bloody in appearance. Which of the following could cause this?
1. The bladder may have been nicked during the surgical procedure.
2. This is a normal response for this type of surgery.
3. The client is probably dehydrated.
4. The client may have a urinary tract infection.

25. During a client's annual gynecological exam, she states that she is concerned about her risk factors regarding ovarian cancer. The nurse reviews which of the following risk factors for ovarian cancer with the client? Select all that apply.
1. Nulliparity.
2. Family history of breast cancer.
3. Use of infertility drugs.
4. Diets high in fat.

26. A 27-year-old client recently diagnosed with cervical polyps appears anxious. The nurse is aware of which of the following about cervical polyps?
1. Cervical polyps are common noncancerous benign growths that may cause premenstrual, postmenstrual, or postcoital bleeding.
2. Cervical polyps are the precursors to the development of cervical cancer.
3. Cervical polyps are very uncommon and may lead to malignancy.
4. Cervical polyps are very common in women who are nulliparas and older than 40 years in age.

27. **The nurse is collaborating with a domestic abuse client and formulating a plan of care. When developing a plan of care for this client, specific expected outcomes will include which of the following? Select all that apply.**
    1. The woman will exhibit embarrassment and shock.
    2. The woman will exhibit passive and hostile behavior.
    3. The woman will formulate a safety plan.
    4. The woman will perceive herself as worthwhile and deserving of respect, not as a victim that is responsible for her abuse.

28. **The nurse providing counseling for a woman diagnosed with HPV (human papilloma virus) should provide which of the following information to the client? Select all that apply.**
    1. HPV is spread by direct contact during oral, vaginal, or anal intercourse.
    2. Treatment will not destroy the HPV virus but will eradicate the wart-like lesions.
    3. Using condoms can reduce the transmission of this disease to the partner.
    4. HPV infection is a very uncommon infection.

29. **A female client that has HSV complains of painful vaginal lesions. The nurse's plan of care for the client includes which of the following? Select all that apply.**
    1. The client should wear loose fitting clothing.
    2. The client should soak in tepid water.
    3. The client should urinate in water if experiencing pain during urination.
    4. The client should apply ice to the perineum.

30. **When writing a sexually transmitted infection teaching plan, the nurse should recall that which of the following is a high-risk sexual behavior for acquiring a sexually transmitted infection?**
    1. Vaginal intercourse with a condom.
    2. Wet kissing.
    3. Vaginal intercourse after anal contact without using a new condom.
    4. Multiple sexual partners.

31. **Effective techniques for sexually transmitted infection counseling include which of the following?**
    1. Asking closed-ended questions when obtaining the health history.
    2. Obtaining a reproductive health history on all women.
    3. Assuming that women in higher socially economic classes are not at risk for sexually transmitted infections.
    4. Assuming that women are aware of the consequences of sexually transmitted infections.

32. **A 40-year-old client presents with complaints of pelvic pain and menorrhagia. She states that she also has pain during intercourse and that she has a lot of clotting during menses. The client complains of tenderness and pain during uterine palpation and examination. The nurse is aware that this is a distinguishing factor when assessing for which of the following?**
    1. Adenomyosis.
    2. Uterine fibroids.
    3. Endometrial hyperplasia.
    4. Uterine cysts/polyps.

33. **The nurse discusses adenomyosis diagnostic testing with the client. Which of the following tests gives the most definitive diagnosis for differentiating adenomyosis from fibroids and malignancy?**
    1. Hemoglobin and hematocrit.
    2. Ultrasound.
    3. MRI.
    4. Endometrial biopsy.

34. An 8-week postpartum client presents with the following signs and symptoms: fatigue, weakness, tremors, hyperreflexia, palpitations, and angina. The client is diagnosed with postpartum thyroiditis. Which of the following may be relevant? Select all that apply.
   1. Presentation of this condition is initially that of hyperthyroidism.
   2. Most women recover spontaneously, but it may reoccur with future pregnancies.
   3. It is a permanent condition with sequelae.
   4. Women with this disorder may be at future risk for thyroid disease.

35. A client asks for information about medical abortion procedures. The nurse provides her with the information. Which of the following facts are correct? Select all that apply.
   1. In the United States, medical abortion is a relatively new method used for pregnancy termination.
   2. Two methods are available: mifepristone and methotrexate, both of which are given in combination with misoprostol.
   3. Efficacy of medical abortion methods increases with gestational age.
   4. Methotrexate is the most common form of medical abortion used in the United States.

36. A 60-year-old woman has been diagnosed with urinary incontinence (UI). The nurse practitioner reviews factors that may provide some symptomatic relief for the woman's UI. Which of the following factors are correct? Select all that apply.
   1. The type and amount of fluid intake may contribute to UI symptoms.
   2. Limiting fluids may cause bladder irritation causing some women to have an increased urge to urinate accompanied by UI.
   3. A high intake of caffeinated beverages improves symptoms of UI.
   4. Artificial sweetener use does not have an effect on UI.

37. A 35-year-old woman presents with pelvic pain, dysmenorrhea, dyspareunia, abnormal menstrual bleeding, and infertility. The nurse practitioner suspects endometriosis and discusses which following gold standard diagnostic procedure with the client?
   1. Ultrasound.
   2. MRI.
   3. Hystersalpingography.
   4. Laparoscopy with biopsy.

38. The nurse is discussing hormone therapy (ET only) with a woman requesting hormone replacement to relieve menopausal symptoms. The nurse reviews absolute contraindications with the client. Which of the following are contraindications to the use of estrogen hormonal replacement therapy? Select all that apply.
   1. A history of dermatitis.
   2. A history of known or suspected cancer of the breast.
   3. A prior or current history of asthma or COPD.
   4. A prior or current history of coronary heart disease or stroke.

39. A woman has been diagnosed with vulvodynea. The nurse provides which of the following information on self-care relief measures to alleviate her symptoms?
   1. The client should increase oxalates in her diet (tea, coffee, and cocoa).
   2. The client should take baths instead of showers.
   3. The client should use unscented toilet paper.
   4. The client should increase the use of latex products.

Child and Adolescent Health

1. **Which of the following is a developmental red flag for a 3-month-old infant?**
   1. The child does not attempt to raise his head when placed on his stomach.
   2. The child does not attempt to sit without support.
   3. The child does not pick up objects with his fingers.
   4. The child has intense stranger anxiety.

2. **The mother of a 2-year-old asks if she should be concerned about the child's temper tantrums. What is the correct response?**
   1. Give the child whatever they want to prevent the temper tantrum.
   2. Temper tantrums are the child's way to try to gain control and power over a situation.
   3. There is a need for a psychological consult.
   4. This is a type of a learning disability.

3. **Thickening formula with rice cereal, burping frequently during feedings, and keeping the infant slightly upright after feedings are all treatment strategies for**

   _____.
   1. Cleft palate.
   2. Esophagitis.
   3. Failure to thrive (FTT).
   4. Gastroesophageal reflux (GER).

4. **An infant born to an HBsAg-positive mother should receive which of the following?**
   1. HBIG.
   2. Hepatitis B vaccine at day 0, 1–2 months, and 6 months.
   3. Hepatitis B vaccine within 12 hours of birth, plus HBIG.
   4. Hepatitis B vaccine within 24 hours of birth.

5. **A 1-month-old with acute otitis media is prescribed Amoxil (amoxicillin) 320 mg PO every 12 hours for 10 days. The suspension comes 400 mg/5 ml. The mother asks how many milliliters (ml) she could administer. Which of the following is the correct answer?**
   1. 3 ml.
   2. 4 ml.
   3. 3.5 ml.
   4. 4.5 ml.

6. **A 2-month-old presents with a history of cough, wheezing, nasal congestion, intermittent fever, difficulty feeding, and two episodes of apnea lasting five seconds each. The most likely cause of these symptoms is which of the following?**
   1. Asthma.
   2. Bronchiolitis/RSV.
   3. Croup.
   4. Epiglottitis.

7. **Congenital heart defects associated with increased pulmonary blood flow include which of the following?**
   1. Coarctation of the aorta.
   2. Patent ductus arteriosis.
   3. Tetralogy of Fallot.
   4. Tricuspid atresia.

8. **A febrile seizure is usually characterized by which of the following?**
   1. Absence of seizure activity.
   2. Complex seizure activity.
   3. Infantile spasms.
   4. Tonic-clonic seizure activity.

9. **The stage when a disease is contagious is known as which of the following?**
   1. The communicability period.
   2. The convalescent period.
   3. The incubation period.
   4. The prodromal period.

10. **You are caring for a 6-month-old infant. Choose an appropriate way to measure pain in this infant.**
    1. FLACC (Face, legs, activity, cry, consolability) pain scale.
    2. Oucher numeric scale.
    3. Wong-Baker faces pain rating scale.
    4. It is not necessary as infants do not feel pain as adults do.

11. **You are sending a child home on an oral medication. Appropriate discharge instructions on giving a medication would include which of the following? Select all that apply.**
    1. How to store the drug.
    2. The name of the medication.
    3. The reason the child is taking the medication.
    4. To stop taking the medication when the child feels better.
    5. Side-effects of the medication.
    6. Use a kitchen spoon to administer the medication.
    7. When to return for the next set of vaccinations.
    8. Written instructions.

12. **At a well-child visit, the child's mother mentions that some of the children at school have head lice. An appropriate response to her concern about head lice would be which of the following?**
    1. It is very easy to catch lice as they can easily jump from head to head.
    2. Instruct your child not to share hats or combs to prevent spread of the lice.
    3. Lice and nits do not survive away from the host.
    4. Your child will not get lice if you wash their hair well and keep it clean.

13. **Accidents, homicide, suicide, cancer, and heart disease are the leading causes of death in which age group?**
    1. Infant.
    2. Pre-school.
    3. School-age.
    4. Adolescent.

14. **Nurses who provide care that minimizes psychological and physical distress of hospitalized children and their families are practicing which type of care?**
    1. Atraumatic care.
    2. Family-centered care.
    3. Parent-professional partnership care.
    4. Therapeutic care.

15. **Erikson's theory on psychosocial development is one of the most widely accepted theories of personality development. Five of the eight stages relate to childhood. Please place them in order from birth through age 18.**
    1. Autonomy vs. shame and doubt.
    2. Industry vs. inferiority.
    3. Identity vs. role confusion.
    4. Initiative vs. guilt.
    5. Trust vs. mistrust.

16. The most common sex chromosome abnormality is known as which of the following?
1. Down syndrome.
2. Fragile X syndrome.
3. Klinefelter syndrome.
4. Turner syndrome.

17. Which of the following is the primary area involved in Kawasaki disease (mucotaneous lymph node syndrome)?
1. Cardiovascular system.
2. Gastrointestinal system.
3. Integumentary system.
4. Respiratory system.

18. Which of the following is an example of a neural tube defect?
1. Cerebral palsy.
2. Hydrocephalus.
3. Muscular dystrophy.
4. Spina bifida.

19. In caring for a child with acute glomerulonephritis, the most important nursing intervention(s) would be which of the following?
1. Daily weight, and blood pressure every four hours.
2. Monitor intake and output.
3. A restricted sodium diet.
4. Strict bedrest.

20. The major nursing priority of a child with suspected bacterial meningitis is which of the following?
1. Administer the antibiotic as soon as it is ordered.
2. Keep environmental stimuli to a minimum.
3. Obtain vital signs.
4. Record accurate intake and output.

21. What is the most common malignant renal and intra-abdominal tumor of childhood?
1. Ewing sarcoma.
2. Osteosarcoma.
3. Neuroblastoma.
4. Wilm's tumor.

22. A 6-month-old with sudden acute abdominal pain, vomiting, distended abdomen, and red currant jelly-like stools is exhibiting the classic signs for which of the following?
1. Appendicitis.
2. Hernia.
3. Intussusception.
4. Pyloric stenosis.

23. A 24-month-old is just diagnosed with celiac disease, or celiac sprue. The mother asks what food would still be acceptable to feed her child. What would your answer be?
1. Barley.
2. Oats.
3. Rice.
4. Wheat.

24. Most children begin to speak their first words at which of the following ages?
1. 6 months.
2. 12 months.
3. 18 months.
4. 24 months.

25. One of the major adjustments a child may experience following the divorce of parents is an adjustment to which of the following?
1. Relatives.
2. Siblings.
3. Synchronicity.
4. Transitions.

26. You are going down the stairs behind a little boy who is placing both feet on each step as he goes while holding the railing. How old is he?
1. 3 years old.
2. 4 years old.
3. 5 years old.
4. 6 years old.

27. By what age do children develop reciprocity in their friendships?

1. 6 years old.
2. 8 years old.
3. 10 years old.
4. 12 years old.

28. Which hormone is responsible for the onset of menstrual flow?

1. Estrogen.
2. Follicle-stimulating hormone (FSH).
3. Luteinizing hormone (LH).
4. Progesterone.

29. Which of the following has the greatest influence on an adolescent's decision to smoke cigarettes?

1. Advertisements showing celebrities smoking.
2. Having friends who smoke.
3. Having good social skills.
4. Having parents who smoke.

30. By what age can children typically ride a 2-wheel bike?

1. 5 years.
2. 7 years.
3. 9 years.
4. 11 years.

31. Which of the following is an example of a 4-year-old's concept of self?

1. "I am a better swimmer than my brother."
2. "I am better at drawing than at coloring."
3. "I like to swim."
4. "People like me because I play fair."

32. At what point after birth do typical infants double their birth weight?

1. 3 months.
2. 6 months.
3. 9 months.
4. 12 months.

33. Place an X on the site where you would give an intramuscular (IM) injection to an 8-month-old.

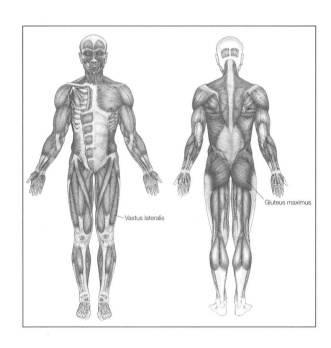

34. Draw a line at the appropriate spot where you would measure head circumference on a 9-month-old.

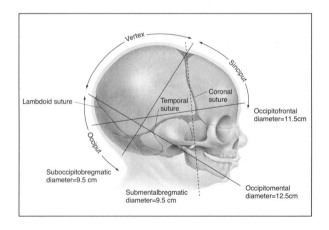

35. A 6-year-old has just been diagnosed with group A beta-hemolytic streptococci (GABHS). A general nursing consideration would be which of the following?

1. Cold or warm compresses to the neck do not provide relief.
2. Continue to take the prescribed antibiotic until symptoms disappear.
3. Discard the child's toothbrush and replace it with a new one after taking the prescribed antibiotic for 24 hours.
4. The child should not return to school for 48 hours after taking the prescribed antibiotic.

36. **Whooping cough or**

_____

is an acute respiratory infection that occurs in children younger than 4 years of age who have not been immunized.

1. Haemophilus influenza.
2. Mycoplasma pneumoniae.
3. Pertussis.
4. Tuberculosis.

37. **A new mother voices concern about sudden infant death syndrome (SIDS). Which of the following would be a correct instruction for her?**

1. Placing her child on the back when sleeping will decrease the risk of SIDS.
2. SIDS is directly correlated to diphtheria, tetanus, and pertussis vaccines.
3. SIDS rates have been rising over the last 10 years.
4. Sleep apnea is the main cause of SIDS.

38. **Congenital aganglionic megacolon or**

_____ **is a mechanical obstruction caused by inadequate motility of part of the intestine. There is absence of ganglion cells in one or more segments of the colon.**

1. Encoporesis.
2. Enterocolitis.
3. Functional constipation.
4. Hirschsprung disease.

39. **What is the calculated absolute neutrophil count (ANC) for the child with the following values: white blood cell (WBC) = 1000, neutrophils = 7%, nonsegmented neutrophils (bands) = 7%?**

1. 14.
2. 140.
3. 1400.
4. 14000.

Mental Health

1. Clozapine (Clozaril) is contraindicated in clients who have which of the following conditions?
   1. Bone marrow depression.
   2. Dry eye syndrome.
   3. Hypertension.
   4. Urinary retention.

2. You are assessing a client on chlorpromazine (Thorazine) for extrapyramidal side effects (EPSEs). EPSEs include which of the following? Select all that apply.
   1. Acute dystonia.
   2. Akasthisia.
   3. Amenorrhea.
   4. Breast secretions.
   5. Dyskinesia.
   6. Parkinsonism.
   7. Sexual dysfunction.

3. A client's psychotropic medication was changed two weeks ago. The nurse finds the client experiencing symptoms of muscle rigidity, hyperpyrexia, and diaphoresis. The nurse recognizes that these are symptoms of a severe life-threatening side effect of all psychotropic medication known as

   _____.

4. When assessing a client taking clozapine (Clozaril) for side effects, what side effects does the nurse see most commonly?
   1. Agranulocytosis and blood dyscrasias.
   2. Anticholinergic symptoms and increased serum prolactin levels.
   3. Dystonias and akasthisia.
   4. Weight gain and sedation.

5. Which statement by a client taking clozapine (Clozaril) indicates that the client needs more teaching about the drug?
   1. "I can continue to smoke without any effects on my medication."
   2. "I should keep my medication in a dry place at room temperature."
   3. "I will report flu symptoms immediately to my psychiatrist."
   4. "If I miss a dose, I will take the next scheduled dose as prescribed."

6. The nurse is evaluating the effectiveness of psychotropic medication on negative symptoms of psychosis. The nurse looks for a decrease in which of the following?
   1. Affective flattening.
   2. Bizarre behavior.
   3. Illogicality.
   4. Somatic delusions.

7. The nurse is administering antidepressant medication to clients. What is a major difference between the selective serotonin reuptake inhibitors (SSRIs) and the tricyclic antidepressants (TCAs)?
   1. SSRIs are more effective than TCAs in relieving depressive symptoms.
   2. SSRIs have more sedative effects than TCAs.
   3. TCAs are lethal in overdose while SSRIs are relatively safe.
   4. TCAs have fewer cardiovascular effects than SSRIs.

8. **The most important nursing intervention for serotonin syndrome is which of the following?**
   1. Administration of an anticonvulsant.
   2. Administration of a muscle relaxant for myoclonus.
   3. Discontinuation of serotonergic drugs.
   4. Immediately initiate body cooling procedures.

9. **The waiting time between stopping a monoamine oxidase inhibitor (MAOI) and starting a tricyclic (TCA) antidepressant is which of the following?**
   1. At least four weeks.
   2. Between four and six weeks.
   3. Determined by taking an MAOI blood level.
   4. Determined by the half-life of the MAOI.

10. **When assessing a hallucinating client, the nurse recognizes that which of the following hallucinations are commonly associated with schizophrenia? Select all that apply.**
    1. Auditory.
    2. Gustatory.
    3. Olfactory.
    4. Somatic.
    5. Tactile.

11. **When assessing a client for presence of alcohol withdrawal delirium, the nurse watches for which of the following? Select all that apply.**
    1. Disorientation.
    2. Distractibility.
    3. Grandiosity.
    4. Paranoid delusions.
    5. Pressure of speech.
    6. Tremors.

12. **When distinguishing between a client condition of depression or anxiety, the nurse recognizes that which of the following appears only in the anxious client?**
    1. Sleep disturbances.
    2. Gastrointestinal complaints.
    3. Irritability.
    4. Seeing some prospect for the future.

13. **The nurse, working with a violent client, assures the client that the staff will not allow the client to hurt herself and/or others. The nurse recognizes the rationale for this assurance is which of the following?**
    1. It empowers the client to use self-control.
    2. It promotes a sense of safety.
    3. It promotes behavior shaping.
    4. It protects self-esteem.

14. **An appropriate goal for a client experiencing Cluster B dramatic-emotional personality disorder (PD) is which of the following?**
    1. Demonstrate a decreased incidence of impulsive acts.
    2. Identify behaviors that maximize social interaction.
    3. Make decisions independently.
    4. Participate in activity groups.

15. **During a family assessment, the nurse finds that the two children are frequently forced to join one or the other of the parents in a coalition against the other. What is this type of coalition existing in the family called?**
    1. Enmeshment.
    2. Disengagement.
    3. Schism.
    4. Skew.

16. **When assessing for the appropriateness of spiritual interventions, the nurse is aware that they are contraindicated in psychiatric care when clients are demonstrating which of the following behavior(s)? Select all that apply.**

1. Delusional.
2. Depressed.
3. Phobic.
4. Psychotic.
5. Suicidal.

17. **A delusional client states, "I can't go to group today. I am expecting a high level official to visit today!" The nurse responds, "I understand, John, but it is time for group and we expect everyone to attend. Let's walk over together." Why is this nurse's response considered therapeutic?**
    1. It clearly articulates what is expected.
    2. It demonstrates empathy.
    3. It sets limits on manipulative behavior.
    4. It uses reflection.

18. **"The client will have a decrease in the urge to sleep." This is an appropriate goal for a client experiencing which of the following?**
    1. Narcolepsy.
    2. Primary hypersomnia.
    3. Primary insomnia.
    4. Sleep apnea.

19. **The nurse is educating an alcoholic client about alcohol withdrawal (prevention, signs, and treatment). What statement indicates that the client understands?**
    1. "I do not expect signs of delirium tremens (DTs) until five days after I stop drinking."
    2. "Disulfiram (Antabuse) will block my craving for alcohol."
    3. "I will keep my fluid intake to 3,000 ml each day."
    4. "I will keep up my vitamins, especially vitamin C."

20. **When are the courts are most likely to uphold a psychiatric client's right to refuse treatment?**

1. When the benefits of the treatment outweigh the risks.
2. When the side effects of the treatment exist but are temporary.
3. When there are religious reasons for the refusal.
4. When the client is competent but involuntarily committed.

21. **Psychiatric mental health nursing advocacy intervention strategies include which of the following?**
    1. Encouraging client feedback about satisfaction with the hospital experience.
    2. Explaining unit rules and policies regarding unacceptable behaviors.
    3. Making sure clients have the necessary knowledge to give informed consent.
    4. Making sure clients understand expectations for client participation.

22. **When planning care for a client experiencing rapid cycling of mania, the nurse recognizes that treatment begins with which of the following?**
    1. An antidepressant and a mood stabilizer.
    2. A mood stabilizer alone.
    3. A mood stabilizer plus an atypical antidepressant.
    4. A mood stabilizer plus a diuretic.

23. **When planning nursing care for the alcoholic client, the nurse realizes that all of the following goals will need to be met. Put the goals in the order you would expect them to be met from short-range to long-range.**
    1. The client will acknowledge alcohol dependence and need for treatment.
    2. The client will rebuild damaged interpersonal relationships.
    3. The client will identify alternative strategies for managing anxiety.
    4. The client will implement alternative strategies for managing anxiety.
    5. The client's withdrawal from alcohol will be managed successfully.

24. Confidential information can be released without the client's written consent in which of the following situations?

1. Commitment proceedings request.
2. Insurance company request.
3. Police request.
4. Previous therapist request.

25. A client has been on a typical antipsychotic fluphenazine (Prolixin) for 12 months. When the client comes into the Community Mental Health Center, the nurse observes that the client has fine, worm-like tongue movements. Which of the following might this behavior indicate?

1. A drug–food reaction, probably to grapefruit juice.
2. The client has missed several doses of medication.
3. Early symptoms of neuroleptic malignant syndrome (NMS).
4. Early symptoms of tardive dyskinesia (TD).

26. A client's blood lithium level is 1.5 mEq/L. The nurse evaluates this lab value to indicate which of the following about the level?

1. It is at the maintenance treatment level.
2. It is at the toxic blood level.
3. It is under the therapeutic treatment level.
4. It is within the therapeutic treatment level.

27. When assessing a crisis situation, the nurse realizes that which of the following important balancing factors are helpful in positively resolving the crisis? Select all that apply.

1. Behavioral reinforcement.
2. Catharsis.
3. Coping mechanisms.
4. Perception of the event.
5. Raising self esteem.
6. Situational support.

28. The Mini Mental State Examination (MMSE) is used to assess which of the following?

1. Delirium.
2. Dementia.
3. Orientation.
4. Thinking.

29. What is an appropriate short-term goal for anxiety control in a client experiencing obsessive compulsive disorder?

1. The client will consistently control the physical effects of anxiety.
2. The client will identify his own patterns of hyperventilation.
3. The client will begin breathing exercising when breaths exceed 14 per minute.
4. The client will use problem-solving rather than worry.

30. Of the following descriptions, which is a piece of family systems data?

1. Descriptions of developmental stages of the family.
2. Descriptions of difficulties for caring for sick members.
3. Descriptions of family alliances.
4. Descriptions of gender, age, religion, and ethnicity.

31. When planning nursing care for a client on a monoamine oxidase inhibitor (MAOI), which of the following should the nurse realize?

1. MAOIs are fairly safe in overdose.
2. The client may have problems with addiction.
3. The client will have a decreased ability to use vitamin B_6.
4. Tolerance to therapeutic effect may occur.

32. **What is true about the reporting of child abuse in most states?**
    1. Abuse evidence must exist.
    2. Reporting is voluntary.
    3. Reporting should occur within 72 hours of discovery.
    4. Suspicion of abuse exists.

33. **A senior nursing student has experienced the sudden death of his wife. He has a 5-year-old son. The student feels paralyzed in his ability to cope with school and family. The type of crisis the student is experiencing is**

    _____.

34. **Benzodiazepines are contraindicated in clients with a history of which of the following?**
    1. Alcohol abuse.
    2. Drug withdrawal.
    3. Seizure disorder.
    4. Suicide attempts.

35. **What statement by the schizophrenic client indicates skill for managing a relapse?**
    1. "I can remember when my hallucinations first began."
    2. "I know which of my hallucinations trigger a relapse."
    3. "I record the number of hallucinations I have each day."
    4. "I will seek out a staff person when I hallucinate."

36. **When assessing a schizophrenic client for memory deficit, what should the nurse look for?**
    1. Concrete thinking.
    2. Difficulty completing a task.
    3. Environmental disinterest.
    4. Time management problems.

37. **Which statement by a schizophrenic client indicates improvement in the core problem of concrete thinking?**
    1. "I know that most problems have more than one solution."
    2. "I need to work on things one step at a time."
    3. "I will try to avoid large crowds."
    4. "I will try to focus on the most important information."

38. **A client professes a deep and everlasting love for his girlfriend. The next day in a college class they both take he ignores her. The nurse recognizes this behavior as displaying which of the following?**
    1. Repression.
    2. Splitting.
    3. Sublimation.
    4. Undoing.

39. **When working with an anxious client, the nurse recognizes that which of the following defense mechanisms is primary and may need to be reinforced by other ego mechanisms of defense?**
    1. Dissociation.
    2. Isolation.
    3. Regression.
    4. Repression.

Unit 6 Answers and Rationales

Test 20 Answers and Rationales

1. **Answer: 4**
   Rationale: Fetal heart tones are best heard directly over the fetal back. The long, smooth surface palpated in the mother's right side is the fetal back. The firm, movable fetal part palpated in the upper portion of the uterus is the fetal head, meaning that the fetus is in a breech position. Therefore, the fetal heart tones would be auscultated in the maternal upper right quadrant.
   Cognitive Level: Application
   Nursing Process: Assessment
   NCLEX-RN Test Plan: HPM
   Reference: Lowdermilk, D. L., & Perry, S. E. (2004). *Maternity and women's health care* (8th ed). St. Louis, MO: Mosby.

2. **Answer: 4**
   Rationale: The effects of progesterone on the GI tract include relaxation of the cardiac sphincter and delayed gastric emptying. Increased pancreatic activity during pregnancy does not cause fat intolerance. Estrogen production causes a decrease in secretion of hydrochloric acid. The growing uterus causes pressure on the stomach and intestines, causing constipation.
   Cognitive Level: Analysis
   Nursing Process: Implementation
   NCLEX-RN Test Plan: HPM
   Reference: Lowdermilk, D. L., & Perry, S. E. (2004). *Maternity and women's health care* (8th ed.). St. Louis, MO: Mosby.

3. **Answer: 1**
   Rationale: 0-1-2-2 describes her present status. She has not carried a pregnancy to term (T); one pregnancy terminated in the preterm (P) birth of twins; two pregnancies ended in abortion (A); and she has two living children (L).
   Cognitive Level: Analysis
   Nursing Process: Analysis
   NCLEX-RN Test Plan: HPM
   Reference: Lowdermilk, D. L., & Perry, S. E. (2004). *Maternity and women's health care* (8th ed.). St. Louis, MO: Mosby.

4. **Answer: 1**
   Rationale: The heart beat is audible by doppler at 12 weeks. At week 20, lanugo covers the entire body and begins to disappear by week 36. The sex of the baby is determined at conception. Feeling the baby move is called quickening, and begins between weeks 16 and 20.
   Cognitive Level: Application
   Nursing Process: Implementation
   NCLEX-RN Test Plan: HPM
   Reference: Lowdermilk, D. L., & Perry, S. E. (2004). *Maternity and women's health care* (8th ed.). St. Louis, MO: Mosby.

5. **Answer: Mark just below the umbilicus**
   Rationale: The uterus rises to just below the umbilicus at about 20 weeks gestation. The uterus may be palpated above the symphysis pubis between the 12th and 14th weeks of pregnancy. It reaches the xyphoid process at term.
   Cognitive Level: Application
   Nursing Process: Assessment
   NCLEX-RN Test Plan: HPM
   Reference: Lowdermilk, D. L., & Perry, S. E. (2004). *Maternity and women's health care* (8th ed.). St. Louis, MO: Mosby.

6. **Answer: 1**
   Rationale: The estimated date of birth is February 11, 2008.

Date of LMP	5	4	2007
	− 3 months	+ 7 days	+ 1 year
EDB	2	11	2008

   Cognitive Level: Application
   Nursing Process: Analysis
   NCLEX-RN Test Plan: HPM
   Reference: Lowdermilk, D. L., & Perry, S. E. (2004). *Maternity and women's health care* (8th ed.). St. Louis, MO: Mosby.

7. **Answer: 1**
   Rationale: Quickening is a presumptive sign of pregnancy. Those feelings may also be associated with gas or peristalsis. Probable signs of pregnancy

include positive serum and urine pregnancy tests, Chadwick's sign, and Goodell's sign. Positive signs of pregnancy include fetal heart tones detected by Doppler and fetal stethoscope, and fetal movements palpated by an examiner. Signs of pregnancy are identified as presumptive, probable, or positive. No signs are identified as possible.

Cognitive Level: Analysis

Nursing Process: Implementation

NCLEX-RN Test Plan: HPM

Reference: Lowdermilk, D. L., & Perry, S. E. (2004). *Maternity and women's health care* (8th ed.). St. Louis, MO: Mosby.

8. **Answer: 2**

Rationale: The client is experiencing symptoms of respiratory alkalosis due to hyperventilation. The client needs to rebreathe carbon dioxide and replace the bicarbonate ion rather than receive more oxygen. It is not necessary to notify the physician at this time. Telling the client to slow her breathing rate will not help relieve her symptoms.

Cognitive Level: Application

Nursing Process: Implementation

NCLEX-RN Test Plan: HPM

Reference: Lowdermilk, D. L., & Perry, S. E. (2004). *Maternity and women's health care* (8th ed.). St. Louis, MO: Mosby.

9. **Answer: 1**

Rationale: This is a late deceleration and is associated with insufficient placental perfusion. This is considered an ominous sign, not benign. Although a scalp electrode may need to be inserted for a more accurate internal assessment, the client's position should be changed first in order to displace the weight of the uterus off the vena cava. This increases maternal circulation to the placenta. Amnioinfusion is indicated for umbilical cord compression, decreased amniotic fluid, or to dilute meconium-stained amniotic fluid.

Cognitive Level: Analysis

Nursing Process: Implementation

NCLEX-RN Test Plan: HPM

Reference: Lowdermilk, D. L., & Perry, S. E. (2004). *Maternity and women's health care* (8th ed.). St. Louis, MO: Mosby.

10. **Answer: 3**

Rationale: According to the gate control theory, pain sensations travel along nerve pathways to the brain. Only a limited number of sensations can travel along these pathways at one time. Distraction techniques, such as massage, reduce or block the nerve pathways transmitting pain. Although the other nursing actions are appropriate for a laboring client who is experiencing discomfort, they do not address the gate control theory.

Cognitive Level: Analysis

Nursing Process: Implementation

NCLEX-RN Test Plan: HPM

Reference: Lowdermilk, D. L., & Perry, S. E. (2004). *Maternity and women's health care* (8th ed.). St. Louis, MO: Mosby.

11. **Answer: 4**

Rationale: Naloxone (Narcan) reverses opioid-induced respiratory depression in the newborn. Beractant (Survanta) is a lung surfactant used to prevent and treat respiratory distress in premature infants due to immature lungs. Fentanyl (Sublimaze) is an opioid analgesic given to the laboring client. Betamethasone stimulates fetal lung maturation by promoting the release of enzymes that enhance the production of lung surfactant.

Cognitive Level: Analysis

Nursing Process: Analysis

NCLEX-RN Test Plan: HPM

Reference: Lowdermilk, D. L., & Perry, S. E. (2004). *Maternity and women's health care* (8th ed.). St. Louis, MO: Mosby.

12. **Answer: 1**

Rationale: Dilation of the cervix is the widening of the cervical opening measured in cm from closed to approximately 10 cm (full dilation). Effacement refers to the shortening and thinning of the cervix. Degree of effacement is stated in terms of percentages from 0 to 100%. Station is the relation of the presenting part of the fetus to an imaginary line drawn between the ischial spines in the maternal pelvis. The degree of descent is noted in centimeters that is either above, below, or at the level of the spines. If the station is −1, then the presenting part is 1 cm above the ischial spines.

Cognitive Level: Application

Nursing Process: Analysis

NCLEX-RN Test Plan: HPM

Reference: Lowdermilk, D. L., & Perry, S. E. (2004). *Maternity and women's health care* (8th ed.). St. Louis, MO: Mosby.

13. **Answer: 4**

Rationale: With the sacrum as the presenting part, the fetus is in a breech presentation. Breech presentation is the most common form of malpresentation, which is considered a complication of labor. A longitudinal fetal lie, general flexion, and gynecoid maternal pelvis are considered normal.

Cognitive Level: Application

Nursing Process: Analysis

NCLEX-RN Test Plan: HPM

Reference: Lowdermilk, D. L., & Perry, S. E. (2004). *Maternity and women's health care* (8th ed.). St. Louis, MO: Mosby.

14. **Answer: 2, 1, 3, 7, 5, 6, 4**

Rationale: The seven cardinal movements of the mechanism of labor that occur in a vertex presentation are engagement, descent, flexion, internal rotation, extension, external rotation, and expulsion.

Cognitive Level: Application

Nursing Process: Analysis

NCLEX-RN Test Plan: HPM

Reference: Lowdermilk, D. L., & Perry, S. E. (2004). *Maternity and women's health care* (8th ed.). St. Louis, MO: Mosby.

15. **Answer: 2**

Rationale: Fetal heart rate is of primary concern because the environment for the fetus has changed. There is an increased risk for prolapse of the umbilical cord immediately after rupture of the membranes. The client's blood pressure and temperature should not be affected by rupture of the membranes. Although frequency of contractions may increase after rupture of membranes, the fetal response is of primary concern.

Cognitive Level: Application

Nursing Process: Implementation

NCLEX-RN Test Plan: HPM

Reference: Lowdermilk, D. L., & Perry, S. E. (2004). *Maternity and women's health care* (8th ed.). St. Louis, MO: Mosby.

16. **Answer: 4**

Rationale: Restricted activity and a quiet environment are employed to decrease stimuli. Reflexes are assessed to determine if there is increased central nervous system activity. Weighing the client will help determine if further edema is occurring. A nonstress test may be performed to establish fetal well-being.

Cognitive Level: Analysis

Nursing Process: Planning

NCLEX-RN Test Plan: HPM

Reference: Lowdermilk, D. L., & Perry, S. E. (2004). *Maternity and women's health care* (8th ed.). St. Louis, MO: Mosby.

17. **Answer: 2**

Rationale: Painless vaginal bleeding is a clinical manifestation associated with placenta previa. Placental attachment is in the lower uterine segment and bleeding is associated with the stretching and thinning of this part of the uterus during the third trimester. Uterine pain and cramping are associated with abruptio placentae and preterm labor. Threatened abortion occurs in the first trimester of pregnancy.

Cognitive Level: Analysis

Nursing Process: Assessment

NCLEX-RN Test Plan: HPM

Reference: Lowdermilk, D. L., & Perry, S. E. (2004). *Maternity and women's health care* (8th ed.). St. Louis, MO: Mosby.

18. **Answers: 2, 3, 4, 6, and 7**

Rationale: Fetal breathing movements, fetal tone, gross body movements, and amniotic fluid index are assessed via ultrasound. A nonstress test indicates a reactive fetal heart rate. These five variables make up a biophysical profile indicating fetal well-being. A contraction stress test is an invasive procedure that is not part of the biophysical profile. Measurement of the biparietal diameter of the fetal skull is used to estimate fetal age.

Cognitive Level: Analysis

Nursing Process: Analysis

NCLEX-RN Test Plan: HPM

Reference: Lowdermilk, D. L., & Perry, S. E. (2004). *Maternity and women's health care* (8th ed.). St. Louis, MO: Mosby.

19. **Answer: 3**

    Rationale: High levels of alpha feto-protein in amniotic fluid help confirm the diagnosis of neural tube defects such as spina bifida. Conditions such as preterm labor, history of cardiac anomaly, and exposure to AIDS do not place a fetus at risk for neural tube defects.

    Cognitive Level: Analysis

    Nursing Process: Analysis

    NCLEX-RN Test Plan: HPM

    Reference: Lowdermilk, D. L., & Perry, S. E. (2004). *Maternity and women's health care* (8th ed.). St. Louis, MO: Mosby.

20. **Answer: 2**

    Rationale: Fetal heart rate should demonstrate two or more accelerations lasting for 15 seconds over a 20 minute period. Accelerations are accompanied by fetal movement. This is considered reactive. If the fetal heart rate does not accelerate or it decelerates, the nonstress test is considered nonreactive. A positive or negative test is interpreted when a contraction stress test is done.

    Cognitive Level: Analysis

    Nursing Process: Evaluation

    NCLEX-RN Test Plan: HPM

    Reference: Lowdermilk, D. L., & Perry, S. E. (2004). *Maternity and women's health care* (8th ed.). St. Louis, MO: Mosby.

21. **Answer: 3**

    Rationale: Ultrasonography will identify placement of the placenta and fetus. This will help to avoid accidental placement of the needle into the placenta or fetus. Although ultrasound may be used to assess the fetus, that is not the purpose of ultrasound prior to an amniocentesis.

    Cognitive Level: Analysis

    Nursing Process: Implementation

    NCLEX-RN Test Plan: HPM

    Reference: Lowdermilk, D. L., & Perry, S. E. (2004). *Maternity and women's health care* (8th ed.). St. Louis, MO: Mosby.

22. **Answer: 3**

    Rationale: Lecithin is the most critical pulmonary surfactant necessary for postnatal lung expansion. It increases after week 24. Sphingomyelin is another surfactant that remains constant. When the L/S ratio

reaches 2:1, the fetal lungs are considered to be mature. The presence, not absence, of another surfactant, phosphatidylglycerol, is also needed for adequate lung maturity. A reactive nonstress test and biophysical profile score of 8 indicate fetal well being, but is not helpful in determining fetal lung maturity.

Cognitive Level: Analysis

Nursing Process: Evaluation

NCLEX-RN Test Plan: HPM

Reference: Lowdermilk, D. L., & Perry, S. E. (2004). *Maternity and women's health care* (8th ed.). St. Louis, MO: Mosby.

23. **Answer: 3**

    Rationale: Evaporation is the loss of heat that occurs when a liquid is converted to a vapor. The newborn's skin is moist with amniotic fluid and blood from delivery and needs to be dried immediately to prevent heat loss due to evaporation.

    Cognitive Level: Application

    Nursing Process: Implementation

    NCLEX-RN Test Plan: HPM

    Reference: Lowdermilk, D. L., & Perry, S. E. (2004). *Maternity and women's health care* (8th ed.). St. Louis, MO: Mosby.

24. **Answer: 2**

    Rationale: The manifestations mentioned are indicative of a positive Moro reflex. The toes hyperextend when the lateral aspect of the sole is stroked to produce a positive Babinksi reflex. When the cheek is stroked, the newborn turns its head toward the stimulus, eliciting the rooting reflex. If the newborn's head is turned to one side, the infant will extend the arm and leg on that side. The opposite arm and leg will flex. This is characteristic of the tonic neck reflex.

    Cognitive Level: Application

    Nursing Process: Evaluation

    NCLEX-RN Test Plan: HPM

    Reference: Lowdermilk, D. L., & Perry, S. E. (2004). *Maternity and women's health care* (8th ed.). St. Louis, MO: Mosby.

25. **Answer: 2**

    Rationale: Caput succedaneum may occur with a vertex presentation due to sustained pressure and compression of local blood vessels. Cephalhematoma is a collection of blood between the skull and periosteum. It does not cross the suture line. Erythema toxicum is a transient newborn rash. Mongolian spots are bluish-black areas of pigmentation that may appear over any part of the exterior surface of the body.

Cognitive Level: Analysis

Nursing Process: Implementation

NCLEX-RN Test Plan: HPM

Reference: Lowdermilk, D. L., & Perry, S. E. (2004). *Maternity and women's health care* (8th ed.). St. Louis, MO: Mosby.

26. **Answer: 1**

Rationale: Maintaining the newborn's body temperature is critical to survival. Measures are taken to prevent cold stress, which forces metabolic and physiologic demands. The respiratory rate increases in response to increased oxygen demands. Heat production, called thermogenesis, occurs by metabolism of brown fat, which is found exclusively in the newborn. Tachycardia may indicate respiratory distress syndrome.

Cognitive Level: Application

Nursing Process: Implementation

NCLEX-RN Test Plan: HPM

Reference: Lowdermilk, D. L., & Perry, S. E. (2004). *Maternity and women's health care* (8th ed.). St. Louis, MO: Mosby.

27. **Answer: 4**

Rationale: A direct Coombs test measures the presence of maternal antibodies in the fetal blood. An indirect Coombs test is performed on the mother's blood to determine if she has developed antibodies to the Rh antigen. Although kernicterus is associated with Rh incompatibility, it is the development of encephalopathy secondary to hyperbilirubinemia.

Cognitive Level: Analysis

Nursing Process: Analysis

NCLEX-RN Test Plan: HPM

Reference: Lowdermilk, D. L., & Perry, S. E. (2004). *Maternity and women's health care* (8th ed.). St. Louis, MO: Mosby.

28. **Answers: 1, 3, 4, and 5**

Rationale: The infant of a diabetic mother is at risk for hypoglycemia, hypocalcemia, hyperbilirubinemia, and polycythemia. A direct Coombs test measures the presence of antibodies against the

newborn's red blood cells which is associated with Rh and ABO incompatibility. The measurement of white blood cell count in newborns is usually performed to determine the presence of infection.

Cognitive Level: Analysis

Nursing Process: Planning

NCLEX-RN Test Plan: HPM

Reference: Lowdermilk, D. L., & Perry, S. E. (2004). *Maternity and women's health care* (8th ed.). St. Louis, MO: Mosby.

29. **Answer: 2**

Rationale: Airway obstruction is always a priority. The newborn needs to maintain an effective breathing pattern in order to survive. Although the other nursing diagnoses need to be addressed when caring for the newborn, oxygenation is a priority.

Cognitive Level: Analysis

Nursing Process: Planning

NCLEX-RN Test Plan: HPM

Reference: Lowdermilk, D. L., & Perry, S. E. (2004). *Maternity and women's health care* (8th ed.). St. Louis: Mosby.

30. **Answer: 8**

Rationale: The Apgar score is 8. The Apgar score is a quick assessment performed at one and five minutes after birth to help determine the need for resuscitation. It is based on five signs that indicated the newborn's physiological state. Heart rate over 100 = 2; respiratory rate of a slow, weak cry = 1; muscle tone with some flexion of extremities = 1; reflex irritability based on crying response to gentle taps on soles of the feet = 2; and pink color = 2.

Cognitive Level: Application

Nursing Process: Analysis

NCLEX-RN Test Plan: HPM

Reference: Lowdermilk, D. L., & Perry, S. E. (2004). *Maternity and women's health care* (8th ed.). St. Louis, MO: Mosby.

31. **Answer: Lochia rubra**

Rationale: Lochia rubra consists of blood and decidual debris lasting about three days after delivery. The lochia then becomes pink or brown and can last up to 22 to 27 days after childbirth. Lochia alba is a yellow to white color drainage. In most women, lochia alba occurs about 10 days after delivery.

Cognitive Level: Analysis

Nursing Process: Analysis
NCLEX-RN Test Plan: HPM
Reference: Lowdermilk, D. L., & Perry, S. E. (2004). *Maternity and women's health care* (8th ed.). St. Louis, MO: Mosby.

32. **Answer: 1**
Rationale: Immediately after delivery, the fundus is about 2 cm below the level of the umbilicus. Within 12 hours, the fundus is approximately 1 cm above the level of the umbilicus. The fundus descends about 1 to 2 cm every 24 hours.
Cognitive Level: Application
Nursing Process: Assessment
NCLEX-RN Test Plan: HPM
Reference: Lowdermilk, D. L., & Perry, S. E. (2004). *Maternity and women's health care* (8th ed.). St. Louis, MO: Mosby.

33. **Answer: 2**
Rationale: The uterus is slightly boggy and displaced due to a distended bladder. Therefore, the client is at risk for hemorrhage. Whether or not the client had anesthesia is unknown. Although options 1 and 4 may be true, they are not specific to the assessment findings.
Cognitive Level: Analysis
Nursing Process: Analysis
NCLEX-RN Test Plan: HPM
Reference: Lowdermilk, D. L., & Perry, S. E. (2004). *Maternity and women's health care* (8th ed.). St. Louis, MO: Mosby.

34. **Answer: 1**
Rationale: The displacement of the uterus is a sign that the bladder is probably distended. Having the client void and reassessing the fundus is the appropriate nursing action. The fundus is firm so there is no need to massage it. The displaced fundus is not considered a normal finding. Ambulating the client will not help the fundus return to midline.
Cognitive Level: Application
Nursing Process: Implementation
NCLEX-RN Test Plan: HPM
Reference: Lowdermilk, D. L., & Perry, S. E. (2004). *Maternity and women's health care* (8th ed.). St. Louis, MO: Mosby.

35. **Answer: 4**
Rationale: Puerperal infection, retained placenta and an unrepaired vaginal laceration may lead to postpartum hemorrhage, but the client's history of an overdistended uterus secondary to a large fetus and an oxytocin-induced labor put this client at risk for uterine atony. Other risk factors for uterine atony include high parity, general anesthesia, and trauma during labor such as forceps, vacuum, or Cesarean birth.
Cognitive Level: Analysis
Nursing Process: Analysis
NCLEX-RN Test Plan: HPM
Reference: Lowdermilk, D. L., & Perry, S. E. (2004). *Maternity and women's health care* (8th ed.). St. Louis, MO: Mosby.

36. **Answer: 3**
Rationale: Vital signs may not be reliable indicators of shock in the immediate postpartum period due to physiologic adaptations that are occurring. First, the fundus needs to be assessed to determine its tone. Further nursing actions will be determined based on assessment of the fundus.
Cognitive Level: Analysis
Nursing Process: Planning
NCLEX-RN Test Plan: HPM
Reference: Lowdermilk, D. L., & Perry, S. E. (2004). *Maternity and women's health care* (8th ed.). St. Louis, MO: Mosby.

37. **Answers: 1, 3, 5, and 6**
Rationale: The nursing diagnoses of acute pain related to postpartum physiologic changes; disturbed sleep patterns related to excitement, discomfort and newborn needs; risk for deficient fluid volume related to uterine atony/hemorrhage; and risk for impaired urinary elimination related to perineal trauma are appropriate for a normal vaginal delivery. There is no need for the client to be on bed rest or to be separated from her newborn. In an uncomplicated vaginal delivery, the client should not experience hemorrhage.
Cognitive Level: Analysis
Nursing Process: Planning
NCLEX-RN Test Plan: HPM
Reference: Lowdermilk, D. L., & Perry, S. E. (2004). *Maternity and women's health care* (8th ed.). St. Louis, MO: Mosby.

38. **Answer: 2**

    Rationale: Caloric requirements are higher during lactation than during pregnancy. An additional 500 kcal is recommended. Folic acid and iron requirements are lower during lactation as compared to pregnancy due to a decrease in maternal blood volume. Calcium needs remain about the same.

    Cognitive Level: Application

    Nursing Process: Implementation

    NCLEX-RN Test Plan: HPM

    Reference: Lowdermilk, D. L., & Perry, S. E. (2004). *Maternity and women's health care* (8th ed.) St. Louis, MO: Mosby.

39. **Answer: 2**

    Rationale: Disseminated intravascular coagulation (DIC) is a clotting disorder that may occur due to conditions such as abruptio placentae, amniotic fluid embolism, and septicemia. Petechiae and bleeding at the IV site are clinical manifestations associated with DIC. Amniotic fluid embolism occurs when particles such as vernix or meconium enter the maternal circulation. Signs and symptoms include respiratory distress and circulatory collapse. Preeclampsia is a syndrome specific to pregnancy associated with gestational hypertension and proteinurea. An elevated temperature of 38°C or more on two consecutive days may indicate puerperal infection, usually due to streptococcal and anaerobic organisms.

    Cognitive Level: Analysis

    Nursing Process: Planning

    NCLEX-RN Test Plan: HPM

    Reference: Lowdermilk, D. L., & Perry, S. E. (2004). *Maternity and women's health care* (8th ed.). St. Louis, MO: Mosby.

Unit 6 Answers and Rationales

Test 21 Answers and Rationales

1. **Answer: 3**
   Rationale: PCOS is treated with oral contraceptives, glucophage (Metformin) and Clomid (Clomiphene). The oral contraceptives are used to treat menstrual irregularities and acne. Glucophage (Metformin) is used to improve insulin uptake by the fat and muscle cells and treats hyperinsulinemia. Ovulation induction agents (Clomid) are used to treat infertility.
   Cognitive Level: Application
   Nursing Process: Planning
   NCLEX-RN Test Plan: PHYS
   Reference: Ricci, S. S. (2007). *Essentials of maternity, newborn, and women's health nursing.* Philadelphia: Lippincott Williams & Wilkins.

2. **Answer: 3 and 4**
   Rationale: The woman should limit her daily fluid intake to 1.5 liters per day. She should also reduce the intake of fluids and foods that may be irritating to the bladder, such as chocolate, caffeine, carbonated beverages, alcohol, orange juice, tomatoes, watermelon, artificial sweeteners, and hot spicy foods. Constipation can be avoided by increasing fiber and fluids in her diet. Performing Kegel exercises will help strengthen the pelvic floor.
   Cognitive Level: Application
   Nursing Process: Implementation
   NCLEX-RN Test Plan: PHYS
   Reference: Ricci, S. S. (2007). *Essentials of maternity, newborn, and women's health nursing.* Philadelphia: Lippincott Williams & Wilkins.

3. **Answer: 1**
   Rationale: Women often exhibit other concerns that may influence their decision to have reproductive surgery. These concerns are categorized as general concerns about surgery and specific concerns about the related gynecological surgery. The nurse needs to assess and explore any issues and concerns with their clients.
   Cognitive Level: Analysis

   Nursing Process: Assessment
   NCLEX-RN Test Plan: PSYC
   Reference: Olds, S. B., London, M. L., Ladewig, P. W., & Davidson, M. R. (2004). *Maternal-newborn nursing & women's health care* (7th ed.). Upper Saddle River, NJ: Pearson Prentice Hall.

4. **Answer: 3**
   Rationale: A pelvic examination consists of two phases: inspection of the vulva, vagina, and cervix using a speculum and palpation of the cervix, uterus, and ovaries via a bimanual examination. A pap smear is also obtained.
   Cognitive Level: Application
   Nursing Process: Implementation
   NCLEX-RN Test Plan: PHYS, PSYC
   Reference: Olds, S. B., London, M. L., Ladewig, P. W., & Davidson, M. R. (2004). *Maternal-newborn nursing & women's health care* (7th ed.). Upper Saddle River, NJ: Pearson Prentice Hall.

5. **Answer: 2**
   Rationale: Coronary artery disease (CAD) is the leading cause of death in American women over the age of 50. The most common presenting symptom of CAD in women is chest pain, which may present as atypical. Women presenting with chest pain, especially premenopausal women, are often diagnosed as anxious or reacting to stress and are denied a full cardiac workup. Symptoms of CAD may be vague and present as nausea, shortness of breath, dizziness, and fatigue, especially during physical activity, and may last only a few minutes. Because a woman's symptoms are often vague, healthcare providers may attribute these symptoms to depression. Depression is very common in women. However, persistent CAD symptoms warrant cardiac evaluation.
   Cognitive Level: Application
   Nursing Process: Implementation
   NCLEX-RN Test Plan: PHYS, PSYC
   Reference: Breslin, E., & Lucas, V. (2003). *Women's health nursing: Toward evidence-based practice.* St. Louis, MO: Saunders.

6. **Answer: 4**

   Rationale: An LDL/HDL ratio of 4 or less is considered acceptable. An LDL/HDL ratio of 6 or higher warrants an aggressive management approach.
   Cognitive Level: Analysis
   Nursing Process: Analysis
   NCLEX-RN Test Plan: PHYS
   Reference: Youngkin, E. Q., & Davis, M. S. (2004). *Women's health: A primary care clinical guide* (3rd ed.). Upper Saddle River, NJ: Pearson Prentice Hall.

7. **Answer: 3**

   Rationale: Modifiable risk factors for coronary artery disease (CAD) in women include cigarette smoking, physical inactivity, hypertension, and hyperlipidemia. Nonmodifiable risk factors for women are family history, age, gender, and diabetes.
   Cognitive Level: Application
   Nursing Process: Implementation
   NCLEX-RN Test Plan: HPM, PSYC
   Reference: Youngkin, E. Q., & Davis, M. S. (2004). *Women's health: A primary care clinical guide* (3rd ed.). Upper Saddle River, NJ: Pearson Prentice Hall.

8. **Answers: 1, 2, and 3**

   Rationale: A thorough pain history and identification of the characteristics of the client's pain will enable the nurse to plan for appropriate interventions. Educating the client about their medications will increase the client's understanding and help promote compliance with medication therapy. The establishment of regular toileting promotes bowel function and evacuation. Clients should be encouraged to increase fluids and fiber in their diet to promote peristalsis.
   Cognitive Level: Application
   Nursing Process: Planning
   NCLEX-RN Test Plan: PHYS
   Reference: Ricci, S. S. (2007). *Essentials of maternity, newborn, and women's health nursing.* Philadelphia: Lippincott Williams & Wilkins.

9. **Answers: 1, 2, and 3**

   Rationale: Kegel exercises strengthens pelvic muscles and prevents further prolapse. Pessories are used to maintain the normal position of the uterus or bladder by exerting pressure and providing sup-

port. Estrogen replacement therapy improves muscle tone and vascularity of supporting tissues in both perimenopausal and postmenopausal women. Lifestyle changes to prevent pelvic prolapse include the avoidance of high impact aerobic exercises and jogging.
   Cognitive Level: Analysis
   Nursing Process: Planning
   NCLEX-RN Test Plan: HPM, PHYS
   Reference: Youngkin, E. Q., & Davis, M. S. (2004). *Women's health: A primary care clinical guide* (3rd ed.). Upper Saddle River, NJ: Pearson Prentice Hall.

10. **Answer: 4**

    Rationale: Pelvic organ prolapse is often asymptomatic. When symptoms do occur, they are related to the site and type of prolapse. Symptoms common to all types of prolapse are a feeling of dragging, a lump in the vagina, or something coming down. Stress incontinence; incontinence of flatus and liquid or solid stool; and dyspareunia are specific site symptoms of prolapse.
    Cognitive Level: Analysis
    Nursing Process: Assessment
    NCLEX-RN Test Plan: HPM
    Reference: Ricci, S. S. (2007). *Essentials of maternity, newborn, and women's health nursing.* Philadelphia: Lippincott Williams & Wilkins.

11. **Answer: 3**

    Rationale: Raloxifene (Evista) is often prescribed for prevention of osteoporosis in postmenopausal women. Alendronate sodium (Fosamax) may be prescribed for women who already have osteoporosis to delay bone loss and increase bone mass. Synthroid is used to treat hypothyroidism, and vitamin E has no effect on bone loss or bone formation.
    Cognitive Level: Analysis
    Nursing Process: Planning
    NCLEX-RN Test Plan: HPM, PHYS
    Reference: Lowdermilk, D. L., & Perry, S. E. (2004). *Maternity & women's health care* (8th ed.). St. Louis, MO: Mosby.

12. **Answer: 3**

    Rationale: Including adequate amounts of calcium in the diet can prevent osteoporosis. Postmenopausal women need 1500 mg of calcium a day.

The body cannot use calcium without the right balance of vitamins and minerals. A combination supplement of calcium and vitamin D aids in the absorption of calcium. Good sources of calcium are dairy products, fish, oysters, tofu, dark green leafy vegetables, and whole wheat bread.
Cognitive Level: Application
Nursing Process: Implementation
NCLEX-RN Test Plan: HPM, PHYS
Reference: Lowdermilk, D. L., & Perry, S. E. (2004). *Maternity & women's health care* (8th ed.). St. Louis, MO: Mosby.

13. **Answer: 4**
    Rationale: Vitamin E 400–800 IU supplements or vitamin E applied directly to the skin can be used to relieve urogenital symptoms of dryness and itching, as an alternative to hormone replacement. Other alternative therapies include valerian to relieve insomnia, and parsley, which is a natural diuretic, to relieve headache. Dietary changes can also be used to decrease nervousness and irritability in menopausal symptomatic women. Walnuts, bran, and brown rice help to contribute to a healthy diet, but have no effect on menopausal symptoms of vaginal dryness.
    Cognitive Level: Application
    Nursing Process: Implementation
    NCLEX-RN Test Plan: HPM, PHYS
    Reference: Lowdermilk, D. L., & Perry, S. E. (2004). *Maternity & women's health care* (8th ed.). St. Louis, MO: Mosby.

14. **Answer: 1**
    Rationale: Most herbal preparations have not undergone testing for safety and efficacy. Benefits and risks are not completely known. Women should always discuss the use of these herbal products with their health care provider before beginning these therapies.
    Cognitive Level: Analysis
    Nursing Process: Planning
    NCLEX-RN Test Plan: HPM, PHYS
    Reference: Lowdermilk, D. L., & Perry, S. E. (2004). *Maternity & women's health care* (8th ed.). St. Louis, MO: Mosby.

15. **Answer: 1**
    Rationale: Bone mineral density measurements are typically used to measure bone density. One of the most common BMD studies is a DEXA scan, which measures bone density in the spine, hips, and forearms. These sites are the most common fracture sites in women. DEXA scans are considered to be the gold standard for diagnosing osteoporosis. Bone biopsy is an invasive test that can be used to differentiate the diagnosis of osteoporosis from osteomalacia, but is not commonly used for diagnosing osteoporosis in women. Spinal X-ray is not a good diagnostic tool for osteoporosis. Osteoporosis cannot be detected by radiographic examination until there has been a loss of 30–50% of the bone mass. CT (computed tomography) is a medical imaging method, which can be used to diagnose osteoporosis and to assess BMD. However, the results do not correlate with a DEXA scan, subjects receive higher levels of radiation, and it is more expensive.
    Cognitive Level: Analysis
    Nursing Process: Assessment
    NCLEX-RN Test Plan: HPM
    Reference: Lewis, S. M., Heitkemper, M. M., & Dirksen, S. R. (2004). *Medical-surgical nursing: Assessment and management of clinical problems* (6th ed.). St. Louis, MO: Mosby.

16. **Answer: 3**
    Rationale: Nonpregnant women with BV are at increased risk for pelvic inflammatory disease (PID), abnormal cervical cytology, postoperative cuff infections after a hysterectomy, and postabortion PID. Symptoms of BV include excessive amounts of thin watery white to gray vaginal discharge with a fishy odor. With endometriosis, endometrial tissue is located outside the uterus in the pelvic cavity. Uterine cancer symptoms usually present as vaginal bleeding, not watery drainage.
    Cognitive Level: Analysis
    Nursing Process: Assessment
    NCLEX-RN Test Plan: HPM
    Reference: Olds, S. B., London, M. L., Ladewig, P. W., & Davidson, M. R. (2004). *Maternal-newborn nursing & women's health care* (7th ed.) Upper Saddle River, NJ: Pearson Prentice Hall.

17. **Answer: 4**
    Rationale: Postprocedure hysteroscopy complications are infrequent. Postprocedure instructions do not usually include special diets such as liquid diets.

Clients should be informed to expect mild cramping or spotting and should not experience heavy bleeding, fever, or vaginal discharge with a foul odor. Douching, tampon use, and sexual intercourse may lead to infection after hysteroscopy and should be curtailed for a few weeks.
Cognitive Level: Application
Nursing Process: Planning
NCLEX-RN Test Plan: PHYS
Reference: Youngkin, E. Q., & Davis, M. S. (2004). *Women's health: A primary care clinical guide* (3rd ed.). Upper Saddle River, NJ: Pearson Prentice Hall.

18. **Answer: 1**
Rationale: A Ca-125 level is not suitable for mass screening for ovarian cancer. This test is only useful if a person has a high risk or if the tumor has suspicious characteristics on imaging because benign conditions (endometriosis) can cause a false positive result. Only certain types of ovarian cancers give elevations of Ca-125. Ca-125 is elevated in only 50% of cases of early stage ovarian cancer.
Cognitive Level: Analysis
Nursing Process: Assessment
NCLEX-RN Test Plan: PHYS
Reference: Condon, M. C. (2004). *Women's health: An integrated approach to wellness and illness.* Upper Saddle River, NJ: Prentice Hall.

19. **Answer: 2 and 3**
Rationale: Reduced rates of ovarian cancer are found in women who have had one or more term pregnancies, have breast fed, used oral contraceptives, and have undergone tubal sterilization or removal of the uterus and ovaries. Risk factors for uterine cancer are obesity, high fat diet, history of infertility, early menarche, late onset of menopause, absence of childbearing, hypertension, and obesity. Exercise has not been associated with uterine cancer risk. Exercise is recognized as a preventative lifestyle measure. Herbal use and diet have not been associated with uterine bleeding. Hyper estrogenic states increase the risk of endometrial hyperplasia, which over time can convert to uterine cancer.
Cognitive Level: Analysis
Nursing Process: Intervention
NCLEX-RN Test Plan: HPM

Reference: Condon, M. C. (2004). *Women's health: An integrated approach to wellness and illness.* Upper Saddle River, NJ: Prentice Hall.

20. **Answers: 1, 2, and 3**
Rationale: Any bleeding in a postmenopausal woman should be evaluated. Women who take unopposed estrogen (no progesterone) are at increased risk for uterine cancer. The use of SERMs (anticancer medications such as tamoxifen) has been associated with uterine cancer.
Cognitive Level: Analysis
Nursing Process: Assessment
NCLEX-RN Test Plan: PHYS
Reference: Condon, M. C. (2004). *Women's health: An integrated approach to wellness and illness.* Upper Saddle River, NJ: Prentice Hall.

21. **Answer: 1**
Rationale: Side effects that have been associated with SERM hormone therapy include hot flashes, bone pain, fatigue, nausea, cough, dyspenia, and headache.
Cognitive Level: Application
Nursing Process: Intervention
NCLEX-RN Test Plan: PHYS
Reference: Condon, M. C. (2004). *Women's health: An integrated approach to wellness and illness.* Upper Saddle River, NJ: Prentice Hall.

22. **Answer: 2**
Rationale: Since the patient was just told about her cancer, fear would be the most appropriate nursing diagnosis. Once the patient has been presented with her options for treatment, the nurse will then need to address the other nursing diagnoses of disturbed body image, the patient's knowledge deficit, and upcoming interrupted family processes.
Cognitive Level: Analysis
Nursing Process: Planning
NCLEX-RN Test Plan: PHYS
Reference: Ricci, S. S. (2007). *Essentials of maternity, newborn, and women's health nursing.* Philadelphia: Lippincott Williams & Wilkins.

23. **Answer: 1**
Rationale: The objective of hormone therapy (use of SERMs) is to block or counter the effect of estrogen. The most widely used SERM is Tamoxifen

(Novadex), which has been associated with an increased incidence of endometrial cancer. There needs to be a balance between treatment and use of SERMs because the side effects may cause quality of life issues for the woman.
Cognitive Level: Analysis
Nursing Process: Planning
NCLEX-RN Test Plan: PHYS
Reference: Ricci, S. S. (2007). *Essentials of maternity, newborn, and women's health nursing.* Philadelphia: Lippincott Williams & Wilkins.

24. **Answer: 1**
    Rationale: Hemorrhage is always a possible complication after surgery. Drainage from any tube postoperatively is assessed for signs of bleeding. Hematocrit is noted and recorded, but increases in hematuria may indicate a bladder nick or trauma to the bladder in postoperative hysterectomy clients. Urinary tract infections rarely occur in the immediate postoperative period. Surgical clients are hydrated during and after surgery with intravenous fluids, therefore, dehydration is uncommon during the immediate postoperative period.
    Cognitive Level: Application
    Nursing Process: Assessment
    NCLEX-RN Test Plan: PHYS
    Reference: Lowdermilk, D. L., & Perry, S. E. (2004). *Maternity & women's health care* (8th ed.). St. Louis, MO: Mosby.

25. **Answers: 1 and 2**
    Rationale: Identified risk factors for ovarian cancer include nulliparity, infertility, previous breast cancer, and family history of breast or ovarian cancers. Research findings with regard to high fat diets and the use of infertility drugs have reported inconclusive findings as they relate to the risk of ovarian cancer.
    Cognitive Level: Analysis
    Nursing Process: Intervention
    NCLEX-RN Test Plan: HPM
    Reference: Lowdermilk, D. L., & Perry, S. E. (2004). *Maternity & women's health care* (8th ed.). St. Louis, MO: Mosby.

26. **Answer: 1**
    Rationale: Cervical polyps form in the mucosa and are the most common benign lesion during the reproductive years. Cervical polyps may cause pre-

menstrual, postmenstrual, and postcoital bleeding and are most common in multiparous women older than 40 years of age.
Cognitive Level: Analysis
Nursing Process: Intervention
NCLEX-RN Test Plan: PHYS
Reference: Lowdermilk, D. L., & Perry, S. E. (2004). *Maternity & women's health care* (8th ed.). St. Louis, MO: Mosby.

27. **Answers: 3 and 4**
    Rationale: Expected outcomes for the abused woman include the development of a safety plan and recognizing that she deserves respect and is undeserving of being victimized. Often women who have been victims of identified abuse may exhibit passive or hostile behaviors or appear embarrassed or shocked because they believe they are at the mercy of the abuser's temper.
    Cognitive Level: Evaluation
    Nursing Process: Evaluation
    NCLEX-RN Test Plan: PSYC
    Reference: Lowdermilk, D. L., & Perry, S. E. (2004). *Maternity & women's health care* (8th ed.). St. Louis, MO: Mosby.

28. **Answers: 1, 2, and 3**
    Rationale: HPV is spread by direct contact and is caused by a slow growing virus of more than 60 strains. It is transmitted via oral, vaginal, or anal intercourse. Treatment only eradicates lesions and does not destroy the HPV virus. The HPV-infected person may be contagious even in the absence of lesions. Therefore, the use of condoms can reduce transmission to the client's partners. In the United States, HPV infection affects about 3 million people annually and is the most common viral sexually-transmitted disease.
    Cognitive Level: Application
    Nursing Process: Intervention and planning
    NCLEX-RN Test Plan: PHYS
    Reference: Condon, M. C. (2004). *Women's health: An integrated approach to wellness and illness.* Upper Saddle River, NJ: Prentice Hall.

29. **Answers: 1, 2, and 3**
    Rationale: Comfort during outbreaks of localized HSV vaginal lesions include instructing the client on comfort measures such as wearing loose fitting

clothing to avoid further irritation. Soaking in warm water and urinating in tepid water to avoid direct urine contact with the lesion will also reduce the pain. Application of ice to the perineal area may cause further trauma to the perineum.
Cognitive Level: Application
Nursing Process: Intervention
NCLEX-RN Test Plan: PHYS
Reference: Lowdermilk, D. L., & Perry, S. E. (2004). *Maternity & women's health care* (8th ed.). St. Louis, MO: Mosby.

30. **Answer: 4**
Rationale: Having multiple sexual partners is a high-risk behavior. Wet kissing and vaginal intercourse with a condom are low-risk behaviors. A possible risk exposure is having vaginal intercourse after anal contact without the use of a new condom.
Cognitive Level: Application
Nursing Process: Intervention
NCLEX-RN Test Plan: HPM
Reference: Lowdermilk, D. L., & Perry, S. E. (2004). *Maternity & women's health care* (8th ed.). St. Louis, MO: Mosby.

31. **Answer: 2**
Rationale: Preventing the spread of sexually transmitted infections is the most effective way of reducing the adverse consequences of sexually transmitted infections in women. A critical first step for the nurse is to obtain a complete health history that includes sexual history, sexual risk behaviors, and drug related behaviors. A technique that is effective in providing sexually transmitted infection prevention is the use of open-ended questions when obtaining a health history. Sexually transmitted infections are among the most common health problems in the United States, affecting 15 million Americans each year regardless of social or economic status. Many women are unaware of the fact that prompt diagnosis and treatment can prevent personal complications and transmission of the infection to others.
Cognitive Level: Application
Nursing Process: Intervention
NCLEX-RN Test Plan: HPM
Reference: Lowdermilk, D. L., & Perry, S. E. (2004). *Maternity & women's health care* (8th ed.). St. Louis, MO: Mosby.

32. **Answer: 1**
Rationale: The presence of pain on examination helps distinguish fibroids and adenomyosis. Fibroids are generally only painful at times of rapid growth or if degenerating, while tenderness to uterine palpation is usually present with adenomyosis. Uterine cysts/polyps are benign overgrowths of tissue found in the uterine lining. They cannot be detected by physical examination. Endometrial hyperplasia is usually painless and may be asymptomatic except for increased vaginal bleeding. This is diagnosed with an endometrial biopsy.
Cognitive Level: Application
Nursing Process: Assessment
NCLEX-RN Test Plan: PHYS
Reference: Schuiling, K. D., & Likis, F. E. (2006). *Gynecologic health.* Sudbury, MA: Jones & Bartlett.

33. **Answer: 3**
Rationale: Hemoglobin and hemocrit is performed to assess the severity of irregular bleeding. Endometrial biopsy is used to evaluate older women with menorrhagia. Ultrasound has limitations—a diffuse adenomyosis lesion may appear as an enlarged uterus and the nodular form of adenomyosis is difficult to differentiate from small uterine fibroids. MRI gives the most definitive picture of adenomyosis and is useful for distinguishing it from fibroids and malignancy.
Cognitive Level: Analysis
Nursing Process: Implementation
NCLEX-RN Test Plan: PHYS
Reference: Schuiling, K. D., & Likis, F. E. (2006). *Gynecologic health.* Sudbury, MA: Jones & Bartlett.

34. **Answers: 1, 2, and 4**
Rationale: Postpartum thyroiditis is a transient condition affecting up to 5% of women. It frequently occurs 8–12 weeks postpartum. The initial presentation is that of hyperthyroidism. Women usually recover spontaneously from postpartum thyroiditis, but it can reoccur in future pregnancies. Women who have this condition may be at risk for future thyroid disease. This condition is not permanent.
Cognitive Level: Analysis
Nursing Process: Assessment
NCLEX-RN Test Plan: PHYS

Reference: Varney, H., Kriebs, J. M., & Gegor, C. L. (2004). *Varney's midwifery* (4th ed.). Sudbury, MA: Jones & Bartlett.

35. **Answers: 1 and 2**
Rationale: In the U.S., medical abortion is a relatively new method used for pregnancy termination. Currently two prominent methods are available—mifepristone and methotrexate—both of which are given in combination with misoprostol. Efficacy has been found to decrease with advancing gestational age. Mifepristone is the most common form of medical abortion in the U.S.
Cognitive Level: Analysis
Nursing Process: Assessment
NCLEX-RN Test Plan: PHYS
Reference: Schuiling, K. D., & Likis, F. E. (2006). *Women's gynecologic health.* Sudbury, MA: Jones & Bartlett.

36. **Answers: 1 and 2**
Rationale: The amount and type of fluid intake may contribute to UI. Limiting fluids may cause bladder irritation and result in an increased urge to urinate in some women. High intake of caffeinated beverages, alcoholic beverages, decaffeinated coffee and tea, carbonated beverages, and artificial sweeteners may play a role in urgency and frequency symptoms.
Cognitive Level: Comprehension
Nursing Process: Assessment
NCLEX-RN Test Plan: PHYS
Reference: Schuiling, K. D., & Likis, F. E. (2006). *Women's gynecologic health.* Sudbury, MA: Jones & Bartlett.

37. **Answer: 4**
Rationale: Laparoscopy with biopsy is the gold standard for the diagnosis of endometriosis. Laparoscopic findings are used to stage the disease and the severity of the endometrial implants and adhesions. There are no laboratory tests for endometriosis. Ultrasound can identify endometriosis but will not demonstrate adhesive changes. MRI can also iden-

tify endometriosis and may detect some endometrial implants, but it is not sufficiently sensitive for diagnosis. Hystersalpingography may demonstrate a tubal obstruction secondary to the adhesive disease.
Cognitive Level: Evaluation
Nursing Process: Planning
NCLEX-RN Test Plan: PHYS
Reference: Schuiling, K. D., & Likis, F. E. (2006). *Women's gynecologic health.* Sudbury, MA: Jones & Bartlett.

38. **Answers: 2 and 4**
Rationale: Absolute contraindications to estrogen use include known or suspected cancer of the breast, estrogen-dependent neoplasia, a history of uterine or ovarian cancer, a history of coronary heart disease or stroke, biliary tract disorders, or undiagnosed abnormal genital bleeding. A history of thrombophlebitis or thromboembolic disorders also contraindicates the use of estrogen therapy. Chronic obstructive pulmonary disease, dermatitis, and asthma have not been identified as contraindications for estrogen replacement therapy.
Cognitive Level: Synthesis
Nursing Process: Implementation
NCLEX-RN Test Plan: PHYS
Reference: Schuiling, K. D., & Likis, F. E. (2006). *Women's gynecologic health.* Sudbury, MA: Jones & Bartlett.

39. **Answer: 3**
Rationale: A diet high in oxalates (teas, coffee, or cocoa) may contribute to vulvdynea. Relief measures include the use of white unscented toilet tissue, wearing loose cotton clothing, using unscented soaps, taking showers instead of baths, and avoiding the use of latex products.
Cognitive Level: Synthesis
Nursing Process: Implementation
NCLEX-RN Test Plan: PHYS
Reference: Varney, H., Kriebs, J. M., & Gegor, C. L. (2004). *Varney's midwifery* (4th ed.). Sudbury, MA: Jones & Bartlett.

Unit 6 Answers and Rationales

Test 22 Answers and Rationales

1. **Answer: 1**

   Rationale: Infants 3 to 4 months of age begin to hold their head up at 45° and then at 90° for sustained periods. Head control becomes stronger. The infant learns to sit without support at 5 to 6 months of age. Fine motor development, such as pincer grasping, and stranger anxiety are not present until 9–10 months of age.

   Cognitive Level: Analysis

   Nursing Process: Analysis

   NCLEX-RN Test Plan: HPM

   Reference: Hockenberry, M. J. (2005). *Wong's essentials of pediatric nursing* (7th ed.). St. Louis, MO: Mosby.

2. **Answer: 2**

   Rationale: Temper tantrums appear during the toddler years. The child is striving to gain control and power over a situation. There are many activities that toddlers want and struggle to do, but are not developmentally ready to perform. The goal is to restore the child's control and calm. This is not achieved by giving the child what they want.

   Cognitive Level: Analysis

   Nursing Process: Analysis

   NCLEX-RN Test Plan: PSYC

   Reference: Hockenberry, M. J. (2005). *Wong's essentials of pediatric nursing* (7th ed.). St. Louis, MO: Mosby.

3. **Answer: 4**

   Rationale: An infant with a cleft palate will have a weak suck and will not be able to nipple thickened formula. An infant with failure to thrive does not have to be kept slightly upright after feeds to gain weight unless the infant has gastroesophageal reflux. Esophagitis is a complication of untreated gastroesophageal reflux. Minimal gastroesophageal reflux is seen in most infants. A small regurgitation of undigested formula or breast milk is usually not of concern and can be treated in the outpatient setting with thickened formula with rice cereal, burping frequently during feedings, and keeping the infant slightly upright after feedings.

   Cognitive Level: Application

   Nursing Process: Implementation

   NCLEX-RN Test Plan: PHYS

   Reference: Hockenberry, M. J. (2005). *Wong's essentials of pediatric nursing* (7th ed.). St. Louis, MO: Mosby.

4. **Answer: 3**

   Rationale: Infants born to HBsAg-negative mothers only require a hepatitis B vaccine at 0–2 months, 1–4 months, and 6–18 months. Infants born to HBsAg-status unknown mothers require hepatitis B vaccine at day 0, 1–2 months, and 6 months (If the mother is found to be HBsAg-positive, the hepatitis B vaccine must be given within 12 hours of birth and HBIG within the first 7 days of life.). Infants born to a known HBsAg-positive mother require the hepatitis B vaccine within 12 hours of birth, and HBIG should also be given at birth.

   Cognitive Level: Application

   Nursing Process: Analysis

   NCLEX-RN Test Plan: HPM

   Reference: Hockenberry, M. J. (2005). *Wong's essentials of pediatric nursing* (7th ed.). St. Louis, MO: Mosby.

5. **Answer: 2**

   Rationale: Amoxicillin is the first-line drug for children with acute otitis media. High dose amoxicillin is given to young children with high fevers (the usual organism is *S. pneumoniae*). If the suspension concentration is 400 mg/5 ml, then 320 mg is equal to 4 ml.

   Cognitive Level: Application

   Nursing Process: Implementation

   NCLEX-RN Test Plan: PHYS

   Reference: Hockenberry, M. J. (2005). *Wong's essentials of pediatric nursing* (7th ed.). St. Louis, MO: Mosby.

6. **Answer: 2**

Rationale: Bronchiolitis/RSV is most common in the infants ages 2 months to 12 months with all of the symptoms listed. A client with asthma would not have a fever and feeding difficulties. Symptoms of croup include stridor, not wheezing; a barky cough; and is most common from 6 months to 3 years. A client with epiglottitis would have drooling, agitation, lethargy, no cough, and prefer to sit in the tripod position.

Cognitive Level: Analysis
Nursing Process: Analysis
NCLEX-RN Test Plan: PHYS

Reference: Hockenberry, M. J. (2005). *Wong's essentials of pediatric nursing* (7th ed.). St. Louis, MO: Mosby.

7. **Answer: 2**

Rationale: The area between the pulmonary artery and aorta remains open, allowing the blood to flow through the patent ductus arteriosis and back to the pulmonary artery and lungs. Coarctation of the aorta is an obstructive congenital heart defect. The aorta is narrowed, obstructing the blood flow. Both Tetralogy of Fallot and tricuspid atresia are congenital defects associated with decreased pulmonary blood flow. In Tetralogy of Fallot, pulmonary stenosis prevents proper pumping of blood from the pulmonary artery. With tricuspid atresia, the absence or closure of the tricuspid valve causes decreased blood flow.

Cognitive Level: Analysis
Nursing Process: Analysis
NCLEX-RN Test Plan: PHYS

Reference: Hockenberry, M. J. (2005). *Wong's essentials of pediatric nursing* (7th ed.). St. Louis, MO: Mosby.

8. **Answer: 4**

Rationale: A febrile seizure has classic tonic-clonic movements associated with a rapid rise in temperature. Symptoms are associated with transient loss of consciousness, staring, and lip smacking. With complex seizure activity, the client will have an aura, be dazed and confused, and suddenly stop activity and stare into space. With infantile spasms, the infant's head will drop suddenly forward and the arms and legs will flex. None of these are associated with a fever.

Cognitive Level: Analysis

Nursing Process: Analysis
NCLEX-RN Test Plan: PHYS

Reference: Hockenberry, M. J. (2005). *Wong's essentials of pediatric nursing* (7th ed.). St. Louis, MO: Mosby.

9. **Answer: 1**

Rationale: The communicability period is the time when the disease can be transmitted to others. The convalescent period is the time between when the symptoms disappear and the client becomes well. The incubation period is the time between when the client is infected by the organism and onset of the illness. The prodromal period is the time between the onset of nonspecific symptoms and the disease-specific symptoms.

Cognitive Level: Analysis
Nursing Process: Analysis
NCLEX-RN Test Plan: HPM

Reference: Hockenberry, M. J. (2005). *Wong's essentials of pediatric nursing* (7th ed.). St. Louis, MO: Mosby.

10. **Answer: 1**

Rationale: The FLACC scale is appropriate to use on infants and children from 2 months to 7 years. A child must be able to count to 100 by ones or tens to use the Oucher numeric scale. The Wong-Baker scale is appropriate for children as young as 3-years-old as they need to be able to point to a face. Infants and children feel pain as adults do and should be treated appropriately.

Cognitive Level: Application
Nursing Process: Assessment
NCLEX-RN Test Plan: PHYS

Reference: Hockenberry, M. J. (2004). *Wong's clinical manual of pediatric nursing* (6th ed.). St. Louis, MO: Mosby.

11. **Answers: 1, 2, 3, 5, and 8**

Rationale: The name of the drug, how to store it, the reason it is taken, and side-effects are all important to know when taking a medication. Written instructions reinforce what has been said. When to return for the next vaccination, while important, is not pertinent to taking the medication. Any medication should be taken for a full course and not discontinued when the client starts feeling better.

Kitchen spoons are different sizes and do not dose out accurately, either over- or underdosing the child.
Cognitive Level: Analysis
Nursing Process: Implementation
NCLEX-RN Test Plan: HPM
Reference: Hockenberry, M. J. (2004). *Wong's clinical manual of pediatric nursing* (6th ed.). St. Louis, MO: Mosby.

12. **Answer: 2**
Rationale: Lice are transmitted via personal items such as hats or combs. They do not fly or jump. An adult louse can stay alive up to 48 hours away from the host. Lice do not discriminate, but can affect anyone of any socioeconomic status. Cleanliness does not prevent lice.
Cognitive Level: Analysis
Nursing Process: Implementation
NCLEX-RN Test Plan: HPM
Reference: Hockenberry, M. J. (2005). *Wong's essentials of pediatric nursing* (7th ed.). St. Louis, MO: Mosby.

13. **Answer: 4**
Rationale: Accidents are a leading cause of death in all age groups, although not first in infants. The leading causes of death in infants are congenital followed by prematurity, SIDS, and complications of pregnancy/birth. Suicide is not a leading cause of death in pre-school and school-age children.
Cognitive Level: Analysis
Nursing Process: Implementation
NCLEX-RN Test Plan: HPM
Reference: Centers for Disease Control. *Health data for all ages.* Retrieved March 13, 2007, from http://209.217.72.34/hdaa/tableviewer/tableview.aspx?reportid=133

14. **Answer: 1**
Rationale: Family-centered care is a philosophy that involves respect, collaboration, and support for the family. A parent-professional partnership is a means of enabling and empowering the family. Therapeutic care includes prevention, diagnosis, and treatment. Pediatric nurses should provide atraumatic care to their patients. Atraumatic care utilizes techniques that eliminate or reduce the psychologic and physi-

cal distress experienced by children and their families while receiving health care.
Cognitive Level: Application
Nursing Process: Assessment
NCLEX-RN Test Plan: SECE
Reference: Hockenberry, M. J. (2005). *Wong's essentials of pediatric nursing* (7th ed.). St. Louis, MO: Mosby.

Wong, D. L., Hockenberry, M. J., Wilson, D., Winkelstein, M. L., & Kline, N. E. (2003). *Wong's nursing care of infants and children.* St. Louis, MO: Mosby.

15. **Answer: 5, 1, 4, 2, 3**
Rationale: Trust vs. mistrust is the first stage from birth to one year. Autonomy vs. shame and doubt encompasses ages 1 to 3 years. Initiative vs. guilt is 3 to 6 years. Industry vs. inferiority is 6 to 12 years and identity vs. role confusion is the final childhood stage at 12 to 18 years.
Cognitive Level: Application
Nursing Process: Assessment
NCLEX-RN Test Plan: PSYC
Reference: Hockenberry, M. J. (2005). *Wong's essentials of pediatric nursing* (7th ed.). St. Louis, MO: Mosby.

16. **Answer: 3**
Rationale: Klinefelter syndrome affects males and is caused by one or more additional X chromosomes. At an incidence of 1:850 live male births, it is the most common of the sex chromosome abnormalities. Turner syndrome affects females and is caused by the absence of one X chromosome; it has an incidence of 1:2500 live female births. Down syndrome is the most common chromosomal abnormality of a generalized syndrome with 95% caused by an extra chromosome 21. Fragile X syndrome is the most common inherited cause of mental retardation and the second genetic cause after Down syndrome. It is caused by an abnormal gene on the longarm of an X chromosome.
Cognitive Level: Application
Nursing Process: Assessment
NCLEX-RN Test Plan: HPM
Reference: Hockenberry, M. J. (2005). *Wong's essentials of pediatric nursing* (7th ed.). St. Louis, MO: Mosby.

17. **Answer: 1**

    Rationale: Kawasaki disease can cause cardiac seque-
    lae in 20% of untreated children. In the early stages
    of the disease, the arteries, veins, and capillaries
    become inflamed. This can progress to coronary
    artery aneurysms in some children. Other symptoms
    of the first phase of Kawasaki disease may include:
    severe redness in the eyes, a rash on the child's stom-
    ach, chest, and genitals, red, dry, cracked lips,
    swollen tongue with a white coating and big red
    bumps, sore, irritated throat, swollen palms of the
    hands and soles of the feet with a purple-red color,
    and swollen lymph nodes. During the second phase
    of the illness, which usually begins within two weeks
    after the first fever, the skin on the child's hands and
    feet may begin to peel in large pieces. The child may
    also experience joint pain and gastrointestinal irrita-
    tion such as, diarrhea, vomiting, or abdominal pain.

    Cognitive Level: Application

    Nursing Process: Assessment

    NCLEX-RN Test Plan: PHYS

    Reference: Hockenberry, M. J. (2005). *Wong's
    essentials of pediatric nursing* (7th ed.). St.
    Louis: Mosby.

18. **Answer: 4**

    Rationale: Neural tube defects occur when the neu-
    ral tube fails to close. Spina bifida occurs when the
    osseous spine fails to close and is the most common
    CNS defect. Cerebral palsy has a number of causes,
    the most common being asphyxia at birth. Muscular
    dystrophies are genetic in origin. Hydrocephalus
    results from an imbalance in production and absorp-
    tion of CSF.

    Cognitive Level: Application

    Nursing Process: Assessment

    NCLEX-RN Test Plan: PHYS

    Reference: Hockenberry, M. J. (2005). *Wong's
    essentials of pediatric nursing* (7th ed.). St. Louis,
    MO: Mosby.

19. **Answer: 1**

    Rationale: Changes in vital signs will signal early
    complications in the disease. The blood pressure is
    frequently elevated and must be monitored. Moni-
    toring intake and output are also important, but a
    daily weight is one of the most useful ways to moni-
    tor fluid balance. Most children do well with a no-
    added-salt diet and it is not necessary to restrict

    sodium. Children do not need strict bedrest and
    should be permitted activities as tolerated as long as
    there are periods of rest.

    Cognitive Level: Application

    Nursing Process: Analysis

    NCLEX-RN Test Plan: PHYS

    Reference: Hockenberry, M. J. (2005). *Wong's
    essentials of pediatric nursing* (7th ed.). St. Louis,
    MO: Mosby.

20. **Answer: 1**

    Rationale: Bacterial meningitis is an acute inflamma-
    tion of the meninges and the CNS. Antimicrobial
    therapy has a marked effect on the course and prog-
    nosis of the illness. Other therapeutic nursing man-
    agement techniques include obtaining vital signs,
    neuralgic signs LOC, recording accurate intake and
    output, and keeping environmental stimuli to a min-
    imum because most affected children are sensitive to
    noise, bright lights, and other external stimuli.

    Cognitive Level: Application

    Nursing Process: Implementation

    NCLEX-RN Test Plan: PHYS

    Reference: Hockenberry, M. J. (2005). *Wong's
    essentials of pediatric nursing* (7th ed.). St. Louis,
    MO: Mosby.

21. **Answer: 4**

    Rationale: Wilm's tumor, or nephroblastoma, is the
    most common malignant renal and intra-abdominal
    tumor of childhood. Ewing sarcoma is the second
    most common malignant bone tumor in children
    and adolescents. It arises in the marrow spaces of the
    bones, such as the femur, tibia, fibula, ulna,
    humerus, pelvis, ribs, and skull. Osteosarcoma is the
    most frequent malignant bone cancer in children
    with a peak incidence between 10–25 years old.
    Neuroblastoma is the most common malignant
    extracranial solid tumor in children.

    Cognitive Level: Application

    Nursing Process: Assessment

    NCLEX-RN Test Plan: HPM

    Reference: Hockenberry, M. J. (2005). *Wong's
    essentials of pediatric nursing* (7th ed.). St. Louis,
    MO: Mosby.

22. **Answer: 3**

    Rationale: Intussusception is one of the most fre-
    quent causes of intestinal obstruction in children 3

months to 3 years old. Clinical manifestations include sudden acute abdominal pain, drawing knees into the chest, screams, vomiting, lethargy, passage of red currant jelly-like stools, tenderness, distended abdomen, and a palpable sausage-like mass in the upper right abdominal quadrant. Symptoms of a hiatal hernia include dysphagia, failure to thrive, vomiting, neck contortions, frequent respiratory problems, and bleeding associated with gastroesophageal reflux. Appendicitis is the most common cause of emergency abdominal surgery in children. Clinical manifestations include right lower quadrant abdominal pain, fever, rigid abdomen, decreased or absent bowel sounds, vomiting, constipation or diarrhea, anorexia, pallor, lethargy, irritability, and stooped posture. Pyloric stenosis occurs when the circumferential muscle of the pyloric sphincter becomes thickened, resulting in elongation and narrowing of the pyloric channel. This produces outlet obstruction with projectile emesis, dehydration, metabolic acidosis, and failure to thrive.
Cognitive Level: Analysis
Nursing Process: Assessment
NCLEX-RN Test Plan: PHYS
Reference: Hockenberry, M. J. (2005). *Wong's essentials of pediatric nursing* (7th ed.). St. Louis, MO: Mosby.

23. **Answer: 3**
Rationale: Celiac disease, or celiac sprue, is characterized by intolerance to the protein gluten found in wheat, barley, rye, and oats. Susceptible individuals are unable to digest the gliadin component of gluten, resulting in an accumulation of a toxic substance that is damaging to the mucosal cells. Corn and rice are used as substitute grain foods.
Cognitive Level: Application
Nursing Process: Analysis
NCLEX-RN Test Plan: HPM
Reference: Hockenberry, M. J. (2005). *Wong's essentials of pediatric nursing* (7th ed.). St. Louis, MO: Mosby.

24. **Answer: 2**
Rationale: Although most words usually are spoken at about 12 months, parents should not be discouraged if language is delayed. The best advice is to watch this phase of development carefully and seek advice if any delay is worrisome.

Cognitive Level: Analysis
Nursing Process: Assessment
NCLEX-RN Test Plan: HPM
Reference: Thies, K. M., & Travers, J. F. (2001). *Quick look nursing: Growth and development through the lifespan.* Thorofare, NJ: Slack Inc.

25. **Answer: 4**
Rationale: Given the current divorce rate, and the rate of divorce following second marriages, children are often shifted from home to home, school to school, etc. These transitions require considerable parental sensitivity, which many parents, given their emotional state, find difficult.
Cognitive Level: Analysis
Nursing Process: Analysis
NCLEX-RN Test Plan: PSYC
Reference: Thies, K. M., & Travers, J. F. (2001). *Quick look nursing: Growth and development through the lifespan.* Thorofare, NJ: Slack Inc.

26. **Answer: 1**
Rationale: At age 3, children can go upstairs using alternating feet, but still descend by placing both feet on each step. By age 4, they descend using alternating feet and holding the railing. At age 6, they are running up and down stairs easily.
Cognitive Level: Analysis
Nursing Process: Assessment
NCLEX-RN Test Plan: HPM
Reference: Thies, K. M., & Travers, J. F. (2001). *Quick look nursing: Growth and development through the lifespan.* Thorofare, NJ: Slack Inc.

27. **Answer: 3**
Rationale: By age 10, the development of a second person perspective allows children to put themselves in the other person's shoes and experience things from another point of view. They expect that friends will do the same for them. Children realize that if they can hide feelings and thoughts, so can others; social appearances can be deceiving. Friendships expand beyond sharing activities to include sharing subjective experiences. Trust means the child does not hurt his or her friend's feelings and that the child understands the desire to be liked and accepted. Consequently, hurting people's feelings is understood to be intentional. Being excluded is painful.
Cognitive Level: Analysis

Nursing Process: Assessment
NCLEX-RN Test Plan: HPM
Reference: Thies, K. M., & Travers, J. F. (2001).
  *Quick look nursing: Growth and development
  through the lifespan.* Thorofare, NJ: Slack Inc.

28. **Answer: 4**
Rationale: Progesterone causes the uterine lining to
mature in preparation for implantation of a fertilized
embryo. It also inhibits the production of FSH,
which would trigger the beginning of a new cycle. If
fertilization does not occur, the increase in progesterone forms the corpus luteum and shuts down LH,
which sustains the corpus luteum itself. As the corpus
luteum begins to disintegrate and progesterone levels
fall, FSH production is no longer inhibited and
begins anew. Without progesterone, the lining of the
uterus cannot be sustained, and it is shed in the form
of the menstrual flow. The cycle begins again.
Cognitive Level: Application
Nursing Process: Analysis
NCLEX-RN Test Plan: HPM
Reference: Thies, K. M., & Travers, J. F. (2001).
  *Quick look nursing: Growth and development
  through the lifespan.* Thorofare, NJ: Slack Inc.

29. **Answer: 4**
Rationale: The best indicator of smoking behavior is
having parents who smoke. The influence of friends
is greater earlier in adolescence than later. Advertisements, especially those that implicate smoking with
thinness in women, also play a role. Adolescents
who are socially skilled are more self-confident, and
less likely to succumb to the influence of peers to
engage in risky behaviors.
Cognitive Level: Analysis
Nursing Process: Analysis
NCLEX-RN Test Plan: SECE
Reference: Thies, K. M., & Travers, J. F. (2001).
  *Quick look nursing: Growth and development
  through the lifespan.* Thorofare, NJ: Slack Inc.

30. **Answer: 2**
Rationale: The organization of the CNS is like that
in adults, contributing to better physical coordination. There is an increase in muscle mass relative to
body weight. Body proportions change during the
school years. Children, at age seven, have a lower
center of gravity. There is also an increase in leg

length, decrease in head size, and decrease in waist
size relative to height. These changes all contribute
to physical agility, so that riding a bike, kicking a
soccer ball, or hiking a mountain trail is easier and
more coordinated.
Cognitive Level: Analysis
Nursing Process: Assessment
NCLEX-RN Test Plan: HPM
Reference: Thies, K. M., & Travers, J. F. (2001).
  *Quick look nursing: Growth and development
  through the lifespan.* Thorofare, NJ: Slack Inc.

31. **Answer: 3**
Rationale: During the preschool years, children's
self-concept is categorical. It includes descriptions of
clothing and hair color, names of siblings and pets,
their school, and prized possessions. They refer to
abilities, likes and dislikes, and emotions: "I can
swim." "I like to play house." "I get mad." Preschool
children can distinguish between how well others
like them (social acceptance) from how well they can
do something (competence): "Sarah likes me, she's
my friend." "I'm good at coloring."
Cognitive Level: Analysis
Nursing Process: Assessment
NCLEX-RN Test Plan: HPM
Reference: Thies, K. M., & Travers, J. F. (2001).
  *Quick look nursing: Growth and development
  through the lifespan.* Thorofare, NJ: Slack Inc.

32. **Answer: 2**
Rationale: The average American newborn weighs
about 3.27 kg. Infants gain 680 grams a month until
about 5–6 months, by which time their weight has
doubled. Birth weight triples by the end of the first
year to about 10 kg.
Cognitive Level: Analysis
Nursing Process: Assessment
NCLEX-RN Test Plan: HPM
Reference: Thies, K. M., & Travers, J. F. (2001).
  *Quick look nursing: Growth and development
  through the lifespan.* Thorofare, NJ: Slack Inc.

33. **Answer: Vastus lateralis**
Rationale: The preferred site for intramuscular
injections in infants is the vastus lateralis. The dor-
sogluteal site is not recommended due to its close
proximity to the sciatic nerve and the gluteal artery.
Cognitive Level: Application

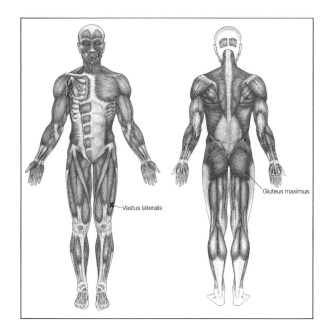

Vastus lateralis

Gluteus maximus

Nursing Process: Implementation
NCLEX-RN Test Plan: PHYS
Reference: Hockenberry, M. J. (2005). *Wong's essentials of pediatric nursing* (7th ed.). St. Louis, MO: Mosby.

34. **Answer: The area directly above the eyebrows to the widest part of the occipital prominence.**
    Rationale: The appropriate measurement area for head circumference in children under 36 months of age is located directly above the eyebrows to the widest part of the occipital prominence.
    Cognitive Level: Application
    Nursing Process: Implementation
    NCLEX-RN Test Plan: PHYS
    Reference: Hockenberry, M. J. (2005). *Wong's essentials of pediatric nursing* (7th ed.). St. Louis, MO: Mosby.

35. **Answer: 3**
    Rationale: To prevent the spread of GABHS, the child should discard their toothbrush and replace it with a new one after they have been taking antibiotics for 24 hours. Cold or warm compresses to the neck may provide some pain relief associated with GABHS. Children with GABHS can return to school after they have been taking antibiotics for a full 24 hour period. If diagnosed with GABHS, you must complete the entire course of the antibiotic prescribed even if symptoms disappear before the course of antibiotics is complete.

Cognitive Level: Application
Nursing Process: Planning
NCLEX-RN Test Plan: PHYS
Reference: Hockenberry, M. J. (2005). *Wong's essentials of pediatric nursing* (7th ed.). St. Louis, MO: Mosby.

36. **Answer: 3**
    Rationale: Whooping cough or pertussis is an acute respiratory infection caused by Bordetella pertussis that occurs mainly in children under 4 years of age who have not been immunized. It is highly contagious and is especially threatening in young infants, who have a high mortality and morbidity rate. Haemophilus influenza, mycoplasma pneumoniae, and tuberculosis are not other names for whooping cough.
    Cognitive Level: Analysis
    Nursing Process: Assessment
    NCLEX-RN Test Plan: HPM
    Reference: Hockenberry, M. J. (2005). *Wong's essentials of pediatric nursing* (7th ed.). St. Louis, MO: Mosby.

37. **Answer: 1**
    Rationale: Sudden infant death syndrome (SIDS) is the sudden death of an infant younger than 1 year of age that remains unexplained after a complete postmortem exam. Mortality rates for SIDS have declined more than 40% since 1992 since the "Back to Sleep" campaign started. SIDS may be related to a brainstem abnormality in the neurologic regulation of cardiorespiratory control. Sleep apnea is not the cause of SIDS. There is no correlation between SIDS and diphtheria, tetanus, and pertussis vaccines. Parents are instructed to put their infants to sleep on their back to prevent SIDS.
    Cognitive Level: Analysis
    Nursing Process: Analysis
    NCLEX-RN Test Plan: HPM
    Reference: Hockenberry, M. J. (2005). *Wong's essentials of pediatric nursing* (7th ed.). St. Louis, MO: Mosby.

38. **Answer: 4**
    Rationale: Hirschsprung disease, or congenital aganglionic megacolon, is a mechanical obstruction caused by inadequate motility of part of the intestine. The primary defect is an absence of ganglion cells in

one or more segments of the colon. Encoporesis is constipation with fecal soiling around the impacted stool. Functional constipation or idiopathic constipation is the major cause for constipation in children. There is no underlying cause for functional constipation. Enterocolitis is inflammation of the small bowel and colon from a variety of causes.

Cognitive Level: Analysis
Nursing Process: Assessment
NCLEX-RN Test Plan: PHYS

Reference: Hockenberry, M. J. (2005). *Wong's essentials of pediatric nursing* (7th ed.). St. Louis, MO: Mosby.

39. **Answer: 2**

Rationale: To calculate the absolute neutrophil count (ANC), you have to determine the total percentage of neutrophils ("polys" or "segs" and "bands"), then multiply the white blood cell count (WBC) by the total percentage of neutrophils.

Example:

7% + 7% = 14%, then 1000 × 0.14 = 140 ANC.

Cognitive Level: Analysis
Nursing Process: Planning
NCLEX-RN Test Plan: PHYS

Reference: Hockenberry, M. J. (2005). *Wong's essentials of pediatric nursing* (7th ed.). St. Louis, MO: Mosby.

Unit 6 Answers and Rationales

Test 23 Answers and Rationales

1. **Answer: 1**
   Rationale: Clients with bone marrow depression have a compromised white blood cell (WBC) count and immune system activity. Agranulocytosis is a life-threatening condition characterized by a marked decrease in the granulated white blood cells. It is the most serious blood-related side effect of psychotropic medication. The risk is highest with clozapine (Clozaril). However, it is also a risk with conventional antipsychotic drugs and benzodiazepines. Clozapine (Clozaril) is not administered unless the WBC is normal. A frequent side effect of clozapine (Clozaril) is orthostatic hypotension, and the drug may increase the effects of antihypertensive drugs. Thus, BP needs careful monitoring. Dry eye syndrome and urinary retention are anticholinergic-related conditions and would most likely not be exacerbated by the drug as anticholinergic side-effects are rare with clozapine (Clozaril).
   Cognitive Level: Application
   Nursing Process: Analysis
   NCLEX-RN Test Plan: PHYS
   Reference: Kneisl, C. R., Wilson, H. S., & Trigoboff, E. (2004). *Contemporary psychiatric-mental health nursing.* Upper Saddle River, NJ: Pearson Prentice Hall.

2. **Answers: 1, 2, 5, and 6**
   Rationale: The extrapyramidal tracts of the central nervous system are involved in the production and control of involuntary and gross motor movements producing acute dystonia, akasthisia, dyskinesia, and parkinsonism. Amenorrhea, breast secretions, and sexual dysfunction are endocrine related side effects.
   Cognitive Level: Application
   Nursing Process: Assessment
   NCLEX-RN Test Plan: PHYS
   Reference: Kneisl, C. R., Wilson, H. S., & Trigoboff, E. (2004). *Contemporary psychiatric-mental health nursing.* Upper Saddle River, NJ: Pearson Prentice Hall.

3. **Answer: Neuroleptic malignant syndrome (NMS)**
   Rationale: About 0.5–1.0% of clients on psychotropic drugs will experience NMS within the first two weeks of medication change or dose increase.
   Cognitive Level: Analysis
   Nursing Process: Analysis
   NCLEX-RN Test Plan: PHYS
   Reference: Kneisl, C. R., Wilson, H. S., & Trigoboff, E. (2004). *Contemporary psychiatric-mental health nursing.* Upper Saddle River, NJ: Pearson Prentice Hall.

4. **Answer: 4**
   Rationale: Of the atypical antipsychotics, clozapine (Clozaril) and olanzapine (Zyprexa, Zydis) have the greatest possibility of causing weight gain and sedation. Agranulocytosis and blood dyscrasias are rare with only a 0.3% occurrence. Anticholinergic symptoms are rare and prolactin elevation is associated with risperidone (Risperdal, Consta). Dystonia and akasthisia are occasional extrapyramidal tract symptoms experienced.
   Cognitive Level: Application
   Nursing Process: Assessment
   NCLEX-RN Test Plan: PHYS
   Reference: Kneisl, C. R., Wilson, H. S., & Trigoboff, E. (2004). *Contemporary psychiatric-mental health nursing.* Upper Saddle River, NJ: Pearson Prentice Hall.

   Stuart, G. W., & Laraia, M. T. (2005). *Principles and practices of psychiatric nursing* (8th ed.). St. Louis, MO: Elsevier Mosby.

5. **Answer: 1**
   Rationale: Antipsychotic medication may interact with nicotine. Medication should not be kept in a room where there is moisture (bathroom) or where temperature fluctuates (in a car). Flu-like symptoms may indicate beginning agranulocytosis, a life-threatening side effect, and should be reported. If a dose is missed, one should not take double extra doses.
   Cognitive Level: Application

Nursing Process: Evaluation
NCLEX-RN Test Plan: PHYS
Reference: Kneisl, C. R., Wilson, H. S., & Trigoboff, E. (2004). *Contemporary psychiatric-mental health nursing.* Upper Saddle River, NJ: Pearson Prentice Hall.

6. **Answer: 1**
   Rationale: Negative symptoms of psychosis involve a diminution or loss of normal functioning. They include affective flattening, alogia (restricted thought and speech), avolution/apathy (lack of behavior initiation), and anhedonia/asociality (inability to experience pleasure or maintain social contacts). Positive symptoms of psychosis involve an excess or distortion of normal functioning. These include psychotic disorders of thinking (delusions) and disorganization of speech (illogicality) and behavior.
   Cognitive Level: Analysis
   Nursing Process: Evaluation
   NCLEX-RN Test Plan: PSYC
   Reference: Stuart, G. W., & Laraia, M. T. (2005). *Principles and practices of psychiatric nursing* (8th ed.). St. Louis, MO: Elsevier Mosby.

7. **Answer: 3**
   Rationale: TCAs are lethal in overdose while SSRIs are fairly safe. Both categories of drugs are equally effective in relieving depressive symptoms. TCAs have more sedative and cardiovascular effects than SSRIs.
   Cognitive Level: Application
   Nursing Process: Implementation
   NCLEX-RN Test Plan: PHYS
   Reference: Stuart, G. W., & Laraia, M. T. (2005). *Principles and practices of psychiatric nursing* (8th ed.). St. Louis, MO: Elsevier Mosby.

8. **Answer: 3**
   Rationale: Serotonin syndrome is a potentially lethal reaction following the use of serotomimetic agents (SSRIs, TCSs) alone or in combination with MAOIs. Treatment is immediate discontinuation of all serotonergic drugs. Anticonvulsants and drugs to counteract specific symptoms (muoclonus) are given as necessary. Symptoms of serotonin syndrome are confusion, mania, agitation, myoclonus, hyperreflexia, diaphoresis, shivering, ataxia, coma, low-grade fever.

Cognitive Level: Application
Nursing Process: Implementation
NCLEX-RN Test Plan: PHYS
Reference: Mohr, W. K. (2003). *Psychiatric-mental health nursing* (5th ed.). Philadelphia: Lippincott Williams & Wilkins.

9. **Answer: 4**
   Rationale: When switching from an MAOI to a TCA or SSRI, the provider should allow a washout period of at least the half-life of the drug. Blood levels of antidepressant drugs are not monitored. However, serum blood levels of the mood stabilizer lithium are closely monitored as there is a narrow window between therapeutic and toxic levels.
   Cognitive Level: Application
   Nursing Process: Planning
   NCLEX-RN Test Plan: PHYS
   Reference: Mohr, W. K. (2003). *Psychiatric-mental health nursing* (5th ed.). Philadelphia: Lippincott Williams & Wilkins.

10. **Answers: 1 and 4**
    Rationale: Auditory and somatic hallucinations are common in schizophrenia. Gustatory and olfactory hallucinations are associated with seizure disorders and tactile hallucinations are associated with acute alcohol withdrawal.
    Cognitive Level: Analysis
    Nursing Process: Assessment
    NCLEX-RN Test Plan: PSYC
    Reference: Kneisl, C. R., Wilson, H. S., & Trigoboff, E. (2004). *Contemporary psychiatric-mental health nursing.* Upper Saddle River, NJ: Pearson Prentice Hall.

11. **Answers: 1, 4, and 6**
    Rationale: Disorientation, paranoid delusions, and tremors are indicators for the presence of alcohol withdrawal delirium. Distractibility, grandiosity, and pressure of speech are diagnostic criteria for a manic episode.
    Cognitive Level: Analysis
    Nursing Process: Assessment
    NCLEX-RN Test Plan: PSYC
    Reference: Stuart, G. (2005). *Handbook of psychiatric nursing* (6th ed.). St. Louis, MO: Elsevier Mosby.

12. **Answer: 4**

    Rationale: Depressed clients see the future as a blank and have given up all hope where the anxious client has not. All other symptoms are shared by clients experiencing the two conditions. Both also experience difficulty concentrating, appetite changes, and nonspecific cardiopulmonary complaints.
    Cognitive Level: Analysis
    Nursing Process: Analysis
    NCLEX-RN Test Level: PSYC
    Reference: Stuart, G. W. & Laraia, M. T. (2005). *Principles and practices of psychiatric nursing* (8th ed.). St. Louis, MO: Elsevier Mosby.

13. **Answer: 2**

    Rationale: This assurance is a limit-setting intervention and promotes a sense of safety to the client. The intervention of discontinuing external limits as soon as the client is able to self-regulate empowers the client to use self-control. The intervention of all staff consistently enforcing limits promotes behavior shaping. Accepting the client while rejecting inappropriate behavior protects self-esteem.
    Cognitive Level: Analysis
    Nursing Process: Implementation
    NCLEX-RN Test Plan: PSYC
    Reference: Kneisl, C. R., Wilson, H. S., & Trigoboff, E. (2004). *Contemporary psychiatric-mental health nursing.* Upper Saddle River, NJ: Pearson Prentice Hall.

14. **Answer: 1**

    Rationale: Demonstrating less impulsive behavior is an appropriate goal for Cluster B PDs including borderline PD (impulsive and unpredictable behavior), histrionic PD (dramatic and reactive behavior), narcissistic PD (grandiose sense of self-importance), and antisocial PD (manipulative behavior in conflict with society). Identifying behaviors that maximize social interactions and participating in activity groups are appropriate goals for Cluster A PDs, which include the odd-eccentric disorders of paranoid PD, schizoid PD, and schizotypal PD. Making decisions independently is an appropriate goal for Cluster C PDs, which includes anxious and fearful disorders such as avoidant PD, dependent PD, and obsessive-compulsive PD.
    Cognitive Level: Application
    Nursing Process: Planning

NCLEX-RN Test Plan: PSYC
Reference: Kneisl, C. R., Wilson, H. S., & Trigoboff, E. (2004). *Contemporary psychiatric-mental health nursing.* Upper Saddle River, NJ: Pearson Prentice Hall.

15. **Answer: 3**

    Rationale: All of the responses represent deviations in adult partners' coalition. In the schismatic pattern, children are forced to join one or the other camp of warring parents. The adult partners belittle and undercut each other as a defense against closeness. In the disengaged coalition, adult members are oblivious to the effects of their actions on others. In the enmeshed pattern, there is one over-controlling adult with high intensity interactions between the partners. In the skew pattern, one mate is severely dysfunctional and the other is passive with regard to the dysfunction.
    Cognitive Level: Analysis
    Nursing Process: Assessment
    NCLEX-RN Test Plan: PSYC
    Reference: Kneisl, C. R., Wilson, H. S., & Trigoboff, E. (2004). *Contemporary psychiatric-mental health nursing.* Upper Saddle River, NJ: Pearson Prentice Hall.

16. **Answers: 1 and 4**

    Rationale: Religious beliefs as a coping pattern decrease the likelihood of major depression, suicide, anxiety, and alcoholism. Ninety percent of Americans consider religion "very or fairly important" in their lives. Spiritual coping strategies that are helpful during illness and crises include prayer, contemplation and meditation, bibliotherapy, and worship rituals. However, these interventions should be avoided if the client is psychotic or delusional.
    Cognitive Level: Application
    Nursing Process: Assessment
    NCLEX-RN Test Plan: PSYC
    Reference: Mohr, W. K. (2003). *Psychiatric-mental health nursing* (5th ed.). Philadelphia: Lippincott Williams & Wilkins.

17. **Answer: 1**

    Rationale: This response acknowledges the need for the false belief while not encouraging it or arguing with the client, clearly states what is expected, and offers self. Empathy is a process in which people feel with one another. Reflection is repeating the client's verbal or nonverbal message. The client is demonstrating delusional thinking, not demonstrating manipulative behavior.

Cognitive Level: Analysis
Nursing Process: Analysis
NCLEX-RN Test Plan: PSYC

Reference: Kneisl, C. R., Wilson, H. S., & Trigoboff, E. (2004). *Contemporary psychiatric-mental health nursing.* Upper Saddle River, NJ: Pearson Prentice Hall.

18. **Answer: 1**

Rationale: Narcolepsy involves brief periods of deep sleep and an irresistible desire to sleep. It is usually associated with cataplexy and sleep paralysis. Primary hypersomnia involves prolonged sleep that interferes with functioning. Primary insomnia is difficulty falling to sleep. Sleep apnea is an absence of breathing usually related to upper airway collapse.

Cognitive Level: Analysis
Nursing Process: Planning
NCLEX-RN Test Plan: PSYC

Reference: Kneisl, C. R., Wilson, H. S., & Trigoboff, E. (2004). *Contemporary psychiatric-mental health nursing.* Upper Saddle River, NJ: Pearson Prentice Hall.

19. **Answer: 3**

Rationale: Many clients in withdrawal are dehydrated. Fluid up to 3,000 ml per day should be encouraged. The peak time of onset of DTs after the last drink is 24–48 hours. Antabuse blocks an enzyme that metabolizes highly toxic acetaldehyde, producing nausea and hypotension. Naltrexone (ReVia, Trexan) blocks the craving for alcohol. Alcohol interferes with the absorption of the B vitamins. Thus, they should be supplemented.

Cognitive Level: Application
Nursing Process: Evaluation
NCLEX-RN Test Plan: PSYC

Reference: Kneisl, C. R., Wilson, H. S., & Trigoboff, E. (2004). *Contemporary psychiatric-mental health nursing.* Upper Saddle River, NJ: Pearson Prentice Hall.

20. **Answer: 3**

Rationale: Religious objections are usually upheld by the courts. When ruling against psychiatric

clients' rights to refuse treatment, courts look for benefits of treatment outweighing risks and side effects that are not permanent. In a case of involuntary commitment of a competent client, a hearing is held before an independent psychiatrist where the client has a right to legal counsel.

Cognitive Level: Analysis
Nursing Process: Analysis
NCLEX-RN Test Plan: SECE

Reference: Kneisl, C. R., Wilson, H. S., & Trigoboff, E. (2004). *Contemporary psychiatric-mental health nursing.* Upper Saddle River, NJ: Pearson Prentice Hall.

21. **Answer: 3**

Rationale: Advocacy is acting in support of a client's rights. Clients have a right to understand and participate in treatment decision-making. Encouraging client feedback, explaining unit rules and policies, and making sure clients understand expectations for participation are strategies for working with clients in a therapeutic environment. Explaining unit rules and policies relates to safety, while encouraging client feedback relates to self-understanding. Clarifying expectations for a client's participation relates to structure.

Cognitive Level: Application
Nursing Process: Implementation
NCLEX-RN Test Plan: SECE

Reference: Kneisl, C. R., Wilson, H. S., & Trigoboff, E. (2004). *Contemporary psychiatric-mental health nursing.* Upper Saddle River, NJ: Pearson Prentice Hall.

22. **Answer: 2**

Rationale: Treatment for severe depression begins with a mood stabilizer and an antidepressant. If psychosis is present in the manic client, treatment begins with a mood stabilizer and an atypical antipsychotic. Diuretics have no role in treatment of mania or depression. If a diuretic is given in combination with lithium, blood lithium levels will increase along with the potential for lithium toxicity.

Cognitive Level: Analysis
Nursing Process: Planning
NCLEX-Test Plan: PSYC

Reference: Mohr, W. K. (2003). *Psychiatric-mental health nursing* (5th ed.). Philadelphia: Lippincott Williams & Wilkins.

23. **Answer: 5, 1, 3, 4, 2**

    Rationale: Withdrawal syndrome is managed first, followed by acknowledging dependence and a need for treatment. The client will then identify alternative strategies for managing anxiety before they can be implemented. Rebuilding relationships will take some time.

    Cognitive Level: Application

    Nursing Process: Planning

    NCLEX-RN Test Plan: PSYC

    Reference: Mohr, W. K. (2003). *Psychiatric-mental health nursing* (5th ed.). Philadelphia: Lippincott Williams & Wilkins.

24. **Answer: 1**

    Rationale: Other situations include criminal proceedings, acting to protect a third party, child custody and abuse situations, and when states have reporting laws. Written client consent is needed in situations 2–4.

    Cognitive Level: Analysis

    Nursing Process: Analysis

    NCLEX-RN Test Plan: SECE

    Reference: Stuart, G. W., & Laraia, M. T. (2005). *Principles and practices of psychiatric nursing* (8th ed.). St. Louis, MO: Elsevier Mosby.

25. **Answer: 4**

    Rationale: These are the first symptoms of TD. Discounting the drug at this point may prevent a full-blown (and irreversible) case of TD. TD includes involuntary choreoathelotic movements of the face and tongue, lip smacking, and foot tapping. Prolixin is compatible with grapefruit juice. Missing several doses of the drug would lead to a return of psychotic symptoms. Symptoms of NMS include severe muscle rigidity and altered consciousness.

    Cognitive Level: Analysis

    Nursing Process: Analysis

    NCLEX-RN Test Plan: PHYS

    Reference: Mohr, W. K. (2003). *Psychiatric-mental health nursing* (5th ed.). Philadelphia: Lippincott Williams & Wilkins.

    Kneisl, C. R., Wilson, H. S., & Trigoboff, E. (2004). *Contemporary psychiatric-mental health nursing.* Upper Saddle River, NJ: Pearson Prentice Hall.

26. **Answer: 4**

    Rationale: The therapeutic treatment level for lithium is 1.0–1.5 mEq/L for initial treatment up to the maintenance level, which ranges from 1.0–1.2 mEq/L. Toxic lithium level is above 1.5 mEq/L.

    Cognitive Level: Analysis

    Nursing Process: Evaluation

    NCLEX-RN Test Plan: PHYS

    Reference: Kneisl, C. R., Wilson, H. S., & Trigoboff, E. (2004). *Contemporary psychiatric-mental health nursing.* Upper Saddle River, NJ: Pearson Prentice Hall.

27. **Answer: 3, 4, and 6**

    Rationale: A realistic perception of the event plus adequate situational support plus adequate coping mechanisms result in positive resolution of the crisis and regaining equilibrium. Behavioral reinforcement, catharsis, and raising self-esteem are examples of techniques the nurse uses when working with individuals and families in a crisis.

    Cognitive Level: Application

    Nursing Process: Assessment

    NCLEX-RN Test Plan: PSYC

    Reference: Stuart, G. (2005). *Handbook of psychiatric nursing* (6th ed.). St. Louis, MO: Elsevier Mosby.

28. **Answer: 3**

    Rationale: The MMSE is used to assess orientation, attention span, recall, and ability to execute simple instructions. Delirium, dementia, and thinking are assessed by the Confusion Assessment Method (CAM), which also assesses acute and fluctuating courses of the condition and altered level of consciousness.

    Cognitive Level: Application

    Nursing Process: Assessment

    NCLEX-RN Test Plan: PSYC

    Reference: Mohr, W. K. (2003). *Psychiatric-mental health nursing* (5th ed.). Philadelphia: Lippincott Williams & Wilkins.

29. **Answer: 2**

    Rationale: Assessment (identification) comes before implementation. Responses controlling the physical effects of anxiety, beginning breathing exercises, and

using problem-solving are implementation activities that are appropriate longer-term goals.
Cognitive Level: Application
Nursing Process: Planning
NCLEX-RN Test Plan: PSYC
Reference: Mohr, W. K. (2003). *Psychiatric-mental health nursing* (5th ed.). Philadelphia: Lippincott Williams & Wilkins.

Kneisl, C. R., Wilson, H. S., & Trigoboff, E. (2004). *Contemporary psychiatric-mental health nursing.* Upper Saddle River, NJ: Pearson Prentice Hall.

30. **Answer: 3**
Rationale: Response 1 collects data on past medical and mental health issues. Response 2 describes family burden. Response 4 collects demographic data.
Cognitive Level: Analysis
Nursing Process: Assessment
NCLEX-RN Test Plan: PSYC
Reference: Fontaine, K. L., Kneisl, C. R., & Trigoboff, E. (2004). *Psychiatric-mental health nursing clinical companion.* Upper Saddle River, NJ: Pearson Prentice Hall.

31. **Answer: 3**
Rationale: MAOIs decrease the body's ability to use vitamin B_6, thus supplements will be necessary. MAOIs may be lethal in overdose. These drugs are nonaddicting and tolerance to their therapeutic effects does not occur.
Cognitive Level: Application
Nursing Process: Planning
NCLEX-RN Test Plan: PSYC
Reference: Stuart, G. (2005). *Handbook of psychiatric nursing* (6th ed.). St. Louis, MO: Elsevier Mosby.

32. **Answer: 4**
Rationale: Since Congress passed the National Child Abuse Prevention and Treatment Act in 1974, many states have passed their own reporting laws. Evidence is not required. Suspicion of abuse is sufficient for reporting. Reporting of child abuse is mandatory in most sates and should occur within 36 hours of discovery.
Cognitive Level: Application
Nursing Process: Implementation

NCLEX-RN Test Plan: PSYC
Reference: Fontaine, K. L., Kneisl, C. R., & Trigoboff, E. (2004). *Psychiatric-mental health nursing clinical companion.* Upper Saddle River, NJ: Pearson Prentice Hall.

33. **Answer: Situational**
Rationale: In a situational crisis, external events upset the client's psychological equilibrium. In developmental or maturational crises, developmental periods in one's life result in psychological disequilibrium that may require role changes.
Cognitive Level: Analysis
Nursing Process: Analysis
NCLEX-Test Plan: PSYC
Reference: Stuart, G. (2005). *Handbook of psychiatric nursing* (6th ed.). St. Louis, MO: Elsevier Mosby.

34. **Answer: 1**
Rationale: Benzodiazepines in combination with alcohol can be fatal. Drug withdrawal and seizure disorders are major indications for use of benzodiazepines. Suicide attempts using benzodiazepines alone are rarely successful. When these drugs are taken alone, they are almost never fatal.
Cognitive Level: Analysis
Nursing Process: Analysis
NCLEX-RN Test Plan: PSYC
Reference: Stuart, G. (2005). *Handbook of psychiatric nursing* (6th ed.). St. Louis, MO: Elsevier Mosby.

35. **Answer: 2**
Rationale: Identifying symptoms that trigger a relapse allows the client and family to take preventative action. Responses 1, 3, and 4 indicate that the client has learned strategies for coping with hallucinations.
Cognitive Level: Analysis
Nursing Process: Evaluation
NCLEX-RN Test Plan: PSYC
Reference: Stuart, G. (2005). *Handbook of psychiatric nursing* (6th ed.). St. Louis, MO: Elsevier Mosby.

36. **Answer: 3**
Rationale: Behaviors in schizophrenic clients related to memory deficit are forgetfulness, disinterest, and lack of compliance. Concrete thinking and time management problems are related to decision mak-

ing deficits. Difficulty completing a task is related to an attention deficit.

Cognitive Level: Analysis
Nursing Process: Assessment
NCLEX-RN Test Plan: PSYC

Reference: Stuart, G. (2005). *Handbook of psychiatric nursing* (6th ed.). St. Louis, MO: Elsevier Mosby.

37. **Answer: 1**

Rationale: Response 1 indicates improvement in the core problem of concrete thinking. Response 2 indicates improvement in the core problem of poor attention span and difficulty completing a task. Responses 3 and 4 indicate improvement in the core problem of being able to distinguish background from foreground information.

Cognitive Level: Analysis
Nursing Process: Evaluation
NCLEX-RN Test Plan: PSYC

Reference: Stuart, G. (2005). *Handbook of psychiatric nursing* (6th ed.). St. Louis, MO: Elsevier Mosby.

38. **Answer: 4**

Rationale: Undoing one act partially negates a previous act. Repression is involuntary exclusion of

thoughts or memories from awareness. Splitting involves a failure to integrate the positive and negative aspects of self and others. Sublimation is substituting a socially approved goal for one that is not socially approved.

Cognitive Level: Analysis
Nursing Process: Analysis
NCLEX-RN Test Plan: PSYC

Reference: Stuart, G. (2005). *Handbook of psychiatric nursing* (6th ed.). St. Louis, MO: Elsevier Mosby.

39. **Answer: 4**

Rationale: Disassociation involves the separating of any group of mental or behavioral processes from the rest of consciousness. In isolation, there is a splitting off of the emotional and thought components of a situation. Regression involves a retreat to behavior characteristic of an earlier developmental period due to stress.

Cognitive Level: Application
Nursing Process: Implementation
NCLEX-RN Test Plan: PSYC

Reference: Stuart, G. (2005). *Handbook of psychiatric nursing* (6th ed.). St. Louis, MO: Elsevier Mosby.

Posttest

Posttest

1. The nurse would discontinue use of a systemic cold application when the client displays which of the following symptoms?
   1. A bounding pulse.
   2. Pink lips and nail beds.
   3. Shivering.
   4. A slow pulse.

2. Which of the following is the most appropriate action by the nurse in caring for a client with a moist heat application?
   1. Assess the skin 30 minutes after application.
   2. Check the temperature of the device.
   3. Leave the device on until the heat has dissipated.
   4. Use medical asepsis for open wounds.

3. A family is requesting a restraint for a client with a feeding tube who is attempting to remove the tube. Which of the following is the best response by the nurse?
   1. "I will increase the stimulation in the environment."
   2. "I will call the doctor and get the order."
   3. "I will check if we can begin oral feedings."
   4. "I will wait and see what the client is going to do with the tube during the night shift."

4. The nurse is caring for a client with congestive heart failure. In which of the following situations should the nurse use gloves?
   1. The nurse draws up the client's medication in a syringe.
   2. The nurse empties the client's Foley catheter drainage bag.
   3. The nurse handles the client's clean linen.
   4. The nurse talks with the client.

5. The nurse is preparing a sterile field. Which of the following actions should be performed first?
   1. Donning clean gloves.
   2. Opening the packages containing sterile items.
   3. Placing the sterile field on the table.
   4. Washing hands using the correct technique.

6. A client is admitted to the unit with methicillin-resistant *Staphylococcus aureus* (MRSA) in an abdominal wound. The nurse enters the room to take the client's pulse. Which action by the nurse is necessary?
   1. Applying gloves and a gown.
   2. Applying gloves and a mask.
   3. Handwashing and applying gloves.
   4. Handwashing and using protective eyewear.

7. The most appropriate nursing diagnosis for a client that is incontinent of urine and stool would be a risk for which of the following?
   1. Altered nutrition is less than the client's body requirements.
   2. Immobility.
   3. Impaired skin integrity.
   4. Risk for falls.

8. **What is the client's total output during an eight hour shift given the following information?**

   _____

   Breakfast of 4 oz. juice and 6 oz. hot tea.
   Voided 450 ml after breakfast.
   IV push pain med 50 cc.
   100 cc ice chips before lunch.
   Lunch of 8 oz. clear broth.
   Vomited 120 cc and voided 600 cc after lunch.
   Jackson Pratt drain emptied at the end of the
       shift for 40 cc bloody drainage.

9. **What is the most effective intervention in preventing complications of bedrest and immobility?**

   _____

   _____

10. **Which of the following is the first step the nurse must do when responding to a client's request for pain medication?**
    1. Completely assess the client's pain.
    2. Prepare and administer the pain medication ordered.
    3. Reposition the client to their specifications.
    4. Use guided imagery or distraction to decrease the pain.

11. **What would be the first priority of the nurse if the client begins choking on food while eating a meal?**

    _____

    _____

12. **Which method best describes teaching a client care in the affective domain?**
    1. Asking the client to perform a return demonstration of the procedure presented.
    2. Discussing the therapeutic action and client response to a medication.
    3. Exploring how the patient feels about having a breast lumpectomy.
    4. Having a family member change an abdominal dressing using sterile technique.

13. **A nurse is assessing an American Indian client who has been admitted for gastrointestinal distress. The nurse is focusing excessively on alcohol intake history and patterns. This behavior by the nurse demonstrates a prejudicial attitude known as**

    _____

14. **When communicating electronically (e-mail) with a client, the nurse recognizes that the only way to protect the computer from viruses is to avoid**

    _____

15. **The nurse is communicating with a client standing with his hands on his hips, his feet apart, and an expressionless, cold stare. The nurse's supervisor evaluates this behavior to be which of the following?**
    1. Aggressive.
    2. Assertive.
    3. Confrontational.
    4. Nonassertive.

16. During an assessment, the client, appearing anxious, states that she is having difficulty remembering if she examined her breasts last month. The nurse replies, "Sometimes, as busy as I am, I have difficulty remembering if I examined my breasts each month." The nurse's response is an application of the therapeutic communication skill of

_____

17. The client's oldest son says to the client, "Gamma's behavior was becoming dangerous. I think you did the right thing by putting her in the nursing home." The nurse evaluates the son's communication to be _____

18. When the nurse is communicating with a client in a nurse-client relationship, which of the following is the least effective type of communication?
1. Nonverbal communication.
2. One-way communication.
3. Open-ended communication.
4. Two-way communication.

19. The nurse is preparing to apply a transdermal medication patch to the client. The nurse should do which of the following?
1. Apply the transdermal patch on the skin of the client's chest as ordered.
2. Cleanse an area of the skin on the client's back and apply the transdermal patch.
3. Locate and remove the previous transdermal patch, then cleanse the area with soap and water, dry the skin, and apply the new patch.
4. Remove the previous transdermal patch and apply the new one.

20. One liter of fluid IV every six hours is ordered for an adult client. Which flow rate indicates the IV calculation is correct if the IV administration set delivers 10 gtts/minute?
1. 22 gtts/minute.
2. 28 gtts/minute.
3. 32 gtts/minute.
4. 36 gtts/minute.

21. A semi-permeable membrane shaped in the form of a disc or patch that contains a drug to be absorbed through the skin is called a

_____

22. The nurse administers eye medication in the form of eye drops. What does the nurse ask the client to do?
1. Look up and the nurse will instill the drops into the center of the conjunctival sac.
2. Look up and the nurse will instill the drops along the upper lid, starting at the inner canthus of each eye.
3. Look down and the nurse will instill the drops along the edge of the lower eyelid.
4. Look down and the nurse will instill the drops into the center of the conjuctival sac.

For the following question, fill in the blank with the correct route (intravenous, intramuscular, oral, rectal, subcutaneous, topical) of administration.

23. _____

Provides the fastest onset of a drug's effect.

24. The nurse is preparing a unit-dose packaged medication for the client. When does the third and final check of the label of the medication occur?
   1. At the client's bedside before administration.
   2. In the medication room where the medicine is obtained.
   3. At the time of documentation.
   4. When removing the medication from the client's medicine cassette.

25. The nurse is just beginning her 11 PM–7 AM shift. Which client should be assessed first?
   1. A four-hour postoperative Cesarean section complaining of pain.
   2. An antepartum patient with pregnancy-induced hypertension with a blood pressure of 130/90.
   3. A one-day postpartum vaginal delivery with no bleeding.
   4. A client that has had a complete abortion earlier in the day and is scheduled for discharge in the morning.

26. What nursing diagnosis takes priority when caring for a client receiving electroconvulsive therapy (ECT)?
   1. Potential for brain damage.
   2. Potential for confusion.
   3. Potential for fracture of the extremities.
   4. Potential for apnea.

27. The registered nurse has a relief licensed practical nurse (LPN) working today and is unsure of the LPN's expertise level in several skills required to provide care. Thus, the registered nurse develops a plan of care where the LPN is responsible for all vital signs and meal tray distribution. The registered nurse will do all treatments and medications. What priority-setting trap has the registered nurse fallen into?
   1. Managing by default.
   2. Path of least resistance.
   3. Squeaky wheel.
   4. Whatever happened first.

28. Which of the following tasks would you assign to the experienced unlicensed assistive personnel (UAP)? Select all that apply.
   1. Bathing a two-day postoperative cardiovascular accident client.
   2. Completing shift input and output totals.
   3. Educating a hypertensive client about a low sodium diet.
   4. Explaining oral hygiene to a chemotherapy client.
   5. Feeding a client.

29. What activity could the nurse on a long-term care unit safely delegate to the licensed practical nurse (LPN)?
   1. Admission of a new client.
   2. Discharge of a client to home.
   3. Giving all medications.
   4. Teaching a client insulin injection.

30. You are the RN returning from dinner. Prioritize the order in which you will complete the following tasks, with 1 being the highest priority and 4 the lowest priority.
   ____ Call the physician about a medication error.
   ____ Restart an IV antibiotic piggyback medication that has infiltrated.
   ____ Suction a patient with copious secretions from a tracheostomy.
   ____ Check the lab results for preoperative patients scheduled for the OR tomorrow morning.

31. **Victims of a disaster may have psychological and physical reactions to a disaster. Which of the following are immediate physical reactions? Select all that apply.**
    1. Shock symptoms, including difficulty breathing, chills, and pale, cold, clammy skin.
    2. Skin reactions.
    3. Teeth grinding.
    4. Chest pain and palpitations.
    5. Hyperventilation.

32. **A community health nurse in a large US city is working with other members of the health department to plan care for community members following a recent flood in the city. What aggravated chronic conditions should this nurse expect to see during this phase? Select all that apply.**
    1. Respiratory problems.
    2. Cardiovascular problems.
    3. Measles, mumps, and rubella.
    4. Immunological problems such as diabetes.

33. **Twenty school-aged children arrive in the emergency department after feeling ill at school. The principal reports that the children ate macaroni and cheese for lunch. Additionally, the heating system furnaces were turned on today due to the chilly outdoor temperatures. Upon arrival, the students' symptoms include nausea and vomiting, headache, dyspnea, and dizziness. This multiple casualty incident was probably caused by which of the following?**
    1. Carbon monoxide inhalation.
    2. Heat stroke.
    3. Food poisoning.
    4. Stress.

34. **Victim of a suspected terror event involving a cutaneous anthrax exposure, a client is brought to the emergency room. The nurse will monitor for major symptoms, including which of the following?**
    1. Respiratory distress would be expected almost immediately upon exposure.
    2. Fever, malaise, headache, and a cough present within hours of inhalation exposure.
    3. Skin lesions progressing from pruritic papules to necrotic ulcers begin appearing within one hour of exposure.
    4. Severe dyspnea, hypoxia, and septic shock follow a prodromal period of malaise, headache, fever, and chills.

35. **In preparing for a mass inoculation program with the smallpox vaccine to a group of health care providers, what would the nurse expect to screen for?**
    1. Past exposure to anthrax.
    2. Potential of pregnancy.
    3. Current medication use of antimicrobials.
    4. A history of heart disease.

36. **In the event of a bioterrorism event, nurses working in schools or community sites may be responsible for implementing "shelter in place" procedures. Which of the following is necessary to accomplish this?**
    1. Occupants of the building will need to first assemble outside the building for directions.
    2. Air conditioning or heating systems will need to be shut down.
    3. Telephone systems will need to be shut down.
    4. Electricity to the building will need to be shut down.

37. The nurse is caring for a client who has a chest tube connected to a water seal drainage (pleura-evac). The nurse knows the system is functioning correctly when she observes which of the following?
    1. The fluctuation of the fluid level within the water seal chamber.
    2. The pleura-evac is even with the chest level.
    3. Continuous bubbling within the water seal chamber.
    4. All chambers have equal amounts of fluid.

38. Effects of tobacco smoke on the respiratory system include which of the following? Select all that apply.
    1. Bronchospasm.
    2. Cancer.
    3. Chronic bronchitis.
    4. Chronic cough.
    5. Decreased incidence of infection.
    6. Decreased secretions.
    7. Increased sense of taste and smell.
    8. Increased cough.

39. The nurse is caring for a client who has a history of asthma. Which medication would be contraindicated for this client due to its side effects of bronchoconstriction?
    1. Beta blockers.
    2. Bronchodilators.
    3. Leukotriene inhibitors.
    4. Steroids.

40. A client complains that her medications smell like "rotten eggs." The nurse explains that the odor is caused by which medication?
    1. Acetylcysteine (Mucomyst).
    2. Acetaminophen (Tylenol).
    3. Potassium iodide (SSKI, Pima).
    4. Terpin Hydrate.

41. Which nursing intervention is essential to the care of a child in severe respiratory distress?
    1. The child should be placed on O_2 @ 3 L per nasal cannula.
    2. The child should be placed in protective isolation.
    3. The child should not be given anything by mouth.
    4. The child should not be allowed visitors.

42. Assuming handwashing is done before and after the procedure, place the following information related to suctioning a tracheostomy tube in order.
    1. Adjust the suction to 120–150 mm Hg and test.
    2. Apply intermittent suction for not longer than 10 seconds.
    3. Apply sterile gloves; designate one hand sterile and one clean.
    4. Assess the baseline SPO_2, heart rate, and rhythm.
    5. Assess and explain the need for suctioning.
    6. Insert the catheter without suction.
    7. Preoxygenation.
    8. Reoxygenate.

43. Which of the following are signs and symptoms of digoxin (Lanoxin) toxicity?
    1. A decrease in urine output, a decrease in potassium (K^+), and an increase in BUN and creatinine.
    2. An increase in heart rate and blood pressure.
    3. Nausea, vomiting, headache, yellow haze vision, and confusion.
    4. Weight gain.

44. A client exhibits the following symptoms: Inflammation of a vein associated with redness, warmth, tenderness, hardness, edema, and pain. What is the client experiencing?

1. Distended neck veins.
2. Pitting edema of the lower extremities.
3. Positive Homan's sign.
4. Thrombophlebitis.

45. **A client is complaining of pain in the chest, neck, and arm. His skin is cool and diaphoretic. What would be the initial intervention of the nurse?**
    1. Administer O_2 by a nasal cannula or nonrebreather mask.
    2. Assess severity of pain using pain scale of 1 to 10.
    3. Ensure a patent airway.
    4. Obtain a 12-lead ECG.

46. **When performing CPR on a client, regardless of the age, the rate of compressions should be**

    _____

47. **A client in the CCU has a ventricular pacemaker. The nurse understands that the pacemaker is functioning properly when which of the following appear on the EKG?**
    1. The pacemaker spikes after each QRS complex.
    2. The pacemaker spikes after each P wave.
    3. The pacemaker spikes before each QRS complex.
    4. The pacemaker spikes before each P wave and before each QRS complex.

48. **Carvedilol (Coreg) is prescribed for a client with CHF. What should the nurse understand regarding the effects of this medication?**
    1. It is contraindicated in clients with bronchial asthma.
    2. It causes an increase in blood pressure.
    3. It may cause an increase in heart rate.
    4. It must be taken on an empty stomach.

49. **The patient complains of intermittent bright red blood in her stools. The doctor orders an occult blood test on three different days. All three tests were negative. Which of the following is a causative factor based on this data?**
    1. Aspirin therapy.
    2. Hemorrhoids.
    3. Pinworms.
    4. Upper GI bleeding.

50. **A client is admitted to the unit with a chief complaint of a dull, aggravating, burning discomfort in the stomach area with tenderness and frequent nausea. Which of the following factors may be related to his complaints?**
    1. A history of bulimia.
    2. An oral temperature of 100°F and a blood pressure of 160/88.
    3. A smoker with an admitted career burnout.
    4. A three pack per day smoker with constipation.

51. **Several client histories are being reviewed for upcoming barium enemas. Which of the following clients may have difficulty with the procedure requirements?**
    1. A 20-year-old male with a hearing deficit.
    2. A 33-year-old blind female.
    3. A 55-year-old amputee.
    4. An 88-year-old with a hearing deficit.

52. **A client admitted with pancreatitis is requesting pain medication. The physician has ordered meperidine (Demerol) 35 mg IM every six hours, as needed. The label on the available Demerol reads 50 mg/ml. To administer the correct dose, how many milliliters should the nurse draw up in the syringe?**

    _____

53. The client admitted with pancreatitis is in severe pain. The nurse develops a plan of care with a main priority being pain management. Once the pain begins to lessen, the nurse realizes the relationship between pain and controlling the pancreatic secretions. Therefore, the nurse must enforce which of the following on the plan of care?
   1. Administer the oral potassium supplement as ordered.
   2. Change the IV medication to oral once the pain is under control.
   3. Keep the pain medication going for at least 10 days to ensure that complete pain relief is obtained.
   4. Maintain NPO status to allow for pancreatic rest.

54. A middle-aged woman with height of 5'8" weighing 85 pounds comes to the emergency department with complaints of severe weakness and continual diarrhea. She has been treated for constipation and depression most of her adult life. Which of the following from her history may contribute to her condition?
   1. She administered two enemas to herself in the last week.
   2. She has lost 30 pounds over two years.
   3. She has suffered from severe depression for nine years.
   4. She has used laxatives on a daily basis for over 10 years.

55. A hemodialysis client has recently had an arteriovenous (AV) graft placed in his left forearm. As a staff nurse, what is the best way to assess the patency of this new graft?
   1. Monitor the client for any increase in BP in the left arm.
   2. Check the capillary refill in the left fingers.
   3. Monitor the client for signs of blood loss from the surgical site.
   4. Listen with the stethoscope over the graft for a bruit.

56. A client is ordered intravenous pyelogram (IVP). Before this procedure, the nurse fills out the health history and consent. She finds which of the following would prevent the client from having the IVP?
   1. The client is diabetic.
   2. The client has an allergy to shellfish.
   3. The client has a history of claustrophobia.
   4. The client has a metal plate in her knee.

57. Which of the following client statements lets the nurse know that the client has knowledge on how to correctly collect a urine specimen?
   1. "I have to wipe back to front with the cleansing cloth."
   2. "I can not collect a urine sample today because I am menstruating."
   3. "I can collect my sample of urine in the morning and drop it off at the lab on my way home from work at 5 PM."
   4. "I need to urinate some in the toilet first before I urinate in the specimen container."

58. Following a kidney transplant, the nurse knows that the most serious complication to the client is which of the following?
   1. Infection.
   2. Hematoma.
   3. Rejection.
   4. Hypertensive crisis.

59. A 45-year-old female client presents to the physician's office with the following symptoms: suprapubic pain associated with bladder filling and urinary urgency. The client states these symptoms come and go but get worse when she postpones urination or is under emotional distress. A urine culture is sent and comes back negative. What would this client's diagnosis be?
   1. Acute pyelonephritis.
   2. Chronic pyelonephritis.
   3. Interstitial cystitis.
   4. Urinary tract infection.

60. **A type of risk factor that contributes to the development of urinary tract calculi would be which of the following?**
   1. Metabolic abnormalities that result in decreased levels of calcium.
   2. Cold climates that cause high urine volume and decreased solute concentration.
   3. A large intake of dietary proteins that increases uric acid excretion.
   4. High fluid intake that causes urine dilution.

61. **In assessing the client with a diagnosis of new onset diabetes insipidus, the nurse would expect to find which of the following?**
   1. Urine with high specific gravity.
   2. Weight gain.
   3. Bradycardia.
   4. Dehydration.

62. **Which of the following dietary modifications are recommended for the patient to control Cushing's disease?**
   1. Decrease potassium intake.
   2. Increase protein intake.
   3. Increase caloric intake.
   4. Decrease fat intake to 5% of total calories.

63. **A client is undergoing thyroid tests (T_3, T_4, TSH) for hyperthyroidism or Grave's disease. Which of the following laboratory test results are indicative of hyperthyroidism?**
   1. Elevated T_3 and T_4 levels and normal TSH.
   2. Normal T_3 and T_4 levels and elevated TSH.
   3. Elevated T_3 and T_4 levels and decreased TSH.
   4. Decreased T_3 and T_4 levels and elevated TSH.

64. **A client is seen in the clinic for testing for hypothyroidism. Which of the following signs and symptoms would the nurse anticipate the client may be experiencing?**
   1. Protruding eyeballs (exophthalamos).
   2. Palpitations.
   3. Weight gain.
   4. Diaphoresis.

65. **A patient presents with the following signs and symptoms: blood glucose of 600 mg/dl, weight loss, polyuria, polydypsia, and polyphasia. The nurse would anticipate administering which of the following?**
   1. Glucocorticoids.
   2. An intravenous infusion of 5% dextrose.
   3. Oral hypoglycemia drugs.
   4. An intravenous infusion of 0.9% normal saline and regular insulin.

66. **A client who is six months pregnant has been newly diagnosed with gestational diabetes. Which statement made by the client indicates a need for more teaching?**
   1. "I plan to closely follow my dietary regimen."
   2. "I will be regularly testing my blood glucose levels and recording the results."
   3. "I will take my oral antidiabetic medication before breakfast and dinner."
   4. "I know this increases my risk for developing Type 2 diabetes."

67. **What should the nurse do when caring for a client admitted with gastrointestinal bleeding whose platelet count is reported as 180,000/mm³?**
   1. Communicate this to the next shift as a platelet count within normal limits.
   2. Communicate this to the next shift as a decreased platelet count.
   3. Communicate this to the next shift as an elevated platelet count.
   4. Immediately initiate bleeding precautions.

68. A healthcare team collaboratively determines that a client has developed a localized hypersensitivity reaction to a medication. The nurse's initial assessment that preceded the diagnosis may have included which of the following symptoms?
    1. Bronchospasm.
    2. Hemolysis.
    3. Urticaria at the injection site.
    4. Allergic rhinitis.

69. When caring for clients with human immunodeficiency virus (HIV) and acquired immunodeficiency syndrome (AIDS), the nurse knows the importance of obtaining which of the following laboratory tests that assess the status and category of HIV infection and AIDS progression?
    1. Viral load and CD4$^+$ cell counts.
    2. Platelet counts.
    3. Renal function tests.
    4. ELISA and Western blot assays.

70. A client with a history of obesity and alcoholism being evaluated for easy bruisability and frequent nosebleeds is found to have a prolonged (elevated) prothrombin time (PT). To which of the following are this client's signs and symptoms most likely related?
    1. Malnutrition.
    2. Increased blood viscosity.
    3. Diabetes.
    4. Cirrhosis of the liver.

71. The nurse is preparing a fact sheet for student nurses on various autoimmune disorders, such as rheumatoid arthritis (RA), systemic lupus erythematosus (SLE), and scleroderma. Information on the fact sheet should state that these disorders originate in which of the following areas?
    1. The musculoskeletal system.
    2. Connective tissue.
    3. The endocrine system.
    4. The peripheral vascular system.

72. A client with DIC is being treated for hypovolemic shock. Which of the following should the nurse identify as the most appropriate type of blood product for this clinical situation?
    1. Frozen washed RBCs.
    2. Platelets.
    3. Fresh frozen plasma (FFP) or albumin.
    4. Packed RBCs.

73. When caring for a client with an open pressure ulcer, which of the following is an important aspect of care?
    1. Applying a heat lamp twice a day.
    2. Cleansing with isotonic saline.
    3. Cleansing with povodone-iodine solution.
    4. Rubbing reddened areas with dressing changes.

74. Antihistamines are frequently prescribed to help with the symptoms of pruritus. In order to minimize the sedative effects of these medications, what should the nurse instruct the client to do?
    1. Gradually increase the dose once tolerance to the effect is reached.
    2. Space the doses evenly throughout the day.
    3. Take most of the daily dose near bedtime.
    4. Take with meals.

75. The nurse is performing an assessment on a client with herpes zoster or shingles. The nurse would expect which of the following findings?
    1. Blisters at the corners of the mouth.
    2. Painful fluid-filled vesicles in the genital area.
    3. Painful vesicles following a nerve pathway.
    4. Papules scattered over the ribcage.

76. Which statement best indicates that the client understands how herpes simplex is transmitted?

1. "I shouldn't have sex if some of those sores are around."
2. "It is okay to share towels as long as it is a family member."
3. "Once I'm over this spell, I won't have to worry about it again."
4. "The only way I can spread this stuff is if I have a lot of sores."

77. Several nurses are assisting with a skin screening at a local dermatologist's office. They are aware that which of the following groups of people are at risk for developing malignant melanoma?

1. Dark-skinned people with regular sun exposure.
2. Dark-skinned people who work indoors.
3. Light-skinned people with regular sun exposure.
4. Light-skinned people who work indoors.

78. When formulating a plan of care for the client with skin lesions, which of the following nursing diagnoses would be least appropriate?

1. Anxiety.
2. Disturbed body image.
3. Disuse syndrome.
4. Social isolation.

79. A client is admitted after chemotherapy treatment with a new diagnosis of aplastic anemia. While preparing to care for this client, the nurse identifies which of the following nursing diagnoses? Select all that apply.

1. Risk for ineffective tissue perfusion.
2. Risk for infection.
3. Risk for injury.
4. Risk for altered level of consciousness.

80. The nurse is assessing a client's knowledge of their cancer, disease stage, and predetermined treatment goals. The nurse is aware that the treatment is palliative and that the physician has documented a clear understanding by the client of the prognosis and treatment plans. What statement by the client indicates they have a clear understanding and acceptance of their prognosis?

1. "I am thinking of getting a second opinion."
2. "I hope this helps with the pain and pressure."
3. "This is making me better every time."
4. "This is not working, I am thinking of stopping treatment."

81. A client with advanced multiple myeloma calls for assistance in moving up in bed. There is no lift under the client and the nurse instructs the UAP to obtain a lift to be placed under the client prior to moving them. The nurse recognizes that this client is at greater risk than most clients for which of the following?

1. Fractures.
2. Immobility.
3. Pressure sores.
4. Shearing injuries.

82. A client was just diagnosed with testicular cancer. Which of the following statements will the nurse include in a discussion with the client?

1. Incidence is greater in African Americans than in White males.
2. It can be familial.
3. It is a rare form of cancer.
4. It occurs in both testicles equally.
5. It occurs in fifteen- to thirty-five-year-olds.
6. Once diagnosed, the sperm is no longer viable.
7. One of the first signs is a painful scrotal lump.
8. Prognosis is generally poor.

83. In individuals age 50 and older, the greatest risk for head and neck cancers is which of the following?

1. Chronic cold sores.
2. Family history.
3. Poor oral hygiene.
4. Prolonged alcohol and tobacco use.

84. Noninvasive cervical cancer is four times more common than invasive cervical cancer. In the past 40 years, there has been a decrease in related deaths. What is the most likely reason for this decrease?

1. Availability of internal radiation.
2. Progressive treatment protocols.
3. Public education and free clinics.
4. Use of magnetic resonance imaging.

85. A client with a herniated disc and in chronic pain is scheduled to have a laminectomy. Which of the following should be done prior to the procedure? Select all that apply.

1 Assess the client's alcohol intake.
2. Assess the client's use of prescribed and nonprescribed medications.
3. Assess the client's recreational drug use.
4. Assess the client's use of herbs and nutritional supplements.
5. Alert the surgeon and anesthesiologist of findings.
6. Be consistent in setting limits while providing pain management.
7. Discontinue opioid analgesics taken at home with vigilant assessment for withdrawal signs and symptoms.

86. The nurse is caring for a client with a left cerebral infarction. Draw the visual pathways and show where you would find hemianopsia.

87. A young male is admitted to the hospital 36 hours after striking his head on the windshield of his auto when he hit a telephone pole. It is not known if he was unconscious. Skull films were negative and he was released from the emergency room with acetaminophen (Tylenol) for his headache. The next day, his complaints of headache persisted and his wife found him wandering around the bedroom after apparently vomiting and being incontinent of urine. What is the priority nursing diagnosis for this client?

1. Ineffective tissue perfusion: Cerebral (ICP).
2. Risk for injury: Seizure and decreased level of consciousness.
3. Impaired gas exchange: Head injury and aspiration.
4. Knowledge deficit: Craniotomy.

88. A nurse assigned to a client with a cerebral aneurysm is making client rounds. Which information should the nurse communicate immediately to physician?

1. The client says, "I have not had a bowel movement for two days and would like a laxative."
2. The client says, "I feel nauseated and do not want any dinner."
3. The client says, "I must have been sleeping and my wet bed linens need to be changed."
4. The client says, "My headache was relieved with the Tylenol (acetaminophen) and I would like to take a nap."

89. **A client is aphasic. The nurse would be correct in telling the family which of the following?**
    1. The client may be responding to nonverbal cues and may understand less than they think.
    2. The client will be able to process information and answer questions with multiple choices rather than yes/no answers.
    3. The client will be able to understand better if the voice volume is high.
    4. The client will respond better to simple "baby-talk".

90. **A client comes into the clinic with a possible diagnosis of myasthenia gravis. The physician orders a Tensilon (edrophonium) test. Which of the following indicates the test is positive?**
    1. There is improvement in their "pill-rolling" tremor.
    2. There is no change in their "pill-rolling" tremor.
    3. There is improvement in muscle strength.
    4. There is no improvement in their muscle strength.

91. **Which of the following drugs is the drug of choice for Paget's disease?**
    1. Bisphosphonates.
    2. Colchicine.
    3. Glucocorticoids.
    4. SERMS.

92. **Which of the following statements best reflects the pathophysiology of osteoarthritis?**
    1. It is characterized by thinning of the articular cartilage, commonly affects weight-bearing joints, and has an asymmetrical distribution.
    2. It is a disease of aging that ultimately results in profound disability. It commonly contributes to pathologic fractures due to increased excretion of calcium and protein by the kidneys.
    3. It is a systemic inflammatory disease that affects many joint structures in a symmetrical fashion and can also involve other body systems.
    4. It is a systemic disease with several phases and is accompanied by hyperuricemia with deposition of urate crystal in joints and other tissues.

93. **Because dizziness may occur, clients should be instructed not to drive or operate heavy machinery until they know the response to which of the following drugs?**
    1. Auranofin (Ridura).
    2. Gold sodium thiomalate (Myochrysine).
    3. Leflunomide (Arava).
    4. Penicillamine (Cuprimine).

94. **What is the basic pathophysiology underlying osteoporosis?**
    1. A decrease in osteoclastic activity.
    2. An imbalance between osteoclastic and osteoblastic activity.
    3. An increase in osteoblastic activity.
    4. Impaired calcium absorption that leads to a decrease in osteoclastic activity.

95. **A client with a symphysis pubis and pelvic rami fractures should be monitored for which of the following?**
    1. A palpable lump in the buttock.
    2. A change in urinary output.
    3. A sudden decrease in blood pressure.
    4. Sudden thirst.

96. Which of the following assessments would be the most appropriate for a client who is in a body jacket cast?
    1. Assessment of the abdomen.
    2. Assessment of pulses.
    3. Assessment of skin integrity.
    4. Assessment of urinary elimination.

97. The preoperative nurse informs the client that nail polish must be removed. When the client questions why, the nurse responds with which of the following statements?
    1. Nail polish impairs the assessment of capillary refill and oxygen saturation.
    2. Nail polish is a source of contamination.
    3. Nail polish might be flammable.
    4. Surgeons do not permit it.

98. A 48-hour postoperative arthroplasty is using a Morphine (morphine sulfate) PCA pump for pain control. The client is complaining of abdominal bloating and vomits after the ingestion of a regular diet. What should the nurse do?
    1. Auscultate and assess the abdomen.
    2. Continue to feed the client.
    3. Discontinue the morphine pump.
    4. Insert a nasogastric tube.

99. Airway obstruction in the immediate postanesthetic period is most commonly caused by which of the following?
    1. Blockage of the airway by the client's tongue.
    2. Laryngeal edema.
    3. Laryngospasms.
    4. Retained secretions.

100. A second day postoperative abdominal surgery client calls for the nurse and tells her he felt something pop. On assessment, the nurse notes that the wound has eviscerated. Which of the following should be the nurse's next step?
    1. Cover the protruding intestine with sterile, moist, saline gauze.
    2. Notify the physician.
    3. Place the client in high fowlers.
    4. Start an IV line.

101. Abdominal assessment of a third day postoperative client reveals absent bowel sounds, abdominal distention, and the inability to pass flatus. Which of the following does the nurse identify as a possibility?
    1. A dietary imbalance.
    2. A medication reaction.
    3. A paralytic ileus.
    4. A prolapsed incision.

102. A spinal headache may result from which of the following?
    1. Increased intake of oral fluids after surgery.
    2. Leakage of spinal fluid.
    3. Lying flat in bed.
    4. Positioning the patient prone.

103. A client is admitted with esophageal varices and severe malnutrition related to alcoholism. Total parenteral nutrition (TPN) is initiated, and on day four the client begins to experience seizures, circumoral and fingertip numbness and tingling, chest pain, and dysrhythmias. The nurse evaluates lab values recognizing that these symptoms are associated with what complication of TPN?
    1. Hyperglycemia.
    2. Refeeding syndrome.
    3. Fluid overload.
    4. Sepsis.

104. A client complains of an excessive ileostomy output for three days with nausea, vomiting, weakness, and headaches. The family reports lethargy, confusion, and warm, flushed skin. The client's blood pressure is 88/54, heart rate is 90, and respirations are deep at 32 bpm. In preparing and planning to initiate infusion therapy, the nurse recognizes that which of the following states best describes this patient?

1. Metabolic acidosis.
2. Metabolic alkalosis.
3. Respiratory acidosis.
4. Respiratory alkalosis.

105. During a multidisciplinary conference with a terminal client and their family, a discussion ensued regarding the client's end of life wishes, which were clearly documented. It was decided life-sustaining therapies would be discontinued and that palliative care therapies, including intravenous pain management, would continue. The family noticed and commented that the .9 saline running at 30 ml/hr with the morphine drip would not be enough fluid to provide hydration and therefore comfort. They were concerned that the client would be thirsty and therefore suffer. The nurse explains the IV fluids are running to ensure delivery of the pain medication but also offers the following additional information:

1. Do not offer sips of water so they are not reminded of their thirst.
2. It is not ethical to provide more treatment than the client desired.
3. More fluids are not necessary to provide comfort if they deny thirst.
4. The doctor will be contacted to discuss your concerns.

106. A client is admitted with congestive heart failure and acute pulmonary edema secondary to an acute myocardial infarction. Emergency medications have been ordered. If given a choice, what type of solution should the nurse select in mixing drips?

1. Isotonic solutions.
2. Hypertonic solutions.
3. Hypotonic solutions.
4. Request meds by IV push.

107. A client with no known medical problems was admitted for observation after a bicycling accident with major bruises all over her body. Laboratory results return with a serum potassium level of 6.0 mEq. What is the most likely cause of the elevated potassium?

1. Acute renal failure.
2. Hemolysis.
3. Metabolic acidosis.
4. New onset diabetes mellitus.

108. A nurse believes that an epidural catheter has migrated through the dura mater and into the intrathecal space. If this has happened, what information regarding epidural and intrathecal pain administration is of most concern to the nurse?

1. Epidural dosing can be given continuously.
2. Intrathecal and epidural doses are different.
3. Inward migration will cause an infection.
4. Pain may occur at the insertion site.

109. You are the RN teaching a client about foods high in potassium. Which food is *not* a high potassium food?

1. Orange juice.
2. Baked potato.
3. Yogurt.
4. Pecans.

110. The nurse discusses the potential drug and food interaction risk for a client who has recently begun anticoagulant therapy. The client should be aware to limit the intake of which food?
    1. Legumes.
    2. Citrus fruit.
    3. Leafy green vegetables.
    4. Seafood.

111. The nurse explains to a burn patient the importance of nutrition in the plan of care. Which vitamins are commonly used to promote wound healing? Select all that apply.
    1. Vitamin A.
    2. Vitamin B_{12}.
    3. Vitamin C.
    4. Vitamin D.
    5. Vitamin E.

112. A mother of 4½-year-old tells the nurse that her son is a "picky eater." Which of the following is the best explanation from the nurse?
    1. The mother should increase the amount of carbohydrates in the daily menu plan.
    2. The mother should administer vitamins twice a day to her child.
    3. The quantity of food is more important than the quality of food.
    4. This is common for preschoolers; their caloric requirements decrease slightly.

113. The recommended kilocalories of carbohydrates consumed for the individual who has diabetes mellitus is which of the following?
    1. 20–25% of the client's diet.
    2. 25–35% of the client's diet.
    3. 45–55% of the client's diet.
    4. 10–20% of the client's diet.

114. Ginseng and ginkgo biloba are contraindicated if the client is taking which type of prescribed drug?
    1. Anticoagulants.
    2. Antidepressants.
    3. Antihistamines.
    4. Hypoglycemic.

115. The nurse in a prenatal clinic is providing health teaching to a client and her partner. Which of the following statements by the nurse is true regarding conception and fetal development?
    1. "Conception takes place in the distal third portion of the fallopian tube."
    2. "Implantation occurs between two and three weeks after conception."
    3. "The fetal stage is the most critical time in the development of organ systems."
    4. "We really are not sure exactly where fertilization occurs."

116. A pregnant woman is at 39 weeks gestation and asks the nurse if there are any signs indicating when she may start labor. The nurse should advise the client that which of the following may occur as a sign preceding labor?
    1. Decreased bloody show.
    2. A surge of energy.
    3. Urinary retention.
    4. A weight gain of 1.5 kg to 2 kg (3 to 4 pounds).

117. Identify which medications may be used for a client experiencing preterm labor. Select all that apply.
    1. Prostaglandin E2 (Cervidil).
    2. Indomethacin (Indocin).
    3. Magnesium sulfate.
    4. Methylergonovine (Methergine).
    5. Oxytocin (Pitocin).
    6. Ritodrine (Yutopar).
    7. Terbutaline (Brethine).

118. Interpret the fetal monitor strip and document your findings.

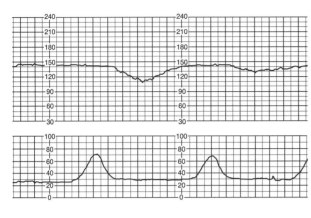

---

119. Which of the following physical characteristics is assessed and recorded as part of the newborn's gestational age assessment?
1. Acrocyanosis of hands and feet.
2. Anterior fontanel soft and level.
3. Plantar creases cover ⅔ of sole.
4. Vernix caseosa noted in creases.

120. A client who delivered 12 hours ago appears excited and talks about her birth experience to her family and friends. She asks the nurse when breakfast will be arriving and does not appear interested in learning about newborn care. The nurse recognizes that this client is in which phase of maternal adjustment?
1. Dependent-Independent: Taking Hold.
2. Dependent: Taking In.
3. Interdependent: Letting Go.
4. Mutually Dependent: Reciprocity.

121. An African American obese woman complains of extreme fatigue and pain in her left jaw. The client believes she may have a bad tooth. The nurse is aware that which of the following is the leading cause of death in women?
1. Cardiovascular disease.
2. Lung cancer.
3. Osteoporosis.
4. Breast cancer.

122. The nurse is assessing a female client for osteoporosis risk. Which of the following data should be collected during the interview? Select all that apply.
1. Menopausal status and date of last menstrual period.
2. Smoking status.
3. Alcohol and soft drink consumption.
4. Employment and educational status.

123. The client asks which test will give the best results when testing for cervical cancer. The nurse responds that the single most reliable method to detect preinvasive cervical cancer is which of the following?
1. A pelvic examination.
2. A pap test.
3. A vaginal ultrasound.
4. An abdominal ultrasound.

124. A four-hour postoperative mastectomy client is admitted to a surgical unit following surgery. Which of the following will be the initial action of the nurse?
1. Observing and emptying the surgical drains as needed.
2. Encouraging the client to turn, cough, and take a deep breath.
3. Assessing the client's pain level and providing pain medication for comfort.
4. Elevating the client's arm on a pillow and placing a sign above the client's bed requesting that no blood pressure or treatment be done on the affected arm.

125. A 15-year-old client presenting at the clinic has been diagnosed with gonorrhea. What is the primary action for the nurse?
1. To teach the client about birth control methods.
2. To notify the client's parents.
3. To obtain information about the client's recent sexual activity and contacts.
4. To obtain parental permission to treat the client.

126. A couple questions the nurse about male factor infertility. The nurse explains that which of the following have been identified as male factor causes of infertility? Select all that apply.
    1. Anatomical and structural problems.
    2. Abnormalities in sperm production.
    3. Genetic conditions and unknown causes.
    4. Diet.

127. A child is admitted to the hospital with a sickle cell crisis. Appropriate nursing management would include which of the following?
    1. Complete bedrest while hospitalized.
    2. Cold compresses to the affected area.
    3. Hydration with IV and oral fluids.
    4. Pain medication every four hours as needed.

128. A 7-year-old has a diagnosis of mild persistent asthma. Which of the following symptoms would you expect to see? Select all that apply.
    1. Continual symptoms.
    2. Daily symptoms.
    3. Nighttime symptoms less than twice a month.
    4. Nighttime symptoms more than twice a month.
    5. Nighttime symptoms nightly.
    6. Peak expiratory flow of 60–80% of the predicted value.
    7. Peak expiratory flow greater than or equal to 80% of the predicted value.
    8. Symptoms more than twice a week.

129. You are instructing the family of a child with a new diagnosis of diabetes on symptoms of high and low blood sugars. What are the symptoms of hypoglycemia? Select all that apply.
    1. Acetone smell.
    2. Flushing.
    3. Hunger.
    4. Polyuria.
    5. Shaky feeling.
    6. Sweating.
    7. Tachycardia.
    8. Thirst.

130. A child with iron deficiency anemia is ordered an oral iron supplement. How should you instruct the mother to give the iron supplement?
    1. With an eight ounce glass of whole milk.
    2. With every meal.
    3. With two ounces of orange juice.
    4. On an empty stomach.

131. What is the best predictor of suicide among adolescents?
    1. A previous attempt of suicide.
    2. Abuse of alcohol or drugs.
    3. Early sexual activity.
    4. Psychiatric disorder.

132. A 2-year-old presents with a fever. The mother is told to give acetaminophen (Tylenol). The child weighs 28 pounds. The amount ordered to administer is 10 mg/kg/dose. The concentration of acetaminophen she has is 120 mg/5 ml. How many milliliters should this mother give her child?
    1. 2.5 ml.
    2. 5 ml.
    3. 7.5 ml.
    4. 10 ml.

133. **Which statement by a client on antidepressant medication indicates that more teaching is needed?**
    1. "I am afraid of addiction, taking the drug so long."
    2. "I should keep my water intake up to 8 glasses a day."
    3. "I need to take the drug for at least 6 to 9 months."
    4. "If I am going to have sexual intercourse, I will dose after."

134. **Nursing care during treatment of acute phencyclidine (PCP) intoxication focuses on which of the following?**
    1. Antiseizure precautions.
    2. Protecting the client and others from injury.
    3. Suicide precautions.
    4. Treatment for autonomic hyperactivity.

135. **When planning discharge teaching for a client of a monoamine oxidase inhibitor (MAOI), the nurse instructs the client to avoid food containing**

    _____.

136. **Place the following activities in sequential order for the nurse for a client receiving electroconvulsive therapy (ECT).**
    1. NPO.
    2. Remove dentures.
    3. Guide extremities to prevent injury.
    4. Witness informed consent.
    5. Place client on side.
    6. Administer short-acting anesthetic and muscle relaxant.
    7. Position client on stretcher.
    8. Perform complete physical exam.

137. **The Mini Mental State Exam (MMSE) would be inappropriate for a client with which of the following conditions?**
    1. A motor movement disorder.
    2. A speech disorder.
    3. Cognitive decline.
    4. Past recall impairment.

138. **What is the most significant factor in the behavioral assessment of the depressed client?**
    1. Anxiety associated with a trigger event.
    2. A sense of worthlessness.
    3. A change in usual patterns.
    4. Despondency in social situations.

Posttest Answers and Rationales

1. **Answer: 3**

   Rationale: Shivering will increase the body temperature, making the cold application less effective. Other adverse effects of cold application include an accelerated, weak pulse and cyanosis of the lips and nails.

   Cognitive Level: Application

   Nursing Process: Assessment

   NCLEX-RN Test Plan: SECE

   Reference: Potter, P., & Perry, A. (2005). *Fundamentals of nursing* (6th ed.). St. Louis, MO: Elsevier Mosby.

2. **Answer: 2**

   Rationale: It is important to check the temperature of the device to avoid burning the skin. The skin should be assessed five minutes after application. The device should be removed after approximately 20 minutes.

   Cognitive Level: Application

   Nursing Process: Implementation

   NCLEX-RN Test Plan: SECE

   Reference: Potter, P., & Perry, A. (2005). *Fundamentals of nursing* (6th ed.). St. Louis, MO: Elsevier Mosby.

   DeLaune, S. C., & Ladner, P. K. (2006). *Fundamentals of nursing: Standards and practice* (3rd ed.). Clifton Park, NY: Thomson Delmar Learning.

3. **Answer: 3**

   Rationale: Alternatives to restraints should be considered. Eliminating a bothersome treatment, such as a feeding tube, can be an alternative. Another alternative is to try to decrease stimuli in the environment to reduce agitation and confusion. Because of a safety issue, the nurse does not want to wait to address this situation.

   Cognitive Level: Analysis

   Nursing Process: Planning

   NCLEX-RN Test Plan: SECE

   Reference: Potter, P., & Perry, A. (2005). *Fundamentals of nursing* (6th ed.). St. Louis, MO: Elsevier Mosby.

4. **Answer: 2**

   Rationale: When emptying a Foley catheter drainage bag, the nurse can potentially be exposed to body fluids; therefore, standard precautions indicate that wearing gloves is necessary. Gloves are not needed when drawing up medication, handling clean linen, or talking with a client as these activities do not involve direct contact.

   Cognitive Level: Application

   Nursing Process: Implementation

   NCLEX-RN Test Plan: SECE

   Reference: Potter, P., & Perry, A. (2005). *Fundamentals of nursing* (6th ed.). St. Louis, MO: Elsevier Mosby.

5. **Answer: 4**

   Rationale: Handwashing should be done first before beginning this procedure. Placing the sterile field on the table and opening packages would be done after handwashing. Clean gloves are not necessary when opening a sterile field.

   Cognitive Level: Application

   Nursing Process: Implementation

   NCLEX-RN Test Plan: SECE

   Reference: Potter, P., & Perry, A. (2005). *Fundamentals of nursing* (6th ed.). St. Louis, MO: Elsevier Mosby.

6. **Answer: 3**

   Rationale: Since the nurse is taking a pulse, it is only necessary to wash hands and wear gloves. Wearing a gown would be necessary only if the nurse anticipates that clothing would have substantial contact with the wound. Wearing a mask and protective eyewear is not necessary.

   Cognitive Level: Application

   Nursing Process: Planning

   NCLEX-RN Test Plan: SECE

   Reference: DeLaune, S. C., & Ladner, P. K. (2006). *Fundamentals of nursing: Standards and practice* (3rd ed.). Clifton Park, NY: Thomson Delmar Learning.

7. **Answer: 3**

   Rationale: The client is at risk for altered epidermis and/or dermis from the enzymes in the stool and acidic urine that can break down the skin. Moisture is a medium for bacterial growth and can cause local skin irritation, softening of epidermal cells, and skin maceration.

Cognition Level: Analysis
Nursing Process: Analysis
NCLEX-RN Test Plan: PHYS
Reference: Potter, P. A., & Perry, A. G. (2005). *Fundamentals of nursing* (6th ed.). St. Louis, MO: Elsevier Mosby.

8. **Answer: Input 590 and output 1210**
Rationale: Input includes all liquids taken by mouth, including through nasogastric or jejunostomy feeding tubes, IV fluids, and blood or its components. Output includes urine, diarrhea, vomitus, and drainage from tubes such as through gastric suction and drainage from postsurgical wounds or other tubes.
Cognitive Level: Analysis
Nursing Process: Evaluation
NCLEX-RN Test Plan: PHYS
Reference: Potter, P. A., & Perry, A. G. (2005). *Fundamentals of nursing* (6th ed.). St. Louis, MO: Elsevier Mosby.

9. **Answer: Turn the client every two hours.**
Rationale: Turning and moving the client relieves pressure on the capillary beds. A pressure site is any skin surface area on which the client is lying or sitting. The force of the pressure can compromise circulation and lead to skin breakdown and ulceration. Tissue areas over bony prominences are more likely to experience skin pressure areas and breakdown. Clients who cannot move or reposition themselves should be put on a routine turning and reposition schedule.
Cognitive Level: Application
Nursing Process: Implementation
NCLEX-RN Test Plan: PHYS
Reference: DeLaune, S. C., & Ladner, P. K. (2006). *Fundamentals of nursing: Standards and practice* (3rd ed.). Clinton Park, NY: Thomson Delmar Learning.

10. **Answer: 1**
Rationale: Assessment of pain includes the collection of subjective and objective data through the use of various assessment tools and the construction of a database for the development of a pain management plan.
Cognitive Level: Application
Nursing Process: Assessment
NCLEX-RN Test Plan: PHYS

Reference: DeLaune, S. C., & Ladner, P. K. (2006). *Fundamentals of nursing: Standards and practice* (3rd ed.). Clifton Park, NY: Thomson Delmar Learning.

11. **Answer: Determine if the client can speak or cough.**
Rationale: Evaluating if the client can speak will determine if it is a partial or total airway obstruction. If the client is making sounds or coughing as some air is passing from the lungs through the vocal cords, it is a partial airway obstruction Gagging and coughing are allowed to clear the airway. A total airway obstruction is present if the client is not able to make sounds. The nurse should then initiate the Heimlich maneuver, which includes using abdominal thrusts to attempt to remove the food from the airway. When trapped air behind an obstruction is forced out, it pushes out the cause of the obstruction.
Cognitive Level: Application
Nursing Process: Assessment
NCLEX-RN Test Plan: PHYS
Reference: DeLaune, S. C., & Ladner, P. K. (2006). *Fundamentals of nursing: Standards and practice* (3rd ed.). Clifton Park, NY: Thomson Delmar Learning.

12. **Answer: 3**
Rationale: Teaching in the affective domain involves the client's emotional and motivational educational needs. Oftentimes the affective teaching is focused on behavioral change. The options addressing teaching of a skill and return demonstration of a skill are teaching in the psychomotor domain. Discussion of the medication action and client responses to the medication are in the cognitive domain of education/patient education.
Cognitive Level: Application
Nursing Process: Implementation
NCLEX-RN Test Plan: HPM
Reference: De Young, S. (2003). *Teaching strategies for nurse educators.* Upper Saddle River, NJ: Prentice Hall.

13. **Answer: Stereotyping**
Rationale: Stereotypes are prejudicial attitudes developed through a person's social and cultural experiences. Subtle intrusion of stereotypical expectations into the nurse–client relationship can result in dis-

torted communication. The expectation that all American Indians abuse alcohol is an example of a stereotype.
Cognitive Level: Analysis
Nursing Process: Assessment
NCLEX-RN Test Plan: PSYC
Reference: Chitty, K. K. (2005). *Professional nursing: Concepts & challenges* (4th ed.). St. Louis, MO: Elsevier Saunders.

14. **Answer: Networking**
Rationale: Networking means opening files that have been on another person's computer. This is how viruses are spread.
Cognitive Level: Application
Nursing Process: Implementation
NCLEX-RN Test Plan: PSYC
Reference: Riley, J. B. (2004). *Communication in nursing* (5th ed.). St. Louis, MO: Elsevier Mosby.

15. **Answer: 1**
Rationale: This response represents an aggressive body stance and eyes.
Cognitive Level: Analysis
Nursing Process: Evaluation
NCLEX-RN Test Plan: PSYC
Reference: Riley, J. B. (2004). *Communication in nursing* (5th ed.). St. Louis, MO: Elsevier Mosby.

16. **Answer: Self-disclosure**
Rationale: In self-disclosure, we reveal our thoughts and feelings and make some of our personal experiences known to others, which helps the client know that we understand them.
Cognitive Level: Application
Nursing Process: Implementation
NCLEX-RN Test Plan: PSYC
Reference: Riley, J. B. (2004). *Communication in nursing* (5th ed.). St. Louis, MO: Elsevier Mosby.

17. **Answer: Giving advice**
Rationale: Giving advice involves telling another what you think should be done.
Cognitive Level: Analysis
Nursing Process: Evaluation
NCLEX-RN Test Plan: PSYC
Reference: Hood, L. J., & Leedy, S. K. (2006). *Conceptual basis of professional nursing* (6th ed.). Philadelphia: Lippincott Williams & Wilkins.

18. **Answer: 2**
Rationale: One-way communication is not therapeutic. It is a highly structured form of communication with the sender being in control and obtaining very little response from the receiver.
Cognitive Level: Application
Nursing Process: Assessment
NCLEX-Test Plan: PSYC
Reference: Christensen, B. L., & Kockrow, E. O. (2003). *Foundations of nursing.* St. Louis, MO: Elsevier Mosby.

19. **Answer: 3**
Rationale: If areas of ointment from previous doses are not removed, the client will be receiving more than the one dose at a time. Cleansing the skin ensures proper absorption of the medication.
Cognitive Level: Application
Nursing Process: Implementation
NCLEX-RN Test Plan: SECE
Reference: Altman, G. (2001). *Delmar's fundamental and advanced nursing skill* (2nd ed.). New York: Delmar Learning.

20. **Answer: 2**
Rationale:
Utilize the formula:

$$\frac{ml/hr}{60\ min/hr} \times \text{drop factor}$$

First need to find ml/hr rate.
You have the following information:
1000 ml in 6 hr
Need to know how many cc's in 1 hr
Set up the following formula:

$$\frac{1000\ cc}{6\ hr} \times \frac{x\ cc}{1\ hr}$$

Cross-multiply:
6x = 1000 cc
x = 166 ml/hr
Use the formula:

$$\frac{ml/hr}{60\ min/hr} \times \text{drop factor}$$

$$\frac{166\ ml/hr}{_6\cancel{60}\ min/hr} \times \cancel{10}^{1}\text{gtts}$$

(You were given this information: "IV set administers 10 gtts/min")

$$\frac{166}{6} = 27.6 = 28\ gtts/min$$

Cognitive Level: Application
Nursing Process: Evaluation
NCLEX-RN Test Plan: SECE
Reference: Potter, P., & Perry, A. (2005). *Fundamentals of nursing* (6th ed.) St. Louis, MO: Elsevier Mosby.

21. **Answer: Transdermal patch**
    Rationale: The nurse needs to understand the components of manufactured medicines to teach the client about prescribed medicines, their effects, storage, and benefits.
    Cognitive Level: Application
    Nursing Process: Implementation
    NCLEX-RN Test Plan: SECE
    Reference: Kozier, B., Erb, G., Berman, A., & Snyder, S. (2004). *Techniques in clinical nursing* (5th ed.). Upper Saddle River, NJ: Pearson Prentice Hall.

22. **Answer: 1**
    Rationale: By looking up, the client reduces the stimulation of the blink reflex and distributes the solution over the conjunctival surface and anterior eyeball.
    Cognitive Level: Application
    Nursing Process: Implementation
    NCLEX-RN Test Plan: SECE
    Reference: Altman, G. (2004). *Delmar's fundamental and advanced nursing skills* (2nd ed.). New York: Thomson Learning.

23. **Answer: Intravenous**
    Rationale: The nurse needs to know the correct route for drug administration for the most effective mode of absorption.
    Cognitive Level: Application
    Nursing Process: Implementation
    NCLEX-RN Test Plan: SECE
    Reference: Mills, E. (2004). *Nursing procedures* (4th ed.). Philadelphia: Lippincott Williams & Wilkins.

24. **Answer: 1**
    Rationale: Medications that come in a unit-dose prepackage form allow the nurse to check the medication a third time at the client bedside before opening the unit-dose package.
    Cognitive Level: Application

Nursing Process: Implementation
NCLEX-RN Test Plan: SECE
Reference: DeLaune, S., & Ladner, P. (2006). *Fundamentals in nursing: Standards and practice* (3rd ed.). Clifton Park, NY: Thomson Delmar Learning.

25. **Answer: 1**
    Rationale: According to Maslow's first level of human needs, physiological needs rank first in priority. Clients with pain, a physiological need, require nursing assessment, judgment, and evaluation. Pain is a high priority client need.
    Cognitive Level: Analysis
    Nursing Process: Planning
    NCLEX-RN Test Plan: SECE
    Reference: Kelly-Heidenthal, P., & Marthaler, M. T. (2005). *Delegation of nursing care.* Clifton Park, NY: Thomson Delmar Learning.

26. **Answer: 4**
    Rationale: Maslow's hierarchy of human needs provides the framework for prioritizing. Apnea represents a life-threatening physiologic need. Freedom from fracture is also a physiologic need, although not life threatening. Confusion represents a safety need and is not life threatening. Brain damage is not related to ECT.
    Cognitive Level: Application
    Nursing Process: Analysis
    NCLEX-RN Test Plan: SECE
    Reference: Mohr, W. K. (2003). *Psychiatric-mental health nursing* (5th ed.). Philadelphia: Lippincott Williams & Wilkins.

27. **Answer: 2**
    Rationale: In this trap, the nurse makes an erroneous assumption that it is easier to do a task personally rather than delegate. In this case, the LPN may have had expertise in some treatment skills. However, the nurse did not assess for this.
    Cognitive Level: Analysis
    Nursing Process: Planning
    NCLEX-RN Test Plan: SECE
    Reference: Marquis, B. L., & Huston, C. J. (2006). *Leadership roles and management functions in nursing: Theory and application* (5th ed.). Philadelphia: Lippincott Williams & Wilkins.

28. **Answers: 1, 2, and 5**
    Rationale: The UAP may complete non-nursing functions such as bathing, vital signs, feeding, and I & O recording. It is the nurse that analyzes the information gathered by the UAP. Nursing activities that rely on the nursing process, patient teaching, specialized knowledge and/or skills, and judgment are never delegated.
    Cognitive Level: Analysis
    Nursing Process: Planning
    NCLEX-RN Test Plan: SECE
    Reference: Marquis, B. L., & Huston, C. J. (2006). *Leadership roles and management functions in nursing: Theory and application* (5th ed.). Philadelphia: Lippincott Williams & Wilkins.

29. **Answer: 3**
    Rationale: Giving medications is within the scope of practice of the LPN. Tasks requiring assessment, teaching, and judgment should not be delegated by the RN.
    Cognitive Level: Application
    Nursing Process: Planning
    NCLEX-RN Test Plan: SECE
    Reference: Ellis, J. R., & Hartley, C. L. (2005). *Managing and coordinating nursing care* (4th ed.). Philadelphia: Lippincott Williams & Wilkins.

30. **Answer: 3, 2, 1, 4**
    Rationale: Airway is the highest priority. Restarting IV antibiotics is the second highest priority in order to maintain therapeutic blood levels of the medication ordered. Next, the nurse should inform the physician of errors, followed by checking lab results for the next day's schedule of patients for the OR. All of the options are RN responsibilities.
    Cognitive Level: Analysis
    Nursing Process: Planning
    NCLEX-RN Test Plan: SECE
    Reference: Carroll, P. (2006). *Nursing leadership and management: A practical guide.* Clifton Park, NY: Thomson Delmar Learning.

31. **Answers: 1, 4, and 5**
    Rationale: Shock symptoms, chest pain, and hyperventilation are immediate reactions. The other physical reactions are usually delayed.

    Cognitive Level: Application
    Nursing Process: Assessment
    NCLEX-RN Test Plan: PHYS
    Reference: Beachley, M. L. (2005). Nursing in a disaster. In F. Maurer & C. Smith (Eds.), *Community/public health nursing practice: Health for families and populations* (496–516). Philadelphia: Elsevier.

32. **Answers: 1, 2, and 4**
    Rationale: Nurses and other healthcare providers often see aggravation of chronic conditions during the impact and recovery stages of a disaster. Communicable disease outbreaks following a disaster are not common in the United States, but may be a problem in another country.
    Cognitive Level: Comprehension
    Nursing Process: Assessment
    NCLEX-RN Test Plan: PHYS
    Reference: Willshire, L., Hassmiller, S., & Wodicka, K. (2004). *Disaster preparedness and response for nurses.* Retrieved April 13, 2006, from http://www.nursingsociety.org/education/case_studies/cases/SP0004.html

33. **Answer: 1**
    Rationale: Clinical manifestations of mild exposure to carbon monoxide include nausea and vomiting, mild throbbing headache, and flu-like symptoms. Moderate exposure to carbon monoxide includes dyspnea, dizziness, and confusion. Symptoms of food poisoning would include abdominal cramping, diarrhea, and fever. Dyspnea would not indicate food poisoning.
    Cognitive Level: Application
    Nursing Process: Assessment
    NCLEX-RN Test Plan: PHYS
    Reference: Schwytzer, D. (2004). Common problems encountered in emergency and critical care nursing. In M. A. Hogan & T. Madayag (Eds.), *Medical-surgical nursing: Reviews and rationales* (pp. 1–44). Upper Saddle River, NJ: Pearson Prentice Hall.

34. **Answer: 3**
    Rationale: Clinical manifestations of cutaneous anthrax exposure include skin-related symptoms occurring within one hour of exposure.

Cognitive Level: Application
Nursing Process: Assessment
NCLEX-RN Test Plan: PHYS
Reference: Veenema, T. G. (2003). *Disaster nursing and emergency preparedness for chemical, biological, and radiological terrorism and other hazards.* New York: Springer.

35. **Answer: 2**
    Rationale: The CDC and ACIP recommend that all pre-event smallpox vaccination programs include pregnancy screening.
    Cognitive Level: Analysis
    Nursing Process: Assessment
    NCLEX-RN Test Plan: PHYS
    Reference: Langan, J. C., & James, D. C. (2005). *Preparing nurses for disaster management.* Upper Saddle River, NJ: Pearson Prentice Hall.

36. **Answer: 2**
    Rationale: Shelter in place procedures secure the building from the outside environment; therefore heating and cooling systems that draw on air from outside will need to be shut down. Communication is essential, phone lines should remain functioning. Electrical supply poses no threat. Assembling persons out in the environment to provide instruction potentially exposes them to the agent.
    Cognitive Level: Application
    Nursing Process: Implementation
    NCLEX-RN Test Plan: SECE
    Reference: Langan, J. C., & James, D. C. (2005). *Preparing nurses for disaster management.* Upper Saddle River, NJ: Pearson Prentice Hall.

37. **Answer: 3**
    Rationale: If no titling is observed with inspiration and expiration, the drainage system is blocked or the lungs are re-expanded. Keep all tubing as straight as possible and coiled loosely below chest level. Do not let patient lie on tubing. Never elevate the drainage system to or above the level of the patient's chest as this will cause fluid to drain back into the lungs. Chest tubes are not clamped routinely.
    Cognitive Level: Application
    Nursing Process: Assessment
    NCLEX-RN Test Plan: PHYS
    Reference: Lewis, S. M., Heitkemper, M. M., & Dirksen, S. R. (2004). *Medical-surgical nursing,*

Assessment and management of clinical problems (6th ed.). St. Louis, MO: Elsevier Mosby.

38. **Answers: 1, 2, 3, 4, and 8**
    Rationale: The effects of smoking also include an *increase* in incidence of infection and cough and a *decrease* in the sense of taste and smell.
    Cognitive Level: Application
    Nursing Process: Evaluation
    NCLEX-RN Test Plan: PHYS
    Reference: Lewis, S. M., Heitkemper, M. M., & Dirksen, S. R. (2004). *Medical-surgical nursing: Assessment and management of clinical problems* (6th ed.). St. Louis, MO: Elsevier Mosby.

39. **Answer: 1**
    Rationale: Nonselective beta blockers block sympathetic nervous stimulation and cause bronchoconstriction. The other choices are medications used to treat asthma. Leukotriene inhibitors and steroids reduce inflammation. Bronchodilators widen airways.
    Cognitive Level: Application
    Nursing Process: Planning
    NCLEX-RN Test Plan: PHYS
    Reference: Crutchlow, E. M., Dudac, P. J., MacAvoy, S., & Madara, B. R. (2006). *Quick look nursing: Pathophysiology.* Sudbury, MA: Jones and Bartlett.

40. **Answer: 1**
    Rationale: Acetylcysteine (Mucomyst) is a mucolytic agent and may release hydrogen sulfide and cause a rotten egg odor. It is also the antidote for Tylenol overdose.
    Cognitive Level: Application
    Nursing Process: Assessment
    NCLEX-RN Test Plan: PHYS
    Reference: Crutchlow, E. M., Dudac, P. J., MacAvoy, S., & Madara, B. R. (2006). *Quick look nursing: Pathophysiology.* Sudbury, MA: Jones and Bartlett.

41. **Answer: 3**
    Rationale: A child with severe respiratory distress, with respirations greater than 60 breaths/min for infants, should not be given anything by mouth to prevent aspiration and decrease the work of breathing.
    Cognitive Level: Analysis
    Nursing Process: Implementation

NCLEX-RN Test Plan: SECE

Reference: Hockenberry, M. J. (2005). *Wong's essentials of pediatric nursing.* St. Louis, MO: Elsevier Mosby.

42. **Answer: 5, 4, 1, 3, 7, 6, 2, 8**

Rationale: Rhonchi and course crackles, moist cough, restlessness, agitation, and a decrease of SPO_2 indicate a need for suctioning. If a client can clear mucous on their own, they do not need routine suctioning. Explaining the need for suctioning may decrease the anxiety associated with air hunger, but it may also cause anxiety if the procedure causes discomfort from incisions or tubes during coughing. Suction should read 120–150 mmHg with the suction tube completely occluded. The hand that handles the catheter (most likely the dominant hand) will remain sterile. The other hand will disconnect client from O_2, hyperoxygenate with an ambu bag and operate suction control. Suction is tested with sterile water. The nurse should determine a baseline SPO_2, heart rate, and rhythm to determine the client's tolerance of the procedure. The client must be hyperoxygenated with 100% O_2 to prevent suctioning residual lung O_2 from the alveoli. The catheter is inserted 5–6 inches or until an obstruction is met. Suction is applied intermittently and withdrawn in a rotating manner. If secretions are copious, continuous suction is applied, but limited to not more than 10 seconds. Reoxygenation of the client is done prior to anything else, including rinsing the catheter.

Cognitive Level: Synthesis

Nursing Process: Intervention

NCLEX-RN Test Plan: SECE

Reference: Lewis, S. M., Heitkemper, M. M., & Dirksen, S. R. (2004). *Medical-surgical nursing* (6th ed.). St. Louis, MO: Mosby.

43. **Answer: 3**

Rationale: Loss of appetite, unusually slow pulse rate, nausea, vomiting, and blurred or "yellow" vision could be signs of digoxin toxicity. Digoxin is contraindicated in clients with low potassium, which will increase the risk for digoxin toxicity.

Cognitive Level: Analysis

Nursing Process: Assessment

NCLEX-RN Test Plan: PHYS

Reference: Karch, A. M. (2005). *2005 Lippincott's nursing drug guide.* Philadelphia: Lippincott Williams & Wilkins.

44. **Answer: 4**

Rationale: Although all of the choices are related to venous abnormalities, the symptoms listed are all symptoms of thrombophlebitis.

Cognitive Level: Application

Nursing Process: Assessment

NCLEX-RN Test Plan: PHYS

Reference: Lewis, S. M., Heitkemper, M. M., & Dirksen, S. R. (2004). *Medical-surgical nursing: Assessment and management of clinical problems* (6th ed.). St. Louis, MO: Elsevier Mosby.

45. **Answer: 3**

Rationale: While all of the choices would be interventions for a client with these symptoms, ensuring a patent airway would be the initial intervention.

Cognitive Level: Analysis

Nursing Process: Implementation

NCLEX-RN Test Plan: PHYS

Reference: Lewis, S. M., Heitkemper, M. M., & Dirksen, S. R. (2004). *Medical-surgical nursing: Assessment and management of clinical problems* (6th ed.). St. Louis, MO: Elsevier Mosby.

46. **Answer: 100**

Rationale: Compressions are to be performed at 100 beats per minute for infants, children, and adults alike.

Cognitive Level: Application

Nursing Process: Implementation

NCLEX-RN Test Plan: PHYS

Reference: Lewis, S. M., Heitkemper, M. M., & Dirksen, S. R. (2004). *Medical-surgical nursing: Assessment and management of clinical problems* (6th ed.). St. Louis, MO: Elsevier Mosby.

47. **Answer: 3**

Rationale: Most pacemakers are designed to pace the ventricles. In this case, a spike will occur before the QRS complex. If the atria is paced, the spike will appear before the P wave.

Cognitive Level: Analysis

Nursing Process: Assessment

NCLEX-RN Test Plan: PHYS

Reference: Wagner, D. W., Johnson, K., & Kidd, P. S. (2006). *High acuity nursing.* Upper Saddle River, NJ: Pearson Prentice Hall.

48. Answer: 1

Rationale: Carvedilol (Coreg) is a beta blocker (thus the suffix 'lol'). Beta blockers are of increasing importance in the management of CHF. Beta blockers block the sympathetic nervous system's negative effects on the failing heart, such as increased heart rate, causing a decrease in heart rate. It will also cause a decrease in blood pressure. Carvedilol (Coreg) is recommended to be taken with food to decrease GI upset. It is contraindicated in clients with asthma and COPD due to the side effect of bronchospasm.

Cognitive Level: Analysis

Nursing Process: Implementation

NCLEX-RN Test Plan: PHYS

Reference: Lewis, S. M., Heitkemper, M. M., & Dirksen, S. R. (2004). *Medical-surgical nursing: Assessment and management of clinical problems* (6th ed.). St. Louis, MO: Elsevier Mosby.

Karch, A. M. (2005). *2005 Lippincott's nursing drug guide.* Philadelphia: Lippincott Williams & Wilkins.

49. Answer: 2

Rationale: Hemorrhoids are inflamed, distended veins at the anus. Therefore the tissue is friable and can get injured and bleed even with defecation. The bleeding would be intermittent and the color will be red. The blood would usually not appear throughout the stool but on the visible edges and/or on the toilet tissue. Bleeding may occur with aspirin therapy if the client develops an ulcer, which is not in this scenario. Pinworms do not cause bleeding. Upper GI bleeding would travel throughout the bowels, therefore, the color takes on a dark appearance and would be consistent.

Cognitive Level: Analysis

Nursing Process: Assessment

NCLEX-RN Test Plan: PHYS

Reference: Pagana, K. D., & Pagana, T. J. (2002). *Mosby's manual of diagnostic and laboratory tests.* St. Louis, MO: Mosby.

Lewis, S. M., Heitkemper, M. M., & Dirksen, S. R. (2004). *Medical-surgical nursing: Assessment and management of clinical problems* (6th ed.). St. Louis, MO: Elsevier Mosby.

50. Answer: 3

Rationale: Nicotine and stress cause an increase in gastric secretions and gastric mobility, which are factors in the development of ulcer disease. Bulimia does not play a role in ulcer formation. The temperature and blood pressure reading are not significant with ulcer disease. While smoking is a factor with ulcers, constipation is not, thus this response is incorrect.

Cognitive Level: Analysis

Nursing Process: Assessment

NCLEX-RN Test Plan: PHYS

Reference: Black, J., & Hawks, J. H. (2005). *Medical-surgical nursing: Clinical management for positive outcomes* (7th ed.). St. Louis, MO: Elsevier Saunders.

51. Answer: 4

Rationale: Bowel prep may be difficult for the elderly. Often they live alone and cannot administer themselves an enema. The remaining clients should not experience difficulty with the requirements of the procedure.

Cognitive Level: Application

Nursing Process: Planning

NCLEX-RN Test Plan: PHYS

Reference: Pagana, K. D., & Pagana, T. J. (2002). *Mosby's manual of diagnostic and laboratory tests.* St. Louis, MO: Mosby.

52. Answer: 0.7 ml

Rationale: The following formula is used to calculate medication dosages:

$$\frac{\text{Dose available}}{\text{Quantity available}} = \frac{\text{Dose ordered}}{X}$$

$$\frac{50}{1} = \frac{35}{X} = 0.7 \text{ ml}$$

53. Answer: 4

Rationale: No food or drink should be administered until the client is largely free of pain. By maintaining NPO status, the nurse is ensuring pancreatic rest since food/drink ingestion increases pancreatic secretion, which may lead to inflammation and pain. There is no set number of days for administration of pain medication.

Cognitive Level: Analysis

Nursing Process: Implementation

NCLEX-RN Test Plan: HPM

Reference: Black, J., & Hawks, J. H. (2005). *Medical-surgical nursing: Clinical management for positive outcomes* (7th ed.). St. Louis, MO: Elsevier Saunders.

54. **Answer: 4**

Rationale: The excessive use of laxatives increases a client's risk for diarrhea since these drugs ruin the normal defecation reflex. Weight loss, weakness, malnutrition, and electrolyte imbalances may occur. The other options may be results of this order.

Cognitive Level: Application

Nursing Process: Assessment

NCLEX-RN Test Plan: PHYS

Reference: Potter, P. A., & Perry, A. G. (2005). *Fundamentals of nursing* (6th ed.). St. Louis, MO: Elsevier Mosby.

55. **Answer: 4**

Rationale: The best way to monitor for patency in an AV graft is to listen with a stethoscope for a bruit over the graft itself. The bruit is created by arterial blood rushing into the vein. BP's should not be performed on the affected extremity because it can cause clotting of the vascular access.

Cognitive Level: Application

Nursing Process: Assessment

NCLEX-RN Test Plan: HPM

Reference: Lewis, S. M., Heitkemper, M. M., & Dirksen, S. R. (2004). *Medical-surgical nursing: Assessment and management of clinical problems* (6th ed.). St. Louis, MO: Mosby.

56. **Answer: 2**

Rationale: Before the procedure, assess the patient for iodine sensitivity to avoid an anaphylactic reaction. Shellfish contain iodine. A diabetic client is able to receive an IVP test done under medical supervision. Claustrophobia and metal plates do not apply in IVP tests.

Cognitive Level: Analysis

Nursing Process: Analysis

NCLEX-RN Test Plan: SECE

Reference: Lewis, S. M., Heitkemper, M. M., & Dirksen, S. R. (2004). *Medical-surgical nursing: Assessment and management of clinical problems* (6th ed.). St. Louis, MO: Mosby.

57. **Answer 4**

Rationale: After cleaning, instruct the patient to start urinating and then continue voiding in the sterile container. The initial voided urine flushes out most contaminants in the urethra and perineal area. For a proper urine sample, the client must wipe front to back and the specimen should be less than an hour old to be processed. A person on their period can have a urine sample taken.

Cognitive Level: Application

Nursing Process: Implementation

NCLEX-RN Test Plan: HPM

Reference: Lewis, S. M., Heitkemper, M. M., & Dirksen, S. R. (2004). *Medical-surgical nursing: Assessment and management of clinical problems* (6th ed.). St. Louis, MO: Mosby.

58. **Answer: 3**

Rationale: The most common and serious complication of transplantation is rejection, which is the leading cause of graft loss. All other answers are also complications of a renal transplant.

Cognitive Level: Analysis

Nursing Process: Evaluation

NCLEX-RN Test Plan: PHYS

Reference: Ignatavicius, D. D., & Workman, M. L. (2006). *Medical-surgical nursing* (5th ed.). St. Louis, MO: Elsevier Saunders.

59. **Answer: 3**

Rationale: Clinical criteria for the diagnosis of interstitial cystitis (IC) include suprapubic pain associated with bladder filling and urinary urgency. The pain varies and is exacerbated by bladder filling, postponing urination, physical exertion, pressure against the suprapubic area, dietary intake of certain foods, or emotional distress. The pain and bothersome voiding symptoms (similar to a urinary tract infection) remit and exacerbate over time. IC is a diagnosis of exclusion. The condition is suspected whenever a client experiences symptoms of a UTI despite the absence of bacteriuria, pyuria, or a positive urine culture.

Cognitive Level: Analysis

Nursing Process: Assessment

NCLEX-RN Test Plan: PHYS

Reference: Lewis, S. M., Heitkemper, M. M., & Dirksen, S. R. (2004). *Medical-surgical nursing:*

Assessment and management of clinical problems (6th ed.). St. Louis, MO: Mosby.

60. **Answer: 3**
Rationale: Types of risk factors for the development of urinary tract calculi include metabolic abnormalities that result in increased urine levels of calcium, oxaluric acid, uric acid, or citric acid; warm climates that cause increased fluid loss, low urine volume, and increased solute concentration in urine; large intake of dietary proteins that increases uric acid excretion; and low fluid intake that increases urinary concentration.
Cognitive Level: Application
Nursing Process: Assessment
NCLEX-RN Test Plan: HPM
Reference: Lewis, S. M., Heitkemper, M. M., & Dirksen, S. R. (2004). *Medical-surgical nursing: Assessment and management of clinical problems* (6th ed.). St. Louis, MO: Mosby.

61. **Answer: 4**
Rationale: Diabetes insipidus is a group of conditions associated with a deficiency of ADH or decreased renal response to ADH. The signs and symptoms of diabetes insipidus include severe polyuria with low specific gravity, fatigue, muscle weakness, irritability, weight loss, dehydration, and tachycardia. A urine specific gravity of less than 1.004 indicates an inability to concentrate urine.
Cognitive Level: Analysis
Nursing Process: Assessment
NCLEX-RN Test Plan: PHYS
Reference: Lewis, S. M., Heitkemper, M. M., & Dirksen, S. R. (2004). *Medical-surgical nursing: Assessment and management of clinical problems* (6th ed.). St. Louis, MO: Mosby.

62. **Answer: 2**
Rationale: Excess glucocorticoids increase catabolism, thereby increasing protein loss. Serum K levels are typically depleted, so potassium rich foods are encouraged. Typically calorie reduction is prescribed to reduce weight. The ADA recommendation for fat in the diet is 20% of total caloric intake.
Cognitive Level: Application
Nursing Process: Planning
NCLEX-RN Test Plan: PHYS

Reference: Lewis, S. M., Heitkemper, M. M., & Dirksen, S. R. (2004). *Medical-surgical nursing: Assessment and management of clinical problems* (6th ed.). St. Louis, MO: Mosby.

63. **Answer: 3**
Rationale: Elevated serum thyroid levels (T_3, T_4) and decreased serum TSH levels are indicative of hyperthyroidism. Decreased serum TSH indicates suppression of TSH secretion due to increased levels of circulation thyroid (T_3, T_4) hormone. This represents a "feedback mechanism."
Cognitive Level: Application
Nursing Process: Analysis
NCLEX-RN Test Plan: HPM
Reference: McCance, K. L., & Huether, S. E. (2006). *Pathophysiology: The biologic basis for disease in adults & children* (5th ed.). St. Louis, MO: Elsevier Mosby.

64. **Answer: 3**
Rationale: With hypothyroidism, the client's metabolism slows. With this decreased metabolism, weight gain is seen. The other options are symptoms of hyperthyroidism (Grave's disease) and are seen as a result of the increased metabolism occurring with hyperthyroidism.
Cognitive Level: Analysis
Nursing Process: Assessment
NCLEX-RN Test Plan: PHYS
Reference: Lemone, P., & Burke, K. (2004). *Medical-surgical nursing: Critical thinking in client care* (3rd ed.). Upper Saddle River, NJ: Prentice Hall.

65. **Answer: 4**
Rationale: Regular insulin is used in the management of diabetic ketoacidosis (DKA), which is what the patient's symptoms suggest. A 5% dextrose solution is added when the blood glucose (BG) level reaches about 250–300 mg/dl. Oral hypoglycemic agents are used in the treatment of Type 2 diabetes mellitus. Glucocorticoids are adrenocortical steroid hormones given primarily for their anti-inflammatory effects.
Cognitive Level: Application
Nursing Process: Planning
NCLEX-RN Test Plan: PHYS

Reference: Lewis, S. M., Heitkemper, M. M., & Dirksen, S. R. (2004). *Medical-surgical nursing: Assessment and management of clinical problems* (6th ed.). St. Louis, MO: Mosby.

66. Answer: 3

Rationale: Gestational diabetes develops during pregnancy and is typically detected at 24–28 weeks gestation. These women are at an increased risk of developing Type 2 diabetes mellitus in the next 5–10 years. Nutritional therapy is the first-line therapy. If nutritional therapy alone is not enough to maintain normal blood glucose levels, insulin therapy is added. Self blood glucose monitoring is done to help achieve normal blood glucose levels. Oral antidiabetic medications are not recommended for use during pregnancy.

Cognitive Level: Application
Nursing Process: Evaluation
NCLEX-RN Test Plan: SECE
Reference: Lewis, S. M., Heitkemper, M. M., & Dirksen, S. R. (2004). *Medical-surgical nursing: Assessment and management of clinical problems* (6th ed.). St. Louis, MO: Mosby.

67. Answer: 1

Rationale: A normal platelet count is generally considered to be between 150,000 and 400,000/mm³. This platelet count is within normal limits. There is no need to initiate bleeding precautions for this client.

Cognitive Level: Analysis
Nursing Process: Implementation
NCLEX-RN Test Plan: PHYS
References: Lewis, S. M., Heitkemper, M. M., & Dirksen, S. R. (2004). *Medical-surgical nursing: Assessment and management of clinical problems* (6th ed.). St. Louis, MO: Mosby.

Smeltzer, S. C., & Bare, B. G. (2004). *Textbook of medical-surgical nursing* (10th ed.). Philadelphia: Lippincott Williams & Wilkins.

Pagana, K. D., & Pagana, T. J. (2002). *Manual of diagnostic and laboratory tests* (2nd ed.). St. Louis, MO: Mosby.

68. Answer: 3

Rationale: Urticaria at a specific site is a local allergic or hypersensitivity reaction. Bronchospasm, hemolysis, and allergic rhinitis are systemic reactions.

Cognitive Level: Analysis
Nursing Process: Assessment
NCLEX-RN Test Plan: PHYS
References: Lewis, S. M., Heitkemper, M. M., & Dirksen, S. R. (2004). *Medical-surgical nursing: Assessment and management of clinical problems* (6th ed.). St. Louis, MO: Mosby.

Smeltzer, S. C., & Bare, B. G. (2004). *Textbook of medical-surgical nursing* (10th ed.). Philadelphia: Lippincott Williams & Wilkins.

69. Answer: 1

Rationale: The status and category of HIV and AIDS can be determined and monitored by laboratory tests that show viral load levels and CD4⁺ counts. Platelet counts and renal function tests do not assess HIV and AIDS disease status. ELISA and Western blot assays assist with diagnosing HIV but not with monitoring its progression.

Cognitive Level: Analysis
Nursing Process: Evaluation
NCLEX-RN Test Plan: PHYS
References: Black, J. M., & Hawks, J. H. (2005). *Medical-surgical nursing: Clinical management for positive outcomes* (7th ed.). St. Louis, MO: Elsevier Saunders.

Lewis, S. M., Heitkemper, M. M., & Dirksen, S. R. (2004). *Medical-surgical nursing: Assessment and management of clinical problems* (6th ed.). St. Louis, MO: Mosby.

Smeltzer, S. C., & Bare, B. G. (2004). *Textbook of medical-surgical nursing* (10th ed.). Philadelphia: Lippincott Williams & Wilkins.

70. Answer: 4

Rationale: Alcoholism is related to liver disease, and the liver affects bleeding times by assisting with the production and utilization of clotting factors. Therefore, liver disease can cause bleeding disorders to occur. Malnutrition can have an effect on bleeding times, but liver disease is a more common cause, especially with this client's history of obesity. Increased blood viscosity can increase the possibility of increased clotting rather than bleeding. Diabetes has no direct effect on bleeding times.

Cognitive Level: Analysis
Nursing Process: Assessment
NCLEX-RN Test Plan: PHYS

References: Black, J. M., & Hawks, J. H. (2005). *Medical-surgical nursing: Clinical management for positive outcomes* (7th ed.). St. Louis, MO: Elsevier Saunders.

Pagana, K. D., & Pagana, T. J. (2002). *Manual of diagnostic and laboratory tests* (2nd ed.). St. Louis, MO: Mosby.

71. **Answer: 2**

    Rationale: RA, SLE, and scleroderma are all autoimmune connective tissue disorders. Although other body systems can be affected by such disorders, the disorders do not originate in the musculoskeletal, endocrine, or peripheral vascular systems.

    Cognitive Level: Application

    Nursing Process: Implementation

    NCLEX-RN Test Plan: PHYS

    References: Black, J. M., & Hawks, J. H. (2005). *Medical-surgical nursing: Clinical management for positive outcomes* (7th ed.). St. Louis, MO: Elsevier Saunders.

    Lewis, S. M., Heitkemper, M. M., & Dirksen, S. R. (2004). *Medical-surgical nursing: Assessment and management of clinical problems* (6th ed.). St. Louis, MO: Mosby.

72. **Answer: 3**

    Rationale: FFP is helpful in replacing essential body fluids and is rich in clotting factors. Albumin is prepared from plasma and acts by shifting fluid from extravascular to intravascular space. Washed RBCs are not frozen. Platelets and packed RBCs are not the first choice of treatment for reversing hypovolemic shock.

    Cognitive Level: Analysis

    Nursing Process: Analysis

    NCLEX-RN Test Plan: PHYS

    References: Black, J. M., & Hawks, J. H. (2005). *Medical-surgical nursing: Clinical management for positive outcomes* (7th ed.). St. Louis, MO: Elsevier Saunders.

    Lewis, S. M., Heitkemper, M. M., & Dirksen, S. R. (2004). *Medical-surgical nursing: Assessment and management of clinical problems* (6th ed.). St. Louis, MO: Mosby.

    Smeltzer, S. C., & Bare, B. G. (2004). *Textbook of medical-surgical nursing* (10th ed.). Philadelphia: Lippincott Williams & Wilkins.

Lilley, L. L., Harrington, S., & Snyder, J. S. (2005). *Pharmacology and the nursing process* (4th ed.). St. Louis, MO: Mosby.

73. **Answer: 2**

    Rationale: A pressure ulcer should be cleansed gently with a nonionic cleanser such as isotonic saline to prevent disruption of healing. Pressure ulcers heal better in a moist environment, so heat lamps are no longer used. Povodone-iodine and rubbing reddened areas may cause the breakdown of fragile healing skin.

    Cognitive Level: Application

    Nursing Process: Application

    NCLEX-RN Test Plan: PHYS

    Reference: Lewis, S. M., Heitkemper, M. M., & Dirksen, S. R. (2004). *Medical-surgical nursing: Assessment and management of clinical problems* (6th ed.). St. Louis, MO: Mosby.

74. **Answer: 3**

    Rationale: Taking most of the dose at bedtime will enable the client to receive a dual benefit from the drug; maximum relief for the pruritus and ability to sleep without symptoms. Tolerance to the drug may be reached in a few weeks of taking the medication but the nurse would never teach a client to change the dose as needed. The sedative effects would not be altered by taking the dose with meals or spreading the dose evenly throughout the day.

    Cognitive Level: Application

    Nursing Process: Implementation

    NCLEX-RN Test Plan: PHYS

    Reference: Lewis, S. M., Heitkemper, M. M., & Dirksen, S. R. (2004). *Medical-surgical nursing: Assessment and management of clinical problems* (6th ed.). St. Louis, MO: Mosby.

75. **Answer: 3**

    Rationale: Herpes zoster (shingles) produces painful, vesicular eruptions along a nerve pathway. Herpes simplex 1 produces cold sores or fever blisters at the corners of the mouth. Herpes simplex 2 produces lesions in the genital area. Herpes zoster is frequently found along one side of the rib cage but the lesions are vesicles not papules.

    Cognitive Level: Analysis

    Nursing Process: Assessment

    NCLEX-RN Test Plan: PHYS

Reference: Smeltzer, S. C., & Bare, B. G. (2004). *Brunner & Suddarth's textbook of medical-surgical nursing.* Philadelphia: Lippincott Williams & Wilkins.

76. Answer: 1

Rationale: Active shedding of the virus and contagion are possible for the first three to five days or while vesicles are present. Sex should be avoided when sores are present. Sharing of towels by anyone should be avoided during an outbreak. Reoccurrence is common because the virus remains dormant until triggered by physical or psychological stressors.

Cognitive Level: Application

Nursing Process: Implementation

NCLEX-RN Test Plan: HPM

Reference: Smeltzer, S. C., & Bare, B. G. (2004). *Brunner & Suddarth's textbook of medical-surgical nursing.* Philadelphia: Lippincott Williams & Wilkins.

77. Answer: 4

Rationale: Malignant melanoma is ten times more common in fair-skinned people who work indoors. This group often experiences severe sunburns and tends to vacation in areas of intense sun exposure. Episodic, intense sun exposure is more damaging than constant exposure.

Cognitive Level: Application

Nursing Process: Assessment

NCLEX-RN Test Plan: PHYS

Reference: Smeltzer, S. C., & Bare, B. G. (2004). *Brunner & Suddarth's textbook of medical-surgical nursing.* Philadelphia: Lippincott Williams & Wilkins.

78. Answer: 3

Rationale: Disuse syndrome results mostly from the complications of immobility and is not usually a problem with most of the skin disorders. Emotional stress can occur for persons who suffer from the various skin disorders. Anxiety, disturbed body image, and social isolation are just a few of nursing diagnoses that frequently apply to these clients.

Cognitive Level: Application

Nursing Process: Analysis

NCLEX-RN Test Plan: HPM

Reference: Lewis, S. M., Heitkemper, M. M., &Dirksen, S. R. (2004). *Medical-surgical nursing: Assessment and management of clinical problems* (6th ed.). St. Louis, MO: Mosby.

79. Answers: 1, 2, 3, and 4

Rationale: Aplastic anemia occurs when there is insufficient number of **all** blood cells due to alterations in the function of the bone marrow. The client is at risk for poor tissue perfusion, including an altered level of consciousness due to a decrease in red blood cells. They are at risk for infection related to inadequate numbers of white blood cells. They are at risk for injury related to bleeding from a decreased number of platelets.

Cognitive Level: Comprehension

Nursing Process: Diagnosis

NCLEX-RN Test Plan: PHYS

Reference: Lewis, S. M., Heitkemper, M. M., & Dirksen, S. R. (2004). *Medical-surgical nursing: Assessment and management of clinical problems* (6th ed.). St. Louis, MO: Mosby.

80. Answer: 2

Rationale: This client is in a palliative stage of treatment when neither cure nor control is possible. The goal of treatment is to control and relieve distressing symptoms of the disease. Stages of the mourning process include shock and denial, anger and bargaining, and depression and acceptance. Understanding that the treatment is to enhance comfort communicates to the nurse an active participation in the treatment plan and progress toward acceptance.

Cognitive Level: Comprehension

Nursing Process: Assessment

NCLEX-RN Test Plan: PSYC

Reference: Lewis, S. M., Heitkemper, M. M., & Dirksen, S. R. (2004). *Medical-surgical nursing: Assessment and management of clinical problems* (6th ed.). St. Louis, MO: Mosby.

81. Answer: 1

Rationale: In multiple myeloma, malignant cells infiltrate and destroy the bone. This results in lytic areas of bone erosion and bone thinning involving the vertebrae, ribs, pelvis, femur and humerus. All clients with chronic illness are at risk for immobility, pressure sores, and shearing injuries.

Cognitive Level: Comprehension
Nursing Process: Planning
NCLEX-RN Test Plan: PHYS
Reference: Lewis, S. M., Heitkemper, M. M., & Dirksen, S. R. (2004). *Medical-surgical nursing: Assessment and management of clinical problems* (6th ed.). St. Louis, MO: Mosby.

82. **Answer: 2, 3, and 5**
Rationale: Testicular cancer accounts for 1% of all cancers. The right testicle is generally affected. It is four times more common in White males than in African American males. It is more common in clients with undescended testes or those with a family history of testicular cancer. Except for 10% who present with acute pain, the first sign is a painless, firm scrotal lump. The client will also complain of scrotal swelling and a feeling of heaviness. With early detection and treatment, 95% of clients have complete remission of the disease. Testicular cancer is the most common type of cancer in 15- to 35-year-olds. It is the treatment that can interfere with erections and fertility, therefore, prior to treatment, fertility and sperm banking is discussed.
Cognitive Level: Knowledge
Nursing Process: Planning
NCLEX-RN Test Plan: PSYC
Reference: Lewis, S. M., Heitkemper, M. M., & Dirksen, S. R. (2004). *Medical-surgical nursing: Assessment and management of clinical problems* (6th ed.). St. Louis, MO: Mosby.

83. **Answer: 4**
Rationale: Head and neck cancers, which include the paranasal sinuses, the oral cavity, the nasopharynx, the oropharynx and the larynx, occur twice as often in males as females. A majority occur in individuals 50 years or older. Prolonged abuse of tobacco and alcohol creates the greatest risk. A positive family history, use of all forms of tobacco, heavy alcohol use, and prolonged use of decongestants and sore throat medications are additional risk factors.
Cognitive Level: Comprehension
Nursing Process: Assessment
NCLEX-RN Test Plan: HPM
Reference: Lewis, S. M., Heitkemper, M. M., & Dirksen, S. R. (2004). *Medical-surgical nursing: Assessment and management of clinical problems* (6th ed.). St. Louis, MO: Mosby.

84. **Answer: 3**
Rationale: The incidence of cervical cancer is greater in African Americans and Hispanics than in the white women. Additionally, there is an increased risk associated with low socioeconomic status, early sexual activity, multiple sex partners, infection with papilloma virus (HPV), and smoking. Community health campaigns to improve dissemination of healthcare information and healthcare access to groups at risk have contributed to prevention of cervical cancer and ultimately a decrease in cervical cancer related deaths. Internal radiation, progressive treatment protocols and magnetic resonance imaging have contributed to the success of treatment regimens after diagnosis.
Cognitive Level: Synthesis
Nursing Process: Intervention
NCLEX-RN Test Plan: PHYS
Reference: Lewis, S. M., Heitkemper, M. M., & Dirksen, S. R. (2004). *Medical-surgical nursing: Assessment and management of clinical problems* (6th ed.). St. Louis, MO: Mosby.

85. **Answers: 1, 2, 3, 5, and 6**
Rationale: Clients with chronic low back pain usually have been taking various analgesics for extended periods and often with unsatisfactory pain relief. The chronicity of pain often causes lifestyle alterations with the use of alcohol and/or drugs. Herbs and nutrition supplements are important pieces of information but they do not impact pain management. Any significant information gathered by the nurse should be communicated to the appropriate individual. All care providers must be consistent in providing effective pain control through pharmacologic and non-pharmacological interventions. Opioids should not be discontinued abruptly, clients should be weaned from opioids by decreasing the dose or frequency to avoid withdrawal syndrome.
Cognitive Level: Analysis
Nursing Process: Assessment
NCLEX-RN Test Plan: SECE
Reference: Lewis, S. M., Heitkemper, M. M., & Dirksen, S. R. (2004). *Medical-surgical nursing: Assessment and management of clinical problems* (6th ed.). St. Louis, MO: Mosby.

86. Answer:

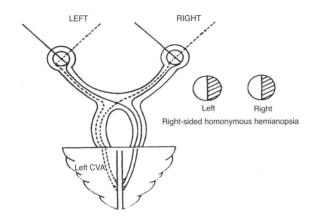

Cognitive Level: Application
Nursing Process: Analysis
NCLEX-RN Test Plan: PHYS
Reference: Phipps, W. J., Monahan, F. D., Sands, J. K., Marek, J. F., & Neighbors, M. (2003). *Medical-surgical nursing: Health and illness perspectives.* St. Louis, MO: Mosby.

87. Answer: 1
Rationale: The number one priority in this head injured client is the prevention of further deterioration in function, identification of specific altered function, and identification of the causative factors responsible for the increased intracranial pressure. Head injury increases the risk of seizures and/or the client may have pre-existing epilepsy that precipitated the accident. Blood gases will need to be maintained to control increased intracranial pressure. There is risk for physical injury due to decreased level of consciousness, and safety will need to be preserved. A craniotomy (an opening into the skull to remove a hematoma or pressure) may need to be performed.
Cognitive Level: Analysis
Nursing Process: Analysis
NCLEX-RN Test Plan: PHYS
Reference: Hickey, J. V. (2003). *The clinical practice of neurological and neurosurgical nursing.* Philadelphia: Lippincott.

88. Answer: 3
Rationale: Clients with aneurysms should avoid straining and are told to take a laxative to prevent constipation. Vomiting unrelated to nausea or eating is a sign of increased intracranial pressure. Increased pressure on cortical cells affects cognition and high level reflex control so the client who thought they had been sleeping and was incontinent needs further evaluation. Headache is associated with increased intracranial pressure, but would be increasing in severity.
Cognitive Level: Analysis
Nursing Process: Assessment
NCLEX-RN Test Plan: PHYS
Reference: Lewis, S. M., Heitkemper, M. M., & Dirksen, S. R. (2004). *Medical-surgical nursing: Assessment and management of clinical problems* (6th ed.). St. Louis, MO: Mosby.

89. Answer: 1
Rationale: General guidelines when communicating with aphasic clients include face-to-face communication with eye contact, and speaking slowly and clearly. It is best to avoid questions with multiple choices and it is not necessary to raise the volume of the voice unless the client has a hearing impairment. It is important to always be respectful of the client.
Cognitive Level: Application
Nursing Process: Implementation
NCLEX-RN Test Plan: PSYC
Reference: Phipps, W. J., Monahan, F. D., Sands, J. K., Marek, J. F., & Neighbors, M. (2003). *Medical-surgical nursing: Health and illness perspectives.* St. Louis, MO: Mosby.

90. Answer: 3
Rationale: Edrophonium (Tensilon) has a rapid onset of action and a short duration. A positive response would be demonstrated by improvement in muscle strength in a previously weakened muscle lasting 5–10 minutes. A "pill-rolling" tremor is a manifestation of Parkinson's disease and would not be affected by the medication.
Cognitive Level: Analysis
Nursing Process: Evaluation
NCLEX-RN Test Plan: PHYS
Reference: Phipps, W. J., Monahan, F. D., Sands, J. K., Marek, J. F., & Neighbors, M. (2003). *Medical-surgical nursing: Health and illness perspectives.* St. Louis, MO: Mosby.

91. Answer: 1

Rationale: Bisphosphonates are the drugs of choice for the pharmacotherapy of Paget's disease. Colchine is used to treat gout, glucocorticoids are used to treat rheumatoid arthritis, and SERMS are used for osteoporosis.

Cognitive Level: Application

Nursing Process: Analysis

NCLEX-RN Test Plan: PHYS

Reference: Adams, M. P., Josephson, D. L., & Holland, L. N. (2005). *Pharmacology for nurses: A pathophysiologic approach.* Upper Saddle River, NJ: Pearson Prentice Hall.

92. Answer: 1

Rationale: Osteoarthritis is caused by wear and tear and trauma, and can occur in middle age as well as in the elderly. The other options describe other forms of arthritis.

Cognitive Level: Application

Nursing Process: Assessment

NCLEX-RN Test Plan: PHYS

Reference: Crutchlow, E. M., Dudar, P. J., MacAvoy, S., & Madara, B. R. (2002). *Quick look nursing: Pathophysiology.* Thorofare, NJ: Slack Inc.

93. Answer: 3

Rationale: Leflunomide (Arava) may cause dizziness and clients should be instructed not to drive or operate heavy machinery until they know the response to the drug. The other drugs are anti-rheumatoid drugs. Auranofin (Ridura) is a gold compound, as is gold sodium thiomalate (Myochrysine). It may take 4–6 months to see therapeutic effects. Penicillamine (Cuprimine) causes taste activity to be altered.

Cognitive Level: Application

Nursing Process: Assessment

NCLEX-RN Test Plan: PHYS

Reference: Herbert-Ashton, M. J., & Clarkson, N. E. (2005). *Quick look nursing: Pharmacology.* Sudbury, MA: Jones & Bartlett.

94. Answer: 2

Rationale: It is a disturbance in the balance between osteoclastic and osteoblastic activity, from a variety of causes, and results in osteoporosis. The other choices are incorrect or incomplete. Osteoporosis can be due to either a decrease in activity of the osteoblasts, which are responsible for bone formation, or an increase in activity of the osteoclasts, which are responsible for bone breakdown. Decreased calcium intake can also lead to osteoporosis.

Cognitive Level: Application

Nursing Process: Assessment

NCLEX-RN Test Plan: PHYS

Reference: Crutchlow, E. M., Dudar, P. J., MacAvoy, S., & Madora, B. R. (2002). *Quick look nursing: Pathophysiology.* Thorofare, NJ: Slack Inc.

95. Answer: 2

Rationale: Due to the fact that a pelvic fracture can damage other organs, assessment of bowel and urinary tract function are important measures to monitor. The other answers are not correct. A palpable lump in the buttock does not occur with a fracture of the pelvis. A sudden decrease in blood pressure could occur in many conditions such as shock. Sudden thirst is not indicative of a pelvic fracture.

Cognitive Level: Application

Nursing Process: Assessment

NCLEX-RN Test Plan: PHYS

Reference: Lewis, S. M., Heitkemper, M. M., & Dirksen, S. R. (2004). *Medical-surgical nursing: Assessment and management of clinical problems* (6th ed.). St. Louis, MO: Mosby.

96. Answer: 1

Rationale: After application of the cast, the client may develop cast syndrome if the body cast is applied too tight and compresses the superior mesenteric artery against the duodenum. The client will complain of abdominal pain and pressure as well as nausea and vomiting. Although assessment of urinary elimination, skin integrity, and pulses is important, due to the location of this cast, the abdomen would be the primary area of concern.

Cognitive Level: Application

Nursing Process: Assessment

NCLEX-RN Test Plan: PHYS

Reference: Lewis, S. M., Heitkemper, M. M., & Dirksen, S. R. (2004). *Medical-surgical nursing: Assessment and management of clinical problems* (6th ed.). St. Louis, MO: Mosby.

97. **Answer: 1**

    Rationale: Assessment of the client's oxygen saturation is essential during surgery. Pulse oximetry is used during surgery for assessment of the client's oxygen saturation level. Nail polish will impair the monitoring ability of the oximeter. Nail polish will not contaminate the surgical field as a source of bacteria and is not capable of igniting a flame. Standards of care follow infection control policies, protocol, and recommendations.

    Cognitive Level: Analysis

    Nursing Process: Implementation

    NCLEX-RN Test Plan: PHYS

    Reference: Lewis, S. M., Heitkemper, M. M., & Dirksen, S. R. (2004). *Medical-surgical nursing: Assessment and management of clinical problems* (6th ed.). St. Louis, MO: Mosby.

98. **Answer: 1**

    Rationale: The abdomen should be auscultated in all four quadrants to determine the characteristics of bowel sounds. Decreased gastrointestinal motility can occur after surgery from the effects of anesthesia and narcotics. The client may also experience abdominal distention from handling and manipulation of the intestine. Nausea and vomiting may result from narcotics, slowed peristalsis, oral intake too soon after surgery, or delayed gastric emptying.

    Cognitive Level: Analysis

    Nursing Process: Implementation

    NCLEX-RN Test Plan: PHYS

    Reference: Lewis, S. M., Heitkemper, M. M., & Dirksen, S. R. (2004). *Medical-surgical nursing: Assessment and management of clinical problems* (6th ed.). St. Louis, MO: Mosby.

99. **Answer: 1**

    Rationale: The most common cause of airway obstruction in the postanesthetic period is the blockage of the airway by the client's tongue. The pharynx is occluded when the base of the tongue falls backward against the soft palate. The other options listed are less common causes.

    Cognitive Level: Analysis

    Nursing Process: Assessment

    NCLEX-RN Test Plan: PHYS

    Reference: Lewis, S. M., Heitkemper, M. M., & Dirksen, S. R. (2004). *Medical-surgical nursing:*

Assessment and management of clinical problems (6th ed.). St. Louis, MO: Mosby.

100. **Answer: 1**

    Rationale: Wound evisceration is an emergency that requires prioritization and prompt treatment. The intestine that has protruded through the wound should be covered with sterile, moist, saline gauze. This will prevent them from drying and will serve as a temporary sterile cover until the doctor can be notified and the client returned to surgery. Changing the client's position may cause the organs to shift or increase the evisceration. An IV line will help with the client's hydration but will not decrease the evisceration.

    Cognitive Level: Analysis

    Nursing Process: Implementation

    NCLEX-RN Test Plan: PHYS

    Reference: Lewis, S. M., Heitkemper, M. M., & Dirksen, S. R. (2004). *Medical-surgical nursing: Assessment and management of clinical problems* (6th ed.). St. Louis, MO: Mosby.

101. **Answer: 2**

    Rationale: These signs and symptoms indicate a paralytic ileus. Altered gastrointestinal motility can lead to postoperative complications. Handling of the intestine during surgery can lead to abdominal distention. Narcotics may alter or impair peristaltic activity. Vomiting can occur if dietary intake was resumed too early after surgery. All other options are incorrect.

    Cognitive Level: Analysis

    Nursing Process: Assessment

    NCLEX-RN Test Plan: PHYS

    Reference: Lewis, S. M., Heitkemper, M. M., & Dirksen, S. R. (2004). *Medical-surgical nursing: Assessment and management of clinical problems* (6th ed.). St. Louis, MO: Mosby.

102. **Answer: 2**

    Rationale: A spinal headache may result after the administration of spinal anesthesia. The leakage of spinal fluid at the injection site has been identified as a causative factor. Increasing oral fluids postoperatively and lying flat for a period of time are interventions that have been implemented to decrease the incidence of headache.

Cognitive Level: Analysis
Nursing Process: Assessment
NCLEX-RN Test Plan: PHYS
Reference: Lewis, S. M., Heitkemper, M. M., & Dirksen, S. R. (2004). *Medical-surgical nursing: Assessment and management of clinical problems* (6th ed.). St. Louis, MO: Mosby.

103. **Answer: 2**
Rationale: In malnourished individuals, stored body fat is the primary source of fuel. When TPN is initiated there is a shift to carbohydrates as the primary fuel source. In response to the rise in carbohydrates, gluconeogenesis (formation of glycogen from fatty acids and proteins) is suppressed and insulin is released at an increased rate. An increase in insulin drives potassium, glucose, and phosphate into the cell causing a decrease in serum levels. Starvation induced serum hypophosphatemia, hypokalcemia as well as hypomagnesemia, after feedings high in glucose alters bioavailability for the Kreb's cycle and for cellular synthesis. Left uncorrected, refeeding syndrome can lead to heart failure, respiratory failure, seizures, red and white blood cell dysfunction, skeletal muscle dysfunction, and acid-base disorders. Symptoms associated with hyperglycemia, fluid overload, and sepsis prior to shock would be detected long before the multisystem involvement that is seen with refeeding syndrome.
Cognitive Level: Evaluation
Nursing Process: Evaluation
NCLEX-RN Test Plan: PHYS
Reference: Mehler, P. S., Kolpak, S., & Padilla, R. (2005). Anorexia nervosa and the use of total parenteral nutrition refeeding. *Current Nutrition and Food Science, 1,* 97–104.

104. **Answer: 1**
Rationale: Large losses of bicarbonate (H_2CO_3) and accumulation of carbonic acid (H_2CO_3) occur with chronic diarrhea, starvation, and malnutrition leading to a state of metabolic acidosis. Central nervous system depression such as lethargy and confusion will occur. The renal and pulmonary systems attempt to compensate for the acid state. Respiratory changes occur as compensatory mechanisms for metabolic acidosis or alkalosis and occur quickly to bring acid base into balance. Respiratory rate and depth increase as the lungs attempt to blow off carbon dioxide (CO_2) to create an alka-

lotic state. To decrease carbonic acid (H_2CO_3), the kidneys excrete hydrogen (H^+) in exchange for sodium (Na^+). In metabolic alkalosis a client would retain bicarbonate and lose carbonic acid, not consistent with that seen with large gastrointestinal fluid loss. As a compensatory mechanism for metabolic alkalosis, the respiratory rate and depth decrease as the lungs attempt to retain carbon dioxide (CO_2) to create an acidotic state. In this client, heart rate, usually decreased in metabolic acidosis, is elevated with a low blood pressure due to hypovolemia related to high ileostomy output and vomiting for three days. In addition to metabolic acidosis, this client is fluid volume deficit and in a state of isotonic dehydration.
Cognitive Level: Analysis
Nursing Process: Assessment
NCLEX-RN Test Plan: PHYS
Reference: LeFever Kee, J., Paulanka, B., & Purnell, L. D. (2004). *Fluids and electrolytes with clinical applications: A programmed approach* (7th ed.). Newark, NJ: Thompson.

105. **Answer: 3**
Rationale: In some cases nutrition and hydration are considered life prolonging and may extend discomfort. Withholding food and fluids in end of life situations is not painful. In some cases, dying persons feel their wishes and their desire to be permitted to die are not being met if fluids and nutrition are continued. In end stages of life, dehydration is not painful. A person's metabolism changes and ketones that form from oxidation of fatty acids produce a mild euphoria. Hunger and thirst are not perceived as a healthy person would imagine. Basic oral care and moisture application to lips and oral mucous membranes should be provided and is considered comfort care.
Cognitive Level: Synthesis
Nursing Process: Implementation
NCLEX-RN Test Plan: PSYC
Reference: Lamer, W. (2006). *Nutrition and dehydration*. Retrieved March 17, 2006 from http://www.hospicefoundation.org/endOfLifeInfo/nutrition_hydration.asp

106. **Answer: 3**
Rationale: Hypotonic fluids will decrease the osmolality of the vasculature. In an attempt to normalize osmolarity on both sides of the capillary membrane,

fluid will move into the interstitial spaces where the osmolality is higher. The vascular volume will decrease. Hypertonic solutions will cause fluid to move across semipermeable membranes by osmosis from interstitial spaces into the vasculature. Without physiological processes or factors affecting osmolality of the vasculature or the interstitial fluids, isotonic fluids will neither cause a shift in nor out of the vasculature. However, isotonic fluids will increase circulatory overload by increasing vascular volume. Some medications can be given by IV push but short-term maintenance doses in acute situations must be given over slow drip.
Cognitive Level: Synthesis
Nursing Process: Evaluation
NCLEX-RN Test Plan: PHYS
Reference: Phillips, L. D. (2005). *Manual of IV therapeutics* (4th ed.). Philadelphia: F.A. Davis.

107. **Answer: 2**
Rationale: Potassium is the major intracellular fluid (ICF) cation. With massive cell and tissue destruction or burns, potassium is released into the serum and levels increase. Potassium would also be increased in acute renal failure, metabolic acidosis, and diabetes mellitus, but this client has no known medical diagnosis.
Cognitive Level: Synthesis
Nursing Process: Diagnosis
NCLEX-RN Test Plan: PHYS
Reference: Corbett, J. (2004). *Laboratory tests and diagnostic procedures with nursing diagnosis* (6th ed.). Upper Saddle River, NJ: Pearson Prentice Hall.

108. **Answer: 2**
Rationale: The intrathecal space is where the cerebral spinal fluid (CSF) is contained and bathes the spinal cord. Intrathecal doses are 10 times less than epidural doses. Inward migration can cause a dangerous and life threatening opioid overdose. Both epidural and intrathecal dosing can be administered continuously. Infections are rare with epidural administration but there is an increased risk with intrathecal routes since the CSF is a medium for bacterial growth. Pain at the insertion site is possible but not of greatest concern at this moment. Inward migration of an epidural catheter requires immediate intervention.
Cognitive Level: Synthesis

Nursing Process: Evaluation
NCLEX-RN Test Plan: PHYS
Reference: Phillips, L. D. (2005). *Manual of IV therapeutics* (4th ed.). Philadelphia: F.A. Davis.

109. **Answer: 4**
Rationale: Orange juice, baked potato, and yogurt are all high potassium foods with greater than 10 mEq of potassium per serving. Pecans are not high in potassium.
Cognitive Level: Application
Nursing Process: Evaluation
NCLEX-RN Test Plan: HPM
Reference: Lewis, S. M., Heitkemper, M. M., & Dirksen, S. R. (2004). *Medical-surgical nursing: Assessment and management of clinical problems* (6th ed.). St. Louis, MO: Mosby.

110. **Answer: 3**
Rationale: Leafy green vegetables are a dietary source of Vitamin K. Anticoagulants are used to prevent clotting. Other options do not interact with the effect of the anticoagulant. Laboratory tests, such as INR and protimes, are monitored to evaluate the drug therapeutic level and identify if food interactions have occurred.
Cognitive Level: Application
Nursing Process: Implementation
NCLEX-RN Test Plan: PHYS
Reference: Lewis, S. M., Heitkemper, M. M., & Dirksen, S. R. (2004). *Medical-surgical nursing: Assessment and management of clinical problems* (6th ed.). St. Louis, MO: Mosby.

111. **Answers: 1, 3, 4, and 5**
Rationale: Vitamins A, D, and E are commonly used to promote wound healing. Other minerals such as zinc, folate, and iron are also used to promote cellular integrity and hemoglobin formation. Vitamin B_{12} (pyridoxine) assists development of red blood cells and maintenance of nerve function.
Cognitive Level: Application
Nursing Process: Implementation
NCLEX-RN Test Plan: PHYS
Reference: Lewis, S. M., Heitkemper, M. M., & Dirksen, S. R. (2004). *Medical-surgical nursing: Assessment and management of clinical problems* (6th ed.). St. Louis, MO: Mosby.

112. **Answer: 4**

    Rationale: The preschooler will be influenced by others' eating habits and demonstrate their likes and dislikes for food preferences. The caloric requirement decreases slightly at this age; it is 90 calories/kg/day. Quality, not quantity, is important. It is not necessary to give vitamins after infancy unless the child is at nutritional risk.

    Cognitive Level: Application

    Nursing Process: Implementation

    NCLEX-RN Test Plan: PHYS

    Reference: Wong, D. (2005). *Wong's essentials of pediatric nursing* (7th ed.). St. Louis, MO: Mosby.

113. **Answer: 3**

    Rationale: The adult with diabetes mellitus is recommended to maintain between 45% and 55% of their total kilocalories as carbohydrates in their daily dietary food intake.

    Cognitive Level: Application

    Nursing Process: Assessment

    NCLEX-RN Test Plan: PHYS

    Reference: Farrell, M., & Nicoteri, J. A. (2001). *Quick look nursing: Nutrition.* Thorofare, NJ: Slack Inc.

114. **Answer: 1**

    Rationale: Ginseng and ginkgo biloba inhibit platelet aggregation. Both have possible drug interactions with anticoagulants. Ginkgo biloba should be used cautiously in people with risk for bleeding. Ginkgo and ginseng have no specific correlation with the other options.

    Cognitive Level: Application

    Nursing Process: Implementation

    NCLEX-RN Test Plan: SECE

    Reference: Lewis, S. M., Heitkemper, M. M., & Dirksen, S. R. (2004). *Medical-surgical nursing: Assessment and management of clinical problems* (6th ed.). St. Louis, MO: Mosby.

115. **Answer: 1**

    Rationale: Fertilization takes place in the outer third of the ampulla of the fallopian tube. Implantation occurs between six and ten days after conception. The embryonic (not fetal stage) is when organ development is taking place.

    Cognitive Level: Analysis

Nursing Process: Implementation

NCLEX-RN Test Plan: HPM

Reference: Lowdermilk, D. L., & Perry, S. E. (2004). *Maternity and women's health care* (8th ed.). St. Louis, MO: Mosby.

116. **Answer: 2**

    Rationale: Signs preceding labor include a surge of energy, increased vaginal discharge, bloody show, a return of urinary frequency as the fetus engages in the pelvis, and weight loss of 0.5 kg to 1.5 kg (1 to 3 pounds). Other signs include lightening, backache, stronger Braxton-Hicks contractions, cervical ripening, and rupture of membranes.

    Cognitive Level: Analysis

    Nursing Process: Implementation

    NCLEX-RN Test Plan: HPM

    Reference: Lowdermilk, D. L., & Perry, S. E. (2004). *Maternity and women's health care* (8th ed.). St. Louis, MO: Mosby.

117. **Answer: 2, 3, 6, and 7**

    Rationale: Indomethacin is a prostaglandin inhibitor that relaxes uterine smooth muscle. Magnesium sulfate is a CNS depressant used to relax smooth muscles of the uterus. Ritodrine (Yutopar) and terbutaline (Brethine) are Beta$_2$-adrenergic agonists that relax smooth uterine muscles and inhibit uterine activity. Cervidil is a prostaglandin E2 given to soften the cervix and also causes uterine contractions. Oxytocin (Pitocin) and Methylergonovine (Methergine) are uterotonic agents given to promote uterine contraction.

    Cognitive Level: Analysis

    Nursing Process: Implementation

    NCLEX-RN Test Plan: HPM

    Reference: Lowdermilk, D. L., & Perry, S. E. (2004). *Maternity and women's health care* (8th ed.). St. Louis, MO: Mosby.

118. **Answer: Late decelerations**

    Rationale: The late deceleration begins after the contraction has started. The lowest point (nadir) of the deceleration occurs after the peak of the contraction. Late decelerations usually do not return to baseline until after the contraction has ended.

    Cognitive Level: Analysis

    Nursing Process: Analysis

NCLEX-RN Test Plan: HPM
Reference: Lowdermilk, D. L., & Perry, S. E. (2004). *Maternity and women's health care* (8th ed.). St. Louis, MO: Mosby.

119. **Answer: 3**
Rationale: Plantar creases are part of the physical maturity assessment of the Ballard Scale for newborn maturity. Acrocyanosis is a slightly cyanotic appearance of the hands and feet due to vasomotor instability. A soft, level anterior fontanel and vernix caseosa noted in creases are normal findings and are not associated with gestational age assessment.
Cognitive Level: Application
Nursing Process: Analysis
NCLEX-RN Test Plan: HPM
Reference: Ballard, J., Novak, K., & Driver, M. (1979). A simplified score for assessment of fetal maturity of newly born infants. *Journal of Pediatrics, 95,* 769–774.

120. **Answer: 2**
Rationale: During the first 24 hours, the postpartum client is in the Dependent: Taking In phase. Her dependency needs predominate over the newborn's needs. By the second to third postpartum day she moves into the Dependent-Independent: Taking Hold phase. This is when the mother begins to focus on care of the newborn. In the Interdependent: Letting Go phase, the mother begins to take charge of the maternal role. In the Mutually Dependent, Reciprocity phase, the body movement or behavior (of the newborn) provides the observer (mother) with cues. The mother interprets these cues and responds to them. This phase usually takes several weeks to develop.
Cognitive Level: Analysis
Nursing Process: Evaluation
NCLEX-RN Test Plan: HPM
Reference: Lowdermilk, D. L., & Perry, S. E. (2004). *Maternity and women's health care* (8th ed.). St. Louis, MO: Mosby.

121. **Answer: 1**
Rationale: Cardiovascular disease is the leading cause of death in women regardless of racial or ethnic group. African American women are more likely to have a higher prevalence of this disease than other

racial groups due to having a higher incidence of CAD risk factors such as obesity, hypertension, diabetes, and physical inactivity. Lung cancer is the leading cause of cancer deaths in women. Lung cancer rarely produces symptoms. The most common symptoms of lung cancer are fatigue, persistent cough, shortness of breath, and chronic chest pain. Osteoporosis is a silent disease that is characterized by low bone mass and structural deterioration of bone tissue. Women are free of symptoms until a fracture occurs. The most common fractures occur in the vertebrae, wrists, and hips. Palpitation of a lump is the most common reason for presentation with breast cancer.
Cognitive Level: Analysis
Nursing Process: Assessment
NCLEX-RN Test Plan: PHYS
Reference: Alexander, L. L., LaRosa, J. H., Bader, H., & Garfield, S. (2004). *New dimensions in women's health* (3rd ed.). Sudbury, MA: Jones & Bartlett.

122. **Answers: 1, 2, and 3**
Rationale: Risk factors for osteoporosis include the loss of estrogen; during the first five to six years after menopause, women will lose bone mass six times more rapidly than men. The women more likely to be at risk are Caucasian or Asian and have small, thin bone structure. Smoking is associated with greater bone mass loss because it decreases estrogen production. Excessive alcohol consumption interferes with calcium absorption and depresses bone formation.
Cognitive Level: Analysis
Nursing Process: Assessment
NCLEX-RN Test Plan: HPM
Reference: Lowdermilk, D. L., & Perry, S. E. (2004). *Maternity & women's health care* (8th ed.). St. Louis, MO: Mosby.

123. **Answer: 2**
Rationale: The pap test will detect 90% of early cervical changes and is the most reliable method to detect preinvasive cancer. Pelvic examination is usually normal except in late stage cancer. Vaginal and abdominal ultrasounds are not used to detect early preinvasive cervical cancer.
Cognitive Level: Application
Nursing Process: Planning

NCLEX-RN Test Plan: HPM
Reference: Condon, M. C. (2004). *Women's health: An integrated approach to wellness and illness.* Upper Saddle River, NJ: Prentice Hall.

124. **Answer: 4**
Rationale: Elevation of the arm will decrease swelling in the extremity. It is possible that the lymphatic system has been altered, therefore no further trauma should occur to this extremity. While all of the options are postoperative concerns, positioning the client's arm takes precedence in the immediate postoperative period.
Cognitive Level: Analysis
Nursing Process: Plan
NCLEX-RN Test Plan: PHYS
Reference: Ricci, S. S. (2007). *Essentials of maternity, newborn, and women's health nursing.* Philadelphia: Lippincott Williams & Wilkins.

125. **Answer: 3**
Rationale: Gonorrhea is a highly communicable disease. Recent (within the past 30 days) sexual partners should be examined and treated. Preventing reinfection and the spread of the disease is a primary prevention strategy and nursing goal. All clients with gonorrhea should be offered confidential counseling and treatment. Parental notification procedures will vary from state to state. Women should be instructed on safe sexual practices and use of birth control.
Cognitive Level: Application
Nursing Process: Planning
NCLEX-RN Test Plan: PHYS, HPM
Reference: Lowdermilk, D. L., & Perry, S. E. (2004). *Maternity & women's health care* (8th ed.). St. Louis, MO: Mosby.

126. **Answers: 1, 2, and 3**
Rationale: Male factor infertility may be caused by anatomic or structural problems, abnormalities in sperm production or function, as well as sexual, hormonal, and genetic conditions. Genetic problems such as Klinefelter syndrome can cause an absence of sperm. Despite many known etiologies, male factor infertility is often idiopathic. To date, diet has not been identified as a factor in male infertility.
Cognitive Level: Synthesis
Nursing Process: Implementation

NCLEX-RN Test Plan: PSYC
Reference: Schuiling, K. D., & Likis, F. E. (2006). *Women's gynecologic health.* Sudbury, MA: Jones & Bartlett.

127. **Answer: 3**
Rationale: A client with sickle cell would need to have some movement to prevent venous stasis and further complications. Cold compresses would promote sickling, not reduce it. Pain medication should be given around the clock to help control the pain. Hydration is appropriate to promote blood flow.
Cognitive Level: Application
Nursing Process: Planning
NCLEX-RN Test Plan: PHYS
Reference: Hockenberry, M. J. (2005). *Wong's essentials of pediatric nursing* (7th ed.). St. Louis, MO: Mosby.

128. **Answers: 4, 7, and 8**
Rationale: In children 5 years and older, mild persistent asthma is described as symptoms more than twice a week but less than once a day, nighttime symptoms more than twice a month, and peak expiratory flow (PEF) greater than or equal to 80% of the predicted value. Continual symptoms would indicate severe persistent asthma. Daily symptoms, nighttime symptoms nightly, and PEF of 60–80% of predicted value indicate moderate persistent asthma.
Cognitive Level: Analysis
Nursing Process: Assessment
NCLEX-RN Test Plan: HPM
Reference: Hockenberry, M. J. (2005). *Wong's essentials of pediatric nursing* (7th ed.). St. Louis, MO: Mosby.

129. **Answers: 3, 5, 6, and 7**
Rationale: Symptoms of hypoglycemia are caused by increased adrenergic activity and impaired brain function. The increased adrenergic activity produces the symptoms of hypoglycemia; nervousness, pallor, tremors, palpitations, sweating and hunger. More severe symptoms, such as, weakness, dizziness, headache, drowsiness, irritability, loss of coordination, seizures and coma, can occur if hypoglycemia is not treated when first recognized due to a decrease of glucose in the CNS. The symptoms may be similar to symptoms of hyperglycemia

at first. The best way to tell whether the blood sugar is high or low is to test the blood sugar level.
Cognitive Level: Analysis
Nursing Process: Analysis
NCLEX-RN Test Plan: PHYS
Reference: Hockenberry, M. J. (2005). *Wong's essentials of pediatric nursing* (7th ed.). St. Louis, MO: Mosby.

130. **Answer: 3**
Rationale: Oral iron should be given between meals. Cow's milk contains substances that bind the iron and interfere with its absorption. Iron supplements should not be given with milk or milk products. A citrus juice or fruit taken with an iron supplement aids in its absorption.
Cognitive Level: Application
Nursing Process: Implementation
NCLEX-RN Test Plan: HPM
Reference: Hockenberry, M. J. (2005). *Wong's essentials of pediatric nursing* (7th ed.) St. Louis, MO: Mosby.

131. **Answer: 1**
Rationale: The comorbidity if alcohol use and emotional disorder, especially coupled with sexual acting out, are powerful predictors of suicidal behavior. However, the best predictor is a previous suicide attempt. Almost 50% of adolescents who die by suicide made a previous attempt.
Cognitive Level: Analysis
Nursing Process: Analysis
NCLEX-RN Test Plan: PSYC
Reference: Thies, K. M., & Travers, J. F. (2001). *Quick look nursing: Growth and development through the lifespan.* Thorofare, NJ: Slack Inc.

132. **Answer: 2**
Rationale: Antipyretics are used to treat fevers and they include acetaminophen and nonsteroidal anti-inflammatory drugs (NSAIDs). The appropriate dose of acetaminophen is 10 mg/kg/dose. The patient weighs 28 pounds or 12.7 kg. If you multiply the weight of 12.7 kg times 10, the result is 127 mg. If there are 120 mg in 5 ml, then 127 mg is equal to 5.3 ml. The closest amount for the mother to draw up and administer is 5 ml.
Cognitive Level: Application
Nursing Process: Analysis

NCLEX-RN Test Plan: PHYS
Reference: Hockenberry, M. J. (2005). *Wong's essentials of pediatric nursing* (7th ed.). St. Louis, MO: Mosby.

133. **Answer: 1**
Rationale: Antidepressants have no potential for abuse. With regard to water consumption, hypotension is a frequent side effect of antidepressants and hydration is recommended. Clients who respond to an initial course of treatment with an antidepressant should continue with the drug for at least 6 to 9 months. Sexual dysfunction is also a side effect to expect and dosing after, not before, intercourse is recommended.
Cognitive Level: Analysis
Nursing Process: Evaluation
NCLEX-RN Test Plan: PHYS
Reference: Stuart, G. W., & Laraia, M. T. (2005). *Principles and practices of psychiatric nursing* (8th ed.). St. Louis, MO: Elsevier Mosby.

134. **Answer: 2**
Rationale: Symptoms of acute PCP intoxication include euphoria, psychomotor agitation, grandiosity, emotional lability, and synesthesias. Nursing care focuses on providing a quiet, safe environment that protects the client and others from injury. Treatment may include antiseizure medication. However, seizure precautions are more of a focus of treatment during amphetamine withdrawal. Suicide precautions are associated with cocaine withdrawal where severe depression is common. Treatment for autonomic hyperactivity is a focus in barbiturate and benzodiazepine withdrawal.
Cognitive Level: Analysis
Nursing Process: Implementation
NCLEX-RN Test Plan: PSYC
Reference: Kneisl, C. R., Wilson, H. S., & Trigoboff, E. (2004). *Contemporary psychiatric-mental health nursing.* Upper Saddle River, NJ: Pearson Prentice Hall.

135. **Answer: Tyramine**
Rationale: When foods containing tyramine and certain medications are taken concomitantly with MAOIs, there is a potential for hypertensive crisis.
Cognitive Level: Application
Nursing Process: Planning

NCLEX-RN Test Plan: PSYC

Reference: Stuart, G. (2005). *Handbook of psychiatric nursing* (6th ed.). St. Louis, MO: Elsevier Mosby.

136. **Answer: 8, 4, 1, 2, 7, 6, 3, 5**

    Rationale: A complete physical is performed to see that the client is a physical candidate for ECT. Informed consent is obtained. The client is NPO the morning of ECT. Before entering the treatment room, dentures are removed. The client is positioned on a stretcher in the treatment room and given a short-acting anesthetist and muscle relaxant. During the seizure phase of treatment, the nurse guides extremities to prevent injury. The nurse should not attempt to restrain the patient. In the recovery room, the client is positioned on the side to prevent aspirations of oral secretions.

    Cognitive Level: Analysis

    Nursing Process: Implementation

    NCLEX-RN Test Plan: PSYC

    Reference: Mohr, W. K. (2003). *Psychiatric-mental health nursing* (5th ed.). Philadelphia: Lippincott Williams & Wilkins.

137. **Answer: 3**

    Rationale: The MMSE was designed to measure cognition. It consists of eleven questions with a maximum score of 30 points. It does not require past recall. The test requires that the responder write and copy a design. Thus, it is an inappropri-ate assessment tool for a client who has a motor movement disorder.

    Cognitive Level: Analysis

    Nursing Process: Assessment

    NCLEX-RN Test Plan: PSYC

    Reference: Fontaine, K. L., Kneisl, C. R., & Trigoboff, E. (2004). *Clinical companion for psychiatric-mental health nursing.* Upper Saddle River, NJ: Pearson Prentice Hall.

138. **Answer: 3**

    Rationale: Behaviors associated with depression are varied. They can be sad and slow or agitated and anxious. A key element in behavioral assessment is change, especially a change in usual patterns of behavior. Anxiety associated with a trigger event is characteristic of phobias. A sense of worthlessness is a cognitive not a behavioral assessment factor associated with depression. Extreme concerns regarding social situations that can lead to despondency and avoidance are associated with social phobia.

    Cognitive Level: Application

    Nursing Process: Assessment

    NCLEX-RN Test Plan: PSYC

    Reference: Stuart, G. (2005). *Handbook of psychiatric nursing* (6th ed.). St. Louis, MO: Elsevier Mosby.

    Townsend, M. C. (2005). *Essentials of psychiatric mental health nursing* (3rd ed., pp. 341–343). Philadelphia: F.A. Davis.

Common Abbreviations

The following is an alphabetized list of common abbreviations utilized in the nursing profession and may also be found on the NCLEX-RN® examination.

a	Before (ante)
AAA	Abdominal aortic aneurysm
ABG	Arterial blood gas
ac	Before meals (ante cibum)
ACE	Angiotensin-converting enzyme
ACTH	Adrenocorticotropic hormone
ADH	Antidiuretic hormone
ADHD	Attention deficit-hyperactive disorder
ADLs	Activities of daily living
AED	Automatic external defibrillator
Afib	Atrial fibrillation
Aflutter	Atrial flutter
AIDS	Acquired immunodeficiency syndrome
AK or AKA	Above-the-knee amputation
AMA	Against medical advice
ANP	Adult Nurse Practitioner
ANS	Autonomic nervous system
A&Ox3	Alert and oriented to person, place, and time
aPTT	Activated partial thromboplastin time
ARC	AIDs-related complex
ARDS	Adult respiratory distress syndrome
ASA	Acetylsalicylic acid (aspirin)
ASAP	As soon as possible
ASD	Atrial septal defect
AVM	Ateriovenous malformation
BK or BKA	Below-the-knee amputation
BM	Bowel movement
BMI	Body mass index
BMR	Basal metabolic rate
BP	Blood pressure
BPH	Benign prostatic hyperplasia/hypertrophy
bpm	Beats per minute
BRP	Bathroom privileges
BUN	Blood urea nitrogen

c̄	With
CABG	Coronary artery bypass graft operation (×1,2,3,...number of grafts)
CAD	Coronary artery disease
CBC	Complete blood count
CCU	Cardiac (intensive) care unit
CDC	Centers for Disease Control
CF	Cystic fibrosis
CHD	Coronary heart disease or Congenital heart disease
CHF	Congestive heart failure
CICU	Cardiac intensive care unit
CMV	Cytomegalovirus
CNS	Central nervous system
c/o	Complaints of
COA	Coarctation of the aorta
COPD	Chronic obstructive pulmonary disease
CP	Cerebral palsy
CPK or CK	Creatine phosphokinase or Creatine kinase
CPR	Cardiopulmonary resuscitation
C&S	Culture and sensitivity
CSF	Cerebrospinal fluid
CSM	Circulation, sensory, and motor
CT	Computerized tomography
CV	Cardiovascular
CVA	Cerebrovascular accident (also known as Brain attack)
CVP	Central venous pressure
D&C	Dilation and curettage
D&E	Dilation and evacuation
DIC	Disseminated intravascular coagulation
DJD	Degenerative joint disease
DKA	Diabetic ketoacidosis
DM	Diabetes mellitus
DNR	Do not resuscitate
DOA	Dead on arrival
DOB	Date of birth
DOE	Dyspnea on exertion
DPT	Diphtheria, pertussis, and tetanus
DRG	Diagnosis-related-group
DTR	Deep-tendon reflex
DTs	Delirium tremens
DVT	Deep vein thrombosis
D_5W/D5W	5% dextrose in water
Dx	Diagnosis
ECF	Extracellular fluid or Extended care facility
ECG	Electrocardiogram
Echo	Echocardiogram

ECT	Electroconvulsive therapy
ED	Emergency department (room) or Erectile dysfunction
EDD	Estimated date of delivery
EEG	Electroencephalogram
EENT	Eye, ear, nose, and throat
EKG	Electrocardiogram
EMG	Electromyogram
EMS	Emergency medical service
EMT	Emergency medical technician
ENT	Ear, nose, and throat
ER	Emergency room
ESR	Erythrocyte sedimentation rate
ETOH	Alcohol (ethanol)
FBS	Fasting blood sugar
FHR	Fetal heart rate
FHT	Fetal heart tones
FNP	Family nurse practitioner
FSH	Follicle-stimulating hormone
FUO	Fever of unknown origin
Fx	Fracture
g	Gram
G	Gravida
GCS	Glasgow coma scale
G&D	Growth and development
GDM	Gestational diabetes mellitus
GERD	Gastroesophageal reflux disease
GI	Gastrointestinal
gm	Gram
gr	Grain
GTT	Glucose tolerance test
gtt(s)	Drop(s)
GU	Genitourinary
GYN	Gynecological
HBGM	Home blood glucose monitoring
HBV	Hepatitis B virus
HCG	Human chorionic gonadotropin
Hct	Hematocrit
HCV	Hepatitis C virus
HDL	High density lipoprotein
HEENT	Head, eyes, ears, nose, throat
Hgb	Hemoglobin
HIB	*Haemophilus influenzae* type B
HIV	Human immunodeficiency virus
HMO	Health maintenance organization

HOB	Head of bed
HPL	Human placental lactogen
HPV	Human papilloma virus
HR	Heart rate
HSV	Herpes simplex virus
HTN	Hypertension
Hx	History
ICP	Intracranial pressure
ICU	Intensive care unit
I&D	Incision and drainage
Ig	Immunoglobin
INH	Isoniazid
I/O or I&O	Intake and output
IPPB	Intermittent positive-pressure breathing
IQ	Intelligence quotient
IUD	Intrauterine device
IV	Intravenous
IVP	Intravenous push or Intravenous pyelogram
JCAHO	Joint Commission on Accreditation of Healthcare Organizations
JRA	Juvenile rheumatoid arthritis
KUB	Kidneys, ureters, bladder (abdominal X-ray)
LDL	Low-density lipoprotein
LGA	Large for gestational age
LLL	Left lower lobe (lung)
LLQ	Left lower quadrant (abdomen)
LMP	Last menstrual period
LOC	Level of consciousness or Loss of consciousness
LPN	Licensed practical nurse
LUL	Left upper lobe (lung)
LUQ	Left upper quadrant (abdomen)
MAOI	Monoamine oxidase inhibitor
MAP	Mean arterial pressure
MCL	Midclavicular line
MD	Muscular dystrophy
MDI	Metered-dose inhaler
Med	Medication
mEq	Milliequivalent
MI	Myocardial infarction
mL	Milliliter
MMR	Measles, mumps, rubella
MOM	Milk of magnesia
Mono	Mononucleosis

MRI	Magnetic resonance imaging
MRSA	Methicillin-resistant *Staphylococcus aureus*
MS	Multiple sclerosis or Mental status or Mitral stenosis or Morphine sulfate
MVR	Mitral valve repair/replacement
NA	Not applicable
NG	Nasogastric
NICU	Neonatal intensive care unit
NPH	Neutral protamine Hagedorn (intermediate acting insulin)
NPO	Nothing by mouth
NS	Normal saline
NSAID	Nonsteroidal anti-inflammatory drug
NSR	Normal sinus rhythm
NST	Nonstress test
N/V	Nausea, vomiting
NVD	Nausea, vomiting, diarrhea
O_2	Oxygen
OB	Obstetrics
OD	Right ear
OFTT	Organic failure to thrive
OOB	Out of bed or Out of breath
O&P	Ova and parasites
OR	Operating room
OS	Left ear
OT	Occupational therapy/therapist
OTC	Over-the-counter
OU	Both ears (left [OS] and right [OD] ears)
P	Pulse (part of TPR)
p	Post (after)
PA	Physician's assistant or Pulmonary artery or Posteroanterior
PAC	Premature atrial contraction
PACU	Postanesthesia care unit
PAO_2	Alveolar oxygen pressure
PaO_2	Arterial partial pressure of oxygen
pc	After meals
PCA	Patient-controlled analgesia (pump) or Patient care assistant
PCP	*Pneumocystic carinii* pneumonia
PDA	Patent ductus arteriosus
PE	Pulmonary embolus or Pulmonary edema
PEEP	Positive end-expiratory pressure
PERRLA(A)	Pupils equally round and reactive to light (and accommodation)
PICU	Pediatric intensive care unit
PID	Pelvic inflammatory disease
PIH	Pregnancy induced hypertension
PKU	Phenylketonouria

PMI	Point of maximum impulse
PMS	Premenstrual syndrome
PNP	Pediatric nurse practitioner
PO	By mouth
PPD	Purified protein derivative (TB skin test) or Percussion & postural drainage
PPN	Peripheral parenteral nutrition
PPO	Preferred provider organization
prn	When necessary
PSA	Prostate-specific antigen
Pt	Patient
PT	Prothrombin time or Physical therapy
PTA	Prior to admission
PTCA	Percutaneous transluminal coronary angioplasty
PTSD	Post-traumatic stress disorder
PTT	Partial thromboplastin time
PUD	Peptic ulcer disease
PVC	Premature ventricular contraction

q	Each, every
qh	Every hour
qid	Four times a day

R	Respirations (in TPR)
RA	Rheumatoid arthritis or Right atrium
RBC	Red blood cell
RDA	Recommended daily/dietary allowances
RDA	Respiratory distress syndrome
RDS	Respiratory distress syndrome
RLL	Right lower lobe (lung)
RLQ	Right lower quadrant (abdomen)
RML	Right middle lobe (lung)
R/O	Rule out
ROM	Range of motion
R	Respirations (in TPR)
RR	Respiratory
RT	Respiratory
R/T	Related to
RUL	Right upper lobe (lung)
RUQ	Right upper quadrant (abdomen)
Rx	Prescription or Treatment

$\bar{s}$	Without
S_1	First heart sound
S_2	Second heart sound
S_3	Third heart sound
S_4	Fourth heart sound
SaO_2	Arterial blood-oxygen saturation
SGA	Small for gestational age

SIADH	Syndrome of inappropriate antidiuretic hormone
SICU	Surgical intensive care unit
SIDS	Sudden infant death syndrome
SL	Sublingually
SLE	Systemic lupus erythematosus
SOB	Shortness of breath
SR	Sinus rhythm
S/Sx	Signs and symptoms
Stat	Immediately
STD(s)	Sexually transmitted disease(s)
Sx	Symptoms
T	Temperature (in TPR)
T&A	Tonsillectomy and adenoidectomy
TB	Tuberculosis
TENS	Transcutaneous electrical nerve stimulation
TIA	Transient ischemic attack
TID	Three times a day
TKO	To keep open
TORCH	Toxoplasmosis
TPA	Tissue plasminogen activator
TPN	Total parenteral nutrition
TPR	Temperature, pulse, and respirations
TSE	Testicular self-examination
TSH	Thyroid stimulating hormone
TURP	Transuretheral resection of prostate
Tx	Treatment
UA	Urinalysis
UAP	Unlicensed assistive personnel
UGI	Upper gastrointestinal
UQ	Upper quadrant (abdomen)
URI	Upper respiratory infection
UTI	Urinary tract infection
UV	Ultraviolet
VD	Venereal disease
Vfib	Ventricular fibrillation
VS	Vital signs
VSD	Ventricular septal defect
w/	With
WBC	White blood cell
WHO	World Health Organization
WIC	Women, infants, and children
WNL	Within normal limits
w/o	Without

References

Lewis, S., Heitkemper, M., & Dirksen, S. (2004). *Medical-surgical nursing: Assessment and management of clinical problems* (6th ed.). St Louis, MO: Elsevier Mosby.

Pagana, K., & Pagana, T. (2006). *Mosby's manual of diagnostic and laboratory tests* (3rd ed.). St. Louis, MO: Elsevier Mosby.

Common Conversions

Listed below is a chart of common conversions utilized in the nursing profession which may also be found on the NCLEX-RN® exam.

Liquid Measure

8 ounces	=	1 cup
2 cups	=	1 pint
16 ounces	=	1 pint
4 cups	=	1 quart
2 pints	=	1 quart
4 quarts	=	1 gallon
1 tsp	=	60 drops (gtts)
3 teaspoons (tsp, t)	=	1 tablespoon (tbsp, T)
2 tbsp	=	1 ounce (oz)
4 tbsp	=	¼ cup
8 tbsp	=	½ cup

US Liquid Measure to Metric System

1 fluid ounce (oz)	=	29 milliliters (ml) or cubic centimeter (cc)
1 cup	=	230 milliliters (ml) or cubic centimeter (cc)
1 quart	=	0.946 liter
1.06 quarts	=	1 liter
0.034 fluid ounce	=	1 milliliter (ml) or cubic centimeter (cc)
3.38 fluid ounces	=	1 deciliter
33.8 fluid ounces	=	1 liter

Dry Measure

2 pints	=	1 quart
4 quarts	=	1 gallon
8 quarts	=	2 gallons or 1 peck
4 pecks	=	8 gallons or 1 bushel
16 ounces	=	1 pound
2000 pounds	=	1 ton

US Dry Measure to Metric System

0.353 ounce	=	1 gram
¼ ounce	=	7 grams
1 ounce	=	28.35 grams
4 ounces	=	113.4 grams
8 ounces	=	226.8 grams
1 pound	=	454 grams
2.2 pounds	=	1 kilogram

Linear Measurement

12 inches	=	1 foot
3 feet	=	1 yard
5,280 feet	=	1 mile
6,080 feet	=	1 nautical mile

US Linear Measure to Metric System

1 inch	=	2.54 centimeters
1 foot	=	0.3048 meter
1 yard	=	0.9144 meter
1 mile	=	16093 meters or 1.6093 kilometers
0.0337 inch	=	1 millimeter
0.3937 inch	=	1 centimeter
3.937 inches	=	1 decimeter
39.37 inches	=	1 meter
3280.8 feet	=	1 kilometer
0.62137 mile	=	1 kilometer

Temperature Conversion

Use the following steps to convert a Fahrenheit temperature to a Centigrade temperature:

Step 1	=	Subtract 32
Step 2	=	Multiply by 5
Step 3	=	Divide by 9

Use the following steps to convert a Centigrade temperature to a Fahrenheit temperature:

Step 1	=	Multiply by 9
Step 2	=	Divide by 5
Step 3	=	Add 32

Common Laboratory Values

The following is a list of common laboratory values utilized in the nursing profession and commonly found on the NCLEX-RN® examination.

Test	Normal Value	Critical Value
Activated partial thromboplastin time (aPTT)	30–40 seconds	> 70 seconds
Partial thromboplastin time (PTT)	60–70 seconds	> 100 seconds
Prostate specific antigen (PSA)	< 4 ng/mL or < 4 mcg/L	
Pulse oximetry	≥ 95%	≤ 75%
Fasting blood sugar (FBS)	< 110 mg/dL	< 50 & > 400 mg/dL
Blood glucose (BG)		
Glycosylated hemoglobin (HbA_{1C})		
Nondiabetic adult	2.2%–4.8%	
Nondiabetic child	1.8%–4.0%	
Good diabetic control	2.5%–5.9%	
Fair diabetic control	6.0%–8.0%	
Poor diabetic control	> 8.0%	
Hematocrit (Hct)		
Male	42%–52%	< 15% or > 60%
Female	37%–47%	
Hemoglobin (Hgb)		
Male	14–18 g/dl	< 5g/dL or > 20g/dL
Female	12–16 g/dL	
Platelet	150,000–400,000 mm^3	< 50,000 or > 1 mill
Red blood cell (RBC)		
Male	4.7–6.1	
Female	4.2–5.4	
White blood cell (WBC)		
Total	5,000–10,000/mm^3	< 2,500 or > 30,000
Differential		
Neutrophils	2,500–8,000	
Lymphocytes	1,000–4,000	
Monocytes	100–700	
Eosinophils	50–500	
Basophils	25–100	

Test	Normal Value	Critical Value
High density lipoprotein (HDL)		
Male	> 45 mg/dL	
Female	> 55 mg/dL	
Low density lipoprotein (LDL)	60–180 mg/dL	
Very low density lipoprotein (VLDL)	7–32 mg/dL	
Cholesterol	< 200 mg/dL	
Triglycerides		
Male	40–160 mg/dL	> 400 mg/dL
Female	35–135 mg/dL	
Calcium (Ca)	9.0–10.5 mg/dL	< 6 or > 13 mg/dL
Chloride (Cl)	98–106 mEq/L	< 80 or > 115 mEq/L
Magnesium (Mg)	1.3–2.1 mEq/L	< 0.5 or > 3 mEq/L
Potassium (K)	3.5–5.0 mEq/L	< 2.5 or > 6.5 mEq/L
Sodium (Na)	136–143 mEq/L	< 120 or > 160 mEq/L

References

Lewis, S., Heitkemper, M., & Dirksen, S. (2004). *Medical-surgical nursing: Assessment and management of clinical problems* (6th ed.). St. Louis, MO: Elsevier Mosby.

Pagana, K., & Pagana, T. (2006). *Mosby's manual of diagnostic and laboratory tests* (3rd ed.). St. Louis, MO: Elsevier Mosby.

Individualized Study Plan Self-Assessment

Content Knowledge Assessment

Pretest Score—**Identify** areas of strength and areas needing more review.

I scored 68% on the pretest—also realize I need a "comfort level" score of 75-80% on my practice tests prior to scheduling my NCLEX-RN exam.

I realize this is only one test so I will continue to analyze these test results as I move through my study plan and continue to take practice tests.

Historical Review—From your educational program, identify content areas of strength and areas needing more review.

Throughout my nursing program coursework, I did best in the following courses—this was indicated by my course grades as well as the topic specific exams we took at the end of each course throughout the program.

> *Medical-Surgical Nursing (Adult)*
>
> *Physical Assessment*
>
> *Fundamental Nursing*

I still will continue to review these areas—but do realize these are my areas of strength and I will prioritize other areas first.

I did good—but not as good in the areas of:

> *Pediatrics*
>
> *Psychiatric/Mental Health*
>
> *Women's Health/ Obstetric Nursing*

I realize I do need additional review in these areas.

I did average in Pharmacology—and need more concentrated review in this area.

In December I took the Diagnostic Readiness Test (DRT) and scored Strong in 5 categories, Relatively Strong in 10 categories, Average in 6 categories and Below Average in 3 categories. This test divided the content into the following areas and identified areas of strength and weaknesses.

The categories are:

Strong:

> *Assessing*
>
> *Adult Health*
>
> *Basic Care & Comfort*
>
> *Safety and Infection Control*
>
> *Endocrine & Renal*

Relatively Strong:

> *Management of Care*
>
> *Health Promotion & Maintenance*
>
> *Evaluating*
>
> *Reduction of Risk Potential*
>
> *Immunological*
>
> *Neurological & Sensory*
>
> *Respiratory*
>
> *Analyzing*
>
> *Implementing*
>
> *Physiological Adaptation*

Average:

> *Planning*
>
> *Gastrointestinal*
>
> *Mental Health*
>
> *Musculoskeletal*
>
> *Psychosocial Integrity*
>
> *Pediatrics / Children's Health*

Below Average:

> *Pharmacological / Parenteral*
>
> *Women's Health*
>
> *Reproductive*

I do see that my scores on this DRT pretty well reflect my course grades and those of my end of course testing exams.

This also reflects how I feel about my knowledge level in each of these content areas. The topics I scored lowest on are the ones I am least comfortable with and those that I scored the best on are the content areas I am most comfortable with.

Data Prioritization—Prioritize your areas of content knowledge with #1 being the content area in which you feel most comfortable/confident of your knowledge. After you have your list, reverse the numbering order so that you begin your study with area #1 being the area in which you feel you need the most study and/or review (use additional pages as needed).

I am next creating a list of content areas and my comfort level with each content area. I have listed them beginning with the areas in which I feel most confident with my knowledge—to the areas I am least confident of my knowledge level.

1. Basic Care & Comfort
2. Safety & Infection Control
3. Adult Health
4. Assessing
5. Endocrine & Renal
6. Reduction of Risk
7. Management of Care
8. Health Promotion & Maintenance
9. Implementing
10. Analyzing
11. Evaluating
12. Respiratory
13. Immunological
14. Nervous & Sensory
15. Physiological Adaptation
16. Planning
17. Gastrointestinal
18. Musculoskeletal
19. Pediatrics—Children's Health
20. Psychosocial Integrity
21. Mental Health
22. Women's Health
23. Reproductive
24. Pharmacology

Now I'll turn my list around so I start studying with the area in which I feel least comfortable with my knowledge (Pharmacology) and save the area I am most confident of my knowledge level (Basic Care & Comfort) for last to review/study.

I also have divided my topic areas into those that need:

*   *Study and review questions/practice tests with review of rationales for each question.*

**   *More review questions and practice tests to see how I do—may need additional study.*

***   *Review questions and practice tests—and will only spend additional time if I find I am having a problem in these areas.*

Prioritized study list

1. *Pharmacology**
2. *Reproductive**
3. *Women's Health**
4. *Mental Health**
5. *Psychosocial Integrity**
6. *Pediatrics/Children's Health**
7. *Musculoskeletal**
8. *Gastrointestinal**
9. *Planning**
10. *Physiological Adaptation***
11. *Nervous & Sensory***
12. *Immunological***
13. *Respiratory***
14. *Evaluating***
15. *Analyzing***
16. *Implementing***
17. *Health Promotion & Maintenance***
18. *Management of Care***
19. *Reduction of Risk***
20. *Endocrine & Renal****
21. *Assessing****
22. *Adult Health****
23. *Safety & Infection Control****
24. *Basic Care & Comfort ****

Study Methods/Skills, Locations, Timeline

Study Methods I have used successfully in the past and will use now:

I have never really enjoyed studying in a group—but do have one friend who I sometimes study with and it seems to work. We are planning to meet once a week on Saturdays from 9:00 am to 11:00 am at a local coffee shop to review for two (2) hours.

We plan to ask each other questions and review specific topic areas for increased comprehension. We will work on Pharmacology first and our plan is to divide the various drug classifications. We will then each develop an outline for our assigned medications and share these with each other. We plan to make note cards for review and can use them as flashcards.

I realize my peak/productive times are in the evening—typically after 7:00 pm. That was the time when I did most of my studying and homework assignments for school. I plan to set this time aside (7:30 pm—9:30 pm) four (4) days as week for review and for my concentrated study of the content areas I need to review the most. I will spend one (1) hour in concentrated study and use the last hour to do review questions and rationales in this book.

I will plan on decreasing my "concentrated" study time and increasing my review questions and rationale time after I complete my study of my target problem areas (the top nine areas on my 'to study' list).

I have completed a calendar identifying my timelines and tentative topics. (See sample week.)

I will continue to evaluate my progress toward 75-80% on the content area tests. If I feel I am improving in a certain area—I will modify my plan and reduce my study time in that content area and replace it with another area— the next on my 'to study list'.

Also, as I am answering questions in the review test if I find an area where I need more review—I will add it to my list of areas to study.

Where I will plan to study:

I will be studying two (2) hours a week at the coffee shop on Saturdays from 8:00 am—10:00 am.

My alone study time will be done in my room at home. I am planning to use my desk in my room as the area where I can keep my review books, textbooks, notes, highlighters, tablets, note cards, and pens/pencils handy. I will not need to waste valuable study time getting my study supplies out each time I am beginning to study and putting them away each time I finish a study session.

I also have a chair in my room and have purchased a small 'laptop table' which will make studying and writing notes more comfortable when I am sitting in the chair.

My study timeline:

Identify the timeframe you will need to completely review your content areas. On the next page is a calendar to schedule appointments for your study sessions and other important events occurring during your preparation timeline for the NCLEX-RN®.

My activity schedule looks like this:

Saturday & Sunday—	Work from 2:00 pm—10:00 pm
Saturday—	Study from 9:00 am—11:00 am at the coffee shop
Monday & Friday—	Nursing Classes—8:00 am—2:00 pm
Tuesday & Wednesday—	Nursing Clinicals—7:00 am—2:30 pm
Monday & Tuesday—	Clinical assignments & preparation—3:00 pm—7:00 pm
Monday & Friday—	Exercise—6:00 am—6:45 am
Thursday—	Exercise—8:00 am—9:00 am
Saturday—	Exercise—7:00 am—8:00 am
Monday—	Study time—7:30 pm—9:30 pm
Tuesday—	Study time—7:30 pm—9:30 pm
Wednesday—	Study time—7:30 pm—9:30 pm
Thursday—	Study time—10:00 am—1:00 pm and 7:30 pm—9:30 pm
Saturday—	Study time—9:00 am—11:00 am

After graduation from nursing school, I will continue with my plan and add additional study time to complete 100 questions and review of question rationales on Monday, Tuesday, Wednesday, and Friday for the four (4) weeks before I am scheduled to take the NCLEX-RN exam.

Month: _____

Sunday	Monday	Tuesday	Wednesday	Thursday	Friday	Saturday
Work from 2:00 pm—10:00 pm	Exercise—6:00 am—6:45 am Nursing Class—8:00 am—2:00 pm or 100 questions and review of rationales Clinical assignment & preparation—3:00 pm—7:00 pm Study time—7:30 pm—9:30 pm	Nursing Clinical 7:00 am—2:30 pm or 100 questions and review of rationales Clinical assignment & preparation—3:00 pm—7:00 pm Study time—7:30 pm—9:30 pm	Nursing Clinical 7:00 am—2:30 pm or 100 questions and review of rationales Study time—7:30 pm—9:30 pm	Exercise—8:00 am—9:00 am Study time—10:00 am—1:00 pm and—7:30 pm—9:30 pm	Exercise—6:00 am—6:45 am Nursing Class—8:00 am—2:00 pm or 100 questions and review of rationales	Exercise—7:00 am—8:00 am Study from 9:00 am—11:00 am Work from 2:00 pm—10:00 pm

Bibliography

Test 1

DeLaune, S. C., & Ladner, P. K. (2006). *Fundamentals of nursing: Standards and practice* (3rd ed.). Clifton Park, NY: Thomson Delmar Learning.

Kozier, B., Erb, G., Berman, A., & Snyder, S. (2004). *Fundamentals of nursing: Concepts, process and practice* (7th ed.). Upper Saddle River, NJ: Pearson Education, Inc.

Lewis, S. M., Heitkemper, M. M., & Dirksen, S. R. (2004). *Medical-surgical nursing: Assessment and management of clinical problems* (6th ed.). St. Louis, MO: Elsevier.

Patient Safety Center of Inquiry & Department of Defense. (2005). *Patient care ergonomics resource guide: Safe patient handling and movement.* Retrieved March 31, 2006, from http://www.visn8.med.va.gov/patientsafetycenter/resguide/ErgoGuidePtOne.pdf

Potter, P. A., & Perry, A. G. (2005). *Fundamentals of nursing* (6th ed.). St. Louis, MO: Elsevier.

Stalhandske, E. (2004). *National center for patient safety 2004 falls toolkit.* Retrieved March 31, 2006, from http://www.patientsafety.gov/SafetyTopics/fallstoolkit/notebook/06_interventions.pdf

Test 2

Bickley, L. S., & Szilagyi, P. G. (2003). *Bates' guide to physical examination and history taking* (8th ed.). Philadelphia: Lippincott Williams & Wilkins.

DeLaune, S. C., & Ladner, P. K. (2006). *Fundamentals of nursing: Standards and practice* (3rd ed.). Clifton Park, NY: Thomson Delmar Learning.

Potter, P. A., & Perry, A. G. (2005). *Fundamentals of nursing* (3rd ed.). St. Louis, MO: Elsevier Mosby.

Test 3

Chitty, K. K. (2005). *Professional nursing: Concepts & challenges* (4th ed.). St. Louis, MO: Elsevier Saunders.

Christensen, B. L., & Kockrow, E. O. (2003). *Foundations of nursing.* St. Louis, MO: Mosby.

Hogan, M. A., Bowles, D., & White, J. E. (2003). *Nursing fundamentals: Reviews & rationales.* Upper Saddle River, NJ: Pearson Education, Inc.

Hood, L. J., & Leedy, S. K. (2006). *Conceptual basis of professional nursing* (6th ed.). Philadelphia: Lippincott Williams & Wilkins.

Mohr, W. K. (2003). *Psychiatric-mental health nursing* (5th ed.). Philadelphia: Lippincott Williams & Wilkins.

Rankin, S. H., Stallings, K. D., & London, F. (2005). *Patient education in health and illness* (5th ed.). Philadelphia: Lippincott Williams & Wilkins.

Riley, J. B. (2004). *Communication in nursing* (5th ed.). St. Louis, MO: Mosby.

Stuart, G. W., & Laraia, M. T. (2005). *Principles and practices of psychiatric nursing* (8th ed.). St. Louis, MO: Elsevier Mosby.

Wright, L. M., & Leahey, M. (2005). *Nurses and families* (4th ed.). Philadelphia: F.A. Davis.

Test 4

Adams, M., Josephson, D., & Holland, L. (2004). *Pharmacology for nurses.* Upper Saddle River, NJ: Pearson Prentice Hall.

Altman, G. (2001). *Delmar's fundamental and advanced nursing skills* (2nd ed.). New York: Delmar Learning.

Curren, A., & Munday, L. (1998). *Dimensional analysis for meds.* San Diego, CA: W I Publications.

DeLaune, S. C., & Ladner, P. K. (2006). *Fundamentals in nursing: Standards and practice* (3rd ed.). New York: Thomson Learning.

Kozier, B., Erb, G., Berman, A., & Snyder, S. (2004). *Techniques in clinical nursing* (5th ed.). Upper Saddle River, NJ: Pearson Prentice Hall.

Mills, E. (2004). *Nursing procedures* (4th ed.). Philadelphia: Lippincott Williams & Wilkins.

Potter, P., & Perry, A. (2005). *Fundamentals of nursing* (3rd ed.). St. Louis, MO: Mosby.

Test 5

Carroll, P. (2006). *Nursing leadership and management: A practical guide.* Clifton Park, NY: Thomson Delmar Learning.

Catalano, J. T. (2006). *Nursing now!* (4th ed.). Philadelphia: F.A. Davis Company.

Ellis, J. R., & Hartley, C. L. (2005). *Managing and coordinating nursing care* (4th ed.). Philadelphia: Lippincott Williams & Wilkins.

Kelly-Heidenthal, P. (2003). *Nursing leadership and management.* Clifton Park, NY: Thomson Delmar Learning.

Kelly-Heidenthal, P., & Marthaler, M. T. (2005). *Delegation of nursing care.* Clifton Park, NY: Thomson Delmar Learning.

Killion, S. W., & Dempski, K. M. (2000). *Quick look nursing: Legal and ethical issues.* Thorofare, NJ: Slack, Inc.

Kneisl, C. R., Wilson, H. S., & Trigoboff, E. (2004). *Contemporary psychiatric-mental health nursing.* Upper Saddle River, NJ: Pearson Prentice Hall.

Marquis, B. L., & Huston, C. J. (2006). *Leadership roles and management functions in nursing: Theory and application* (5th ed.). Philadelphia: Lippincott Williams & Wilkins.

Mohr, W. K. (2003). *Psychiatric-mental health nursing* (5th ed.). Philadelphia: Lippincott Williams & Wilkins.

Stuart, G. W., & Laraia, M. T. (2005). *Principles and practices of psychiatric nursing* (8th ed.). St. Louis, MO: Elsevier Mosby.

Test 6

Beachley, M. L. (2005). Nursing in a disaster. In F. Maurer & C. Smith (Eds.), *Community/public health nursing practice: Health for families and populations* (pp. 424–444). Philadelphia: Elsevier.

Department of Health and Human Services Centers for Disease Control and Prevention. (2002). *Fact sheet: Anthrax information for health care providers.* Retrieved April 15, 2006, from http://www.bt.cdc.gov/agent/anthrax/anthrax-hcp-factsheet.asp

Goodwin Veenema, T. (2003). *Disaster nursing and emergency preparedness for chemical, biological, and radiological terrorism and other hazards.* New York: Springer.

Hassmiller, S. B. (2003). Disaster management. In M. Stanhope & J. Lancaster (Eds.), *Community & public health nursing* (6th ed., Chapter 20). St. Louis, MO: Mosby.

Langan, J. C., & James, D. C. (2005). *Preparing nurses for disaster management.* Upper Saddle River, NJ: Prentice Hall Health.

Lehne, R. A. (2004). *Pharmacology for nursing care* (5th ed.). St. Louis, MO: Saunders.

Lewis, S. M., Heitkemper, M. M., & Dirksen, S. R. (2004). *Medical-surgical nursing: Assessment and management of clinical problems* (6th ed.). St. Louis, MO: Elsevier.

Mauer, F. A., & Smith, C. M. (2005). *Community and public health nursing practice: Health for families and populations.* St. Louis, MO: Elsevier Saunders.

Romig, L. E. (n.d.). *Combined Start/Jumpstart Triage Algorithm.* Retrieved April 26, 2005, from http://www.jumpstarttriage.com/JumpSTART_and_MCI_Triage.php

Schwytzer, D. (2004). Common problems encountered in emergency and critical care nursing. In M. A. Hogan & T. Madayag (Eds.), *Medical-surgical nursing: Reviews and rationales* (Chapter 17). Upper Saddle River, NJ: Prentice Hall Health.

Stanhope, M., & Lancaster, J. (2005). *Community and public health nursing* (6th ed.). St. Louis, MO: Mosby.

Willshire, L., Hassmiller, S., & Wodicka, K. (2004). *Disaster preparedness and response for nurses.* Retrieved April 13, 2006, from http://www.nursingsociety.org/education/case_studies/cases/SP0004.html

Test 7

Crutchlow, E. M., Dudac, P. J., MacAvoy, S., & Madara, B. R. (2002). *Quick look nursing: Pathophysiology.* Thorofare, NJ: Slack Inc.

Hockenberry, M. J. (2005). *Wong's essentials of pediatric nursing.* St. Louis, MO: Elsevier Mosby.

Karch, A. M. (2005). *2005 Lippincott's nursing drug guide.* Philadelphia: Lippincott Williams & Wilkins.

LeFever Kee, J., Paulanka, B., & Purnell, L. D. (2004). *Fluids and electrolytes with clinical applications: A programmed approach* (7th ed.). Newark, NJ: Thompson.

Lewis, S. M., Heitkemper, M. M., & Dirksen, S. R. (2004). *Medical-surgical nursing: Assessment and management of clinical problems* (6th ed.). St. Louis, MO: Elsevier Mosby.

Phillips, L. D. (2005). *Manual of i.v. therapeutics* (4th ed.). Philadelphia: F.A. Davis.

Potts, N. L., & Mandleco, B. L. (2002). *Pediatric nursing: Caring for children and their families.* Clifton Park, NY: Delmar.

Wagner, D. W., Johnson, K., & Kidd, P. S. (2006). *High acuity nursing* (4th ed.). Upper Saddle River, NJ: Pearson Prentice Hall.

Test 8

Baird, M. S., Keen, J. H., & Swearingen, P. L. (2005). *Manual of critical care nursing: Nursing interventions and collaborative management* (5th ed.). St. Louis, MO: Elsevier Mosby.

Crutchlow, E. M., Dudac, P. J., MacAvoy, S., & Madara, B. R. (2002). *Quick look nursing: Pathophysiology.* Thorofare, NJ: Slack Inc.

Karch, A. M. (2005). *2005 Lippincott's nursing drug guide.* Philadelphia: Lippincott Williams & Wilkins.

Lewis, S. M., Heitkemper, M. M., & Dirksen, S. R. (2004). *Medical-surgical nursing: Assessment and management of clinical problems* (6th ed.). St. Louis, MO: Elsevier Mosby.

Spratto, G. R., & Woods, A. L. (2003). *PDR nurses drug handbook.* Clifton Park, NY: Thomson Delmar Learning.

Wagner, D. W., Johnson, K., & Kidd, P. S. (2006). *High acuity nursing* (4th ed.). Upper Saddle River, NJ: Pearson Prentice Hall.

Test 9

Black, J., & Hawks, J. H. (2005). *Medical-surgical nursing: Clinical management for positive outcomes* (7th ed.). St. Louis, MO: Elsevier Saunders.

Brown, M., & Mulholland, J. (2004). *Drug calculations and problems for clinical practice* (7th ed.). St. Louis, MO: Mosby.

Hodgson, B. B., & Kizior, R. J. (2006). *Saunders nursing drug handbook 2006.* St. Louis, MO: Elsevier Saunders.

Lewis, S. M., Heitkemper, M. M., & Dirksen, S. R. (2004). *Medical-surgical nursing: Assessment and management of clinical problems* (6th ed.). St. Louis, MO: Mosby.

Lutz, C. A., & Przytulski, K. R. (2006). *Nutrition and diet therapy: Evidence-based application* (4th ed.). Philadelphia: F.A. Davis.

Munden, J. (Ed.). (2006). *Fluids and electrolytes.* Philadelphia: Lippincott Williams & Wilkins.

North American Nursing Diagnosis Association. (2005). *Nanda nursing diagnoses: Definitions and classification 2005–2006.* Philadelphia: NANDA International.

Pagana, K. D., & Pagana, T. J. (2002). *Mosby's manual of diagnostic and laboratory tests.* St. Louis, MO: Mosby.

Potter, P. A., & Perry, A. G. (2005). *Fundamentals of nursing* (6th ed.). St. Louis, MO: Elsevier Mosby.

Test 10

Baumberger, H. M. (2005). *Quick look nursing: Fluid and electrolytes.* Sudbury, MA: Jones and Bartlett.

Corbett, J. V. (2004). *Laboratory tests and diagnostic procedures* (6th ed.). Upper Saddle River, NJ: Pearson Prentice Hall.

Herbert-Ashton, M. J., & Clarkson, N. (2005). *Quick look nursing: Pharmacology.* Sudbury, MA: Jones and Bartlett.

Ignatavicius, D. D., & Workman, M. L. (2006). *Medical-surgical nursing* (5th ed.). St. Louis, MO: Elsevier Saunders.

LeFever Kee, J., Paulanka, B. J., & Purnell, L. D. (2004). *Fluids and electrolytes with clinical application* (7th ed.). Clifton Park, NY: Thomson Delmar Learning.

Lewis, S. M., Heitkemper, M. M., & Dirksen, S. R. (2004). *Medical-surgical nursing: Assessment and management of clinical problems* (6th ed.). St. Louis, MO: Mosby.

Potter, P. A., & Perry, A. G. (2005). *Fundamentals of nursing* (6th ed.). St. Louis, MO: Mosby.

Skidmore-Roth, L. (2004). *Mosby's 2004 nursing drug reference.* St. Louis, MO: Mosby.

Test 11

Lemone, P., & Burke, K. (2004). *Medical-surgical nursing: Critical thinking in client care* (3rd ed.). Upper Saddle River, NJ: Prentice Hall.

Lewis, S. M., Heitkemper, M. M., & Dirksen, S. R. (2004). *Medical-surgical nursing: Assessment and management of clinical problems* (6th ed.). St. Louis, MO: Mosby.

McCance, K. L., & Huether, S. E. (2002). *Pathophysiology: The biologic basis for disease in adults and children* (4th ed.). St. Louis, MO: Mosby.

Pagana, K. D., & Pagana, T. J. (2005). *Mosby's diagnostic and laboratory test reference* (7th ed.). St. Louis, MO: Elsevier Mosby.

Smith, S., Duell, D., & Martin, B. (2000). *Clinical nursing skills: Basic to advanced skills* (5th ed.). Upper Saddle River, NJ: Prentice Hall.

Springhouse nurse's drug guide. (2007). Philadelphia: Lippincott Williams & Wilkins.

Test 12

Ackley, B. J., & Ladwig, G. B. (2004). *Nursing diagnosis handbook: A guide to planning care* (6th ed.). St. Louis, MO: Mosby.

Black, J. M., & Hawks, J. H. (2005). *Medical-surgical nursing: Clinical management for positive outcomes* (7th ed.). St. Louis, MO: Elsevier Saunders.

Brown, M., & Mulholland, J. M. (2004). *Drug calculations: Process and problems for clinical practice* (7th ed.). St. Louis, MO: Mosby.

Kozier, B., Erb, G., Berman, A., & Snyder, S. J. (2004). *Fundamentals of nursing: Concepts, process, and practice* (7th ed.). Upper Saddle River, NJ: Pearson Prentice Hall.

Lewis, S. M., Heitkemper, M. M., & Dirksen, S. R. (2004). *Medical-surgical nursing: Assessment and management of clinical problems* (6th ed.). St. Louis, MO: Mosby.

Lilley, L. L., Harrington, S., & Snyder, J. S. (2005). *Pharmacology and the nursing process* (4th ed.). St. Louis, MO: Mosby.

Lutz, C., & Przytulski, K. (2006). *Nutrition and diet therapy: Evidence-based applications* (4th ed.). Philadelphia: F.A. Davis Company.

Pagana, K. D., & Pagana, T. J. (2002). *Manual of diagnostic and laboratory tests* (2nd ed.). St. Louis, MO: Mosby.

Smeltzer, S. C., & Bare, B. G. (2004). *Textbook of medical-surgical nursing* (10th ed.). Philadelphia: Lippincott Williams & Wilkins.

Test 13

Lewis, S. M., Heitkemper, M. M., & Dirksen, S. R. (2004). *Medical-surgical nursing: Assessment and management of clinical problems* (6th ed.). St. Louis, MO: Mosby.

Smeltzer, S. C., & Bare, B. G. (2004). *Brunner & Suddarth's textbook of medical-surgical nursing.* Philadelphia: Lippincott Williams & Wilkins.

Test 14

Arnaout, W. S., & Demetriou, A. A. (2006). Hepatic failure: Approach to patient with liver failure. *ACS Surgery online.* Retrieved June 18, 2007, from http://www.medscape.com/viewarticle/535479

Bourdeanu, L., Loseth, D. B., & Funk, M. (2005). Management of opioid-induced sedation in patients with cancer. *Clinical Journal of Oncology Nursing, 9*(6), 705–711.

Corbett, J. (2004). *Laboratory tests and diagnostic procedures with nursing diagnosis* (6th ed.). Upper Saddle River, NJ: Pearson Prentice Hall.

Hogan, M. A., & Hill, K. (2004). *Pathophysiology reviews and rationales.* Upper Saddle River, NJ: Prentice Hall.

LeFever Kee, J., Paulanka, B., & Purnell, L. D. (2004). *Fluids and electrolytes with clinical applications: A programmed approach* (7th ed.). Newark, NJ: Thompson.

Lewis, S. M., Heitkemper, M. M., & Dirksen, S. R. (2004). *Medical-surgical nursing: Assessment and management of clinical problems* (6th ed.). St. Louis, MO: Mosby.

Phillips, L. D. (2005). *Manual of i.v. therapeutics* (4th ed.). Philadelphia: F.A. Davis.

Weinstein, S. (2001). *Plumer's principles and practice of intravenous therapy* (7th ed). Philadelphia: Lippincott.

Test 15

Aschenbrenner, D., Cleveland, L. W., & Venable, S. (2002). *Drug therapy in nursing.* Philadelphia: Lippincott.

Curren, A. M. (2002). *Dimensional analysis for meds.* Clifton Park, NY: Thomson Delmar Learning.

Hickey, J. V. (2003). *The clinical practice of neurological and neurosurgical nursing.* Philadelphia: Lippincott.

Lewis, S. M., Heitkemper, M. M., & Dirksen, S. R. (2004). *Medical-surgical nursing: Assessment and management of clinical problems* (6th ed.). St. Louis, MO: Mosby.

Phipps, W. J., Monahan, F. D., Sands, J. K., Marek, J. F., & Neighbors, M. (2003). *Medical-surgical nursing: Health and illness perspectives.* St. Louis, MO: Mosby.

Swearingen, P. L. (2003). *Manual of medical-surgical nursing care: Nursing interventions and collaborative management.* St. Louis, MO: Mosby.

Test 16

Adams, M. P., Josephson, D. L., & Holland, L. N. (2005). *Pharmacology for nurses: A pathophysiologic approach.* Upper Saddle River, NJ: Pearson Prentice Hall.

Crutchlow, E. M., Dudar, P. J., MacAvoy, S., & Madora, B. R. (2002). *Quick look nursing: Pathophysiology.* Thorofare, NJ: Slack Inc.

Herbert-Ashton, M. J., & Clarkson, N. E. (2005). *Quick look nursing: Pharmacology.* Sudbury, MA: Jones & Bartlett.

Hodgson, B., & Kizior, R. (2006). *Saunders nursing drug handbook 2006.* St. Louis, MO: Elsevier.

Lemone, P., & Burke, K. (2004). *Medical-surgical nursing: Critical thinking in client care.* Upper Saddle River, NJ: Prentice Hall.

Lewis, S. M., Heitkemper, M. M., & Dirksen, S. R. (2004). *Medical-surgical nursing: Assessment and management of clinical problems* (6th ed.). St. Louis, MO: Mosby.

Tamparo, C. D., & Lewis, M. A. (2005). *Diseases of the human body.* Philadelphia: F.A. Davis.

Test 17

Gray Morris, D. (2006). *Calculating with confidence* (4th ed.). St. Louis, MO: Mosby.

Lewis, S. M., Heitkemper, M. M., & Dirksen, S. R. (2004). *Medical-surgical nursing: Assessment and management of clinical problems* (6th ed.). St. Louis, MO: Mosby.

Spry, C. (2005). *Essentials of perioperative nursing* (3rd ed.). Sudbury, MA: Jones and Bartlett.

Test 18

Baumberger-Henry, M. (2005). *Fluid and electrolytes.* Sudbury, MA: Jones and Bartlett.

Corbett, J. (2004). *Laboratory tests and diagnostic procedures with nursing diagnosis* (6th ed.). Upper Saddle River, NJ: Pearson Prentice Hall.

Gordon, D. B., Dahl, J., Phillips, P., Frandsen, J., Cowley, C., Foster, R. L., Fine, P. G., Miaskowski, C., Fishman, S., & Finley, R. S. (2004). The use of 'as-needed' range orders for opioid analgesics in the management of acute pain: A consensus statement of the American Society for Pain Management Nursing and the American Pain Society [Electronic version]. *Pain Management Nursing.* 5, 53–58. Retrieved March 17, 2006, from http://www.ampainsoc.org/pub/bulletin/jul04/consensus1.htm

Hogan, M. A., & Hill, K. (2004). *Pathophysiology reviews and rationales.* Upper Saddle River, NJ: Prentice Hall.

Infusion Nurses Society. (2006). *Infusion nursing standards of practice.* Norwood, MA: Lippincott.

Josephson, D. (2004). *Intravenous infusion therapy for nurses: principles & practice* (2nd ed.). Clifton Park, NJ: Delmar.

Lamer, W. (2006). *Nutrition and dehydration.* Retrieved March 17, 2006 from http://www.hospicefoundation.org/endOfLifeInfo/nutrition_hydration.asp

LeFever Kee, J., Paulanka, B., & Purnell, L. D. (2004). *Fluids and electrolytes with clinical applications: A programmed approach* (7th ed.). Newark, NJ: Thompson.

Lewis, S. M., Heitkemper, M. M., & Dirksen, S. R. (2004). *Medical-surgical nursing: Assessment and management of clinical problems* (6th ed.). St. Louis, MO: Mosby.

Mehler, P. S., Kolpak, S., & Padilla, R. (2005). Anorexia nervosa and the use of total parenteral nutrition refeeding. *Current Nutrition and Food Science, 1,* 97–104.

Murray, B. E. (2005). Clinical implications of glycopeptide use: Pros and cons [Electronic version]. *Clinical Updates in Infectious Diseases, 8,* 1–4. Retrieved November 18, 2006, from http://www.nfid.org/pdf/id_archive/glycopeptides.pdf

Phillips, L. D. (2005). *Manual of i.v. therapeutics* (4th ed.). Philadelphia: F.A. Davis.

Weinstein, S. (2001). *Plumer's principles and practice of intravenous therapy* (7th ed.). Philadelphia: Lippincott.

Test 19

American Society of Health-System Pharmacists Inc. (2006). *Atorvastatin.* Retrieved November 18, 2006, from http://www.nlm.nih.gov/medlineplus/druginfo/medmaster/a600045.html

Farrell, M., & Nicoteri, J. A. (2001). *Quick look nursing: Nutrition.* Thorofare, NJ: Slack Inc.

Lewis, S. M., Heitkemper, M. M., & Dirksen, S. R. (2004). *Medical-surgical nursing: Assessment and management of clinical problems* (6th ed.). St. Louis, MO: Mosby.

Lulinski, B. (1999). *Creatine supplementation.* Retrieved November 18, 2006, from http://www.quackwatch.org/01QuackeryRelatedTopics/DSH/creatine.html

State of Ohio Board of Nursing. (2006). *Chapter 4723-13: Delegation of nursing tasks.* Retrieved November 18, 2006, from http://nursing.ohio.gov/PDFS/NewLawRules/4723-13DelegationbyLicensedNurses.pdf

The Liquid Vitamin C Supplements Store. (n.d.). Retrieved November 18, 2006, from http://www.vitamin-supplements-store.net/vitamins/vitamin-c.html

Wong, D. (2005). *Wong's essentials of pediatric nursing* (7th ed.). St. Louis, MO: Mosby.

Test 20

Ballard, J., Novak, K., & Driver, M. (1979). A simplified score for assessment of fetal maturity of newly born infants. *Journal of Pediatrics, 95,* 769–774.

Lowdermilk, D. L., & Perry, S. E. (2004*). Maternity and women's health care* (8th ed). St. Louis, MO: Mosby

Test 21

Alexander, L. L., LaRosa, J. H., Bader, H., & Garfield, S. (2004). *New dimensions in women's health* (3rd ed.). Sudbury, MA: Jones & Bartlett.

Breslin, E., & Lucas, V. (Eds.). (2003). *Women's health nursing: Toward evidence-based practice.* St. Louis, MO: Saunders.

Condon, M. C. (2004). W*omen's health: An integrated approach to wellness and illness.* Upper Saddle River, NJ: Prentice Hall.

Lewis, S. M., Heitkemper, M. M., & Dirksen, S. R. (2004). *Medical-surgical nursing: Assessment and management of clinical problems* (6th ed.). St. Louis, MO: Mosby.

Olds, S. B., London, M. L., Ladewig, P. W., & Davidson, M. R. (2004). *Maternal-newborn nursing & women's health care* (7th ed.). Upper Saddle River, NJ: Pearson Prentice Hall.

Ricci, S. S. (2007). *Essentials of maternity, newborn, and women's health nursing.* Philadelphia: Lippincott Williams & Wilkins.

Schuiling, K. D., & Likis, F. E. (2006). *Gynecologic health.* Sudbury, MA: Jones & Bartlett.

Varney, H., Kriebs, J. M., & Gegor, C. L. (2004). *Varney's midwifery* (4th ed.). Sudbury, MA: Jones & Bartlett.

Youngkin, E. Q., & Davis, M. S. (2004). *Women's health: A primary care clinical guide* (3rd ed.). Upper Saddle River, NJ: Pearson Prentice Hall.

Test 22

Hockenberry, M. J. (2005). *Wong's essentials of pediatric nursing* (7th ed.). St. Louis, MO: Mosby.

Hockenberry, M. J. (2004). *Wong's clinical manual of pediatric nursing* (6th ed.). St. Louis, MO: Mosby.

Centers for Disease Control and Prevention, National Center for Health Statistics. (2007). Health Data for All Ages. Retrieved June 18, 2007, from http://www.cdc.gov/nchs/health_data_for_all_ages.htm

Thies, K. (2006). *Quick look nursing: Growth and development through the lifespan.* Sudbury, MA: Jones & Bartlett.

Test 23

Fontaine, K. L., Kneisl, C. R., & Trigoboff, E. (2004). *Psychiatric-mental health nursing clinical companion.* Upper Saddle River, NJ: Pearson Prentice Hall.

Kneisl, C. R., Wilson, H. S., & Trigoboff, E. (2004). *Contemporary psychiatric-mental health nursing.* Upper Saddle River, NJ: Pearson Prentice Hall.

Mohr, W. K. (2003). *Psychiatric-mental health nursing* (5th ed.). Philadelphia: Lippincott Williams & Wilkins.

Stuart, G. (2005). *Handbook of psychiatric nursing* (6th ed.). St. Louis, MO: Elsevier Mosby.

Stuart, G. W., & Laraia, M. T. (2005). *Principles and practices of psychiatric nursing* (8th ed.). St. Louis, MO: Elsevier Mosby.

NCLEX-RN Review: 1,000 Questions to Help You Pass
by Patricia McLean Hoyson and Kimberly Serroka

Pre-Test Answers and Rationales

Below are the answers to the Pretest: The rationales for each question are located within the book at the page number indicated.

1. Answer: 4; pg 69
2. Answer: 3; pg 70
3. Answer: 1; pg 72
4. Answer: 3; pg 73
5. Answer: 4; pg 77
6. Answer: 2; pg 78
7. Answer: 4; pg 80
8. Answer: 2; pg 81
9. Answer: 1; pg 85
10. Answer: 4; pg 86
11. Answer: 4; pg 87
12. Answer: 1; pg 88
13. Answer: 1; pg 91
14. Answer: 4; 92
15. Answer: 4; pg 94
16. Answer: Oral; pg 95
17. Answer: 4; pg 113
18. Answer: 1; pg 114
19. Answer: 4; pg 116
20. Answer: 4; pg 117
21. Answer: 4; pg 119
22. Answer: 3; pg 120
23. Answer: 4; pg 122
24. Answers: 1, 3, 4, and 6; pg 123
25. Answer: 2; pg 187
26. Answer: 3; pg 188
27. Answer: 2; pg 190
28. Answers: 1, 2, and 3; pg 192
29. Answer: 3; pg 195
30. Answer: 2; pg 196
31. Answer: 4; pg 198
32. Answer: 4; pg 199
33. Answer: 1; pg 201
34. Answer: 2; pg 202
35. Answer: 4; pg 204
36. Answer: 2; pg 205
37. Answer: 4; pg 207
38. Answer: 3; pg 208
39. Answer: 4; pg 210
40. Answer: 2, 3, 1, 4; pg 212
41. Answer: 3; pg 215
42. Answer: 3; pg 216
43. Answer: 1, 5, 8, 2, 4, 6, 7, 3; pg 218
44. Answer: 2; pg 219
45. Answers: 1, 2, 3, 4, 5, and 7; pg 223
46. Answer: 3; pg 225
47. Answer: 2; pg 228

48. Answer: 3; pg 229
49. Answer: 2; pg 233
50. Answer: 1; pg 234
51. Answer: 2; pg 237
52. Answer: 2; 238
53. Answer: 3; pg 241
54. Answer: 2; pg 243
55. Answer: 2; pg 245
56. Answer: 4; pg 247
57. Answer: 1; pg 251
58. Answer: UMN: Use reflex emptying 30 minutes after a meal. LMN: Use manual stool removal and small volume enemas; pg 253
59. Answer: 3; pg 255
60. Answer: 1; pg 256
61. Answer: 4; pg 259
62. Answers: 1, 2, 3, and 4; pg 260
63. Answer: 2; pg 262
64. Answers: 2, 3, and 4; pg 263
65. Answer: 3; pg 287
66. Answer: 1; pg 288
67. Answer: 4; pg 291
68. Answer: 1; pg 292
69. Answer: 2, 4, 5, 8, 7, 3, 1, 6; pg 295
70. Answer: 3; pg 297
71. Answer: 3; pg 301
72. Answer: 1; pg 302
73. Answer: 4; pg 305
74. Answer: 2; pg 306
75. Answer: 2; pg 308
76. Answer: 1; pg 310
77. Answer: 1; pg 339
78. Answer: 4; pg 340
79. Answer: 2; pg 342
80. Answer: Lochia rubra; pg 343
81. Answer: 3; pg 347
82. Answer: 3; pg 348
83. Answer: 1; pg 351
84. Answer: 2; pg 352
85. Answer: 3; pg 355
86. Answers: 1, 2, 3, 5, and 8; pg 356
87. Answer: 2; pg 359
88. Answer: 3; pg 360
89. Answer: 4; pg 363
90. Answers: 1, 4, and 6; 364
91. Answer: 1; pg 367
92. Answer: 3; pg 368